The Fourth International Symposium on the History of Anaesthesia

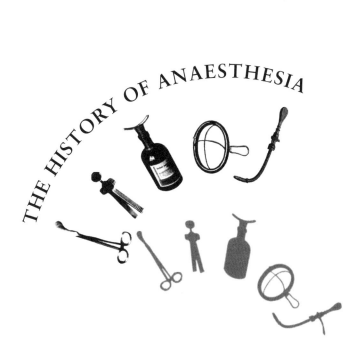

The Fourth International Symposium
on the History of Anaesthesia

Proceedings

Edited by
Jochen Schulte am Esch
Michael Goerig
with 334 Figures and 82 Tables

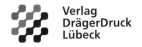

Die Deutsche Bibliothek – CIP-Einheitsaufnahme

**International Symposium on the History of Anaesthesia
< 4, 1997, Hamburg >:**
Proceedings / The Fourth International Symposium on the History of
Anaesthesia : with 82 tables / ed. by Jochen Schulte am Esch ;
Michael Goerig. - Lübeck : Dräger, 1998.
(The history of anaesthesia)
ISBN 3-925402-00-4

Impressum:

*Proceedings of the Fourth International Symposium
on the History of Anaesthesia (FISHA) Hamburg*
Hamburg, 26th – 29th April 1997

edited by
Jochen Schulte am Esch, M.D.
President of the German Society of Anaesthesiology
and Intensive Care (DGAI),
Professor and Chair of the Clinic of Anaesthesiology,
University Hospital Eppendorf, Hamburg, Germany

and
Michael Goerig, M.D.
Chairman of the "Arbeitskreis für Geschichte der Anästhesie",
Clinic of Anaesthesiology University Hospital Eppendorf,
Hamburg, Germany

Printed by: DrägerDruck GmbH & Co., Lübeck
ISBN 3-925402-00-4

Table of Contents:

Preface 7

Organizing 8

Papers presented 9

Text of Papers 21

List of Contributors 855

Index of Persons 863

Index of Topics 873

Preface:

It has been about one year that the Fourth International Symposium on the History of Anaesthesia (FISHA) took place in Hamburg, Germany in April 1997. We are now proud to present this volume containing the symposium proceedings to all our colleagues with an interest in the history of anaesthesia.

More than 250 participants from all around the world attended this meeting where more than 150 papers as well as posters were presented within three days reviving important historical events in the development of anaesthesia and pain management. Similar to earlier symposia in Rotterdam in 1982, London in 1987 and in Atlanta 1992, we have tried to arrange all the presentations around specific topics including "Special Lectures", an "Early-Bird-Session" as well as two "Plenary Sessions". This volume contains 130 articles representing a wide of interrelated topics on the history of anaesthesia. The articles in this issue appear according to their order in the symposium program, the tables and addresses are given in alphabetical order. A detailed subject index enables the reader to quickly find topics and persons.

In order to bring some uniformity into the structure of the papers, we felt free to edit them concerning style and content with the help of an international team. We would like to thank Dr. F.E. Bennetts (UK), Dr. G. Zeitlin (USA) and Dr. K. Agarwal from our department for valuable contribution completing this task. In addition we added some interesting pictures to selected articles.

Without the committed involvement of many people, the completion of this book would have been unthinkable. We are especially thinking of the engagement of the staff of the Clinic of Anaesthesiology of the University Hospital Eppendorf, Hamburg, which was a "conditio sine qua non" for bringing out this book.

Also, we would like to thank the Dräger Druck company for the excellent print of this book which is of the same quality as the catalogue for the exhibition during the symposium. Namely, we are grateful to Peter Arndt for his active support and ready cooperation. We are particularly indepted to the Dräger Company for their generous support that enabled us to edit these proceedings.

We hope that the reader will enjoy going through the various articles as much as we enjoyed compiling them.

Hamburg, April 1998

Jochen Schulte am Esch
Michael Goerig

The Fourth International Symposium on the History of Anaesthesia

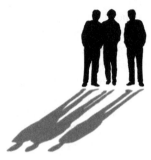

IN COOPERATION WITH ARBEITSKREIS GESCHICHTE FÜR ANÄSTHESIE (GERMANY), HISTORY OF ANAESTHESIA SOCIETY (UK) AND ANESTHESIA HISTORY ASSOCIATION (USA)

Chairman: J. Schulte am Esch
Co-Chairman: M. Goerig
Secretary: J. Scholz

Scientific Board:
R. Atkinson (UK)
J. A. Bennett (UK)
J. M. Horton (UK)
L. E. Morris (USA)
J. Rupreht (NL, Slovenia)

National Committee:
H. Böhrer (Heidelberg)
C. Nemes (Pfaffenhofen)
W. Röse (Magdeburg)
H. Stoeckel (Bonn)
J. Wawersik (Kiel)

International Committee:
M. Andreen (Sweden)
D. Bacon (USA)
S. M. Basu (India)
M. T. Cousin (France)
E. Damir (Russia)
R. J. Defalque (USA)
A. Franco (Spain)
E. Frost (USA)
G. Gurman (Israel)
M. Kus (Poland)
W. List (Austria)
J. R. Maltby (Canada)
A. Matsuki (Japan)
O. Mayrhofer (Austria)
C. Parsloe (Brazil)
J. Pokorny (Czech Rep.)
L. Rendell-Baker (USA)
J. E. Steinhaus (USA)
M. S. Takrouri (Saudi Arabia)
M. Tekeres (Hungary)
R. Westhorpe (Australia)
D. J. Wilkinson (UK)

Table of Contents:

Special Lecture I   Seite

International symposia on the history of anaesthesia (1982-1992): with particular emphasis on the first one	J. Rupreht, W. Erdmann	21
Pain and analgesia for operative interventions - from the beginning up to 1846	T. Boulton	35
Pain and analgesia for operative interventions - from 1847 up to 1997	L. Morris	57

Forgotten pioneers of early vapour administration

W. G. Atherstone: A pioneer anaesthesist in South Africa	R. Haridas	73
Unknown facts about Johann Friedrich Dieffenbach (1792 - 1847)	D. Wessinghage	79
Who introduced nitrous oxide into French practice?	M. Zimmer	87
How the French were informed and implemented surgical anaesthesia in 1846	M. Cousin	97

Biographic reminescences

Rudolf Frey's unfinished historical legacy	J. Rupreht, W. Erdmann	101
From the beginning of anaesthesia to the first chair of anaesthesia in Innsbruck (1959) - The contribution of Bruno Haid to this development	H. Benzer	109
Who was Dr. Reuben Wade?	D. Wilkinson	113
Jochen Bark, a German pioneer of modern anaesthesiology	H. Menzel	117
Robert Reynolds Macintosh - Life before anaesthesia	A. Baker, C. Mck Holmes	123

Miscellaneous I

François Magendie: the apostel of pain?	C. Parsloe	127
The Cushing tradition	J. Horton	131
The history of neuroanaesthesia	I. Kiss	135
The introduction of lidocaine	M. Andreen-Sachs	139
Development of anaesthesiology and intensive therapy in Czechoslovakia after the second World War	J. Pokorný	145
Walter Kausch – an unknown German pioneer of parental nutrition	K. Stinshoff	153

Plenary Session I

Early reports on deaths under anaesthesia where – when – why – who and its consequences

Early reports on deaths under anaesthesia	C. N. Adams	157
Death under anaesthesia in the Middle East	M. S. M. Takrouri	167
Early reports on death under anaesthesia in the German speaking countries	H. Petermann, M. Goerig	171
Early mortality from general anesthesia	D. Cope	179
Early reports on death under anaesthesia in the XIXth century in Spain	A. Franco, J. C. Diz	191

Historical reports of anaesthetic complications

An early chloroform death in Berlin	B. Panning, H. G. Kloes, S. Piepenbrock	195
Gurlt's report "Zur Narkotisierungstechnik" in 1847 – an early contribution to quality assurance in anaesthesia	W. Röse	199

The circulatory risks of anaesthesia in Leiden before 1930	M. van Wijhe	205
The Lahey explosion	G. Zeitlin	209
The Wooley and Roe case – 1. The anaesthetist's thoughts	J. Maltby	213
The Wooley and Roe – case 11; an explanation	C. Hutter	219

Anaesthesia spreads through Europe

Karl E. Hammerschmidt (1801 - 1874): humanist, scientist and anaesthesia pioneer	W. List, A. Kernbaumer	223
First surgical anaesthesia in Czech countries	J. Pokorný	227
The first surgery operation using ether in Lisbon/Portugal	A. Fortes-Espinheira	229
Chloroform anaesthesia in the practice military surgery in 1849 in Hungary	M. Tekeres	231
The role of the "Societas Medicorum Germanicorum Parisiensis" for the spread of anaesthesia in Europe	M. Goerig, C. Nemes, A. Straimer	235

Early steps of inhalation anaesthesia in Germany

Some remarks on the first etherization in Germany	U. von Hintzenstern, W. Schwarz, H. Petermann	247
"Der schöne Traum..." German publications on ether and chloroform narcosis in 1847	H. Petermann	251
Robert Ritter von Welz (1814 - 1878) and the first experiences of ether anaesthesia at Würzburg	C. Weißer	259
Was the "Rauschnarkose" born in Hamburg?	R. Defalque, B. Panning, A. J. Wright	265

Early Bird Session

Historical development of anaesthesia during the times of Austrian-Hungarian monarchy and the decade after the first World War	H. Eiblmayr	267
Pain relief during surgery in the Middle Ages and in the early modern times	Ch. Maier	279

Special Lecture II

Historical aspects of resuscitation	P. Safar	287
Misleading developments in anesthesia techniques as an impediment of progress in surgical anaesthesia	E. Frost	311

Forgotten pioneers of local anaesthetic techniques

Albert Niemann and the cocaine research in Göttingen	U. Braun, Th. Riedl	321
Spinal block for surgery above the diaphragm	R. Atkinson	327
Ryszard Rodziński – a pioneer of combined spinal-epidural anaesthesia	K. Duda, A. Kubisz, M. Ziętkiewicz	329
Kirschner's "Spinal zone anaesthesia placed at will and dosage individually granded" – technique; recent importance	C. Weißer	333

Unknown facts about well respected personalities

Delay in the introduction of anaesthesia	A. Adams	339
From ether to chloroform – the beginnings of chloroform anaesthesia in France	M. Cousin	343
From Simpson to Livingstonia	A. McKenzie	347
Doctor Charles Thomas Jackson's aphasia	R. Patterson	353

Early encounters with a stranger	L. Morris	359
Helmut Schmidt – an early protagonist of professionalized anaesthesia in Hamburg	M. Goerig, J. Schulte am Esch	367

Resuscitation through the centuries

Cardio – pulmonary resuscitation in Egypt 3000 years ago?	A. Ocklitz	379
Pulmonary resuscitation in ancient Egypt	W. Maleck, K. Koetter	383
Franz Koenig and Friedrich Maass: protagonists of closed chest cardiac massage	H. Böhrer, M. Goerig	389
Historical remarks on medicamenteous therapy in emergency medicine	U. von Hintzenstern, M. Goerig	395
Continuing medical education in American anesthesiology 1905 - 1940	D. Bacon	401
Eisenmenger's biomotor – predecessor of active compression – decompression resuscitation?	K. Kötter, W. Maleck, G. A. Petroianu	405

Plenary Session II

Alternative analgesic and anaesthetic techniques

Alternative analgesic and anaesthetic techniques	R. Westhorpe	421
The alternative patients	B. M. Q. Weaver	425
The technique of thermoetherization of Dr. Antonio Morales	J. C. Diz, A. Franco	431
Alternative analgesic and anaesthetic techniques	H. Baar	437

Technique and anaesthesia

Who introduced the rebreathing systems into clinical practice?	J. Baum	441

The closed anaesthesia system: 1946 - 1996. A 50 years perspective	C. Parsloe	451
Nathan Zuntz (1847 - 1920) and his contributions to the history of anaesthesia	H. Gunga	455
Mal-constructions in anaesthetic apparatus and respirators	J. Stoffregen	461

Anaesthesia in operative gynecology

Answers to opponents of obstetric anaesthesia 1847 - 1850	J. Maltby, Ch. K. Davies	473
Anaesthesia in gynaecology and obstetrics at the turn of the century up to 1935 – documents of "Landesfrauenklinik Oberösterreich"	H. Eiblmayer	477
Pain relief for childbirth in 1930's Britain	S. Williams	483
Joseph Sebrechts and the spinal anaesthesia in Belgium	P. Desbarax	493
Flavio Kroeff-Pires and his contribution to intravenous regional anaesthesia	H. Nolte †	505

Airway management in anaesthesia

Reconstruction of the ancient Egypt mouth-opening instrument the practice of artificial respiration 5000 years ago	A. Ocklitz	507
Experiments with the "laryngoscope" from Papyrus Hunefer in a mannequin	K. Kötter, W. Maleck	511
Separation of the airways - historical aspects	K. Wiedemann, E. Fleischer, P. Dressler	517
The story of the Wendl-tube and its use	J. Wendl	531

The men behind the technique

Automobile & medical engineer: Captain G.T. Smith Clarke chief engineer: Alvis car & engineering company 1922 - 1956	A. Padfield	535
Louis Ombrédanne and his inhaler. The man and his contribution to anaesthesia in Central Europe viewed today and in his time	J. Plötz	539
The Ombrédanne inhaler and its modifications: 1908 - 1950	C. Parsloe	543
Russian modifications by Sadevenko and Gersch of Ombrédanne's inhaler (1908)	J. McIntyre †	547
The "Göttinger Modell" – A trichlorethylene vaporizer created by Hosemann / Hickel	P. Ahrens, U. Braun	549
Forgotten Jewish pioneers of German anaesthesia	M. Goerig, J. Schulte am Esch	553

Miscellaneous II

The importance of collaborative research to American academic anesthesiology	D. Bacon	567
Stethoscopy during anaesthesia: past, present and future	J. McIntyre †	571
Preoperative fasting 1846 - 1996	J. Maltby	579
The contribution of anaesthesiology to the development of palliative care in Germany	T. Krause, B. Wiedemann	583
The impact of the Copenhagen Anaesthesiology Centre on the practice of anaesthesiology in the Czech and Slovak Republics	B. Dworaczek, M. Buroš, J. Pokorný	587

Special Lecture III

History of blood gas analysis	J. Severinghaus, P. Astrup	591
Historical interactions of pharmacology and anesthesia	J. Parascandola	597

Plenary Session III

More than 100 years anaesthesia related research by companies

Development of skeletal muskle relaxants	R. Hughes	607
More than 100 years development of analgesics and general and local anaesthetics at hoechst: a historical review	R. Muschaweck	617

Poster-Presentations

Postspinal headache – its prevention over the decades	St. Wilhelm, M. Goerig, Th. Standl	631
Had the beginning of modern anaesthesia been possible in the 16th century?	H. Petermann	635
A quantitative analysis of newspaper reports a on the introduction of anaesthesia	H. Connor	641
Notes on the history of anaesthesia for cardiac surgery in Southern Moravia	I. Čundrle	647
From Boston, Mass. to Timişoara, Febr. 5, 1847: The first surgical use of anaesthetic ether in today Romania	S. Ghişoiu	649
Introduction of ether anaesthesia into Japan	A. Matsuki	655
Priority to whom? Who was the first in applications of inhalation of ether	H. Petermann	659
The first day of chloroform anaesthesia in Spain	J. Diz, A. Franco J. Alvarez, J. Cortés	663

The search for the holy grail	C. McLaren	667
Where have all the bellows gone? 10 manual respiratory devices reviewed	K. Kötter, W. Maleck, G.A. Petroianu	671
The oesophageal detector device (ODD)	W. Maleck, G.A. Petroianu, K. Kötter	675
Some notes on the history of capnometry, its use for detection of oesophageal intubation and hand-held-capnometers	W. Maleck, G.A. Petroianu, K. Kötter	679
Using things right out of home. Apparatus for inhaling ether and chloroform in 1847	H. Petermann	683
Administration of ether anaesthesia per rectum in Spain	J. Diz, A. Franco, J. Alvarez, J. Cortés	689
James Young Simpson and American women in medicine	S. Harrison-Calmes	693
Pioneers and innovators in anesthesia	L. Rendell-Baker, J. A. Mayer, G. Bause	697
Arthur Läwen – his work on the field of anaesthesia	U. Ziegler, B. Kohlweyer, B. Wiedemann	725
Ernst Jeger – a nearly forgotten pioneer in cardiovascular surgery and in thoracic anaesthesia	H. J. Klippe	727
Paul Frenckner – Swedish pioneer in bronchology and in thoracic anaesthesia	H.J. Klippe	733
Eric Carlens – skiful Swedish pioneer in bronchology and thoracic medicine	H.J. Klippe	737
Heliodor Święcicki, the inventor of modern analgesia for delivery	W. Jurczyk, J. Kroll, P. Kroll	741
Fritz Lotsch – a forgotten pioneer in German anaesthesia	W. Röse	745
Narcosis and nightshade	A. Carter	749

Anaesthesia in German military practice during World War II – A comparison	M. Wollbrück, G. Giese, G. Hempelmann	757
S.E.E. (Skophedal), the Wehrmacht's "miracle" drug	R. Defalque	763
CODIC - an universal therapeutic system, p.e. for auto-matically controlled general anaesthesia by infusion	J. Stoffregen	767
Johann Sigismund Elsholtz: Clysmatica Nova 1665	J. McIntyre †	771
Paraphrasing Descartes – a personel perspective on the history of anaesthesia	F. Magora	779
An international study of educational programs for nurses providing anesthesia care	J. Kelly	783
A census of copies of the original edition of John Snow's "On the inhalation of the vapour of ether in the surgical operations"	A. Matsuki, J. McIntyre †	797
The use of curare in Poland – a historical outline	M. Szymanska-Kowalska	805
From transportation to prehospital care – the emergency medical system in Hamburg 1946 - 1996	H.R. Paschen	811
Heinz Wohlgemuth and Otto Roth: The men behind the technique	M. Goerig, E. Schaffner	815
Did the introduction of anaesthesia influence the indication for surgical procedures at the University of Erlangen?	W. Schwarz, U. v. Hintzenstern	823
Tracheostomy in ancient Egypt – myth or reality?	W. Maleck, U. v. Hintzenstern, K. Koetter	827
Management of difficult airways in 1898: E. Tschudy (Zürich) forgotten pioneer of orotracheal intubation	H. Wulf, H. Gockel, J. Wawersik	837
Dr. CT Jackson's inductive discovery	R. Patterson	841

The "Cough Pistol", Hustenpistole or Tussomat	J. Stoffregen	847
A non-rebreathing system used with the Takaoka-ventilator ("Modell Göttingen", "ANE 2000")	J. Stoffregen	851
Stanislaw Przybyszewski's drawing which became an inspiration of Carl Schleich's discovery	J. Kroll	853

International Symposia on the History of Anaesthesia (1982-1992);
With Particular Emphasis on the First One

J. Rupreht* and W. Erdmann**
* University of Ljubljana, Institute of Anaesthesiology, Slovecia
** Erasmus University Rotterdam, Department of Anaesthesiology, The Netherlands

Introduction

Books have been written over passage of time only a day long and one who is supposed to give an overview of a years-long process, such as the backgrounds to the International Symposium on the History of Anaesthesia (ISHA), this one realizes that it is not an easy task. One can present a formal skeleton of events devoid of the turgor which is inherent to the growth of every living thing. However, when memory goes back to facts of one's own experience, one is close to re-experience the whole process. The story becomes unacceptably long and would no more serve any reasonable informative purpose. History, indeed, becomes re-experience of human existence. For practical reasons, the author will try to be informative, the history of ISHA will become a collection of dry herbarium specimens, representing events which once have flourished. In this way, history is conservation of human experience, confirmed by dry facts. However, even stored facts can spread the perfume of the day when events occurred and they can testify to the power of growth at their origin.

Purpose of this Overview.

Two abstracts, dealing with the pre-history of ISHA and with the first ISHA were sent to the organizers of the 4th ISHA, Hamburg, April 26-29, 1997. At a later stage the authors were approached to melt the two stories and present an introductory overview. No easy task when one is not a politician or a tragic hero. The first one captures the audience with niceties attuned to the times. The other one may leave the stage like Shakespeare's Hamlet, Prince of Denmark: "Had I but time, - as this fell sergeant, death, is strict in his arrest, - O, I could tell you - But let it be". An amateur anaesthesia historian, however, does his best to do what is possible - he does what he can under given circumstances. If he succeeds to capture and enthuse the audience with only a few of dry facts remains to be seen. No doubt, with the audience already knowledgeable in the topic and drilled in discerning a fact from the fable, the amateur may succeed in picturing the history of ISHA's even in a short time allotted.

Method of Compilation of this Short Overview.

The collection of documentation in Rotterdam, pertaining to the ISHA's and organizations of the history of anaesthesia is considerable, to say the least. Predominantly in chronological order documents will be mentioned to testify to the things past. Personal reminiscences have proved to be surprisingly unreliable and will, therefore, be kept at a minimum. The most significant shortcoming of a lapidary presentation certainly is that it cannot do justice to all those who were on the stage when events occurred. Thanks to them one now talks history and tries to preserve something which we lived together.

It is hoped that all those involved in the history of the history of anaesthesia will get the just tribute at some more permitting opportunity; the place which every individual has in the dry and dusty collection of the documents representing the facts of the past. Every attempt was made not to put oneself into picture more than one would like to do so. Notwithstanding this attitude, overexposure, if any occurs, is the result of one's being at a certain place at a given time in the past. Those who prefer personal testimony to at random chosen facts will be pleased more than those who do not.

The Earliest Indication for a Rotterdam Meeting on the History of Anaesthesia.

In the programme of academic meetings called "Erasmus Anaesthesiological Proceedings" for year 1982 announcement was made for an "International Symposium: Modern History of Anaesthesia: This document[1] is not dated but must have been produced in February 1981 or before.

Early international publicity is documented by a letter from J. Rupreht and W. Erdmann of Rotterdam to R. Calverley of San Diego, California, dated 29th April 1981. The reason for writing the letter[2] was Calverley's interesting article about the Patron Saint of Anaesthetists, St. René. A part of the letter reads: "Next year at the beginning of May, exactly when the whole Holland is one luxurious tulip garden, we shall hold a Symposium Modern History of European Anaesthesiology (Britain and the Continent). The meeting takes place in a series: "Erasmus Anaesthesiological Proceedings".

The international publicity and advertising resulted in several encouraging incoming letters, personal or official. Jean Horton, then the Secretary of The Association of Anaesthetists of Great Britain and Ireland wrote[3] on 18th June 1981, in response to W. Erdmann's letter of 7th May 1981: *"The As-sociation would be pleased to help you in any way with suggestions for invitations to the nestors of the British anaesthesia"* and on 12th August 1981: *"The Council of The Association of Anaesthetists of Great Britain and Ireland have nominated Dr. D. Howat as the official representative of the Association"*[4].

More International Support for the History of Anaesthesia Meeting in Rotterdam.

A separate line of support and intent to attend resulted from correspondence which Prof. D. Soban of Ljubljana sent on 26th June 1982 to: Bunatian (USSR), to Denmark (W. Dam, O. Secher, H. Ruben) and to Britain (D. D. C. Howat, W. W. Mushin). All these letters[5] were answered within September '81, many with a request for instructions concerning the topic we asked for. Table 1 shows different titles for the meeting before the big and mini posters with *"Erasmus writing" (by A. Dürer)* were produced.

From the changes of the name for the Symposium which occurred between April and December 1981, one can see that the scope grew from European situation towards the world meeting. In the course of 1981 it became clear that the meeting was unique in its international aspect and that it was not possible to cover all what is of historical interest in anaesthesia. It was sensed that more meetings would have to follow and therefore "The first" was printed on posters and other materials. No one objected to the aims of the meeting which were publicized: *"The symposium intends to cover development, spread and affirmation of anaesthesiology, resuscitation and intensive care, after World War II. Most original contributors will take an active part at the symposium. This symposium serves as come-together of teachers and students. It is a unique opportunity to pay tribute to nestors and pioneers of anaesthesiology".*

Table 1. **Evolution of the Name for the Anaesthesia History Symposium**

1. Modern History of European Anaesthesiology (Britain and the Continent)	W. Erdmann - J. Rupreht	**April 29, 1981**
2. Congress on Modern History of Anaesthesiology	J. Rupreht	**June 18, 1981**
3. Symposium on the History of Modern Anaesthesia in Europe	D.D.C. Howat	**June 18, 1981**
4. Symposium on the Modern History of European Anaesthesia	D.D.C. Howat	**July 2, 1981**
5. History of Modern Anaesthesia	Sir Robert Macintosh	**October 2, 1981**
6. Congress "History of Modern Anaesthesia"	W.W. Mushin	**October 25, 1981**
7. The International Symposium: "History of Modern Anaesthesia"	J. Rupreht - W. Erdmann	**December 1981**
8. The First International Symposium on the History of Modern Anaesthesia	J. Rupreht - W. Erdmann	**December 1981**
9. Second International Symposium on the History of Anaesthesia	T. B. Boulton R. S. Atkinson	**London, 1987**

In retrospect, the stress on "modern" was very usefull as was the emphasis on coming together of people who contributed so much to what anaesthesia now is. Strictly academically, Sir Robert of Oxford was correct in remarking "What is this so-called modern anaesthesia"? Indeed, the word "modern" was rightly dropped from the title of the 2nd Symposium, London 1987.

The 1981-Response to the Planned Symposium

Judging from the impressive volume of correspondence during the second half of 1981, the prospective participants for the history meeting liked the idea very much. It should be quite clear that British colleagues helped beyond measure and that many Scandinavians were actively involved in shaping of the contents of the meeting. A very special tribute however, is due to Prof. D. Soban of Ljubljana whose support re-enforced interest in U.K. and Scandinavia.

The underlying strength of the planned symposium was individual approach to potential participants and a well-informed request for the topics they should present. We never dreamt to simply mail an announcement and wait and see what would happen. Once the mass mailing went out, we could advertise the fact that contributors would be deserving and knowledgeable individuals from all over the world. A long and impressive list of these names was printed on page 5 of the preliminary programme. Among them, Sir Robert, Sir Geoffrey, Thomas E. Keys, J. A. Lee, Hans Killian and Hideo Yamamura.

In several journals advertisements were placed: *Anaesthesia, The Japanese J. Anesth., Japanese J. Clin. Anesth. and Anesthesiology*. Whether they had any effect is not known but one famous anaesthesia historian may so have been alerted, the 1996-First Laureate of the History of Anaesthesia, Gwenifer Wilson of Australia. Besides having the cream of anaesthesia past for the meeting in 1982 more stature for the event was hoped for, without avail. The European Academy of Anaesthesiology refused patronage because the symposium was not their idea. An attempt to gain patronage from the royalty resulted in a negative letter of response when the meeting was already over.

Call for abstracts worked very well regardless of absence of FAX, and time constraint. The dead line was extended from 31st January 1982 to the end of February when a lovely Final Programme booklet was mailed[8]. This booklet set the tone, on the first page with a passage from as yet unpublished Sir Robert's reminiscences of his trip to Germany in 1937 and of anaesthesia there[9].

A difficult choice was made to accept all 120 abstracts for oral presentation which resulted in five simultaneous sessions. This draw-back and criticism which followed payed off when, from the 120 manuscripts, the Springer-Verlag produced a beautiful book of *Anaesthesia: Essays on Its History*[10]. The "Abstracts" book for the 1982 meeting has by now become a much wanted collector's item[11].

The well-known professors H. Killian and R. Frey from Germany had intended to participate, both pioneers of anaesthesia in their own right. Following R. Frey's death, the 1st Symposium was dedicated to his memory and a memorial service was held, on the opening day, at the famous Pilgrim's Church at Delfshaven of Rotterdam. Professor Killian had also died before symposium. In his last letter written to the organizers, "from the horizontal" of the hospital bed, he announced his absence and the fact that the collection of his paintings would not be brought to the symposium.

**The Happy Days,
5-8 May 1982 at Rotterdam**

The conventional course of events of the Rotterdam meeting can be reconstructed from the Programme and Abstract books[8,11]. Behind the screens video-interviews were made, champagne birthday party was held for J. Severinghaus, the presentations were audiorecorded and photographers were busy. Several exhibits were of interest, among them a unique presentation of Dräger apparatus. Participants enjoyed Rotterdam and Holland and the tulip season. Numerical data are given in Table 3.

**The Immediate Echo
of the Rotterdam Meeting**

Response to the meeting was overwhelming and is surprisingly well documented. Within 3 weeks dozens of enthusiastic and appreciative letters testified that participants enjoyed the meeting and hoped for another one after some time. Remarks from these letters are presented in Table 2.

In order to give a historically justified impression of the 1st International Symposium on the History of Anaesthesia one should refer to A. R. Hunter's Editorial "Rotterdam Meeting on the History of Anaesthesia"[12] and to G. Wilson's "A Significant Occasion"[13]. Both texts deserve to be quoted in full as an

Table 2. **Participants about the 1st International Symposium on the History of Modern Anaesthesia (May 5-8, 1982; Rotterdam)**

	Aphorism	Author	Date
1.	"I think it is a splendid idea and I hope that it receives the support it deserves".	D.A.B. Hopkin	09-11-1981
2.	"I've dispatched my abstracts for the meeting at Rotterdam. I'm looking forward to that trip more than any other professional meeting for many years".	R. Calverley	Dec. 1981
3.	"The happiest meeting ever".	J. Rees	May 1982
4.	"This meeting was in itself a significant step in the history of anaesthesia"; "A significant occasion".	G. Wilson	1982
5.	"Never have I attended so happy an anaesthetic congress".	J. A. Lee	09-05-1982
6.	"And I have never met so many happy participants as in Rotterdam".	B. Lind	11-05-1982
7.	"A most successful and pleasant symposium".	I. Lund	13-05-1982
8.	"Such a splendid meeting".	I. McLellan	May 1982
9.	"Symposium was such a success".	R. Mansfield	June 1982
10.	"The meeting in Rotterdam was the very best and most enjoyable I have ever attended, and one I'll certainly remember the longest".	R. Calverley	11-07-1982
11.	"Still I would not have traded the experience for the world".	R. Calverley	02-09-1982
12.	"It was a marvellous opportunity to meet so many people who have contributed much to modern anesthesia".	B. J. Bamforth	07-10-1982
13.	"Wonderful abstract issue; the very textbook of the history of modern anaesthesiology".	A. Matsuki	07-10-1982
14.	"Schenkte die Tagung das unvergängliche Erlebnis, in die Weltfamilie der Anästhesisten eingeordnet zu sein".	H. Schoepner	15-08-1982

15.	"Appreciation for the excellent symposium"; "hope that the first symposium devoted to the history of our specially will not be the last".	L. Couper	**19-07-1982**
16.	"Outstanding Symposium". "Your gathered together all the 'giants'".	R. Binning	**11-05-1982**
17.	"As Professor Gray said at the end, it really was a very happy meeting".	D.D.C. Howat	**20-05-1982**
18.	"An exceptionally successful first meeting in the history of modern anaesthesia".	R. Calverley	**28-12-1982**
19.	"Such an enjoyable four days. You and your committee have set a very high standard for the 2nd symposium to follow".	D. Wilkinson	**02-05-1982**
20.	"The whole symposium was a tremendous success".	J. Davenport	**June 1982**
21.	"Vôtre réunion a eu beaucoup de succès et je vous en félicite. Je ne m'attendais pas à un nombre aussi élevé de participants".	H. Reinhold	**07-06-1982**
22.	"Fabulous symposium"; "impressive, initiating accomplishment".	P. Safar	**14-05-1982**
23.	"This important meeting".	J. E. Steinhaus	**29-01-1982**
24.	"The meeting was by any standard a very considerable success, but for me it was a pinnacle of enjoyment"; "such a fine week for all of us".	J. W. Severinghaus	**14-05-1982**
25.	"This highly significant symposium".	J. E. Steinhaus	**22-01-1982**
26.	"It would be a great pleasure to contribute in some small way to the symposium".	D. Wilkinson	**02-02-1982**
27.	"A really first class event".	T. B. Boulton	**31-05-1983**
28.	"Your venture was of interest to many".	G. Wilson	**18-08-1983**
29.	"Timely to organize this meeting"; "so many outstanding members of our profession".	H. Yamamura	**May 1985**
30.	"Your brain child".	T. B. Boulton	1986
31.	"Had you not accepted my papers for Rotterdam, I would not have appeared on the world stage"!	G. Wilson	**08-11-1995**

illustration of the beginning of the anaesthesia history symposia (Appendix I and Appendix II). They were written with impressions from Rotterdam still fresh in mind and convey the sight of two prominent authors about the intrinsic value of the meeting. Anaesthesia became more than the doctor patient interaction and professor Hunter sensitively pointed out that a nurse-anaesthetist and a secretary also contributed to the first symposium. G. Wilson stressed that history of the specialty is indispensable for the anaesthetist's self-esteem and for the insight needed to head for the future.

Table 3. **International Symposia on the History of Anaesthesia**

Number, Date & Place	nr. Participants	nr. Papers	Printed Books & Publishers
1. May 5-8, 1982 Rotterdam	210 29 countries	120 Exhibits Video & Interviews	400 Abstracts books 2000 (Essays) *Springer-Verlag*
2. July 20-23, 1987 London	over 500 25 countries	100 free papers Extra sessions Exhibits	2000 soft cover & hard bound volumes *The Roy. Soc. Med.*
3. March 27-31, 1992 Atlanta	175 (450) 20 countries	97 Exhibits	2000 soft cover & 200 hard cover *The Wood-Library Museum*
4. April 26-29, 1997 Hamburg	255 20	150	1500

Table 3 gives a comparison of numerical facts of the Rotterdam meeting with subsequent events in London (1987) and Atlanta (1992) and Hamburg (1997). The information about numbers of registered delegates in Rotterdam and London are correct, but there is doubt about number of delegates in Atlanta and Hamburg. From those taking part it has been suggested that Atlanta gathered about 220 and Hamburg about 200 delegates interested in the history of anaesthesia, participating actively or passively. Numbers may be higher if one adds accompanying persons and those representing the trade.

Importance of ISHA's cannot be judged solely from the number of participants. The impact created would be more realistic if one were to multiply the delegates number with the number of books they had authored and only then compare the impact with a conventional meeting of anaesthesiologists. The lasting importance and effect of the first ISHA at Rotterdam is largely due to people who attended and contributed to it.

In the Wake of the first Symposium

Of the 120 papers read at the 1st ISHA manuscripts were not received of all. There was difficulty in finding the very best international publisher. The Elsevier refused to undertake the task to print the proceedings of a remarkable meeting, failing to recognize the 1st ISHA as such. Later, the Springer-Verlag decided to print a book of a selected number of edited contributions on a limited number of pages. The Editor in Chief expressed his worries of dissatisfied authors whose papers were not included. The Co-Editor, Dr. J. A. Lee wisely remarked: *"My dear chap, being an editor is making enemies"*. About 80 manuscripts were printed in 1985 entitled *"Anaesthesia: Essays on Its History"*[10]. The book soon became a collector's item. And a reprint has long been overdue and is due 1998.

Organisations of Anaesthesia History

Already during the Rotterdam meeting, on May 7, 1982, delegates from the USA gathered informally, inviting also the Secretary General of the 1st ISHA, and discussed the need "to get organized". This ad hoc meeting was followed by the Las Vegas 1982 meeting where decision was taken to establish *The Association of History of Anaesthesia (AHA)*.

Another far stretching event was discussion between Dr. J. A. Lee and Dr. J. Rupreht at the Rotterdam Airport, on May 9, 1982, concerning establishment of an international society of the history of anaesthesia. The early past of societies of the history of anaesthesia deserves and requires a separate study.

An attempt was also made to continue the ISHA-event at Rotterdam by requesting lasting support from The University to hold the successful meeting at regular intervals. The response was negative. Another request, to the major of the city, to co-sponsor purchase of Kaare Nygard's statue *"Victory over Pain"* also fell on deaf ears.

From the First to the Second ISHA

The Rotterdam ISHA gave much pleasure to all participants and remarkably many of them pondered aloud about the next such meeting. Some suggested to hold the meeting in Rotterdam at regular intervals. The other option of organizing the symposium in different countries gained grounds as time went on and no intent for the Second Symposium was announced from Rotterdam. On May 14th, 1982, Dr. I. McLellan of Leicester wrote: *"I would like to thank you and to congratulate you for such a splendid meeting. I am sure that all participants thoroughly enjoyed the First International Symposium on The History of Modern Anaesthesia. We are still thinking about the organization for the Second Symposium"*[14].

In the following months leading towards the memorable 6th European Congress of Anaesthesiology, in London, there was much correspondence between the participants to the First Symposium. Predominant topic was the need of anaesthesia historians to organize, followed by inquiries about publication of the proceedings and about the possibility of a Second Symposium. Dr. R. S. Atkinson wrote on 27th September 1982: *"As I understand it, there are a number of British anaesthetists who are interested in holding another symposium to follow on from your successful meeting in Rotterdam, but perhaps not for a number of years. In fact, 1987 has been mentioned as a possible time. I am sure that any such symposium would be international in flavour and that you want to be associated with it"*[15].

Already in December 1982 *"Anesthesia History Association Newsletter"* included a report from England: *"There are plans for a second international symposium on the history of anaesthesia in 1987"*[16]. By May 1983, the Council of the Association of Anaesthetists of Great Britain and Ireland resolved to follow the Rotterdam example and appointed dr. T. B. Boulton as chairman of the organizing committee for the second symposium in 1987. Only later, London was chosen as the place and the date was adjusted close to the 50th anniversary of the foundation of the Nuffield Chair of Anaesthetics, at the Oxford University[17]. Other members of the Organizing Committee were: J. F. Baskett, M. Rosen, R. S. Atkinson, R. H. Ellis, M. T. Inman, I. McLellan, G. M. C. Patterson, P. Thompson, R. S. Vaughan, D. Wilkinson and J. S. M. Zorab[18]. They worked very efficiently and with advertising phantasy. In a letter to Dr. Mainzer of March 1, 1984, Dr. Rupreht wrote: *"It is good to see how efficiently and dedicatedly Dr. Boulton works on the Second International Symposium on the History of Anaesthesia. I am including a poster"*[26].

The Second ISHA, London, July 20-23, 1987

The History of Anaesthesia Society was inaugurated on June 7, 1986 at Reading, England, with Dr. J. A. Lee as President. This Society and the Association of Anaesthetists were the main and powerful sponsors of the 2nd ISHA, in contrast to the solitary action of the Department of Anaesthesiology at the Erasmus University Rotterdam sponsoring the first event.

The word "modern" had been dropped from the name of the second ISHA; appropriately so as the scope of the meeting was enlarged to accommodate complete history of anaesthetic endeavour. The meeting in London certainly surpassed the first one in glamour, venue site, social events, number of participants and patronage. It was a great success by any standard and the organizers deserve every one's gratitude. A special feature were presentations of prominent pioneers of anaesthesia. Manuscripts of the 2nd ISHA were aptly edited by T. B. Boulton and R. S. Atkinson and were published by the Royal Society of Medicine (Table 3)[19]. The 1987-ISHA demonstrated again that meetings of anaesthesia historians are good humoured, agreeable and of high scientific interest. It is hoped that an extended monograph about this meeting will be written by one of the organizers.

The Third ISHA, Atlanta, Georgia, March 29 - April 2, 1992

Following the resounding success of the 2nd ISHA[20], the Anaesthesia History Association (AHA); inaugurated October 9, 1983, Atlanta, Georgia) opted for the 1992 - venue to be Atlanta, Georgia. The Organizing Committee (J. Steinhaus - Chairman, M. Albin, R. Calverley, E. Frost, C. R. Stephen and J. Walter) distributed leaflets already during the London meeting and the 3rd ISHA was to coincide exactly with the 150th anniversary of Crawford Long's anaesthetic use of ether, on 31st March 1832. The chief sponsor was AHA in collaboration with Georgia Medical Association and Atlanta Society of Anaesthesiology. The American Society of Anesthesiologists was intrinsically not involved, this in contrast to the London meeting.

The 3rd ISHA was again a symposium to be remembered[21], although one would have hoped for greater participation from the U.S.A., so rich in the history of anaesthesia. A remarkable feature was the expedient collecting and editing of manuscripts by Dr. B. Raymond Fink, resulting in beautiful Proceedings in 1993[22]. This volume was published by the Wood-Library Museum, Park Ridge, Illinois.

During the 3rd ISHA, the two societies of the history of anaesthesia played a major role for the first time (AHA and the History of Anaesthesia Society, HAS). Besides niceties being exchanged, a semi-structured attempt took place to designate the venue of the next ISHA. The bid was from Hamburg, Germany and from Israel. It was decided to continue to advertise events such as ISHA through the channels of the WFSA (World

Federation of Societies of Anaesthesiologists) but to remain independent from other anaesthesiological groups. The Hamburg bid was accepted later during the ad hoc meeting of anaesthesia historians, in 1992, during the Xth World Congress of Anaesthesiologists, at The Hague[24].

The ISHAs and the World Federation of Societies of Anaesthesiologists (WFSA)

In the wake of the Rotterdam successful 1st ISHA and in the fervour towards the 2nd ISHA at London, dr. J. S. M. Zorab, Secretary, WFSA, mailed a memorandum to all member societies of the WFSA, proposing a mechanism for selection of ISHA future venues[23]. The idea was that the member societies wishing to organize an ISHA were to apply to the WFSA whereupon a small panel of advisers sould submit an evaluation to the Executive Committee of the WFSA. Thus, national societies or affiliated anaesthesia history societies could become candidates for organization of history symposia.

Surprisingly, the independent Anaesthesia History Association was left out as would be the History of Anaesthesia Society (inaugurated in 1986).

It is not known what impact the memorandum had and whether decision to place 3rd ISHA to Atlanta had anything to do with it. Opinion is still divided whether the attempt was correct to use the WFSA channels for the purpose of anaesthesia historians. Most anaesthesia historians have wished to remain independent of existing establishment within anaesthesiology, both on national and international level.

Incidentally, study of the WFSA-past led some anaesthesia historians to suggest to the WFSA that archives of this big organization should be collected and then kept at one place. Indeed, Dr. Zorab was later instrumental in arranging that WFSA-Archives are now kept at the Wood-Library Museum, Illinois.

The Hague Meeting Concerning ISHA - Venue

Along with numerous events of the jubilee 10th World Congress of Anaesthesiologists at The Hague, 1992, anaesthesia historians deliberated about a mechanism for deciding on the venue of future ISHA's. It was decided that the 4th ISHA would take place at Hamburg, 1997. There was such interest in ISHA, bids forthcoming from countries like Czechoslovakia, Poland, Israel, Australia, Spain that it was decided to hold the meeting quadrennially but so that it would not coincide with major international events in anaesthesia[24,25].

During this meeting in The Hague the need for an international federation of societies of the history of anaesthesia was discussed and tabled as premature. The main concern against such a federation was the wish of AHA and HAS to remain independent whereas other national anaesthesia history groups were merely sections of national societies.

The Hamburg Meeting on the ISHA - Venue

As of 1997, the current mechanism to decide on future venues of ISHA is a meeting of ISHA - Venue Committee (IVC). The IVC consists of one representative of previous ISHA - organizers, of one representative of AHA and HAS, the latter two representing organized anaesthesia historians and their choice of future venues. An Australian delegate has been adopted to IVC because of remarkable anaesthesia history activity in their land.

At Hamburg, the IVC heard bids for 5th ISHA from Israel, Bohemia and Spain. It was decided to organize the 2001 - ISHA in Santiago de Compostela, Spain. The IVC will be closely monitoring all aspects of future IS-

HA's, including finances. Fund raising will start in order to be able to contribute to the overall success of these meetings. Publication of Proceedings has become a must.

The IVC decided to formulate and adopt ISHA-venue criteria and the code of conduct concerning individual ISHA's. The final decision was to hold the quadrennial ISHA also in event of no national bids. This move, apparently, is the most optiminiscic indicator that ISHA's will continue to contribute to the anaesthesiological profession.

References:

1. Programme, 1 page, Erasmus Anaesthesiological Proceedings 1981-2; Anaesthesia Archives, Rotterdam, The Netherlands.
2. Letter to R. Calverley of 29th April 1981. Idem 1.
3. Letter, Jean Horton to W. Erdmann, of 18th June, 1981. Idem 1.
4. Letter, Jean Horton to W. Erdmann, of 12th August, 1981. Idem 1.
5. Letters, Prof. D. Soban, six in number, of 26th June, 1981, Copies. Idem 1.
6. Poster for the 5-8 May 1982 Symposium, December 1981. Idem 1.
7. Preliminary programme; The First International Symposium on the History of Modern Anaesthesia. Dec. 1981. page 5. Idem 1.
8. Final Programme. The First I.S.H.A.; February 1982. Idem 1.
9. Macintosh, R: Some examples of how attitudes to anaesthesia, in Germany and Austria alone, have changed over the past thirty-forty years. Manuscript, 2 pp. December 1981. Idem 1.
10. Anaesthesia: Essays on Its History. J. Rupreht et al. Eds. Springer-Verlag; Heidelberg, Berlin, New York, Tokyo, 1985.
11. Abstracts. The First International Symposium on the History of Modern Anaesthesia, Rotterdam, April 1982. Idem 1.
12. Hunter, A R: Editorial. Rotterdam Meeting on the History of Anaesthesia. Br J Anaesth., 54: 797, 1982.
13. Wilson, G A: A Significant Occasion: The First International Seminar on the History of Modern Anaesthesia. Erasmus University, Rotterdam 5th - 8th May, 1982. Anaest. Intens. Care, 1982: 10:370.
14. McLellan, I. A letter, 14th May, 1982. to Dr. J. Rupreht. Idem 1.
15. Atkinson, R. S. A letter, 27th September, 1982, to Dr. J. Rupreht. Idem 1.
16. Anaesthesia History Association Newsletter, Vol. 1., nr. 1., p. 2., December 1982.
17. Boulton, T. B. A letter, 31st May, 1983, to Dr. J. Rupreht. Idem 1.
18. Anaesthesia, Annual Report of the Council 1982-1983; 1984: 39, p. 96.
19. The History of Anaesthesia. R. S. Atkinson and T. B. Boulton, Eds. Internat. Congress and Symp. Series Nr. 134. Royal Society of Medicine Services, Ltd. London, New York, 1989.
20. Stephen, C R: Second International Symposium on the History of Anaesthesia. Anaesthesia History Association Newsletter, 5 : 4 : p. 2, Oct. 1987.
21. Stephen, C R: A symposium to remember. Anaesthesia History Association Newsletter, 10 : 3 : p.1, July 1992.
22. The History of Anaesthesia. Third International Symposium. Proceedings, B. Raymond Fink, Ed. Wood-Library Museum of Anesthesiology, Park Ridge, Illinois, 1992.
23. Zorab, J S M: Memorandum to all member Societies, WFSA. October 25, 1985. Idem 1.
24. Morris, L E: Minutes of an ad hoc Committee to discus future Symposia on the History of Anaesthesia: Sunday, June 14, 1992, Congress Center, Den Haag, Holland. Minutes available on July 14, 1992. Idem I.
25. Letter, L. E. Morris to J. Rupreht. February 14, 1997. Idem I.
26. Letter J. Rupreht to J. Mainzer. March 1, 1984. Idem I.

Appendix I

Editorial
Rotterdam Meeting on the History of Anaesthesia

Henry Ford of Ford Motors is credited with the aphorism that history is bunk and A. J. P. Taylor with the suggestion that the only lesson to be learned from history is that the fact than men never learn the lessons of history. Nonetheless it is, to say the least of it, interesting to learn the facts concerning the introduction of new anaesthetic drugs and those who were responsible for them, and especially to meditate on the times when such advances were made and what was the ethos thereof.

The history of anaesthesia really falls into two sections. First there is the ether and chloroform era which began with Morton's administration of ether in Boston, in 1846, and extended until about the beginning of the 1939-45 War. About this time, however, there was a revolution in the practice of anaesthesia and a large number of those who were involved are still alive, but in the nature of things cannot expect to survive beyond the biblical three score and ten years. It was therefore singularly appropriate to bring together those who were pioneers of modern anaesthesia so that the stories of what happened during the critical years could be recorded. At a conference on the History of Modern Anaesthesia, in Rotterdam on May 5-8 of this year, more than 150 contributors participated. In general presentations were concerned with people who had been active in the development of anaesthesia, with the way in which anaesthesia developed in certain specific locations (sometimes countries, sometimes cities) and with the drugs that became available over the years.

Not only was it desirable that the stories should be recorded - it was salutary for those who entered anaesthesia at a later date to learn something of the now forgotten difficulties which beset the pioneers.

The history of our own Journal found a place in the programme, as did an account of the UEMS and the World Federation of Societies of Anaesthesiologists. An opportunity was given to a nurse anaesthetist to present her view of their place in current practice and in the future, and the secretary of the Department of Anaesthetics at St Thomas's Hospital in London, who had served in this capacity for some 30 years, presented a "worm's eye" view of the specialty.

It is not possible within the compass of an editorial to do justice to the numerous papers which were read, but it is planned there will be a publication of the Proceedings of the Congress.

In the meantime we offer our congratulations to Dr. J. Rupreht and his colleagues who conceived the idea of holding the conference and carried it through so successfully.

A. R. Hunter

Appendix II

A Significant Occasion:
The First International Seminar on the History of Modern Anaesthesia
Erasmus University, Rotterdam, 5th-8th May, 1982

For some years various Societies of Anaesthetists and Faculties of Anaesthesia have occasionally included in their meeting programmes a session, or part session, on the history of the specialty. These programmes have indicated a growing interest in this aspect of the study of anaesthesia. Such interest is usually a sign of the maturation of a specialty from the early stages of the struggle for recognition to the calm contemplation of the steps which have led to this success.

It is to the Department of anaesthesiology, Erasmus University, Rotterdam, that we owe recognition of this awakened enthusiasm, and the organisation of the First International Seminar on the History of Modern Anaesthesia, held in the Medical School of the Erasmus University, from 5th-8th May, 1982. This meeting was in itself a significant step in the history of anaesthesia.

Though every form of anaesthesia and intensive care received due recognition, the emergent themes of discussion were "Pioneering in Anaesthesia" and "The Spread of Modern Anaesthesia around the World". This was natural, since the organising committee had made a point of inviting not only the known pioneers of methods and equipment, but also those who had led the establishment of the specialty in countries all around the world.

The list of participants was a microcosm of anaesthetic history, for although such men as Harold Griffith of Canada and Ivan Magill of England were physically unable to be present, many other pioneers read fascinating papers describing in person their early experiences with methods and apparatus taken or granted by today's anaesthetists. Sir Robert Macintosh and Dr. Lucien Morris aroused great interest with their papers on the postgraduate training schools, whilst Ibsen of Denmark very truly pointed out that it was a result of his work with Lassen during the poliomyelitits epidemic in Copenhagen in 1952 that the anaesthetist, as he said, "was taken out of the operating theatre".

As the only Australian present, I must pay tribute to the Australian Society of Anaesthetists and the Faculty of Anaesthetists, Royal Australian College of Surgeons. Due to the policy of annual invitation of a distinguished anaesthetist from overseas to lecture in all states and attend meetings, I found myself among many old friends, who made eager enquiries about other anaesthetists in Australia, and sent their good wishes to you all.

As well as the papers, there were a number of excellent demonstrations; a magnificent series of illustrations of German apparatus throughout the 136 years of anaesthetic history; Dr. Morris' "family tree" of noted anaesthetists in descent from Ralph Waters of Madison, Wisconsin, the pioneer of postgraduate training; as small but elegant exhibit by the Netherlands Society which included St. René, the patron saint of anaesthesia (of whom I'd never heard); and the "quiz" demonstration, that is, "Name this piece of apparatus".

It was to be anticipated that this first meeting should have been perhaps too brief for the number of papers offered, which led to tantalising decisions as to which of several simultaneous sessions to attend, when one really wanted to hear them all, but the organisers are to be congratulated on their initiative and enthusiasm in inaugurating this progressive movement.

Dr. Erdmann, Professor of Anaesthesiology, Eramus University was Chairman of the Symposium. He and his wife were most gracious hosts. As with every meeting, the secretary is the lynch-pin. Dr. Rupreht was excellent in this role.

Gwen Wilson*
D. A., F.F.A.R.R.C.S., Honorary Historian
to the Faculty of Anaesthetists, Royal
Australasian College of Surgeons.

Pain and Analgesia for Operative Interventions from the Beginning to 1846

Th. B. Boulton
United Kingdom. Past President History of Anaesthesia Society.

Summary

The public demonstration by Morton of ether anaesthesia at the Massachusetts General Hospital on 16 October 1846, to the right audience, at the right time, resulted in the worldwide acceptance of general anaesthesia; however the event was the culmination of a search for a means of allaying surgical pain extending over many centuries!

B.C. to c1500. A locally applied technique may have been used c.2300 B.C. during circumcision; certainly freezing with ice was used during the medieval period. Oral and rectal herbal preparations, including cannabis, opium and mandragora, were employed from the first century A.D. and possibly earlier, and throughout the medieval period.

c.1500 to c.1750. Renaissance surgeons were wary of using unstandardised herbal preparations because of the possibility of fatal accidents and association with the capital crime of witchcraft. Paré (France) used nerve compression during amputations but condemned the use of potions to control pain.

c.1750 to c.1800. The "age of enlightenment" brought the development of science and humanitarianism; in the U.K. Priestley discovered oxygen and nitrous oxide, Beddoes attempted to treat disease by the inhalation of gases and vapours, and his assistant Davy demonstrated the inebriating and analgesic properties of nitrous oxide.

c.1800 to 1842. Many techniques were tried in the effort to control surgical pain including nerve compression, asphyxiation, hypnosis and local refrigeration. Ether and nitrous oxide were inhaled for recreational inebriation.

1842. William Clarke (medical student of New York State) and Crawford Long (general practitioner of Georgia USA), inspired by prior personal recreational use, independently gave ether by inhalation for minor surgical procedures.

11 December 1844. Horace Wells, a dentist of Hartford, Connecticut, prompted by attendance at a stage demonstration of its properties by the popular lecturer Quincy Colton, himself inhaled nitrous oxide successfully for a dental extraction.

January 1845. Partial failure of a demonstration of nitrous oxide anaesthesia by Wells in Boston witnessed by Morton.

16 October 1846. W.T.G. Morton, Boston dentist and former partner of Wells, after use in his own practice, gave the first public demonstration of ether anaesthesia by inhalation.

Introduction.

The era of modern anaesthesia is, almost universally and correctly, dated from the successful public demonstration of the use of ether vapour for allaying the pain of surgery by the dentist William Thomas Green Morton just over 150 years ago, on Ether day 16 October 1846.[1] Morton did not "discover" anaesthesia however, nor was he the first person in history to relieve, or seek to relieve, surgical pain, nor the first to use inhaled ether for that purpose; but his professional conviction and his successful administration of the right agent, before the right people, at the right moment in history, ensured that the news of his success spread rapidly throughout the world and led to a revolution in the practice of surgery.[1-3]

At least one philosopher has chosen the introduction of surgical anaesthesia as the greatest event in medical history.[4] I would not go that far, but, in my view, at the time of its discovery only Paré's revolutionary treatment of wounds (c.1540), and Jenner's vaccination (1798) preceded it.[1,2,5]

The title of this presentation, which was provided by the organisers of the Symposium, rather implies that the word "analgesia" simply means the relief of surgical pain, whether the patient remains conscious or is rendered unconscious. In this presentation the term "anaesthesia" or "general anaesthesia" indicates the relief of pain by rendering the patient unconscious, and "analgesia" the relief of pain in the conscious patient and, further, that "analgesia" can either be "local", by blocking the peripheral nervous system, or "central" by direct action on the higher brain centres, but short of producing unconsciousness.

Early attempts at local analgesia.

Nunn[7] pointed out during the Second International Symposium in 1987 that the first illustration of an attempt to relieve the pain of surgery by a locally applied method was possibly that on the tomb of Ankhmahor, vizier or principal officer of state of the Egyptian Pharaoh Teti the first, about 2300 B.C. The hieroglyphics suggest that one medical attendant is applying something to numb the pain of circumcision at the operation; though what that might be is obscure; probably not ice as ice was not known in Egypt at that time.[1,7]

Local refrigeration analgesia with ice or snow has however been practised from the earliest time, the first known reference being in an Anglo-Saxon manuscript in the eleventh century. Marco Aurelio Severino in Venice in the 17th century was cunning enough to disguise the snow hwich he used, by colouring it red.[1,8]

Benjamin Richardson employed the evaporation of ether to numb the skin for surgical analgesia when the introduced his "ether spray" in 1866.[9] This was two decades after Morton's demonstration in 1846, and refrigeration with ice was used for amputation of gangrenous limbs in poor risk patients as late as the nineteen fifties.[1,10] Morton's demonstration of inhalational general anaesthesia with ether in 1846, of course, predated the introduction of reversible pharmacological local analgesia by Koller in 1884 by nearly four decades.[11]

Centrally acting oral and rectal herbal preparations.

If we now turn back to the early use of centrally acting oral and rectal herbal preparations capable of producing unconsciousness of indifference to pain in the centuries immediately before and after the birth of Christ, they included cannabis, opium, and the extracts of plants of the Solanaceae family including the mandrake or mandragora. The principal alkaloids in the extracts are hyocine and hyocyamine. How far these extracts were used for the relief of surgically inflicted pain in the pre-Christian millenium is uncertain; but Hippocrates recommended a draught of mandragora juice in wine before surgical intervention in the fourth century BC, and Cicero wrote a diatribe against surgeons who did not use drugs to allay the pain of surgery in the first century BC.[1,2,7,8,12-14] Two of the herbs, the mandrake root and the seed boxes of the opium poppy are depicted in the coat of arms of the Association of Anaesthetists of Great Britain and Ireland.[14,15] The use of the soporific sponge (spongia somnifera) is considered below separately.

There are more specific references to the relief of surgical pain by oral and rectal preparations in the first century AD. Both the Roman Pliny the Edler and the Greek Plutarch were familiar with the use of drugs for this purpose, but most information can be gained from the writings of Pedanius Dioscorides, the Greek who was sometime surgeon to the armies of the Roman Emporer Nero.[1,2,8,12,13] Dioscorides published a *Materia Medica* which remained a standard work for many centuries. He was the first to use the word "anaesthesia" in its modern meaning[12] some eighteen hundred years before Morton's Boston contemporary, the physician and author Oliver Wendell Holmes, independently recommended its use for the process of etherisation.[16]

Dioscorides administered oral and rectal extracts of the mandrake root in wine to relieve the pain of surgery.[12] Dioscorides can be regarded as the first anaesthetist to give a "balanced anaesthetic"! He combined extract of mandragora with extract of Hemlock, which contains the muscle relaxant coniine, in order to avoid the muscular spasms associated with mandragora administrations.[13]

The oral administration of wine to which soporific herbal extracts such as those of the mandrake had been added are known to have been offered as an act of mercy to those about to undergo crucifixion. Christ himself was offered but refused such a draught on the way to his crucifixion, and he had a sea sponge on a reed held to his lips after he had been crucified for several hours when he complained of thirst. This sponge was traditionally soaked in vinegar containing hyssop. Extracts of *Hysopus officinalis* itself are merely aromatic and astringent, but the term "hyssop" is used more generically of herbal preparations in Biblical writings, and a soporific, such as mandrake, might also have been included.[14,17]

Witchcraft and the Mandrake. Considerable mythology which gradually grew up around the mandrake was partly because of the resemblance of the root to the human form. The plant was supposed to scream when pulled out of the ground and for a human to hear the screams was fatal; consequently the leaves were tied to a dog's tail for uprooting and the herbalist kept well out of the way, and it was the dog that died. Some herbalists were however less superstitious than others about the dangers of the procedure![1,18]

The use of these herbal concoctions began to decline after the thirteenth century. The main reason was because the use of the unstandardised extracts was very dangerous and often proved to be fatal. This was unfortunate for the patient, but also dangerous for the physician who was liable to be executed. The herbs fell into the hands of wise women or witches who used them both to proceduce sleep and as fertility drugs and for anyone, particularly physicians, to be associated with witches and the herbs, particularly mandragora, was a capital crime.[1,13]

One of the charges of heresy made by the English against St. Joan of Arc, the Maid of Orleans, before they burnt her at the stake as a witch in 1431, was that she "possessed a mandrake", but, if true, for what purpose is open to question.[1,13] It must be appreciated that, though pain was regarded as a divine punishment, pain relief as an act of redemption was not necessarily a sin; to appreciate this one has only to recall the superlative record of medieval monasteries in caring for the sick and injured. In the case of the mandrake it was its association with witchcraft which led to the capital charges. Ambroise Paré, the great sixteenth century French military surgeon, was a critic of the use of soporific herbal extracts to relieve the pain of amputations, but he used nerve compression for the purpose; similarly the near contemporary burning of Eufaine MacCalzean in

Edinburgh was not, as is sometimes asserted, because she endeavoured to relieve the pain of childbirth, but because she employed witchcraft for the purpose.[1,8]

Use and investigation of herbal preparations in the nineteenth century. The Japanese surgeon Seishu Hanaoka very successfully used an oral preparation of herbs of the Solanaceae family as anaesthesia for western style surgery half a ce century before the so-called "period of isolation" of Japan was ended by the action of the American Navy in 1854 eight years after Morton's Boston demonstration of ether by inhalation. Hanaoka probably learnt his surgical skills and the knowledge of the herb *Datura alba,* which is closely related to Mandrake, from Dutch traders who had limited contact with Japanese ports during the years of isolation.[1,19]

Benjamin Ward Richardson (1828-1896), the friend and biographer of John Snow (1813-1858), the first professional anaesthetist, demonstrated experimentally the effectiveness of mandragora extract prepared in the manner described by Dioscorides as "a general anaesthetic of the most potent quality" in 1888.[14] It was however with the discovery and isolation of the active agents morphia and hyocine, which could be administered in accurate dosage by the syringe and hollow needle,[20] that secopolamine (hyocine) combined with morphia found its use in anaesthesia. First as an anaesthetic administered by multiple injection, both in the technique of "twillight sleep" for obstetrical pain and for operative surgery, in an effort to produce safer anaesthesia at the height of the peak incidence of chloroform deaths at the turn of the century; and nowadays, of course, as a combination which is widely used as a premedicant.[14]

The mysterious soporific sponge (spongia somnifera).

Written references to the use of the soporific sponge to relieve the pain of surgery occur from the ninth century to the sixteenth century1, and there are two rather strange references to its use, one in a modified form before, and the other just after the news of Morton's demonstration reached France in 1847.[14]

The soporific sponge was soaked in extracts of opium, mandragora and other herbs and reconstituted prior to use. It is said that the sponge was held close to the patient's nose and inhaled. Modern attempts to produce anaesthesia in this way have failed. It may be that the fluid from the sponge was absorbed from the nasal mucous membrane or even ingested.[1,22]

Smilie's use in Boston from 1844 onwards, before Morton's demonstration is fascinating. He was endeavouring to relieve surgical pain by having the patient inhale opium. There is no doubt he was successful! This is not surprising as the solvent he had chosen was ether.[1,21] Anthony Carter has recently drawn attention to the curious claim of Dauriol in a provincial French journal to have successfully used inhalation from a herbal sponge to relieve surgical pain as an alternative to ether seven months after Morton's demonstration.[14] This is hardly credible: hypnosis seems to be the only explanation. (Stex)[1]

Attitudes to pain in the seventeenth and eighteenth century.

There were those who continued to commend the use of drugs to relieve pain in the seventeenth and eighteenth century but, for the most part, surgery was conducted amidst indescribable agony;[23] but, by the end of the eighteenth century, in the era we call "the age of enlightenment" more humanitarian attitudes developed.[1,24,25] Surgeons of the period are often represented as brutes rejoicing in the infliction of pain, but many were distressed about the suffering which they inflicted on their patients. Speed of operating and the way they made their incisions was their only resource.[1,25]

Joseph Priestley (1733-1804).

The age of enlightenment also brought with it scientific discovery. The amazing theologian and self-taught scientific genius Joseph Priestley prepared and elucidated the physical and physiological properties of carbon dioxide, oxygen and nitrous oxide and other oxides of nitrogen in the seventeen seventies.[1,8,26-28] The inhalation of diluted ether vapour was already well established as a method of treating lung diseases including quite correctly, or at least symptomatically, asthma. Priestley, though not a physician himself, suggested that the inhalation of the inorganic gases might be used to treat lung diseases such as tuberculosis and asthma. He was living in Birmingham in the seventeen eighties and nineties and was associated with a number of scientists and physicians who acted upon his suggestions, and pneumatic medicine was born.[1,28]

Thomas Beddoes (1760-1808) and the Pneumatic Institute.

Prominent among the advocates of pneumatic medicine was Thomas Beddoes, a Bristol physician, who in 1798 founded the Medical Pneumatic Institute with the express purpose of evaluating the therapeutic value of the inhalation of gases and vapours.[1,8,27-30]

Humphry Davy (1778-1829) and nitrous oxide.

Beddoes chose as his superintendent of the pneumatic institute Humphry Davy, a twenty year old surgeon's apprentice from Penzance who was much more interested in chemistry than surgery. Davy's early research work on inhalation with makeshift apparatus had been brought to the attention of Beddoes. Davy had demonstrated by animal and self administration that nitrous oxide could be inhaled safely. This was contrary to the gloomy prognostications of some physicians who believed that the prolonged inhalation of this particular gas might be fatal or even cause them to contract plague.[1,28,29]

Davy worked at the Institute for just two years from 1798-1800. So far as curing lung disease was concerned the inhalation of the gases was, or course, a failure; however Davy, conducted a series of brilliant experiments, which exhaustively evaluated the physics and physiological of nitrous oxide, and he conducted experiments of its effect, both on himself and animals. Davy was particularly intrigued with the stimulating and inebriating effect of nitrous oxide. Many members of the fashionable Bristol circle came to experience the exciting and pleasurable effects of inhaling the gas including poets Southey and Coleridge.[1,27-29]

Davy made his now famous observation about the analgesic properties of nitrous oxide while cutting a wisdom tooth and, as a consequence, made his equally well known suggestion about its possible use to relieve surgical pain, while he was at the Pneumatic Medical Institution.[1,27-29]

Davy published his observations in 1800 in his classic book *Researches chemical and philosophical; chiefly concerning nitrous oxide or dephlogisticated nitrous air, and its respiration,* in which occurs the much quoted passage:- "As nitrous oxide in its extensice operation appears capable of destroying physical pain, it may probably be used with advantage during surgical operations in which no great effusion of blood takes place."[31]

Davy's much debated and rather cryptic remark about the desirability of there being "no great effusion of blood" has probably been best explained by Cartwright. Davy possibly believed that, since the nitrous oxide was dissolved in the blood, its effect would rapidly be lost to the body after the single dose administration which he envisaged, if there was severe haemorrhage.[27]

Davy was head hunted to become the Lecturer in Chemistry at the recently founded Royal Institution soon after his book was published.[1,27]

It is important to stress that Davy placed his emphasis on the stimulatory effects of nitrous oxide. This led Beddoes to hope and believe for a time that the inhalation of nitrous oxide might be a treatment for various forms of paralysis. Nitrous oxide inhalation became a stimulatory recreational drug amongst scientists who knew how to prepare it, and, more important, a drug of entertainment in public demonstrations of the laughing gas. It was this stimulating effect, and not Davy's incidental observations about its analgesic properties, which ultimately led to its use as an anaesthetic by Wells some forty years after Davy published his *Researches* volume.[28]

Attempts at the relief of surgical pain in the late eighteenth and the first half of the nineteenth century.

The late eighteenth century and the first half of the nineteenth century was a period when methods for the relief of surgical pain were being actively considered. It is important philosophically to emphasise that the goal of most of these early nineteenth century pioneers was the relief of surgical pain, and not necessarily oblivion to the fact that surgery was being undertaken. That is they aimed to produce "analgesia" as we have defined it, rather than "general anaesthesia". Physical methods of producing local anaesthesia were studied. These included the revival of interest in both refrigeration analgesia and nerve compression.[32] The use of nerve compression by Dr. James Moore for amputations by John Hunter is particularly interesting in view of Hunter's attitude to pain as an inevitable but reprehensible consequence of surgery.[2,24,32,33]

Baron Larrey, Napoleon's brilliant military surgeon who was responsible for so many advances in the surgery of trauma, is sometimes also credited with the reintroduction of refrigeration anaesthesia;[8] sadly this is not the case. Larrey's observation was that frozen gangerous limbs were also free from pain.[34] James Arnot, a physician in Brighton, England did however practise refrigeration techniques for minor procedures immediately prior to Morton's demonstration in 1846.[35]

Henry Hill Hickman, (1800-1830) suspended animation, and carbon dioxide.

The life history of Henry Hill Hickman, a compassionate and thoughtful general practitioner from Shropshire, England, and his success in relieving experimental pain in small animals in the eighteen twenties, has been comprehensively reviewed by Denis Smith[20] and also by Cartwright.[27] So far as we know Hickman never attempted to anaesthetise a human subject, and his experiments are not directly relevant to the line of development of pharmacological general anaesthesia.[1]

Hickman's purpose was to undertake very rapid surgery under the state of extreme but reversible oxygen deprivation just short of permanent damage to the brain.[1,27,28] This state of so called "suspended animation" was well known to Hickman and his contemporaries because of the prevalent interest in reviving the apparently dead after drowning and other causes of asphyxia. In some of his experiments in small animals and birds Hickman set them to exhaust the oxygen in a bell jar starting with ambient air, in others air to which chemically generated carbon dioxide been added, and in a third group in a atmosphere of his own expired air containing carbon dioxide. He did make the observation that the animals became unconscious more rapidly when carbon dioxide was present at the start of the experiment, but he does not seem to have made the deduction that CO_2 might be an anaesthetic, and there is no evidence that he was aware of Davy's observation of the analgesic properties of nitrous oxide. Hickman's largely unsuccessful attempts to interest the British Scientific establishment, headed by the now famous but rather arrogant Humphry Davy, and the French Academy, in the possibility of the relief of surgical pain make a poignant story. Cartwright's assessment of Hickman's contribution is undoubtedly correct:- "His glory lies in the idea which lies behind his work .... for he, the first of all men, set out to banish pain by means of experimental investigation".[1,27,28]

Hypnosis and the relief of surgical pain.

Hypnosis was another method used successfully to reduce surgical pain by isolated practitioners during this period of searching for a means of relieving surgical pain in the first half of the nineteenth century. Knowledge of the means of production of the hypnotic state dates back beyond recorded history, long before it was popularised by Mesmer (1734-1815) in the mid eighteenth century.[1,36]

Mesmer himself did not try to use hypnosis to control surgical pain but others did;[36] notable amongst these was John Elliotson (1791-1868), physician to the North London hospital, which is now known as the University College Hospital, and his pupil James Esdaile (1808-1859), surgeon to the East India Company in India, just before Morton's ether demonstration.[1,8,29,36] Elliotson was successful but, like Mesmer himself, he allowed his enthusiasm to overcome cautions optimism in his claims for hypnotism as a therapeutic agent in general and, because mesmerism was considered to be mysterious and not quite respectable by the orthodox medical profession, he was forced to resign his appointment at the North London Hospital.[1,8,29,36] The use of hypnosis to overcome the pain of dentistry and plastic surgery was revived in the nineteen fifties.[37]

The "discovery" and early medical use of ether.

Ether which was known and prepared by Paracelsus and Valerius Cordus in the sixteenth century in an impure form as "sweet oil of vitriol" - a mixture of ether alcohol and water; and was fed by them to hens to induce reversible sleep. Ether was purified and given the name "aether" by Froben in the eighteenth century.[1,8,38]

The agent then became a popular surface application for headaches, an oral medication for gastric complaints and, by nasal sniffing, for nervous diseases.[1,30] More prolonged inhalation followed for lung diseases, and subsequently, when its intoxicating properties were appreciated, it became an easily obtainable recreational drug. It was used to some extent orally in Scotland, but mainly by inhalation, particularly amongst medical students both in the United Kingdom and North America.[1,24,33,38]

It was therefore common knowledge that there were two inhalation and relatively safe recreational drugs available (nitrous oxide and ether). This was particularly the case amongst the medical and scientific community of the United States. Ether was the more readily available of the two drugs and it was known that if pushed to the limit it could render a person stuporous.[1]

The use of ether by inhalation for the relief of surgical pain by William E. Clarke (New York State) and Crawford W. Long (Georgia, USA) in 1842.

William E. Clarke (1809-1880) a medical student of Rochester, New York State, had experienced the recreational use of ether and he, almost casually applied his knowledge of the drug as an inhalational anaesthetic in 1842.[1,8,39]

Clarke, aged 33 and still a medical student, suggested to a Miss Hobbie, a young lady friend of his who was nervous of having a dental extraction to try having it under ether, in January 1842. Clarke successfully administered the ether and the dentist Elijah Pope extracted the tooth painlessly; however Clarke's tutor, Professor E. M. Moore, having learnt of the event, believed that the young lady might have been in a hysterical state and he cautioned Clarke about further experiments with ether. Clarke heeded the advice. He became a well known physician and lived until 1880 but always seems to have been reluctant to admit his part in the discovery of surgical anaesthesia.[1,40]

Crawford William Long (1815-1879) was the son of a comfortably off Georgian plantation owner. He had received an exceptionally thorough medical education for the period and, by 1842 aged 27, was established as a general practitioner and surgeon in Jefferson, Georgia.[40] Like Clarke, Long had a patient who dreaded having surgery. Both Crawford Long and his patient had also had experience of inhaled ether as a recreational drug. It thus came about that Long excised one sebaceous cyst from the neck of James Venables under ether on 30 March 1842 and a second cyst on the following 6 June.[1,11,41]

Long continued to use ether occasionally in his practice thereafter but he did not publish his cases until 1849 when the controversy over the priority for the introduction of general anaesthesia was at its height after Morton's demonstration in 1846.[41] The reason for this reticence has caused much debate.[41,42] Long was in an isolated country practice and he was not sure of the nature of the process he had introduced (he too suspected at one time that he might merely have produced the condition of hypnosis).[1,41,42] A very potent reason was however given by his daughter many years later; that was that some superstitious members of the local rural public believed that Long might be reckless or mad, and that he had a mysterious medicine with which he could put them to sleep and then cut them to pieces. Long's friends warned him that in the event of a fatality, he might be lynched. Such an attitude and possible course of action echoed what we have already noted, and dates back to the belief in witchcraft in the middle ages.[40]

One other interesting speculation is contained in a surviving letter from Long written many years later. He states that, shortly after his first use of ether, an itinerant dentist visited his isolated community to practice his profession for a short period, as was not uncommon in those pioneering days.[11] Long wondered whether this could have been Wells who was to give the first anaesthetic with nitrous oxide in 1844 or, less likely, Morton. Either of these individuals might have been given food for thought by learning of Long's use of general anaesthesia![1]

The dentists of New England in the 1840s and the birth of modern anaesthesia.

Be that as it may we must now turn to the circumstances which led to that first use of nitrous oxide as an anaesthetic for dental extraction by Horace Wells in New England in 1844.[1,23,24]

Why indeed should fate decree that this pioneering event should take place in Hartford, Connecticut in New England at that particular time, and why should this first nitrous oxide anaesthetic be for a dental extraction? Both Greene[24] and Vandam[23] have studied this question extensively. Firstly New England was the most sophisticated and enlightened area in the United States, and its intelligentsia were in close contact with centres of culture and scientific development in Europe. On the other hand New Englanders were less liable to be bound by academic tradition, and thus more likely to be innovative and receptive to new concepts. Then again dentistry was more highly developed in New England than in Europe or in any other part of the world, and was fast developing into a profession from its previous status as a trade practised by unqualified artisan tooth-pullers. Lastly, dental extraction was the most common surgical procedure before the introduction of anaesthesia; dentists were thus more frequently inflicting pain than surgeons who were restricted to body surface procedures and, furthermore, any reduction of the pain of extractions would not only facilitate dentistry but also have considerable commercial advantages.[1]

Horace Wells and the first use of nitrous oxide for anaesthesia in 1844.

Horace Wells (1815-1849), 29 years of age in 1844, was typical of the new breed of educated professional dentists. He was born in Hartford, Vermont of a well-to-do landowning family and, by coincidence, practised in Hartford Connecticut. He had received an excellent basic, and, by the standards of the day, a sound dental education. Wells was locally regarded as a leader of his profession in Hartford, Connecticut and was much sought after as a teacher. Morton was one of his pupils and, later became his partner for a short while. Horace Wells was a sensitive man with an inventive brain. He originated several advances both in dentistry and other fields.[1,11,29,43-45]

It has already been noted that there is a possibility that Wells had already heard of Long's anaesthetics using ether,[11] whether that is true or not there is certainly compelling evidence that he knew of Humphry Davy's descriptions of the ability of nitrous oxide to cause inebriation followed by insensibility before the events on 10 and 11 December 1844 which led up to the first dental extraction under nitrous oxide; he was however probably not specifically aware of the very short passages in Davy's *Researches* on analgesia under nitrous oxide. It is also certain that Wells had been considering the possibility of using either ether or nitrous oxide to eliminate the pain of dental extraction for some time before 10 October 1844.[28,44,45]

The event which finally made up the mind of Wells to employ nitrous oxide as an anaesthetic was the visit to Hartford of the popular lecturer and entertainer Gordon Quincy Colton (1814-1898), a former medical student who had had to abandon his studies for financial reasons. His lectures included demonstrations of the amusing effects of nitrous oxide intoxication on members of an audience.[28] Either at Colton's public entertainment on the evening of 10 October 1846 at which Wells inhaled the gas and was afterwards reproved by his wife for making an exhibition of himself or, more likely, at a private demonstration to professional colleagues on the next morning. Wells observed that the young man Samuel Cooley injured himself by knocking against furniture while throwing himself about under the influence of the nitrous oxide but was unaware that he had damaged himself until he sat down afterwards.[1,8,11,28,29,44-46]

Wells made up his mind. He invited Colton to bring an oil silk bag of nitrous oxide round to his surgery and after Wells himself inhaled the gas, had a painful tooth extracted by his partner John Rigg under its influence; when Wells had come round Colton reports that Wells declared "It is the greatest discovery ever made. I didn't feel it as much as a pin prick"; another version, possibly apocryphal, says that he added that it was "a new era in tooth pulling".[44,46]

Colton taught Wells how to prepare nitrous oxide and then went on his way.[46] Wells then anaesthetised between twelve and fifteen more patients successfully; after which he felt ready to announce his discovery to his medical and dental colleagues.[47] To this end Wells went to Boston in January 1845 and called on the leading surgeon of the time John Collins Warren (1778-1856),[33,48] on Charles Thomas Jackson (1805-1880)[11,43] the eminent physician and chemist, and on his erstwhile partner Morton.[28,44,45,47] Warren had already been interested in the possibility of relieving pain for some years; he had tried large doses of opium and hypnosis.[33,48] Warren invited Wells to demonstrate the use of nitrous oxide for an amputation; unfortunately the amputation was cancelled and a robust student for a dental extraction was substituted. The demonstration took place before a crowded audience of physicians, surgeons, and medical students, the patient was only partially anaesthetised and cried out during the extraction. Wells was hissed from the room as a humbug.[11,47]

It must be remembered that Wells had only previously administered nitrous oxide in the quiet of his own surgery where calm words of suggestion had doubtless aided induction.[11,47] He had also used the small bag similar to the one used by Colton in his entertainments. This contained only two litres of nitrous oxide, whereas those who later used nitrous oxide clinically for dental extractions, before apparatus with cylinders of nitrous oxide became available, used bags containing up to 30 litres.[11,49]

The explanation put forward by Wells for the phenomenon of anaesthesia is interesting. He cites stimulation rather than depression ("an individual when much excited from ordinary causes, may receive severe wounds without manifesting severe pain; as for instance the man who is engaged in combat"). This is, of course compatible with the theories of Beddoes and Humphry Davy.[1,47]

Wells returned to Hartford straight away after his unfortunate demonstration. He was immediately plunged into a state of pathological depression, and, he ceased to practice for over eight months. He began again in September 1845 and continued to use nitrous oxide. He also tried ether in cooperation with the surgeon Edward Marcy as a substitute for nitrous oxide, but found it unsatisfactory for his purposes and returned to the use of nitrous oxide. Wells therefore used ether before Morton's demonstration the following year. He abandoned practice altogether in December 1845 to pursue various artistic enterprises connected with business interests.[44,45,47]

The eclipse and revival of the use of nitrous oxide for anaesthesia.

Nitrous oxide was completely eclipsed for nearly two decades by Morton's demonstration of ether anaesthesia in 1846 and the discovery of chloroform in 1847. It was Colton who revived it. Colton was once again in Hartford on one of his periodic lecture tours in 1862. He was persuaded to demonstrate the manufacture and use of nitrous oxide for dental extraction to a dentist named Dunham. Dunham had successfully anaesthetised 600 cases by the time Colton returned to Hartford a few months later. Colton, a shrewd business man, saw the potential of nitrous oxide with its rapid recovery for dental extractions, and indeed, its superiority for this purpose at that time over ether and chloroform for short outpatient procedures. He returned to New York and opened the very successful New York Dental Institute solely for the administration of nitrous oxide for the extraction of teeth. This commercial organisation completed 97,000 cases by 1877 without fatality. Colton was a good business man but the also appears to have been a likeable and honest individual. He took no part, as he might well have done, in the controversy about priority that followed Morton's ether demonstration. Nitrous oxide was taken up by many American dentists - especially after cylinders became available in the late sixties - and its use quickly spread to Europe thereafter.[29,46]

Inhalation anaesthesia in the period 1842-1846 before Morton's demonstration at the Massachusetts General Hospital in 1846.

The period leading up to Morton's seminal demonstration of ether anaesthesia in 1846 which alerted the world to the reality of ether anaesthesia, thus included at least three other independent instances of the intentional use of ether as an anaesthetic, by Clarke,[39] Long[41] and Wells[47], and one unintentional use of the agent by Smilie[21] using an etherial solution of opium, as well as the introduction of nitrous oxide anaesthesia by Wells.[29,47]

William Thomas Green Morton and the events leading up to "Ether Day" 16 October 1846.

William Thomas Green Morton (1819-1868) was the youngest of the major originators of modern anaesthesia. He was 27 at the time of his demonstration at the Massachusetts General Hospital on 16 October 1846. He came from a family of Scottish origin in Charlton, Massachusetts but started his adult working life in business, first as an employed of a printing firm, and then in a business of his own which failed. In 1840 he entered the Baltimore College of Dental Surgery (the first such institution in the world) but left without taking a diploma in 1841 to become apprenticed to Horace Wells. He remained on good terms with Wells and continued to benefit from discussion of the latter's advanced techniques which Wells practised after he set up on his own, first in Farmington and then in Boston. He was briefly in legal partnership with Wells to promote methods of prosthetic dentistry developed by Wells including a cement endorsed by the ubiquitous Professor Charles Jackson the Chemist and Physician, but the partnership did not prove to be lucrative to either party and was dissolved amicably just two months before the first use of nitrous oxide by Wells in 1844.[1,29,43-45,47]

1844 was an important year for Morton. His practice in Boston prospered and he had his own apprentices. He enrolled as a medical student continuing to practice dentistry, and he married in May. The young couple then lodged with Charles Jackson, who was one of Morton's tutors, until January 1845.

Morton had a clinical problem; although, undoubtedly influenced by Wells, he had developed skills in prosthetic dentistry including the fixing of crowns, he had no means of making the necessary preliminary procedures painless. Morton himself recorded later that he discussed the problem with Jackson while he lodged with him in 1844. Jackson advised the local application of ether to the gums and, as an unconnected issue they discussed the intoxicating properties of ether.[29,50]

Morton was very much less well educated than Wells and certainly did not have the considerable academic knowledge of Charles Jackson. He therefore had to glean information about chemistry and pharmacology from others, and, incidentally, he had a deep respect for their superior knowledge. Morton probably had little, if any, knowledge of Davy's work. Morton was present and intensely interested in the failed demonstration by Wells in January 1845.[1] Morton is also known to have consulted Wells about the practicalities of the preparation of nitrous oxide in July 1845 at a time when Wells himself was interested in ether as an alternative. It is possible, indeed probable, that it occurred to Morton at this stage that readily available ether might be a better solution to his clinical problems than nitrous oxide, which had at that time to be manufactured in house by the administrator.[47,49,50]

Morton had certainly become seriously interested in the possibility of using ether inhalation for dental extractions by the middle of 1846. This was at a time when the consensus view was that, though short periods of inhalation of ether for recreation and the treatment of conditions such as asthma was relatively safe, prolonged inhalation would probably be fatal; by June 1846 Morton's practice was doing sufficiently well for him to be able to engage a locum and conduct a series of experiments at the farm he had bought at West Needham (now Wellesley). Not surprising his experiments with worms and insects were inconclusive, but he then succeeded in reversibly anaesthetising his dog and finally inhaled ether himself. Morton did not lose consciousness, but convinced himself that he had become stuperose enough for a tooth to be extracted with little pain; again we may note that the aim was analgesic freedom from pain rather than unconscious general anaesthesia.[1,29,50]

Morton's first supply of ether was exhausted. He obtained a fresh supply from a different supplier and then returned to his practice and induced several of his apprentices and assistants to inhale it; to Morton's surprise they all became wildly inebriated, as he did himself when he inhaled the new supply of ether. Morton determined to consult someone with superior knowledge of ether, and quite naturally he chose Jackson. This interview tok place on 30 September 1846.[50]

The interview between Morton and Jackson on 30 September 1846.

What exactly happened at that prolonged interview between Morton and Jackson became a critical factor in the dispute about priority which followed Morton's seminal demonstration at the Massachusetts General Hospital on the following 16 October 1846.[29,50,51]

Morton's version of the interview with Jackson appears to be honest and down to earth and there therefore seems little reason to doubt it. Morton was aware of the reputation Jackson had of claiming other workers discoveries as his own despite his eminence in his own field. He therefore states that he asked Jackson for the loan of a gas bag which he said he intended to fill with air and then attempt to persuade a patient by hypnotic suggestion that it contained nitrous oxide and that inhalation from it would consequently relieve the pain of an extraction. Jackson was said to have condemned this idea on the grounds that Morton would be thought to be as big a humbug as Wells. Morton then describes how he casually introduced the topic of obtaining the most stimulating results of the recreational use of ether by inhalation. Jackson emphasised that the best effects were only possible if the purest rectified ether was used. Jackson also gave Morton a flask with a cork with a glass tube through it which he stated wuld be a better way of inhaling ether than by pouring the fluid into a gas bag, which was a common method.[29,50]

Jackson later maintained during the dispute about priority that it was at this interview that he had put the idea of using ether to combat the pain of surgery into Morton's mind. This is manifestly untrue however, as there is no doubt whatever that Morton had already been experimenting with the inhalation of ether for several months beforehand.[29,50]

The use of ether by Morton for a dental extraction and its consequences.

Morton realised that his difficulties had arisen because his second supply of ether had not been pure. He obtained a supply of pure rectified ether from his original supplier and shut himself up in his office alone. He then inhaled ether first from Jackson's flask which was not effective and then from a handkerchief. This time he became unconscious but, although very frightened when he regained consciousness, he demonstrated analgesia by pinching himself.[50,51]

The same evening (30 September 1846) an emergency patient named Eben Frost presented himself with toothache. Morton anaesthetised him with ether and extracted the offending tooth in the presence of his assistants and his colleague Greville Hayden.[29,50,51]

Morton was certainly anxious to capitalise commercially on his new technique but, at the same time protect his discovery. The very next day (1st October 1846) he inserted a report of Eben Frost's extraction in the form of an advertisement in the *Boston Daily News* and consulted the lawyer and Patent Commissioner Richard Eddy about the possibility of obtaining a patent.[29]

The news of the advert of painless dentistry spread throughout Boston and many patients presented at Morton's practice to avail themselves of its benefits. The medical and dental establishment (including Charles Jackson) were sceptical or positively condemnatory. The administrations varied in their perfection. Morton experimented with a number of different methods of inhalation and inhalers.[50]

There is definite evidence that surgeon Henry J. Bigelow, aged 28 and, who had been recently appointed to the staff of the Massachusetts General Hospital, went to Morton's practice to see the miracle for himself and witnessed a number of his ether anaesthetics.[1,52] It is also highly probable that it was Henry Bigelow who suggested to his senior colleague John Warren that Morton should be asked to demonstrate his new method of relieving pain at the Massachusetts General Hospital for a surgical operation rather than a mere dental extraction.[52,53]

"Ether Day" 16 October 1846.

Warren issued the invitation.[29,52,53] The scene has been described by several of those who were actually present. The patient was Gilbert Abbot, a young printer agend 20 with a vascular congenital tumour of the left side of the neck. The operating theatre was crowded at 10.00 am on 16 October 1846. Morton was late. He had in fact been delayed while the instrument maker Chamberlain finished off his latest inhaler. Warren raised derisory laughter by remarking "I presume Morton is otherwise engaged", and took up the knife to proceed without the aid of etherisation, when Morton burst into the room accompanied by Eben Frost, his first dental patient, who he had brought with him to give supporting evidence. Warren then remarked "Well Sir your patient is ready". Morton spoke to the patient and persuaded him to inhale the ether. In four or five minutes he appeared to be asleep. Morton withdrew the inhaler and turning to Warren declared "*Your* patient is ready, Sir".[29,48,52,53]

The well known picture by Robert Hinckley is, as far as we can tell, a reasonable if somewhat stylised representation of the scene, but it was painted in the eighteen eighties some 35 years after the event and only Henry Bigelow of the senior figures was alive to advise.[54,55] Hinckley took a great deal of trouble to ensure that the likenesses of the principal participants were as they were in 1846 and Bigelow expressed himself as generally satisfied. Both Vandam[54] and Wolfe[55] have analysed the picture; one or two of the peripheral participants are missing, and again one or two of those who were not present on the first occasion of the use of ether on 16 October 1846, although they attended at the second session of surgery under anaesthesia the following day.[54,55]

The patient phonated during the procedure and he was aware of the blunt dissection of the tumour but did not feel pain; again we note that only analgesia had been produced as in so many early cases.[48]

It is to Warren's great credit that he had the vision to pronounce the demonstration a success ("this is no humbug" he asserted): even though a number of those present were not entirely convinced.[56] Henry Bigelow was quite sure however, and indeed it was his pen which was destined to send the "good news round the world".[52,53,56]

Morton's inhaler.

Simple inhalers were familiar items of medical equipment, for the inhalation of steam, ether and other medicaments for the treatment of chest diseases, in the middle of the nineteenth century.[1,57] Both Morton and John Snow (1813-1858), of London, the first professional physician anaesthetist[58] based their inhalers on such devices.[1,2,24,27,57,59]

Bryn Thomas established that the device used on 16 October was quite simple without valves thus facilitating "to and fro" vaporisation of the ether to a concentration of 24%.[49] Ether is or was a very safe agent but the difficulty with its use as a sole agent is the slow induction requiring a high initial concentration. John Snow's vaporiser which he developed in the following year (1847) was capable of delivering a concentration over 40%.[2,49]

Morton's patent.

Morton administered ether successfully at the Massachusetts General Hospital on the 16th and 17th October; but Warren and his fellow surgeons, under pressure from the Massachusetts Medical Society, placed an embargo on its use.[48] This was because the nature of the fluid had not been disclosed and because Morton, being a dentist and therefore not governed by the Massachusetts Medical Society, was applying for a patent for both the fluid and his vaporiser.[29]

Morton's motives for applying for a patent were not entirely commercial. There is no doubt that he was also concerned that the possible consequences of etherisation were not fully understood and that the process might be abused in "nefarious" or criminal hands. He was supported in this to a large extent by Henry Bigelow.[52,53]

Morton conceded the free use of his preparation and the inhaler to the surgeons of the Massachusetts General Hospital on 5 November 1846, and he admitted that the fluid was ether before the next surgical operation under anaesthesia on November 7th, just before the next use of ether at the Massachusetts General Hospital for an amputation which finally convinced the medical profession in Boston of its efficacy. Both these concessions were made before Morton's United States patent was granted on 12 November.[1,29,50]

The patent was granted in the names of both Morton and Jackson. Jackson was not present at the first administration on 16 October but, as soon as etherisation appeared to be successful, he claimed that it was he who had given the idea to Morton, and pestered him to have hin name included for 10% of any profits. Morton was naturally reluctant but, on the advice of his lawyers, conceded, because it was believed that the endorsement of the eminent Jackson would stifle criticism.[1,29,50]

It is not true, as is often stated, that Morton concealed the identity of his preparation with the name "Letheon" from the time of the first administration on 16 October 1846. The name was decided upon at a meeting which Morton had with Henry Bigelow and Oliver Wendell Holmes officially representing the Massachusetts General Hospital in November 1846.[1,29,50] It may be that, having been granted the free concession from Morton for the use of the preparation and vaporiser at the Massachusetts Hospital, and also the knowledge that Morton was being generous to other hospitals in the United States they were content for Morton to pursue the enforcement of his patent abroad.[1] A patent was, in fact, granted in London on 21 December 1847 but it could not be enforced.[1,29]

Morton's fate.

Morton continued to administer ether in and around Boston during 1847, but, realising that his patent was not enforcable anywhere in the world, he then retired to pursue a prolonged legal claim for an award from the United States Congress in competition with

Jackson.[3,50] Morton gallantly anaesthetised casualties during the American Civil War,[60] but died in Washington D.C. from a cerebral vascular accident on a stifling hot day in July 1868 while visiting the capital in an attempt to contest Jackson's latest claim. He was 43.[29,51] Jacob Bigelow Professor of Materia Medica in Boston and father of the surgeon H.J. Bigelow described Morton on the inscription on his tomb as "inventor and revealer of anaesthetic inhalation".[49] "Inventor", perhaps not, "revealer", certainly.[1]

The claim of Charles Thomas Jackson.

The extent of Jackson's advice to Morton before his demonstration at the Massachusetts General Hospital, and his insistence of joining with him in the granting of the patent has already been considered.[1,29,50]

Jackson also sent a sealed letter by steamer addressed to the French Academy outlining what he claimed to be his discovery of etherisation on 1 December 1846 without mentioning Morton by name. This was to be opened if, and only if, the news of the successful use of the technique reached France. This was common practice with new discoveries in the scientific world at that time.[29,61-63] The letter was in fact dramatically opened on 18 January 1847 when the Academy debated the successful use of etherisation in Paris and; for a time Jackson was credited with priority in France.[8] This was later contested by both Wells and Morton; the Academy hedged their bets by granting each a share in the origination of the discovery and a share in a monetary prize. Morton purchased a gold medal with his share and had it suitably inscribed much to the annoyance of Jackson.[29]

Jackson revoked his share in Morton's patent as soon as it was obvious that it would not be enforced, because he said that he had a "tender conscience" over the matter.[29,50]

The competing claims of Jackson and Morton for the recognition of the United States Congress occasioned an increasingly expensive legal battle and negated one another. Jackson even tried to enlist the aid of Crawford Long in a joint claim in 1852, but Long would have none of it.[1,42] Jackson did give some anaesthetics in the years following Morton's demonstration and he wrote a reasonably practical manual on etherisation in 1861 for the benefit of naval and military surgeons in the Civil War, although it also contained his familiar diatribe about his claim.[32] As already mentioned Morton died in 1868. Jackson became increasingly paranoid and he was ultimately confined to a mental asylum and died in 1880 at the age of 75.[1,43]

The claim and fate of Horace Wells.

We have considered the relevant facts of the involvement of Horace Wells in the events which led up to Morton's demonstration on 16 October 1846. Flushed with success Morton wrote to Wells on 19 October describing the successful use of his "preparation" and inviting Wells to go to New York as his agent to promote the patent.[29] Wells visited Morton on 25 October and Morton demonstrated the use of ether to him. Wells was at first dismissive (perhaps Morton's anaesthetics were not yet perfected at that time), but later became angry when he learned that Morton and Jackson had taken out a patent.[50] He then started a claim to establish his priority, with increasing ferocity in communications both to the public and profession and the press.[44,45]

Wells had, of course, at that time ceased to practise dentistry. He left Boston for Paris at the end of December 1846 in pursuit of his latest business venture which involved the buying and selling of artistic paintings. He arrived in Paris in February 1847 at the height of the controversy in the French Academy over the counter claims of Morton and Jackson for priority, but he had no written evidence of his prior use of nitrous oxide and ether with him. Wells returned to Boston and prepared a memorandum supported by testimonials and sent it to the Academy.[27,28] He then attempted to set up practice as an extractor of teeth without pain in New York in January 1848 but, by that time, he had become addicted to chloroform which James Young Simpson had introduced in Edinburgh, Scotland in November 1847.[29] Wells was becoming increasingly deranged, he sprinkled chloroform on the clothes of a prostitute as a condemnatory gesture and was arrested. He committed suicide while in prison by severing his femoral artery with a razor on 23 January 1848. He was 29 years old when he first inhaled nitrous oxide and had his tooth extracted, and just 33 when he died.[44,45] Ironically he was elected to Honorary Membership of the Paris Faculty of Medicine posthumously in March 1848 partly because Hickman's submission to the Academy on anaesthesia by inhalation in 1826 was recalled. There is a statue of Wells in Paris, the inscription of which acknowledges him as the discoverer of anaesthesia.[27,28,44,45]

The modesty of Crawford Long.

Crawford Long continued as a much loved and respected general practitioner; being a Southerner he was almost ruined by the American Civil War but tended the wounded of both sides with devotion. He died after he suffered a stroke while attending a confinement at the age of 62. His last words were a request to his assistants asking them to look after the baby.[1,42]

The news of etherization spreads to the United Kingdom.

Cable and wireless telegraphy were, of course, unknown in 1846. Written evidence of the "good news" of Morton's demonstration at the Massachusetts General Hospital was conveyed to Europe by the Cunard paddle steamers which operated a regular service from Boston, Massachusetts to Liverpool, England. The precise details were elucidated in a brilliant piece of research by my colleague the late Richard Ellis.[62,64]

Morton was quick off the mark. The *Caledonia* which sailed on November 1st had a letter from the Boston patent agent Eddy to a London lawyer which resulted in the granting of Morton's patent in London on 21 December 1846.[64]

The *Brittania,* which departed on November 16th, conveyed a letter from Edward Everett, Principal of Harvard University to Dr. Henry Holland, a fashionable London physician. This letter gave a preliminary account of Morton's demonstration, but Holland does not seem to have been impressed and did not take any action.[64]

The *Acadia* sailed on December 1st. It carried several letters describing the use of ether as an anaesthetic which was by then the talk of Boston's professional and public communities. There were letters from Edward Everett to Boott, an expatriate American physician living in Gower Street, London and to Robert Liston the leading London surgeon of the time.[64] Both these letters were important factors in initiating the events which led to the first anaesthetics in London; however, the vital letter was one written to Boott by Jacob Bigelow who was a prominent physician and pharmacologist in Boston, and the father of Henry Bigelow. Everett also wrote another letter to Holland and one to Brodie a famous London surgeon and scientific researcher. Brodie had already experimented with ether on animals with fatal results and was not enthusiastic.[64]

There was however a human messenger on the *Acadia* in the person of William Fraser, who was acting as ships surgeon. Fraser went north to Dumfries his home town in Scotland as soon as the *Acadia* docked in Liverpool on 16 December 1846; on arrival in Dumfries he told his friend William Scott, the Dumfries surgeon, about Morton's use of ether.[65,66] Scott then carried out an operation under ether at the Dumfries and Galloway Royal Infirmary on 19 December 1846. Records of the exact nature of this operation do not exist but, having studied Thomas Baillie's careful account, the present writer has no doubt that it took place; in addition, the claim for precedence was substantiated later by none other than Professor James Young Simpson after careful investigation.[65,66] There is circumstantial evidence to suggest that the surgical procedure was an amputation and that the postoperative outcome might have been fatal; this may explain Scott's reticence in not publicising the case for many years.[65,66]

The letter sent by Dr. Jacob Bigelow, father of Henry Bigelow the surgeon, was delivered to Doctor Francis Boott in Gower Street London on 17 December 1846.[62,64] Boott was an American who had come to England as a botanist and become quite well known in that field before obtaining British medical qualifications in Edinburgh and practising in London.[67]

Bigelow senior enclosed a paper with his letter which his son Henry had written for the Boston Medical and Surgical Journal.[52,64] This gave professional details of the events of ether day. Boott received a letter from Edward Everett endorsing the discovery of etherisation at the same time.[64]

The first ether anaesthetics in England.

Boott lost little time in communicating the information to the dentist James Robinson who also practised in Gower Street which was then in the area of London which had the highest concentration of doctors and dentists. James Robinson was one of the few professional dentists in England at that time.[68] Robinson in the presence of Boott administered ether to a Miss Lonsdale at Boott's house on 19 December 1846 (the same day as the Dumfries anaesthetic) and extracted a troublesome tooth.[29,68]

The improvised apparatus which Robinson used was constructed from a Nooth's apparatus (designed for producing carbon dioxide by dropping hydrochloric acid on calcium carbonate for impregnating water).[68]

Robinson and Boott invited Liston, the senior surgeon of the North London (now University College) Hospital also in Gower Street, to a further session of etherisation for dental extractions. The administrations were not entirely satisfactory but Liston, who had also received a letter from the eminent Edward Everett,[64] was convinced that the use of ether for anaesthesia was a practical proposition.[69]

Liston accompanied by James Squire a medical student then went to the workshop of Squire's uncle William Squire, an instrument maker in Cavendish Square, and commissioned him to make an apparatus similar to Robinson's. They tried the apparatus on a dental case but the patient refused to inhale any more ether after a few breaths.[69]

Despite this setback Liston proceded next day to carry out his now famous and very well attended amputation on the patient Churchill, a butler, with James Squires as the anaesthetist; at the conclusion of the operation he is said to have exclaimed "his Yankee dodge beats mesmerism hollow".[29,70] If this is true he was doubtless recalling the activities of Elliotson.[29,36]

The only other recorded use of ether anaesthesia in 1846 outside of the United States was in Paris when Jobert de Lamballe successfully used the process for a surgical operation on 24 December 1846 after an abortive attempt on 22 December.[3,71]

The more events in the ongoing history of anaesthesia in December 1846.

Two important events in London in December 1846 must be added to the chronology of

51

the history of anaesthesia. Firstly Professor James Young Simpson (1811-1872), Professor of Obstetrics, Edinburg) happened to be in London in connection with his appoitment surgeon to the household of Her Majesty Queen Victoria in Scotland. Simpson visited Liston and heard about his success.[65,69,72] He returned to Scotland and first used ether for the relief of pain in childbirth on 17 January 1847, and subsequently introduced chloroform in November of that year.[2,29] Secondly John Snow (1813-1858)[2,58] a leading London general practitioner, later epidemiologist of the cholera epidemics in the eighteen fifties, visited Robinson and witnessed one of his demonstration of ether anaesthesia on 28 December 1846.[69] Snow was impressed and inspired and became the first professional physician anaesthetist and the first to study the effects of ether and later chloroform scientifically. It was largely due to his careful research and consummate clinical ability that first ether, and then chloroform anaesthesia became accepted worldwide by the members of the medical profession and their patients.[2,29,58,73,74]

Conclusion.

Henry Bigelow's prediction that knowledge of the discovery of ether anaesthesia would "go round the world"[52] was fulfilled with a rapidity which even he could not have foreseen as the late Ole Secher so diligently researched.[3] The news went up and down the North and South American continents from Boston, along the trade routes of the British Empire from London (as Gwen Willson eloquently describes in her recent book),[75] and throughout Europe largely through Paris; by the end of 1847 there were few areas where Europeans originated or had settled where the first administrations of ether had not been given.[3]

This paper has traced the development of modern anaesthesia from the earliest times through the direct line of the work of Priestley, Davy, Long, Wells and Morton to "Ether day" to the end of 1886. It is worth remembering however that the operations for which ether was administered in the quarter of a century following Morton's demonstration were chiefly those body surface procedures which were undertaken before the introduction of etherisation, although, no doubt, more effectively.[2] Surgery required other discoveries besides anaesthesia before it could progress. These were notably the introduction of Lister's antisepsis and subsequently aseptic technique before the abdomen could be opened with impunity, and later advances in anaesthetic technique including controlled ventilation and curarisation before cardiothoracic surgery could develop.[16]

References:

1. Boulton TB, Wilkinson DJ: The Origins of Modern Anaesthesia. In: Healy TEJ, Cohen PJ (Eds). A Practice of Anaesthesia, 6th edn. Edward Arnold, London, 1995, p.3-35

2. Snow J: On Chloroform and other Anaesthetics. Churchill, London, 1858

3. Secker O: Forty-six "first anaesthetics in the world". Acta Anaesthesiologica Scandinavica 1990; 34: 552-556

4. Joad CEM: The Recovery of Belief, 1953

5. Lyons AS, Petrucelli RJ: Medicine. An illustrated History. Abrams, New York, 1987: 380-1 and 492-493

6. The Bible: Genesis 2: xxi and 3: xvi

7. Nunn JF: Anaesthesia in ancient Times - Fact or Fable. In: Atkinson RS, Boulton TB (eds). The History of Anaesthesia. International Congress and Symposium Series No 134. Royal Society of Medicine, London 1989 p 21-26

8. Davison MHA: The Evolution of Anaesthesia. Sherratt and Son, Altrincham (UK): 1996

9. Richardson BW: On a new and ready mode of producing local anaesthesia. Medical Times and Gazette 1866; 1: 115-117

10. Helliwell PJ: Refrigeration analgesia. Anaesthesia 1950; 5: 58-66

11. Keys TE: The History of Surgical Anaesthesia. New York: Dover Publications, 1945: 3-193

12. Morch ET, Major RH: "Anaesthesia". Early use of the word. Res. Anesth. Analg. 1954; 33: 64-68

13. Moser HHP: Early Anaesthesia. Anaesth. 1949; 4: 70-75

14. Carter AJ: Narcosis and nightshade. Br Med J 1996; 313: 1630-1632

15. Boulton TB: Heraldry and Anaesthesia. In: Barr AM, Boulton TB, Wilkinson DJ. (eds.) Essays on the History of Anaesthesia. International Congress and Symposium Series 213. London: Royal Society of Medicine, 1996: 185-190

16. Holmes OW: Letter to EL Snell 1893. In: Keys TH. The History of Anaesthesia. New York: Dover publications, 1962

17. The Bible. St. Mark 16: xxiii and St. John 19: xxviii

18. Bowes JB: Mandrake in the History of Anaesthesia. In: Atkinson RS, Boulton TB. (eds.) The History of Anaesthesia. International Congress and Symposium Series No 134. London: Royal Society of Medicine, 1989: 26-28

19. Ogata T: Seishu Hanaoka and his anaesthesiology and surgery. Anaesth 1973; 28: 645-652

20. Boulton TB: Alexander Wood MD (1817-1884) and the use of the syringe and hollow needle for parenteral medication. Survey of Anesthesiology, 1984; 28: 346-354

21. Smilie ER: Insensibility produced by the inhalation of the vapour of the ethereal solution of opium. Bost. Med. Surg. J. 1846; 35: 263-264

22. Infusino M, O'Neill YV, Calmes S: Hog beans, Poppies and Mandrake leaves. A Test of the Efficacy of the Medieval Soporific Sponge. In: Atkinson RS, Boulton TB. (eds.) The History of Anaesthesia. International Congress and Symposia Series No 134. London: Royal Society of Medicine, 1989: 29-33

23. Vandam LD: The Start of Modern Anaesthesia. In: Atkinson RS, Boulton TB. (eds.) The History of Anaesthesia. International Congress and Symposium Series No 134. London: Royal Society of Medicine, 1989: 64-69

24. Greene NM: Annals of Anaesthetic History. A consideration of factors in the discovery of anaesthesia and their effects on its development. Anesthesiology 1971; 35: 315-322

25. Caton D: The secularisation of pain. Anesthesiology 1985; 62: 485-501

26. Haeger K: The Illustrated History of Surgery. London: Starke, 1989: 9-288

[27] Cartwright FF: The English Pioneers of Anaesthesia (Beddoes), Davy, Hickman). Bristol: Wright, 1952: 1-338

[28] Smith WDA: Under the Influence. A History of Nitrous Oxide and Oxygen Anaesthesia. Macmillan, London: 1982: 1-188

[29] Duncum BM: The Development of Inhalation Anaesthesia. Oxford: University Press, 1946: 1-640

[30] Slatter EM: The evolution of anaesthesia. 4: Pneumatic medicine. Br Med J Anaesth 1960; 32: 194-188

[31] Davy H: Researches Chemical and Philosophical Chiefly Concerning Nitrous Oxide, or Dephlogisticated Nitrous Air, and Its Respiration. London: Johnson, 1800: 1-580

[32] Sykes WS: Essays on the First Hundred Years of Anaesthesia. Vol 2. Edinburgh: Livingstone, 1961: 1-187

[33] Warren JC: Address of the President. The influence of anaesthesia. Transactions of the American Surgical Association 1897; 15: 1-25

[34] Wilkinson DJ: History of Trauma Anaesthesia. In: Grande M. ed. Textbook of Trauma Anaesthesia. St. Louis: Mosby, 1993: 1-34

[35] Bird HM: James Arnott MD (Aberdeen) 1797-1883. A pioneer in refrigeration anaesthesia. Anaesthesia 1949; 4: 10-17

[36] Gould A: A History of Hypnotism. Cambridge: University Press, 1992: 1-738

[37] Mason AA: Surgery under hypnosis. Anaesthesia 1955; 10: 295-299

[38] Cartwright F: The early history of ether. Anaesthesia 1960; 15: 67-69

[39] Stetson JB: William E Clarke and his 1842 use of ether. In: Fink R. (ed.) The history of anaesthesia. Third International Symposium. Atlanta, Georgia, 1992: 400-407

[40] Stone RF: Biography of Eminent Physicians and surgeons. Indianapolis: Carlton and Hillenbeck, 1894: 286

[41] Long CW: An account of the first use of sulphuric ether as an anaesthetic for surgical operations. Southern Medical Journal 1849; 5: 705-713

[42] Sykes WS: Ellis RH. ed.: Essays on the First Hundred Years of Anaesthesia. Vol 3. Edinburgh: Churchill, 1982: 1-272

[43] Sykes WS ed: Essays on the First hundred Years of Anaesthesia. Vol 1. Edinburgh: Churchill, 1960: 1-171

[44] Wells CJ: Horace Wells. Anesth Anal. 1935; 14: 176-189

[45] Archer WA: Chronological history of Horace Wells, discoverer of anaesthesia. Bull Hist Med 1939; 7: 1140-1169

[46] Colton CQ: Anaesthesia. Who made and developed this great discovery? A statement "delivered during the mellowing of occasion". New York: Sherwood, 1866: 3-15

[47] Wells H: A history of the discovery of the application of nitrous oxide gas ether and other vapors to surgical operations. Hartford: Gaylord Wells, 1847: 1-14

[48] Warren JC: Etherisation with surgical remarks. Boston: Ticknor, 1848: 1-100

[49] Thomas KB: The Development of Anaesthetic Apparatus. A History based on the Charles King Collection of the Association of Anaesthetists of Great Britain and Ireland. Oxford: Blackwell Scientific Publications, 1975: 1-268

[50] MacQuilty B: The battle for oblivion. London: Harrap, 1969: 1-200

[51] Rice NP: Trials of a public benefactor. As illustrated in the discovery of etherization. New York: Pudney and Russell, 1859: 13-460

[52] Bigelow, HJ: Insensibility during surgical operations produced by inhalation. Bost Med Surg J. 1846; 35: 309-317

[53] Bigelow HJ: Etherization. A compendium of its history, surgical use, dangers and discovery. Boston Medical and Surgical Journal, 1848; 37: 229-245 and 254-266

54. Vandam LD: Robert Hinckley's "The first operation with ether". Anesthesiology 1980; 52: 62-70

55. Wolfe RJ: Robert Hinckley and the recreation of the first operation under ether. Boston: Countway Library, 1993: 1-182

56. Ayer W: The discovery of anaesthesia by ether; with an account of the first operation performed under its influence, and an extract from the record book of the hospital. Occidental Medical Times 1896; 10: 121-129

57. Slatter EM: The evolution of anaesthesia 2. The first English inhalers. Br Med J 1960; 15: 35-45

58. Shephard DAE: John Snow. Anaesthetist to a Queen and epidemiologist to a Nation. Prince Edward Island: York Point Publishing, 1955: 1-373

59. Jeffreys J: On artificial climates, for the restoration and preservation of health. London Medical Gazette 1841-1842; 1: 814-822

60. Morton WTG: The first use of ether as an anaesthetic. At the battle of wilderness in the Civil War. JAMA 1904; 42: 1068-1072

61. Gould AB: Charles T. Jackson's claim to the discovery of etherization. In: Ruprecht J, Lieburg MJV, Lee JA, Erdman W. (eds.) Anaesthesia. Essays on its history. Berlin: Springer Verlag, 1985: 384-387

62. Ellis RH: The introduction of ether anaesthesia to Great Britain. 1. Boston Massachusetts to Gower Street, London. Anaesthesia 1976: 31: 766-777

63. Trent J: Surgical anaesthesia 1846-1946. Journal of the History of Medicine 1946; 1: 505-514

64. Ellis RH: Early Ether Anaesthesia. The news of anaesthesia spreads to the United Kingdom. In: Atkinson RS, Boulton TB, (eds.) The history of Anaesthesia. International Congress and Symposium Series No 134. London: Royal Society of Medicine, 1989: 69-78

65. Baillie TW: The Dumfries ether diary. The first surgical use of ether in the old world. Dumfries: Solway offset services, 1996: 1-72

66. Baillie TW: The first European trial of anaesthetic ether. The Dumfries claim. Br Med J 1965; 37: 952-954

67. Ellis RH: The introduction of ether anaesthesia to Great Britain. 2. A biographical sketch of Dr. Francis Boott. Anaesthesia 1977; 32: 197-208

68. Robinson J: A Treatise on the Inhalation of the Vapour of Ether for the Prevention of Pain in Surgcial Operations. London: Webster, 1847. In: Ellis RH. (ed.) James Robinson on the inhalation of the vapour of ether. Eastbourne: Baillieère Tindall, 1983: 1-63

69. Ellis RH: Early Ether Anaesthesia. The enigma of Robert Liston. In: Barr AM, Boulton TB, Wilkinson DJ. (eds.) Essays on the history of anaesthesia. London: Royal Society of Medicine, 1996: 23-30

70. Dawkins CJM: The first public operation carried out under an anaesthetic in Europe. Anaesth 1947; 2: 51-61

71. Tirer S: Rivalries and controversies during early ether anaesthesia. Can J Anaesth 1988; 35: 605-611

72. Kellar RJ: Sir James Young Simpson. Victo Dolore. Journal of the Royal College of Surgeons of Edinburgh 1966; 12: 1-13

73. Ellis RH. eds: On Narcotism by the Inhalation of Vapours by John Snow. London: Royal Society of Medicine, 1991: 1-112

74. Ellis RH. (ed.): The Case Books of John Snow. Medical History, Supplement No 14. London: Wellcome, 1994: 1-633

75. Wilson G: One Grand Chain. The History of Anaesthesia in Australia 1846-1962. Melbourne: Australia and New Zealand College of Anaesthetists, 1996: 1-657

76. Boulton TB: T. Cecil Gray and the "Disintegration of the nervous system". The development of the concept of the Triad of Anaesthesia. Survey of Anesthesiology 1994; 38: 239-252

Pain and Analgesia for Operative Interventions: From 1847 up to 1997

L. E. Morris
University of Washington, Seattle, Washington

Summary
Pain and Analgesia for Operative Interventions from 1847 to 1997

This presentation includes a discussion of some changes in concept and will emphasize selected contributions, events, and factors which had important impact in promoting the growth and development of anesthesiology as a medical specialty. Environmental situations, previous experiences, and common patterns of human response often lead to acceptance or rejection of new ideas and concepts.

Recognition of complications led to a desire for improvement. However, good ideas sometimes languished or were rejected, perhaps because of poor publicity, inadequate concepts, or simply resistance to change. On the other hand, some ideas and practices which were originally embraced with enthusiasm were later recognized as not being in the best interest of the patients.

Some extraneous changes affected the evolutionary course of development. Included in these were the advent of compressed gases, transfusions, antibiotics, heat sterilization, and concepts of asepsis, recognition of need to maintain proper ventilation, and for avoidance of respiratory dead space, as well as an increased ability for measurement of such things as gas and vapor concentration, blood gases and acid/base balance have all played major roles. Most important of all in the widespread improvement of standards has been the dissemination of knowledge through postgraduate education of physicians in the principles of safe practice of clinical anesthesia.

There is a need to recognize that available written accounts do often represent only a small fraction of the total picture; that indeed for any given slice of time there has been a wide disparity of thought and standards between the leading individuals and centers as compared to what was offered elsewhere to the general public.

Symposium participants are invited to enjoy the sessions of this meeting in a receptive spirit, to absorb new ideas and gain perspective. All are urged to document current and personally known recent history, so that there will be less opportunity for future misinterpretation.

Introduction

It was with mixed feelings of trepidation and challenge that I prepared my thoughts to share with you today. In these sesquicentennial years, I have given a number of lectures on the history of anesthesia, some to physicians in training, some to practicing anesthesiologists, some to the lay public. But I find that it is quite different talking before a group of historians, many of whom even as amateur historians know as much or more than I about the subject. I now understand the saying that "it is easier to preach to strangers than to a group of peers". There is however, no merit in preaching to those already persuaded so it is today not my intent to preach, but I do hope to remind you of some fascinating aspects of the heritage of anesthesiology and to offer you some challenges. My qualifications for doing this include the fact that, after a career in anesthesiology which dates back more than fifty years, I am a survivor who still takes an active interest in teaching and research. Although I have not been as peripatetic a traveler as Sir Robert Macintosh and some others, it has been by privilege to make anesthesia related visits to all six populated continents and to do or view anesthetics in many differing environments. Like some of the senior members of this audience I've had the good fortune to number among my professional friends and acquaintances many of the legendary figures of our profession, including such as Arthur Guedel, Dennis Jackson, Wesley Bourne, Harry Shields, and Digby Leigh of North America; William Mushin, Edgar Pask, Olive Jones, and Geoffrey Organe of the United Kingdom; Harry Daley, Geoffrey Kaye, Mary Burnell, and Gilbert Brown in Australia, and many more too numerous to mention by name, including some colleagues and friends in this room. I am sure that to some degree each of these contacts has molded my ideas and altered my views, but I take full responsibility for all of the choices, challenges, thoughts and perspectives which I will now share with you today.

The limited time allotted for the scope of the assigned topic will allow only the briefest mention of the many noteworthy developments within these years. Forty minutes for one hundred and fifty years is less that 2.7 minutes per decade. Books, monographs, and libraries have been devoted to both this overall topic and to segments of its fascinating aspects. Even if I were as talented in rapid speech as the renowned and redoubtable Virginia Apgar, which I am not, it would be obviously necessary to be highly selective in the choice of subjects and areas of discussion for the ensuing discourse. My selections will include what appears most interesting to me, and will not include all that all of you may think important. I will call attention to some observed patterns, changing concepts, and specific contributions with longrange effects, as well as some unheeded suggestions and missed opportunities. Areas which I may neglect or only allude to in passing may be covered in some detail in other sessions in this Symposium.

The history of medicine like all history is a chronology of recorded events - and the contributions and innovations of people. I believe it is important to emphasize that the response or reaction by an individual to any new idea or concept depends upon environmental factors and previous experience of that individual as well as concurrent levels of knowledge and social consciousness. As said not too long ago by Professor Ole Secher, one of our own anesthesia historians: "It is interesting reading to learn how they were thinking and what they knew in the older days. Not everything has been invented in our days." We could add that since many good ideas are initially rejected, or languish and lie dormant, a careful perusal of historical papers provides opportunity for re-discovery and development.

As one looks at the chronicles of struggles during these one hundred and fifty years it is evident that progress in anesthesia has been sporadic and halting. This was particularly true during the first seventy-five years after the first credible demonstration of surgical anesthesia by Morton. Anesthesia is a good example of the fact that it is often a long time from the inception of a useful idea to the practical implementation of that idea and still further until it becomes the accepted practice in general usage.

For our purposes today it may be useful to divide this historical review into three separate eras of approximately fifty years each. (Table 1) There is between these some everlap in content and activity, but there are also distinct differences, which may justify separate characterization helpful to our understanding.

First Era 1847-1897	Second Era 1897-1947	Third Era 1947-1997
Trial and Error with Inhalation Anesthesia - Limited Concepts of Use. How to use? Analgesia; Short Surgery; Complications and Deaths. Discovery of Local Anesthesia	Exploration and Development New Drugs and Equipment; New Ideas Organization of Societies; Post Graduate Education	Expanding Knowledge Research Publications Society Meetings WFSA Standards Qualifications Safety Monitoring Changing Scope

Table 1. Three Eras in the development of Anesthesiology:
a) Era of Etherists and Chloroformists, 1847-1897.
b) Era of Anaesthetists, 1897-1947.
c) Era of Anesthesiologists, 1947-1997.

1847-1897 Era of the Etherists and Chloroformists

The first era began with the introduction of general anesthesia by inhalation and continued through the discovery and introduction of local and regional anesthesia. This was a time of limited concepts, and of trial and error. As users of the anesthetic agents gained experience, and sometimes unwarranted confidence, there were complications and deaths. (But deaths were commonplace before anesthesia and from many other causes throughout the 19th century.) Operations were still relatively few, procedures brief, anesthesia light - often only analgesia - with usual duration of only a very few minutes.

Contributions of Physicians in England

When word of the new discovery of inhalation anesthesia reached England, through communications to the expatriated American, Francis Boot, it was received with interest which gradually turned to enthusiasm. Among those who became most active in the new concept of abolishing the pain of surgery was the inquisitive, innovative, and methodical physician John Snow. Over the next eleven years, before the end of his short life, this scholarly physician became not only the acknowledged leading anaesthetist in London but also the world's first physician specialist in anaesthetics. Snow's research expanded basic information about the anaesthetic effects of ether, chloroform and some other agents. Indeed, Snow was the first of several British physicians who became specialists in the practice of surgical anesthesia over the next several decades (Table 2). Best remembered of those who followed was Joseph T.

Physician Specialists in Britain	
1847-1858	John Snow Clinician, investigator, author
1860-1880	Joseph T. Clover Clinician, inventor, writer
1885-1915	Frederick Hewitt Clinician-teacher, textbook author

Table 2. English physicians most prominent in the early development of Anaesthesia.

Clover who made several important contributions, but who also unfortunately abrogated several of the principles which John Snow had enunciated. Most egregious was Clover's advocacy of asphyxial rebreathing techniques, which others followed. Both Snow and Morton had used non-rebreathing valves on their inhalers. Clover designed several inhalers for use with ether and nitrous oxide-ether as well as an ingenious method for limiting the maximum concentration of chloroform offered to patients, whereby he filled a reservior back pack with four percent chloroform in air. There is also a famous pictures of Clover, with the pack on his back, clearly monitoring the pulse of a patient being given an anaesthetic. By the close of the nineteenth century, and after Clover's death, Frederick Hewitt had become the most prominent clinical anaesthetist in London and had authored a textbook on anaesthetics.

At various times, Snow, Clover and Hewitt were all called upon to anaesthetize members of the royal family. The early open support by British Royalty for use of anaesthesia to prevent pain of surgery and obstetrics was a strong recommendation for less prominent members of society.

In contrast to the generally receptive atmosphere gradually attained in Britain the use of anaesthesia for surgical procedures in areas of the United States apart from Boston was not an unqualified immediate success. The slow acceptance may have been partly due to a well established rivalry and lack of trust between medical centers, and partly due to physician annoyance with Morton's attempted secrecy about the agent he called "Letheon", and the subsequent squabbles between Morton, Jackson and Wells as to priority for the credit of discovering anesthesia.

It is interesting that although the discovery of anesthesia was certainly an American contribution to the history of world medicine, much of the exploration, innovation and progress during the following several decades was done by physicians in Britain rather than emanating from the United States.

Contributions of Dentistry

When one reviews the total history of anesthesia, the very real role of dentistry in its introduction and further early development becomes apparent. (Table 3) Indeed the dentists seem to have been the principal group to recognize the significance and potential of this new concept of relief from acute pain of surgical procedures. As one considers the social background at the time of introduction of anesthesia, it seems probable that serious pain associated with caries and/or extraction of teeth was more frequently observed than any other single cause in the public awareness. Dental procedures were actually much more frequent than other types of surgery. One can imagine that many patients would have deferred or avoided the trip to the dentist because of anticipated pain. Both the dentists

Involvement of Dentistry	
1840's-	Clarke, Wells, Morton → Robinson (U.K.) → Europe and elsewhere.
1860's	G. Q. Colton, T. Evans, Coleman
1900-1930	Charles Teter, Jay Heidbrink, McKesson (Development of Equipment)
1920's	Nitrous Oxide reintroduction - Led by dentists in many countries.

Table 3. Contributions by Dentistry to the development of Anesthesia continued through the first and second Eras.

and the patients would have readily welcomed something that assured avoidance of pain, and for the dentists it would have been an economic benefit as well.

The primary individuals who had been involved in the Boston demonstrations were dentists. Again, it was John Robinson, a dentist, who administered the introductory Ether anesthetics in England and who wrote the first known monograph about Ether anesthesia. So also for the same reasons, dentists elsewhere were quick to act on receipt of the new information and contributed to the introduction of inhalation anesthesia in Europe and other parts of the world including Australia. Dentistry continued to publicize the benefits of anesthesia and to make contributions to the practice of anesthesia in all countries during much of the first hundred years. Most notable was the re-appearance of Gardner Quincy Colton whose entertainment lecture on nitrous oxide had first excited Horace Wells about the potential benefit of nitrous oxide in pain relief for his patients. Colton, after a digression to the California gold fields, returned to the East Coast and established the Colton Dental Association which set up several painless dentistry clinics, each provided with a means for making nitrous oxide, and by so doing returned attention to the use of nitrous oxide gas as an anesthetic. The Colton technique was brief exposures of pure nitrous oxide without benefit of dilution with air or oxygen, certainly a method with a large component of asphyxia. Colton continued to promote nitrous oxide including an 1867 demonstration of its effects at an international medical congress in Paris following which T. W. Evans, an American dentist with a carriage trade in Paris, went across to London and introduced the use of nitrous oxide to dental colleagues in England. The subsequent interest in nitrous oxide led to the provision of pressurized gas in tanks, which in turn led to the development of anesthesia machines.

Again some of these machines were designed by dentists. The most prominent of these was Charles Teter of Cleveland, Ohio. Nitrous oxide had several subsequent re-introductions or surges of popularity, the timing of which was different in various countries depending on a reduction in cost, improved local availability or local manufacture. With the subsequent advent of agents suitable for local anesthesia, the dentists were once again quick to adopt these in their practice.

Numbing Effects of Cocaine

In 1860, Albert Niemann purified and named the alkaloid Cocaine which Gaedicke had previously isolated from coca leaves. In 1884, Carl Koller, a young ophthalmologist in Vienna, was the first to publish his recognition of the significance of the numbing effects of Cocaine on mucus membranes, a phenomenon which had been noted by other observers but not applied to clinical practice. His abstract report of the numbing effect of Cocaine on the cornea was read for him by a friend on September 15, 1884, at an ophthalmology congress in Heidelberg. Koller's discovery was a boon to ophthalmic surgery but it was also quickly shown by others to be useful when applied to all mucous membranes; also for infiltration and block of the nerves to head and neck, and extremities. (Table 4) William Halsted, the subsequently famous American surgeon, was among the first elsewhere in the world to recognize the importance of the anesthetic effects produced by Cocaine. He and a colleague, Richard Hall, began experiments on themselves with Cocaine, not realizing its addictive potential. In December of 1884, they described blocks of the sensory nerves of the face and arm.

The first spinal anesthesia was in 1885, done by a New York neurologist, John Leonard Corning, who had obtained most of his education including a medical degree in Germany. Corning's interest was in the possible

	Local Anesthesia
1855	- Frederick Gaedicke isolated Cocaine.
1860	- Albert Niemann purified Cocaine.
1884	- Carl Koller - Corneal Analgesia with Cocaine. William Halstead - block of Mandibular Nerve with Cocaine.
1885	- John Leonhard Corning performed epidural injection of Cocaine (spinal?).
1891	- Heinrich Quincke described Lumbar Puncture.
1892	- Carl Ludwig Schleich introduced Infiltration Analgesia. Heinrich Braun introduced Conduction Anesthesia.
1898	- August Bier - Spinal Anesthesia with cocaine. Théodor Tuffier popularized Spinal. Anaesthesia.
1899	- Dudley Tait and Guido Caglieri Spinal Anesthesia in San Francisco.
1904	- Alfred Einhorn synthesized Procaine.
1905	- Heinrich Braun popularized Procaine.
1908	- August Bier described I. V. Regional Analgesia.
1947	- Torsten Gordh used Lignocaine.

Table 4. Highlights in the discovery and introduction of Local Anesthesia.

use of Cocaine for therapy of neurologic disease, but the did suggest after experimental observation of injecting Cocaine in one dog and seeing a similar effect in one patient, that spinal anesthesia might be a substitute for etherization in neurologic procedures and some other kinds of surgery. It was in 1898 that August Bier, using the lumbar puncture technique described by Irenaeus Quincke, did the first *planned* spinal anesthetic with cocaine. The news of spinal anesthesia with cocaine was received with great interest and soon the technique was applied in Paris, New Orleans, San Francisco, and elsewhere in the world before enthusiasm was tempered by realization of the drug's toxicity.

There were during these years, some ancillary changes which helped the progress of surgery. Most important was the concept of asepsis and the correlated heat sterilization which reduced the likelihood of post-surgical infection.

1897-1947 – Era of Anesthetists

Procaine Introduced

The second era began with a strong emphasis on the benefits and use of "local", regional, and spinal anesthesia. Among the substitutes eventually provided in lieu of the relatively toxic Cocaine, was a new agent - Novocaine (procaine), described by Alfred Einhorn (first used in 1904) and popularized by Heinrich Braun, who in 1905 published his classic textbook on "Local Anesthesia". In 1908 August Bier described the use of intravenous procaine peripheral to a tourniquet for regional block anesthesia of the extremities. The technique was re-introduced thirty-five years ago by C. McK. Holmes of New Zealand using xylocaine as the agent. Procaine remained as the standard drug for local anesthesia for more than forty years, until it was eventually replaced at mid-twentieth century by the amide-linked Lignocaine which was first used by Torsten Gordh of Sweden.

Early Anesthesia Machines

The availability early in the 20th century of pressurized bottled gases (oxygen and nitrous oxide) prompted the design and manufacture of equipment to control flow and administer these gases. Rotameters were first used in 1908 on an anesthesia machine built in Aachen, Germany for Maximillian Neu. It was decades later that rotameters were built into modern anesthesia machines. In spite of the availability of several models of early anesthesia machines, many general anesthetics of that time continued to be given by the simpler open drop mask techniques.

Hewitt's Airway

A most notable and important contribution to the safety of patients was the publication in 1908 of an article by Frederick Hewitt in which he described an oropharyngeal tube. This was the precursor of today's oral airway. In retrospect, it is somewhat amazing that this simple, effective idea was delayed in appearance for a full sixty years after the introduction of anesthesia. It was preceded by tracheal intubation and cuffed tracheostomy tubes for anticipated airway obstruction during surgical anesthesia, and came long after head lift and jaw thrusting maneuvers had been advocated to control pharyngeal obstruction caused by the relaxed tongue during anesthesia.

Early Specialty Organizations

In London the Society of Anaesthetists, founded by Frederick Silk in 1893, published transactions of its meetings from 1898 to 1907, after which it evolved into the Section on Anaesthetics as it joined with other specialty groups to form the Royal Society of Medicine. A separate Section of Anaesthetics appeared on the program of the annual scientific meeting of the British Medical Association for the first time in 1926. In the United States, a section for anesthesia was initially rejected by the American Medical Association in 1911, and despite subsequent repeated requests, this was not granted until 1940.

On any listing of individuals prominently associated with organizations of anesthetists during the first third of the 20th century, the name of Francis Hoeffer McMechan has received and deserves special mention. (Table 5) In spite of disabling arthritis, Dr. McMechan was the driving force in the founding of many sectional anesthesia societies in the United States and Canada, and ultimately of the International Anesthesia Research Society (IARS), for which he was the Secretary General and editor of its journal which we have come to know as Anesthesia and Analgesia, the oldest journal devoted to anesthesia literature and continuously published since 1922. McMechan had been the editor of the Quarterly Supplement of Anesthesia and Analgesia published with the American Journal of Surgery from 1914-1922. He was also the editor of the Yearbook of Anesthesia, published as bound volumes in 1915 and 1917. These were the first efforts to collate current anesthesia literature for publication in a single place. During these years textbooks, manuals, and other publications began to appear, which all served to improve communication between members of the slowly growing groups of physician anesthetists. The meetings and congresses of the several anesthesia societies supported a needed feeling of identity and community of interests. The Long Island Society of Anesthetists, started in 1905 by Adolph Erdmann, expanded in 1911 to become the New York State Society of Anesthetists which gradually became national in character and under the aegis of its longtime Secretary Paul Wood, the name was changed in 1936 to the American Society of Anesthetists. In 1940 this fledgling national society began publishing Anesthesiology, which rapidly became a leading journal for the specialty throughout the world. Still later in 1945, the Society name was changed again to American Society of Anesthesiologists.

	Organizations
1893 -	Society of Anaesthetists (London) In 1908 this became Anaesthetics Section, Royal Society of Medicine.
1905 -	Long Island Society of Anesthetists In 1911 the Long Island Society became New York State Society of Anesthetists.
1911-1923	F. H. McMechan stimulated organization of many state and sectional Societies in the U.S. and Canada.
1919 -	National Anesthesia Research Society formed. (Later became IRAS.)
1922 -	B.M.A. Section of Anaesthesia authorized.
1923 -	American Society of Regional Anesthesia.
1932 -	Associated Anaesthetists Great Britain and Ireland.
1936 -	New York State Society became American Society of Anesthetists.
1944 -	Name of ASA changed: Anesthetists to Anesthesiologists.
1955 -	First Congress, World Federation of Societies of Anesthesiologists.

Table 5. Organized groups supported specialty interests.

Pioneers of the Early Twentieth Century

One of the most innovative figures of early 20th century anesthesia was Elmer McKesson, anesthetist, physiologist, and manufacturer from Toledo, Ohio. Although very controversial because of his advocacy of what was clearly an hypoxic use of nitrous oxide, McKesson was internationally known as a charismatic leader in anesthesia affairs as well as being prominent in his home community. McKesson was a keen observer and a strong believer in the merits of careful recording of events and vital signs during anesthesia. As a result of his urging, the IARS made available a standard anesthesia record format available for use for all its members. Those who learned to use the anesthesia graphic charts found them to be an important aid to self-education.

Ivan Magill in England, another innovator, pioneered the use of wide bore endotracheal tubes. Magill had designed a larygoscope but was especially adept at blind nasal intubation. Because of Magill's growing reputation as an anaesthetist skilled in techniques he developed for use with thoracic surgery, there were frequent visitors to watch him work and to learn his methods of intubation. But he was reputed to be very clever at diverting attention, so that the visitor rarely if ever actually saw the maneuvers of introducing the tube. After all, this professional skill was a reason for many of his referrals and a part of his livelihood, so why teach potential competitors?

It is appropriate at this juncture to recognize the fact that our host institutions, Eppendorf Hospital and the Medical School of Hamburg University have, from the beginning of the 20th century, a history of individuals with particular interests in the field of anesthesia. Hermann Kümmell, Chairman of Surgery at the Eppendorf Hospital and a founder of the medical school in Hamburg University, was a leading protagonist of general anesthesia and a strong advocate for the use of perioperative fluid replacement as well as being an enthusiast for the administration of Ether anesthesia by intravenous infusions. Two of his pupils, Sudek and Schmidt, deserve special mention. Early in his career while still assistant to Professor Kümmell, Paul Sudeck described a technique of Ether analgesia used for minor operations and even amputations in the elderly and very ill. More than fifty years later a similar technique was described by Joseph Artusio for use in cardiac operations. Sudek became Chairman of Surgery at Hamburg in 1923, but his interest and support of anesthesia continued. Paul Sudek and his younger colleague Helmut Schmidt were instrumental in the reintroduction of nitrous oxide anesthesia to central Europe. Together with the Dräeger Company they developed apparatus to be used with nitrous oxide, oxygen and ether vapor. Their apparatus featured an early clinical circle system for carbon dioxide absorption, to help in conservation of the imported expensive nitrous oxide. These machines are said to have been in daily use at the Eppendorf Hospital from early 1925. By 1928, Helmut Schmidt had persuaded the Hoechst-IG-Farben Company to start production of nitrous oxide, which up to that time had been imported from England and too expensive for routine use. Helmut Schmidt ultimately became the first German surgeon to be appointed Professor of Surgery because of his contributions to anesthesia. Helmut Schmidt traveled to the United States in 1928, visited a number of medical centers and attended a congress of the IARS in Minneapolis. It is significant I think that the Australian, Geoffrey Kaye, writing of people in anesthesia that he observed in a 1930 tour of the United Kingdom, Europe and the United States, mentions Helmut Schmidt as one of only two individuals prominent for anesthesia in Germany, the other being the eminent Hans Killian of Freiburg.

Many of the various early prototypes of anesthesia machines were designed by practicing anesthetists as aids and expedients to meet their own recognized needs. Some of these individuals who were of entrepreneurial inclination engaged in manufacture of equipment, but most sought help with development of their ideas from established suppliers. Among these the most receptive and helpful were Dräeger of Lübeck, Charles King of London and Richard von Foregger of New York City. Foregger was a particularly good listener and built his company on a reputation for cooperation with the physicians.

Indeed it is worth reminding all of us that throughout our history, progress in the growth and development of all aspects of anesthesiology have not resulted solely from the efforts of the physician specialists involved, but also through the many friendly assists from interested individuals in various areas including business, clinical medicine and surgery, basic sciences, and even institutional administration.

Intravenous Barbiturates

Over the years the intravenous route had been tried for many drugs but none had been really satisfactory. The era of useful intravenous contributions to anesthesia began in 1932 with the introduction of Hexobarbitone by Hellmut Weese. This was the first of a series of ultra-short acting barbiturates. Hexobarbitone was very quickly replaced by Thiopentone (synthesized by E. H. Volwiler in 1932). Thiopentone, which was tried first by Ralph Waters in 1934 but actively promoted by John Lundy in the United States and by Ronald Jarman in Britain, was not suitable as a sole anesthetic but its role for induction and intermittent supplement to nitrous oxide oxygen has assured a continued measure of popularity for sixty years.

Cyclopropane

1934 was the year in which a new gaseous anesthetic agent, cyclopropane, was cautiously introduced by Ralph Waters after extensive studies by the Wisconsin group. Cyclopropane in contrast to nitrous oxide was a fully potent anesthetic gas with which maximum anesthetic effect could be obtained without encroachment on the amount of oxygen in the respired gas mixture, but it was also expensive, flammable and potentially explosive, which required use of a closed carbon dioxide absorption system which had been previously introduced into clinical practice by Waters. As a result, all physicians of that time who wished to use cyclopropane anesthesia became familiar with the closed carbon dioxide absorption systems, which with cyclopropane was used extensively over the subsequent twenty-five years. Cyclopropane was a versatile anesthetic agent providing quick induction, prompt recovery, and allowing rapid changes in depth of anesthesia in accord with surgical needs. The easily produced deep anesthesia of cyclopropane was accompanied by marked depression of spontaneous respiration. Because of this, physicians learned to keep respiratory exchange more nearly normal by intermittent manual compression of the anesthesia breathing bag. In this way, hypoventilation and the consequent hypercarbia could be avoided.

Introduction of Curare

We give due credit to the temerity, judgement and vision of Harold Griffith for the use, in 1942, of intocostrin, an extract of "arrow poison", as an adjuvant to cyclopropane anesthesia. Intocostrin was the first of several intravenous muscle relaxants introduced into clinical practice. Actually much had been previously known about curare; Claude Bernard in 1850 had shown the action of curare to be at the myo-neuronal junction, while Charles Waterton and Benjamin Brodie had earlier demonstrated in 1814 on a donkey that poisoning with extract of curare need not be fatal provided artificial ventilation of the lungs was maintained throughout whatever the duration of the curare effect. In fact extracts of crude curare had been tried in Germany for surgical anesthesia by Arthur Läwen in 1912, and in London by F. P. de Caux in eight surgical cases in 1928. Clinical use did not continue because of variable effects from the non-standard crude extracts of curare which were used. Consequently, it was Harold Griffith's report of twenty-five cases in which curare was used with cyclopropane which got the attention of his colleagues. In retrospect it was somewhat fortuitous that the introduction of curare into regular use in the operating rooms did not occur until after clinical anesthetists were well versed in laryngoscopy, endotracheal intubation, and support of ventilation during anesthesia.

Reaction to New Ideas and Concepts

At this point I would like to digress again to share with you some brief thoughts about patterns of response to new concepts and ideas. (Table 6) These either receive uncritical acceptance, perhaps because of apparent convenience; or more likely are viewed with suspicion and rejected. Many examples of either can be found in medical practice. Rejection is frequently capricious, sometimes simply resistance to change. Conversely, many poor ideas have been embraced without due consideration of the potential complications. Fortunately, rejected good ideas often re-surface and sometimes find a more receptive audience. In considering the resurgence of ideas it is interesting to look at the matter of adding oxygen to anesthetic atmospheres. (Table 7) This was first recommended by Duroy in 1850. He suggested to the French Academy of Sciences that if oxygen were added to anesthetic atmospheres it would tend

Patterns
1) Given the same facts and environment, individuals of similar intelligence and experience will reach similar conclusions in about the same time.
2) Uncritical acceptance - popularity waxes and wanes.
3) Good ideas often rejected (or some factor missing).
4) Delayed acceptance - (not my idea).

5) Doubt it is true;
   - perhaps true but unimportant;
   - important - but anyone could do it.

6) Resurgence of ideas.

Table 6. Patterns of response to the introduction of new ideas.

Oxygen	
1850 -	Duroy suggests use oxygen in anesthesia.
1868 -	C. E. Andrews advocates Oxygen with Nitrous oxide for anesthesia.
1870-1880	Compressed gases become available in some centers.
1887 -	First Gas Machine with Nitrous oxide and Oxygen.
1910 -	McKesson machine with percentage mixtures of Oxygen with Nitrous oxide.

Table 7. Although suggested early, the need for oxygen to be used in all anesthetic administrations was recognized very slowly.

to ameliorate all the difficulties associated with inhalation anesthesia. Edmond Andrews suggested in 1868 that oxygen should be routinely added with the administration of nitrous oxid, but for the next several decades nitrous oxide continued to be used in Britain and the United States without benefit of dilution with oxygen. Fortunately, most of these asphyxial episodes were of only very short duration because of the brevity of sugery. McKesson made anesthesia machines for accurate mixtures of nitrous oxide and oxygen but in usage advocated hypoxic mixtures in order to get a greater effect from the nitrous oxide. Oxygen was rarely if ever added during use of the open drop technique despite reduction of the respired oxygen concentration by the presence of carbon dioxide and a high percentage of ether vapor in the dead space under the mask. So, except for a few enlightened medical centers, Duroy's admonition to add oxygen to anesthetic atmospheres was not routinely employed during the first hundred years of anesthesia. Indeed, it was not until oxygen measurement was fairly conveniently available that there was realization of how frequently encroachment upon normal inspired oxygen levels occurred. I invite your attention to a lecture on oxygen measurement by Professor Sugioka on Monday afternoon.

Academic Anesthesia began at Wisconsin

It is my belief that the most notable accomplishment of the second era of anesthesia was in the area of education. For this we must turn our attention again to Ralph Waters and the model program for post-graduate education which he started in 1928 at the University of Wisconsin Hospital in Madison, Wisconsin. Ralph Waters was the initiator or instigator of many significant contributions and changes related to the practice of modern anesthesiology. He was involved in the early organization and leadership of several societies of anesthetists, the development of new techniques and equipment, the introduction of new drugs, and the negotiations which resulted in the credentialing of competence and the establishment of the American Board of Anesthesiology, for which he was the first president of the Board of Directors. Any one or more of these would have earned an honored place in our history.

However, Dr. Waters' major contributions as an educator were of even greater importance and longer lasting in impact.

Waters' original academic goal at Wisconsin was to include the science of anesthesia in the curriculum for the basic medical education of all medical students and to set up what would be the world's first academic anesthesia program for post-graduate education of physicians, with intent for the trainees not only to gain knowledge, clinical skills and experience, *but also to learn effective methods for teaching the specialty.* Visitors came to see the way that things were done at Wisconsin, to learn about teaching methods for anesthesia, were charmed by Waters' projected enthusiasm and, intrigued with his program, went home resolved to emulate his model for study and teaching of clinical anesthesia to the extent possible in their own environments. Dr. Waters accomplished his goals at the University of Wisconsin and in doing so began to fill a great need in what up to then was a neglected area of medicine. His personal dynamics, enthusiasm, and professional skill won the respect of his faculty colleagues and attracted students and post-graduate trainees. Two thirds of his residents did go on to teach at other centers. Most eminent was Emery Rovenstine at Bellevue Hospital, New York University.

Among the many international visitors to the Waters program at Wisconsin was Robert R. Macintosh, who was appointed in 1936 as the initial Professor and Chairman of the Nuffield Department of Anaesthetics at Oxford University in England. This was the first professorial appointment for anaesthetics in the United Kingdom and for all of Europe. The establishment of an academic anaesthesia program in the Nuffield Department at Oxford was an achievement in itself noteworthy, with far reaching impact because of the prestige of Oxford University. For this we owe much to the perspicacity of William Morris the car manufacturer, better known as Lord Nuffield, who not only recognized the need for education of physicians in anesthesia but was able to negotiate establishment of anaesthetics as one of the first four endowed departments in a new post-graduate medical centre at Oxford. Also, contrary to all university protocol, Lord Nuffield chose Robert Macintosh as the man for appointment as professor and leader of what was then a unique department in Europe.

From these modest beginnings in the U.S. and U.K. have sprung all the world's academic centers for teaching and research of anesthesiology. It was the original educational efforts of Waters, his students and admirers which started the process of putting the specialty of clinical anesthesiology on an equal basis with other academic branches of medicine. All current anesthesiologists of this world are in debt and owe a daily thought of gratitude to Ralph Milton Waters, his vision, and the dynasty of teachers which he established for physicians entering the specialty of anesthesiology.

1947-1997 – Era of the Anesthesiologist, Perioperative Care, and Pain Management.

The Changing Image of Anesthesia

In the third Era, the further enhancement and spread of post-graduate education continued as the most important theme.

Anesthesia had been a part of surgery for the first hundred years. It was considered a technical and originally a somewhat menial exercise which could be assigned to and learned easily by junior house officers or technicians. Consequently, it was in many parts of the world done by nurse technicians under the presumed and usually remote supervision of the surgeon. In the third era, certified physician anesthesiologists began to assume a role of partnership with the surgeons. In the years immediately following the Second World War there was a dramatic surge of interest in anesthesia by large numbers of physicians returning from wartime service who recognized the potential of anesthesiology practice and the personal satisfactions to be had in spite of what was then a poor economic return. Many American surgeons who had been exposed to physician control of military anesthesia, also recognized the merits and advantages of shared responsibilities in the operating room and relinquished their dominant role, albeit sometimes grudgingly. Whatever the assault on surgical ego, there was a growing demand for better quality anesthesia care which could be best provided by dedicated attention of skilled physicians certified in the specialty of anesthesiology. The result was a proliferation of post-graduate programs in hospitals and medical schools, especially in North America and the United Kingdom, with a gradual increase in numbers of autonomous academic medical school departments of anesthesia in various parts of the world. This resulted in a steady flow of trained physicians into the practice of anesthesiology. As numbers of certified specialists increased to reach a critical mass, their impact on institutions, organizations and even government became more apparent. This did much to change the image and improve the status of the practice of anesthesiology.

In 1948 the Council of the Royal College of Surgeons in England established the Faculty of Anaesthetists which would set the educational standards, examine and certify those candidates qualifying for the specialty. Four decades later that Faculty of Anaesthetists evolved into an independent College of Anaesthetists which a short few years later attained Royal College status. Similar changes have occurred in some other parts of the world, following to some extent the U.K. pattern and reflecting the gradual changes in recognition.

In 1948 also another significant event occurred with the introduction in the U.K. of a National Health Service in which anaesthesia was recognized as a specialty with consultants of fully equal status to those of all other medical and surgical specialties.

Increased Educational Efforts

In the years immediately after World War II, the World Health Organization (WHO), in cooperation with the Unitarian Service Committee, had sponsored medical teaching missions to Eastern Europe, Middle Eastern countries and Japan. Anesthesiologists were included on each of these missions. Concerned about the needs of less favored and developing countries, the WHO had also established in Copenhagen a center for teaching anesthesiology to physicians. These educational efforts did much to spread the current information about the scientific basis of anesthesiology and its safe clinical practice.

In the early 1950's there was also formation of many new national anesthesia societies with consequent increases in group meetings and congresses for exchange of ideas and increased general awareness of progress among member physicians. Some of the larger of the new societies have sponsored their own journals with intent to improve communication for their members. Most notable of these were initiated in Canada, Scandinavia, Germany, Belgium, and Australia - New Zealand.

World Federation Established

Concurrently, there was an alliance of national societies in the formation of the World Federation of Societies for Anesthesiologists (WFSA). Prominent in the support and promotion of the WFSA was quite appropriately the IARS, originally founded and nurtured by Frank McMechan; much credit should be given to the organizing committee for the World Federation, chaired by Harold Griffith (Montreal) famed for his introduction of curare. Other members of the original interim committee included Torsten Gordh (Stockholm), Jacques Boureau (Paris), John Gillies (Edinburgh) and A. Goldblat (Brussels). From the WFSA came world congresses and additional interposed regional or continental congresses as well. The WFSA also set up teaching centers for improvement of anesthesiology in Asia and South America. More recently, an outreach of teaching effort from some of the established Western societies for benefit of developing countries has occurred in various parts of the world including Southeast Asia, Nepal, Africa, the Pacific Islands and Latin America. The sum total of all these educational efforts has been a marked improvement in the standard of anesthesia care available throughout much of the world.

Developments, Changes and Challenges

This third era is a time with which most of us at this Symposium are familiar by having participated in it. Nonetheless, it may be useful to mention what I consider in retrospect to be the important events and changes in concept worthy of particular historic interest. A plethora of new agents has been offered in what appears to be a never-ending procession. Each has had its sponsors and enthusiasts, in spite of the fact that some have had seemingly minimal or no advantage over predecessors. The somewhat surprising report of clinical anesthesia produced by the pharmacologic action of the costly rare gas Xenon, which is a minimal component of Earth's atmosphere, excited academic interest and provoked discussion about theoretical considerations of the mechanisms of general anesthesia. Meantime, the versatile cyclopropane, which during its popularity had to some extent displaced the original volatile liquid ether, was in turn, because of its inherent hazards of flammability and possible explosion, superseded by vaporized fluorinated liquid agents, notably fluothane and subsequently isoflurane. I find it interesting that nitrous oxide, the first to be originally rejected, continues to survive. It is also evident that inhalation anesthesia is still strongly entrenched, despite groups of enthusiasts who have advocated only intravenous anesthesia or regional anesthesia. Synthetic relaxants which have supplanted the original extracts of curare seem to be ensconced permanently in the anesthesiologist's armamentarium and many would support the idea that the advent of intravenous relaxants was the most important change in clinical anesthesia practice during the 20th century.

In the post war years, there was a continuing development of increasingly complicated and sophisticated types of surgical operations including extensive cardiovascular, oncologic, thoracic and open heart valve procedures, as well as various endoscopies, reconstructive surgery, and organ transplants. All of these were matched and facilitated by equally sophisticated changes and developments in the conduct and management of anesthesia and the perioperative care of patients.

Some of the knowledge and clinical skills developed by anesthesiologists have found their way into wider use in such areas as resuscitation, respiratory therapy, pain management and intensive care. From this also came emergency room care and ultimately public education efforts in cardio-pulmonary resuscitation (CPR) and advanced life support.

Improved Patient Safety

A recurring theme throughout the decades of the third Era has been a multi-faceted approach for increased emphasis on patient safety. In addition to the all important organized effort in several countries toward improvement of post-graduate education and the certifying of qualified anesthesiologists, specific steps were taken to correct recognized hazards associated with anesthesia equipment. This started with pin indexing of pressurized small cylinders and coded connections for large tanks and pressure lines to prevent unintended mis-connections and wrong use of piped gases. Standards committees worked hard to eliminate known incompatibility and recognized risks by standardizing design, sizes, and connections of equipment while trying to avoid undue interference with potential innovation. The addition of aids for monitoring anesthetized patients started with devices for continuous tracings of the electrocardiograms and for automatic, intermittent blood pressure. These were followed by systems for intermittent and/or continuous sampling of respired gases and anesthetic vapors. Currently models of this type equipment are now available in which the information is shown on a screen for continuous observation by the anesthesiologists. The most important monitoring device that has become a standard part of anesthesia equipment in recent years is the pulse oximeter.

The various societies have made an issue of safety by establishing committees to examine details of untoward events so that educational attention may be directed toward elimination of the causes of identified complications. This extends the purpose of the morbidity and mortality conference originally introduced in the Wisconsin teaching program as an educational tool, to the sharing of such events with a wider audience.

The Impact of Out Patient Surgery

No one can deny that in recent years outpatient or "Day Surgery" has made a tremendous impact on cost and conduct of anesthesia and surgery. This has altered also the management of all patients admitted to hospital for elective surgery, who now even for major procedures are most likely to arrive in hospital only an hour or so before surgery rather than the night before. This has modified the approach to medical care, reduced opportunity for pre-operative evaluation by the anesthesiologist, and restricts opportunity for clinical research studies, which again is a loss to patient, profession and society.

Day Surgery clinics made their appearance in the United States as a popular, sustainable entrepreneurial enterprise adapted from an old idea tried thirty to forty years earlier. The original most successfully developed of these had been "the downtown anesthesia clinic" as initiated and described in 1919 by Ralph M. Waters. (There's that name again!)

Ethical Considerations

Along with all of these changes, including progress in CPR and our ability to maintain vital functions for the prolongation of life, have come important ethical questions to confront Anesthetists in all aspects of their work: - in critical care, pain management, and perioperative care, as well as in the traditional necessary dedicated attention to care of anesthetized patients. Ethical concerns, many of which have been related to organ transplants, are so frequent that at least one of our leading departments (NDA, Oxford) has found it expedient to appoint an ethicist as educator and consultant for these problems. In this regard a rather noteworthy event occurred in 1957 when Professor Bruno Haid, Department of Resuscitation and Anesthetics at Innsbruck, Austria, personally asked a direct question of the Pope about whether there is obligation to maintain artificial respiration when there is no evidence of returning function. The succinct answer indicated that physicians are under no obligation to undertake prolonged life support by extraordinary means.

Comment

It is worth pointing out that there was probably a marked difference between what was generally perceived or experienced at any particular time in the history of anesthesia versus what we read about and assume today was the practice and understanding then. The leaders who wrote about and published their ideas and methods were often in marked contrast to the other ninety percent. Advances are slow to catch on and to be implemented.

There has always been and continues to be a wide disparity in the stages of development between areas. This is not just the developed countries versus the developing, nor the west versus the rest, but also within each country a wide disparity of standards and service. This difference exists between the teaching centers and the non-teaching, the trained and the untrained individuals, but also sometimes even between individuals or presumed comparable professional standards and training working in similar environments.

Conclusion

History is a dynamic including the past, present and future. We are all a part of anesthesia history. One hundred and fifty years sounds like a long time, yet the time spanned by the lives of many individuals in this audience is one third to one half or more of that time. Some few of us have had up to fifty years of clinical experience and may have known personally the prominent leaders of earlier times and certainly those of current times. I urge you to each take the time and make the effort to document your unique view of past events with supporting vignettes or anecdotes. All such memoirs help to make future historic evaluation more realistic and less likely to misrepresent what you believe to be the correct interpretation.

Now I did promise you a challenge. There are a lot of younger colleagues who have little or no knowledge about anesthesia history. This makes a deficit in their professional attitudes and understanding as they confront present and future problems. *You and I have both opportunity and obligation* to correct this deficit by actively sharing our interests in history with younger colleagues and trainees. I urge you all to walk the walk, talk the talk; do your bit - get history into the curriculum for post-graduate education, and as a regular feature of society meetings and congresses.

Finally, I invite you to take advantage of all aspects of this Symposium. Many of the participants are a part of the living history of anesthesia. In the audience today are a surprising number of teachers, contributors and innovators whose efforts set the stage for the high standards of clinical anesthesiology which is available in much of the world today. Get to know some of these people. Make some new friends. Enjoy! Thank you very much.

Dr. WG Atherstone:
A Pioneer Anaesthetist in South Africa

R. P. Haridas
Department of Anaesthetics, University of Natal,
Durban, South Africa.

Dr. William Guybon Atherstone was probably first doctor in South Africa to administer ether for a surgical procedure. This article will present details of the life and career of this pioneering doctor and scientist, and discuss how he might have obtained news about ether anaesthesia. Also included is the text of a remarkably detailed newspaper report of the first ether anaesthetic that he administered.

Biographical details

Dr. Atherstone was the eldest son of Dr. John Atherstone and his first wife Elizabeth Damant. He was born on 27 May 1814, at Sion Hall, Nottingham, UK and came to the Cape with his parents in 1820 on the ship *Ocean*. After his schooling in Grahamstown and Uitenhage he was apprenticed to his father, and also did some medical work with the army. In 1836 Atherstone enrolled in Dublin for his medical studies. He also spent time in Paris and Heidelberg, and received his MD from the University of Heidelberg in 1839. While overseas, he married Catherine Handel Atherstone (his first cousin), and returned to Grahamstown in 1839 to join his father's practice. He became the District Surgeon of Albany after his father's death in 1853 and continued as such until 1878. He stopped medical practice in 1887 because of failing eyesight.

Atherstone had wide interests outside medicine - in geology, botany and natural history. He helped establish the Scientific, Literary and Medical Society (now the Albany Museum) and the Botanic Gardens in Grahamstown. He was also the founder and first medical officer of the Albany Hospital. In 1864, he was elected a Fellow of the British Geological Society. In March 1867, he identified as a diamond, a stone which was found near Hopetown. The stone was sent to him as he was regarded as "the country's leading mineralogist". This discovery sparked off the Diamond Rush of the 1870s. He was a Member for Grahamstown in the Cape Parliament from 1881-1890. Atherstone was also the first vice-president of the South African Geological Society in 1895. He died in Grahamstown on 26 June 1898.

Ether anaesthesia

News of ether anaesthesia first reached South Africa on the P & O iron paddle steamer *Pekin,* which left Southampton on her maiden voyage on 15 February 1847, and arrived in Table Bay on 1 April 1847. The news was carried by Dr. Thomas Bell, the ship's surgeon, and in newspapers. Mr. Alfred Raymond, who practiced as a dentist, first used ether for a dental extraction on 17 April 1847. The report of this in *"De Verzamelaar, id est: The Gleaner"* on Tuesday, 20 April 1847 is the earliest known report of the successful use of ether for anaesthesia-analgesia in South Africa. Raymond was initially overlooked by some medical historians[1-2]. Much of what is known of Raymond was provided by Couper at a previous Symposium[3] and in his thesis[4].

Atherstone stated in 1897 that he received the news of the use of ether "direct from the U.S. by sailing vessel *en route* for England. I had no details whatever supplied me, and knew nothing of Simpson's work in Edinburgh"[5]. Atherstone administered it by means of a "hubble-bubble" type of apparatus (which resembled a Turkish narghile), which he had constructed (Figure 1). His first patient was Mr. Frederick Carlisle, the Deputy Sheriff of Albany, who had a painful, chronic ulcer associated with a contracture of his leg. Atherstone performed an above knee amputation on Wednesday, 16 June 1847, assisted by his father Dr. John Atherstone (who was the District Surgeon of Albany), and two army surgeons, Dr. Hadaway and Dr. Irwin. The *Graham's Town Journal* of 19 June reported the event, while the issue of 26 June carried a report of the procedure written by Atherstone, and a sketch of the apparatus that was used.

Atherstone wrote the first detailed case report by a medical practitioner of a procedure under ether in South Africa. At the time he did not claim to be the first in South Africa or the first outside Europe and America to administer ether. He made no mention of Raymond's anaesthetics - reports of Raymond's anaesthetics, and a mention of the use of ether in India were reprinted in Grahamstown newspapers in April and May. In one newspaper report Atherstone mentions warming ether, which he probably picked up from the English papers.

It is not clear how Atherstone obtained the news "direct from the U.S.", and the nature of his early experiments with ether are also unknown. His medical casebook for that period has dated entries between 1842-1857, but there are no notes on Mr. Carlisle or a mention of ether (Medical Casebook No. 4 *in* Killie Campbell Library, Durban). This is a remarkable omission as part of this casebook was also used as a notebook. There are lists of books and equipment ordered, and notes on fossils, sea shells, stones and rainfall. He may have received the news together with the books that he frequently ordered, or through his relatives in the United States (personal communication, Mrs N. Mathie, Grahamstown). The Cape Town and Grahamstown newspapers of April and May had at least 12 references to the use of ether for surgery, including 3 reports of the use of ether by Raymond in Cape Town, and Atherstone must have also been aware of these.

Newspaper reports

Below are some extracts from the first article in the *Graham's Town Journal* and the complete text of the second article. The text of the second article has been rearranged into paragraphs.

Notable features include mention of experiments of an unknown nature, trial inhalation by the patient on the day before the operation, the emphasis on the absence of pain rather than the need to be asleep for the procedure, the duration of inhalation of ether being about three minutes, and the desirability of using an inhaler with a low resistance to breathing.

Graham's Town Journal, 19 June 1847.

Painless operation by means of Ether.

On Tuesday a very successful surgical operation was performed by Dr. A. G. Atherstone, - the patient, Mr. F. Carlisle, Deputy sheriff of Albany, being at the time under the influence of Ether, ... was quickly thrown into a state of stupor, partially conscious of what was going on, and yet the sense of pain entirely absent. The limb was most ably amputated by Dr. Atherstone, ... In our next we hope to give the report of the operator, as the humanity, as well as the advancement of science, alike demand that this subject should have the widest publicity. ... The same process has, we learn from late papers, been introduced into medical practice in British India, ...

Graham's Town Journal, 26 June 1847.

Sulphuric Ether.

We now redeem the promise made in our last to state some additional facts, relative to the surgical operation recently performed by Dr. W. G. Atherstone in the case of Mr. F. Carlisle, he being at the time in a state of stupor, caused by the inhalation of ether. The following particulars, interesting alike to the lover of science and friend of humanity, have been furnished by the operator :

The first opportunity I had of testing the efficacy of ether in surgical operations was on Mr. F. Carlisle, Deputy Sheriff of Albany. This gentleman about 27 years ago lost almost the whole of the calf of his leg from erysipelas, terminating in gangrene, which nearly proved fatal. From this very great contraction of the leg resulted, and for the last few years there has been an irritable ulcer, extending up into the bend of the knee, being a constant source of such continual pain and annoyance that he would gladly have got rid of the useless limb years ago if it could have been removed without pain. After several experiments with different kinds of apparatus, with and without valves, which it is unnecessary for me to describe, I succeeded in producing the requisite degree of insensibility to pain by means of a simple contrivance as shown in the following sketch: (Fig. 1)

The patient being satisfied as to the powerful effects of ether at length consented to have his leg removed, stipulating that the operation should not be commenced till he himself gave the word, and the following day (Wednesday, 16th inst.) I amputated the thigh in its lower third, assisted by my father, Mr. J. A. District surgeon, Dr. Hadaway, 91st and Dr. Irwin, 27th Regt.

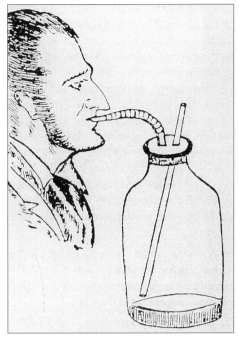

Fig. 1: Sketch from Graham's Town Journal, 26 June 1847 of the apparatus used for inhaling ether.

After ten or twelve inhalations of the ether the patient put down his hand and pinched himself to ascertain what degree of sensibility there was. He then continued inhaling for a short time longer, when he again pinched himself and immediately said "I am drunk enough now - you may begin." The tourniquet was immediately tightened and at the same instant the first plunge of the knife effected without the least motion or sign of suffering on the part of the patient, who at this stage appeared perfectly unconscious, and continued inhaling the ether, mechanically opening and closing his nostrils with his own hand. So perfect was the insensibility that Dr. Irwin, who had placed his hand on the patient's arm, thinking he might start, finding not the slightest resistance during the first incision, removed his hand altogether, as did also an assistant who had taken hold of the leg, and for the rest of the operation the patient lay perfectly free and motionless on the bed. At the second incision, which divided the large nerves and vessels, he uttered an involuntary shriek, although not the slightest movement was perceptible or other symptom of pain. As soon as the leg was off the ether bottle was removed, the patient still holding his nose and becoming very talkative and even humourous as he gradually recovered from the stupefying effects of the ether. The time during which the ether was inhaled was about three minutes.

When the arteries were taken up and the dressing being applied, the following dialogue took place between the patient and one of the medical gentlemen present :

Patient - "It's very odd, do you know I fancy I am *still* holding my nose!"

Dr. I - "Well, so you are, most energetically too!"

"Then why remove the vapour?"

"Because the operation is all over - your leg has been off some time now."

"Now don't talk nonsense to me - I'm a reasonable man you know - explain why the bottle is gone."

"You don't want it any longer - your leg is off, Mr. Carlisle."

"What! my leg taken off? impossible - I can't believe it - let me see for myself - and, on seeing the stump he burst out "God be praised! It's the grandest discovery ever made, - we must erect a monument to this fellow's memory, - It's the greatest boon ever conferred on man, I have been totally unconscious of everything - the sound of that horrid saw still grates upon my ear as if heard in a dream from which you have just awoke me, but as for pain I have not felt the slightest."

He has since stated that the impression on his mind was that he was present at an amputation performed upon some other person, - he has a vivid recollection of hearing the scream, and pitied the poor fellow from his heart, but had no conception that the poor fellow he so commisserated was in reality *himself*!

The ether should be inhaled *cold*. I found that rapid vaporisation from *extent of surface* is much preferable to vaporisation by heat. The vessel, as shown in sketch, in which the ether is placed should be of such a size as to contain sufficient vapour to induce *rapid* insensability, success appeared to depend in a great measure on the *rapidity* with which it acted. The tube through which the ether is inhaled should be sufficiently large to offer no resistance whatever to free inspiration, and the respiration should be slow and prolonged so that the lungs are well filled with the vapour which should be retained for a few seconds before being expired again. The apparatus on the present occasion consisted of a large wide mouthed bottle, capable of holding two quarts, which had two apertures on the cork, through one of which passed a glass tube, $1/2$ inch in diameter, reaching to within $1/4$ inch of the surface of the ether; in the other aperture an elastic tube with ivory mouth piece was fixed for inhaling the vapour. About two ounces of ether being poured down the glass tube, both tubes were stopped for some minutes to allow the vapour to fill the bottle before inhaling. Assuming the quantity of air taken into the lungs at each inspiration to be 20 cubic inches, which is about the average, a bottle of this size will contain vapour for about $5 1/2$ inspirations. These experiments have fully satisfied me as well as the other medical gentlemen who attended the operation, that the inhalation of ether is perfectly safe, and unattended by any unpleasant consequences when properly administered, and that it is capable of producing complete insensibility to pain and prostration of muscular power.

Conclusion

Atherstone was one of the great scientific minds in South Africa in the last century, and his contributions to science and the development of Grahamstown are unrivaled. He was probably the first medical practitioner in South Africa to administer ether for a major surgical procedure. His success was published in the *Graham's Town Journal* and in some of the Cape Town newspapers (e.g. *South African Commercial Advertiser* on 30 June 1847; *De Zuid-Afrikaan* on 1 July 1847), and did not elicit any report or claim to any prior use of ether by other medical practitioners. It is therefore reasonable to assume that no major operations were successfully performed under ether in Cape Town between Alfred Raymond's first use of ether for a dental extraction on 17 April 1847 and Atherstone's use of ether for an amputation on 16 June 1847.

Acknowledgement

I would like to acknowledge the help that I received from the Late Professor JL Couper. His extensive research on early ether anaesthesia in South Africa provided much new information on Alfred Raymond, who was initially overlooked as the first person to use ether for anaesthesia in South Africa.

References:

[1] Burrows EH A History of Medicine in South Africa. A.A. Balkema, Cape Town, 1958

[2] Laidler PW, Gelfand M. South Africa. Its Medical History. 1652 - 1898. A Medical and Social Study. C. Struik (Pty) Ltd., Cape Town, 1971

[3] Couper JL. Putting the record straight - The first ether administration in South Africa. In: Atkinson RS, Boulton TG, eds. The History of Anaesthesia (Proceedings of the Second International Symposium on the History of Anaesthesia, London, July 1987). International Congress and Symposium Series, Number 134. Royal Society of Medicine Services, Ltd., London, 1989, 149-153

[4] Couper JL The Introduction of Ether into South Africa. PhD Thesis, Medunsa, Pretoria, 1990

[5] Atherstone WG Reminiscences of medical practice in South Africa fifty years ago. South African Medical Journal 1897; 4: 243-247

Some little known Aspects of Johann Friedrich Dieffenbach's Life and Death

D. Wessinghage
Rheuma-Zentrum, Bad Abbach, Germany

Dieffenbach's life was a long journey, beginning with his early attempts at transplanting single eyebrow hairs into the arm, doing free skin transplantations and dealing with spur in wounds of cocks' combs, and reaching its peak with his reconstructive surgery - the many and varying -plasties and -raphies in the head and neck and ano-genital regions [2-6,7,8,10,11,17-19,20].

Johann Friedrich Dieffenbach (Fig.1) was born in 1792 in Königsberg, East Prussia, the city of the first Prussian King, Friedrich 1st, and of Immanuel Kant (1724-1804). While studying theology, Dieffenbach, like many German students at the time, felt bound to fight against Napoléon between 1812 and 1814. After the war he met Johanna Motherby and fell in love with her. At the time she was married to Dr. William Motherby (1778-1847), the son of a Scottish family of merchants who had lived in Königsberg for a lot of years. After qualifying in Edinburgh, Motherby was the first to bring Jenner's smallpox vaccination to East Prussia. After divorcing from William, Johanna married Dieffenbach in 1824; he, meantime, had gone to Bonn University to study under the surgeon Philipp Franz von Walther (1782-1849). Dieffenbach then went to France, spending some time in Paris and meeting the celebrities of the time in French medicine - Baron Guillaume de Duypuytren (1777-1835), Dominique Jean Larrey (1766-1842), Alexis Boyer (1757-1833), François Magendie (1783-1855), Jacques Delpech (1777-1832) and others. After com-

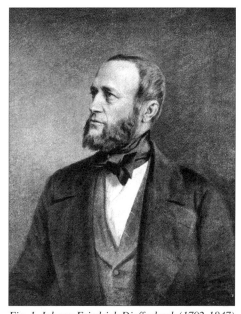

Fig. 1 Johann Friedrich Dieffenbach (1792-1847)

pleting his studies at Würzburg Dieffenbach settled in Berlin in 1823, calling himself "Arzt und Operateur"[8].

Dieffenbach gained a considerable reputation by performing and describing a number of new operations. In May 1829, when 37 years old and having until then mainly worked in his Berlin consulting rooms, he was appointed "Charitéarzt bei der chirurgischen Station". He was still subordinate to the head of the surgical department of the Charité Hospital, the leading Prussian surgeon, Johann Nepomuk Rust (1775-1840), who was no longer practising to any great extent. In 1831 Dieffenbach founded the first school for male

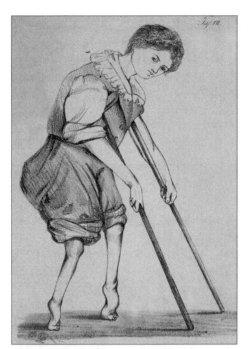

Fig. 2 A case for orthopaedic surgery

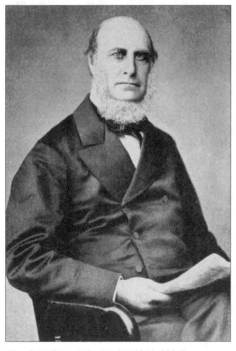

Fig. 3 William John Little (1810-1894)

and female nurses in Berlin and for this he wrote "Anleitung zur Krankenwartung" (A Manual of Nursing) dedicated to the famous "Vater Heim", the most popular practitioner in Berlin, Dr. Ernst Ludwig Heim (1747-1834)[7]. Dieffenbach became "extra-ordinary" professor in 1832 and from then gave courses on surgical procedures using cadavers (Operationskurs an der Leiche). He also introduced infusion and transfusion therapy and gave defibrinated human blood to exsanguinated patients.

During the second period of his active life he turned towards orthopaedics and orthopaedic surgery (Fig. 2). Initially he was concerned with congenital deformities of fingers and toes - especially with syndactily. Even at that time he emphasised that surgery should not be performed too early, but only, in spite of the insistence of parents, on the older child . He started treating deformities of the feet, but only with moderate success even though he performed subcutaneous tenotomies and did redressings in plaster. After some serious complications took place, he became more cautious and sent a patient, William John Little (1810-1894) (Fig.3)- an English physician studying in Berlin [14,15]- to his friend and respected colleague in Hannover, Georg Friedrich Louis Stromeyer (1804-1876), for treatment of his club foot (Fig.4).

Stromeyer used to treat this deformity by tenotomy of the Achilles tendon, following a method developed by Dr. Johann Friedrich Sartorius[12] (1750-1812) who had studied at Herborn[17]. When the patient returned ten weeks later, Dieffenbach and his interns were astonished; the operated foot looked almost normal, the cavus deformity had diminished, the calf was prominent, the leg was of normal length and the sole touched the floor completely[14,15].

The young physician-patient, later an orthopaedic surgeon himself and founder of the Royal Orthopaedic Hospital in London in

1839, was so impressed by the result of Stromeyer's surgery that in 1837 he wrote a dissertation[9] at the Berlin Friedrich-Wilhelm-University on his own medical history and surgical procedure (Fig. 5). Out of gratitude to Stromeyer, he even called his second son John Stromeyer Little after his godfather. Because of this good relationship, Stromeyer gave his godson, the younger Little, a copy of his autobiography with a hand-written dedication (Fig. 6a, 6b, 6c). For decades, the success of this operation fostered international goodwill, especially in German-English relations, and the friendship of surgeons from the two countries (Fig. 7).

Dieffenbach, convinced about Sartorius' and Stromeyer's procedure, recalled all his patients who had had unsatisfactory results from earlier surgery. In addition, he induced his juniors and nursing staff to look for children with club feet in the streets of Berlin. In his memoirs, Stromeyer describes street children pretending to be deformed in order to get a few pfennigs. They would disappear just before the time of operation. This method of obtaining patients was soon extended from club feet to torticollis and many other deformities. One beggar argued against being cured by surgery because his club feet were his best feature and he earned his living with them - and without the necessity of working!

At that time the Berlin street urchins used to sing:

"Wer kennt nicht Dr. Dieffenbach -
Den Doktor der Doktoren? -
Er schneidet Arm und Beine ab
- macht neue Nas' und Ohren"

"Who doesn't know Doc Dieffenbach -
Doctor of all Doctors? -
He cuts off arms and legs
[as everybody fears]
and adds on nose and ears"

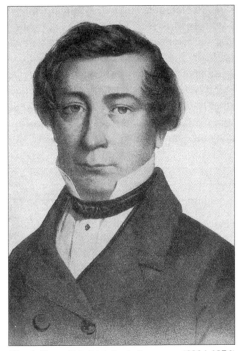

Fig. 4 Georg Friedrich Louis Stromeyer (1804-1876)

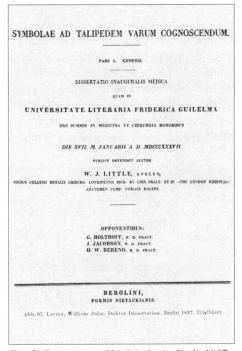

Fig. 5 Cover page of Little's thesis, Berlin 1837

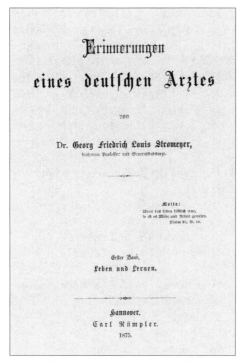

Fig. 6a Cover page of Stromeyer`s autobiography[13]

ted and improved, but we, today, can study his life's work in his book "Die Operative Chirurgie" which shows his detailed and comprehensive knowledge of the subject. The book was partly edited after his death by his nephew Johann Julius Bühring[1], an "orthopaedic surgeon", as Julius Wolff (1836-1902) had already called himself[18].

It is to the credit of Dieffenbach's first wife Johanna, that she tried to keep him on the straight and narrow path of duty and to curb his excessive love of experimentation. However, Dieffenbach divorced the wife he had previously adored and contracted a further happy marriage in 1831 with Emilie Heydecker, the daughter of a physician of Bad Freienwalde. Dieffenbach became "extraordinarius" at the Friedrich-Wilhelm-Universität of Berlin in 1832, soon succeeding the famous Carl Ferdinand von Graefe (1787-1840) as "ordinary" Professor of Surgery. For years he continued to work as an inspired physician, teacher and scientist - widely celebrated and highly esteemed.

Due to his increasing experience and equipment for after-treatment, Dieffenbach achieved greater and greater success with his tenotomics. He extended the indication to the treatment of torticollis, squint, ankylosis and even to stammer - here with moderate success. Not only did his patients bear witness to the variety of procedures he initia-

On 9th of November 1846 the first scientific description of etherisation performed by William Morton (1819-1868) on 16th of October of that year, was published by Henry Jacob Bigelow (1818-1890). The technique quickly became known in Europe. The first anaesthetic with ether in Germany was carried out on 10th of January 1847 by

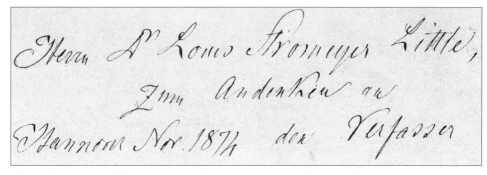

Fig. 6b Handwritten dedication to his godson John Stromeyer Little, working as a surgeon in China[13]

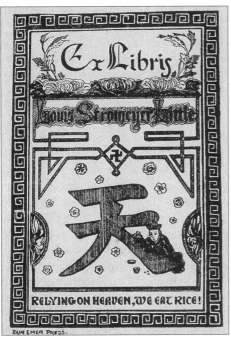

Fig. 6c "Ex libris" of John Stromeyer`s Little`s exemplar of Stromeyer`s autobiography book

Johann Ferdinand Heyfelder (1789-1869), a surgeon of Erlangen[16]. On 10th of February 1847, Dieffenbach introduced ether anaesthesia for major operations in the Berlin Charité Hospital. He managed the technique with care and critically considered the unknown biological mechanisms involved and the likely affects of the agent on the lungs of the patients. In that same year, he discussed these problems in his last published book: "Der Aether gegen den Schmerz" (Fig. 8a, 8b, 8c).

In this he wrote that during long operations etherisation is able to completely prevent severe pain. This means great relief for the suffering patient, but for the surgeon it causes difficulties. He believed that, while many operations can only take place when the patient is under the influence of ether, others should not be attempted by this means and for some, particularly minor procedures, it is unnecessary. However, while it is clear that he perceived the great advance that anaesthesia would provide for suffering humanity, he still asked where this development could lead and was unable to provide an answer. He warned, from his own experience, that anaesthesia with ether can actually increase the sensation of pain and may be followed by madness. It could give rise to apoplexy, haemorrhage and other severe complications. Overdosage led to death.

"Der Aether gegen den Schmerz" was the first monograph on ether anaesthesia to be published in German speaking countries and Dieffenbach should be considered as a pioneer in establishing a new branch of medicine - anaesthesia - in a similar way to Wilhelm Conrad Röntgen (1845-1923) who, 50 years later, revolutionised diagnosis and treatment to the benefit of physici-

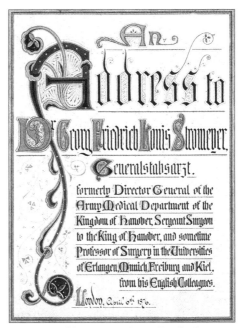

Fig. 7 An address to Dr. Georg Friedrich Louis Stromeyer from his English colleagues, London, April 6th 1876, anniversary of his Doctor's jubelee book

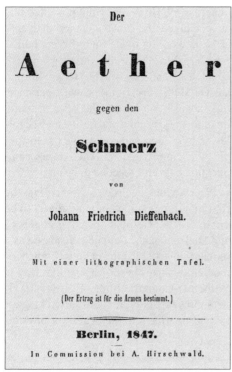

Fig. 8a Cover page of Dieffenbach's textbook "Der Aether gegen den Schmerz"

ans and patients. Dieffenbach died in a way which might be envied by many academic teachers, in the lecture theatre while presenting a priest who had been cured by surgery. One of his students, de la Pierre, a young doctor from Berlin attempted and described resuscitation with the methods of the time - applying stimuli such as hot and cold water, irritating the larynx with a feather or rubbing with ether. It was later suggested that Dieffenbach's death might have been related to self-medication with ether[7].

The epitaph of de la Pierre following the death of his great teacher on 11th of November 1847, reads: "Dieffenbach ist todt. Ernst und kalt sind seine Zuege, das edle Haupt liegt schwer auf den Schultern eines neben ihm sitzenden Arztes. Die Nächsten springen hinzu, um durch Lösung des Anzugs die vermeintliche Ohnmacht vorüber zu führen. Im selben Augenblicke sind die Kleider von seinen Armen gerissen, nein, es ist keine Ohnmacht; zwei Lanzetten dringen in seine Adern, und es fliesst das Blut nicht mehr! Jetzt stürzt Alles von Sitzen herbei mit dem Schmerzensruf, er ist todt. In einem Augenblick liegt er entblösst in den Armen seiner Schüler und Alles drängt sich um ihn. Glühender Siegellack wird auf seine Brust geträufelt, sie reiben, sie bürsten in krampfhafter Verzweiflung den geliebten Lehrer. Blutig werden seine Glieder. Kaltes Wasser wird auf die Herzgrube gespritzt, mit einer Feder der Kehlkopf gereizt, Aether wird vorgehalten, Aether wird auf die Brust gegossen. Alles, Alles ist vergebens. Jetzt klammert sich

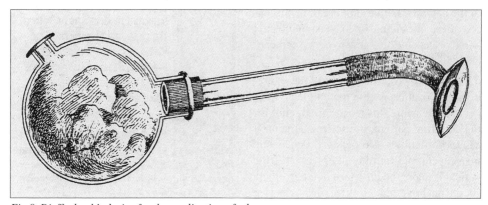

Fig 8 Dieffenbach's device for the application of ether

der letzte Gedanke der hinsterbenden Hoffnung an ein heisses Bad. Im Nu haben seine Schüler Wasser und eine Wanne herbeigetragen, der theure Leib wird schnell hineingesenkt, man bürstet, man reibt ihn aufs Neue; kein Lebenszeichen mehr, kein Atemzug, kein Zucken - er ist dahin. Vor 20 Minuten trat er mit freundlichen Gruss vor seine harrenden Schüler. In Entsetzen und hilflos hatte greise Priester das Auditorium verlassen, und wir trugen nun verwaist die Leiche des Geliebten aus dem Saal".

He died the 11th of November 1847.

In summary, an outstanding and popular surgeon of his time, Dieffenbach contributed to the rapid expansion of pain-free surgery by publishing in 1847 - the year of his death - his book "Der Aether gegen den Schmerz" on his experience with ether anaesthesia.

Schlussfolgerungen.

Nach dem was wir bis jetzt über die Anwendung der Aetherdämpfe bei chirurgischen Operationen erfahren haben, sind wir zu folgenden Schlüssen berechtigt.

Die Aetherisation ist im Stande, den höchsten Schmerz bei den gröfsten chirurgischen Operationen vollständig aufzuheben.

Die Aetherisation ist daher für den Kranken die gröfste Erleichterung. Dem Arzte (mit Ausnahme bei Verrenkungen) immer eine Erschwerung.

Die Aetherisation kann aber auch Steigerung des Schmerzgefühls und Tobsucht zur Folge haben.

Die Aetherisation ist lebensgefährlich bei Neigung zum Schlagflufs, Blutsturz und manchen anderen Zuständen.

Uebertreibung der Aetherisation kann augenblicklichen Tod herbeiführen.

Fig. 8c The summury of Dieffenbach concerning the use of ether for pain relief during surgical procedures

References:

[1] Bühring J J: Vorwort zu "Die operative Chirurgie" von J. F. Dieffenbach. F A B Brockhaus, Leipzig 1848

[2] Dieffenbach J F: Die Transfusion des Blutes und die Infusion der Arzneien in die Blutgefäße. Th Ch F Enslin, Berlin 1828

[3] Dieffenbach J F: Über die Durchschneidung der Sehnen und Muskeln. A Förstner, Berlin 1841

[4] Dieffenbach J F: Über das Schielen und die Heilung desselben durch die Operation. A Förstner, Berlin 1842

[5] Dieffenbach J F: Die operative Chirurgie. Bd. 1 u. 2, F A B Brockhaus, Leipzig 1845

[6] Dieffenbach J F: Der Aether gegen den Schmerz. Hirschwald, Berlin 1847

[7] Genschorek W: Wegbereiter der Chirurgie: Johann Friedrich Dieffenbach und Theodor Billroth. Hirzel-Teubner, Leipzig 1983

[8] Lampe R: Dieffenbach. Barth, Leipzig 1934

[9] Little W J.: Symbolae ad talipedem varum cognoscendum. Diss. Berlin 17.1.1837

[10] Meier Th : Vorträge in der chirurgischen Klinik der königlichen Charité. Gehalten von Dieffenbach. A Dunchker, Berlin 1840

[11] Rohlfs H: Die chirurgischen Classiker Deutschlands, 4. Abth., 2. Hälfte: Johann Friedrich Dieffenbach. CL Hirschfeld, Leipzig 1885

[12] Sartorius J F: Glückliche Herstellung eines verkrümmten Fusses durch die Durchschneidung der Achillessehne. JB v Siebold's Sammlung seltener und auserlesener chirurgischer Beobachtungen. III, Hildebrand. Arnstadt 1812, 258

[13] Stromeyer G F L: Erinnerungen eines deutschen Arztes, Bd. I und II; C Rümpler. Hannover 1875

[14] Valentin B: Dieffenbach an Stromeyer. Briefe aus den Jahren 1836 bis 1846. J A Barth, Leipzig 1934

[15] Valentin B: Geschichte der Orthopädie. Thieme, Stuttgart 1961

[16] Walser H H.: Zur Einführung der Äthernarkose im deutschen Sprachgebiet im Jahre 1847. Sauerländer, Aarau 1957

[17] Wessinghage D: Die Hohe Schule zu Herborn und ihre Medizinische Fakultät - The high School of Herborn and its Medical Faculty: 1584-1817-1984. Schattauer, Stuttgart 1984

[18] Wessinghage D: Reprints Medizinhistorischer Schriften, Nr. 4: Julius Wolff - Das Gesetz der Transformation der Knochen. Schattauer, Stuttgart 1991

[19] Wessinghage D: 200. Geburtstag von Johann Friedrich Dieffenbach - Wegbereiter der plastischen und der orthopädischen Chirurgie. Orthopädische Praxis 1994; 30: 329-334

[20] Wolff H: Zum 200. Geburtstag von Johann Friedrich Dieffenbach. Zbl f Chir 1992; 117 : 238 - 243

Who Introduced Nitrous Oxide into French Practice?

M. Zimmer
Dental Surgeon, Strasbourg, & DEA, Ecole Pratique des Hautes Etudes, Paris, France

The merit of popularising the use of nitrous oxide as an anaesthetic undoubtedly owed to Gardner Quincy Colton (1814-1898) twenty years after Horace Wells (1815-1848) misfortune in January 1845 at the Massachusetts Hospital. Yet, it is interesting to examine the use of nitrous oxide gas as an anaesthetic in dental and head surgery in the early years of its introduction.

Horace Wells letter[1], addressed to the Lancet mailed by Galignanis Messengers Paris, on February 18th, 1847, certifies that Wells had administered nitrous oxide gas and the vapour of ether to about fifty patients since these substances had been discovered. Wondering why the number of patients is this small, one has to mention, that he suffered from an illness, which immediately ensued on his return home from Boston, in January 1845.

Early use of nitrous oxide.

However, according to Samuel S. White[2], between December 1844 and 30th September, 1846, the Hardfords dentists John B. Terry, John Braddock, and E.E. Crowfoot used nitrous oxide gas.

In the hospitals, nitrous oxide was used in January 1847 in the First Surgical Division of the New York Hospital for an operation of an ectropion[3]. According to Pickwey W. Ellsworth[4], and John Murray Carnochans reports[5], E. E. Marcy used nitrous oxide anaesthesia for the removal of a scirrhous testicle in the hospital of Hartford on August 17th, 1847, and Ellsworth performed an amputation of a thigh on January 1st, 1848. In both cases it was Horace Wells who administered the gas. On January 4th, 1848, S. B. Beresford of Hartford, removed an adipose tumor from the shoulder of an adult. According to Ira Manley[6], Horace Wells administered nitrous oxide to Kearney Rodgers(1793-1851) patient in a blepharoplastic operation because of an ectropium, without any pain. This last testimony is very interesting because Wells committed suicide on January 24th 1848, a week after Ira Manley saw him giving anaesthesia at the Hospital of New York.

Eighteen months after William Green Mortons (1819-1868) ether anaesthesia at the Massachusetts General Hospital, Henry J. Bigelow[7,8] (?-1890) inhaled nitrous oxide himself and administered it for the first and only time to a 45 year old woman on April 27th, 1848. The removal of the mammal tumor could be performed without poblems or unpleasant sensations for the patient, but as Bigelow stated: *anaesthesia by nitrous oxide was then abandoned, in view of the livid surface and muscular rigidity, both doubtless due to asphyxia, but also on account of the inconvenience of the preparation of the gas on a large scale, and especially from the bulk of the apparatus required for its administration.* The manufacturing of sulphuric ether was easier, not so cumbersome; chloroform and ether anaesthesia then divided the surgeons for years.

It took until May 1863[9], i.e fifteen years on, to find people taking a new interest in the extraction of teeth and fangs under nitrous oxide anaesthesia again. Gardner Quincey Colton, just like a showman as Collins[10], had traveled all around the United States, organizing popular lectures and demonstrations on the effects of laughing gas, the so called frolics at which the gas was inhaled for the pleasant reactions it produced[11]. *Colton administered the gas for ordinary entertainment, save that the patient was sitting and the inhalation was continued much longer* wrote J. S. Latimer[12] in August 1863. *Two minutes were required to induce complete anaesthesia, when half the fangs were quickly removed and three minutes from the commencement of inhalation, the patient was completely conscious.* As Truman Smith[13] reports in a deposition made in March 1864, 3929 teeth were extracted between June 1863 and March 1864.

After July 1863, Colton moved to New York and established an anaesthetic institution downtown. The technique was quickly adopted by the dental surgeons in New York, especially as A. W. Sprague invented his gazometer[14]. *For inhalation, nitrous oxide should be made from the purest nitrate of ammonia, thoroughly washed by straining through several washers, confined over water, and inhaled in its purity through a valved inhaler,* he[15] said. The reason why this technique was not immediately adopted in Europe according to by Richard Cooper Hopgood[16] was that: *one of the principal drawbacks to the use of nitrous oxide in England has been the time and trouble required to be expended in its manufacture.* In the United States, there was a different development: as soon as October 1863, the apparatus for manufacturing nitrous oxide in larger quantities could be obtained at dental depots.

In London Samuel Lee Rymer (1833-1909) decided to investigate the matter, and even in Paris, the American dental surgeons were interested in nitrous oxide anaesthesia, since most of them had brothers who practiced as dental surgeons and medical doctors in New York or in the Western urban areas.

James Marion Sims[17] (1813-1883), a surgeon of the Womens Hospital in New York, and a honorary fellow of the Obstetrical Society of London, wrote in 1868, that: *Almost all the American dentists in Paris have apparatus for making it (the gas). Dr. Crane was the first to use it here. He has been using it for four years; Dr. Préterre for more than two years. Then followed Dr. Parmly, Dr. Rottenstein, and Dr. Lond, and now it has received a new impetus in the hands of Dr. Evans and Dr. Colton.* This means that the method was introduced in France by Dr. John W. Crane (1836-?) as early as 1864, and that it became wide spread in Paris because of Apolloni Pierre Préterre (1821-1893), after December 1865.

Who was Dr. Crane?

Dr. John W. Crane was the son of John W. Crane (1799-1870), a medical doctor, graduated from Castleton Medical College, in Vermont, Connecticut. The father's biodata helps to understand why the son was concerned with nitrous oxide anaesthesia. In the first years of his professional life, John W. Cranes father practiced for some time in Hartford, the town where Horace Wells was to establish his office in 1836. After a few months, he decided to study dentistry with A. G. Cogswell and Josuah Foster B. Flagg (1804-1872) in Boston. Josuah Flagg was the first dentist of American nationality, the first author of the first number of the Dental News Letter in October 1847, probably the first to discover and to make known that Mortons letheon was sulphuric ether, and one of the first in Philadelphia to turn its administration in dental and surgical practice into a speciality[18]. After his studies in Boston, John W. Crane returned to Hartford, practising dentistry until 1834. Then he moved to New-York, where he opened an office in Park Place that existed for more than forty years. He was one of the Committee officers of the New York Dental Society and its Librarian after 1834[19]. If we consider that he died in Hartford, on April 11th, 1870, it is easy to imagine that he had contacts with colleagues in Hartford and perhaps that he met Horace Wells. He definitely was familiar with the experience of the latter, who was teaching in Hartford as early as 1838.

Another member of the Crane family, Samuel LeGrande Crane (1830-1912), and who was practising dentistry in Hartford, might have been John W. Crane Juniors brother, but unfortunately this could not be officially confirmed. The obituary[20] of Samuel LeGrande Crane indicates that he was one of the first dental practitioners to use nitrous oxide as an anaesthetic during dental operations.

Therefore, it is not astonishing that John W. Crane Jr., who practiced dentistry in Paris since 1858, was interested in the technique of giving nitrous oxide gas. His address, 41 Boulevard des Capucines, Paris, can be found on the list of the participants of the FDI Congress in1900. His father was in a position to supply him with the latest news from New York, and it is not surprising that Crane had equipped his office with a gazometer as early as 1864. John W. Crane Jr. not having published any articles, it is quite difficult for the historians to find his name in literature. However, the father of orthodontics, Norman W. Kingsley[21] (1829-1913) stated that John W. Crane Jr. had rendered him most valuable aid as he had visited the asylums and hospitals in Paris in order to examine the teeth of three to four hundred handicapped people. His brother, Charles Kingsley (1819-1874), had been associated with Crane for many years[22]. As Thomas Evans (1823-1897) created the American Dental Club of Paris, on October 13th, 1890, John Crane was one of the founding members. On November 21st, 1908, the same Association gave a banquet in memoriam of Cranes fiftieth anniversary of practice in Paris. At that time he was 72 years old. He also was a honorary member of the W. D. Miller Club of Berlin.

Apolloni Pierre Préterre and nitrous oxide anaesthesia.

Dental historians know Apolloni (also named Apollonie or Apoléonie) Pierre Préterre because he was the first person in France in 1857, along with his operator Fowler, to put the journal l'Art Dentaire into print. Apolloni Préterre had three brothers living in the United States. Eugène (1817-?) and Peter A. (1812-1870) were dental surgeons too. Eugène Préterre established a dental office in the Bowery in New York as early as 1838. Peter A. Préterre, M.D., D.D.S., practiced dentistry since 1847; he graduated from Pennsylvania College of Dental Surgery in 1865 and then worked in New Orleans. Adolphe P. Préterre (1824-1886) was a medical doctor, who had graduated from New York College of Physicians and Surgeons, class of 1849. Adolphe then studied in Paris for three years, but in 1852, he returned to New York and built up a partnership with his brother Eugène.

Apolloni Pierre Préterre was a scientist keeping an eye on every new invention. In 1864, his brother Adolphe carried out experiments on birds, keeping them under the influence of nitrous oxide. L. Figuier wrote in the journal La Presse, Année Scientifique et merveille des Sciences that in 1864, *several American physicians and in particular Adolph P. Préterre from New-York, and brother of Préterre from Paris, have again conducted experiments with nitrous oxide gas.* Apolloni Préterre confirmed this statement himself[23]. Adolphe was convinced that nitrous oxide was a helpful agent and that the gas would be adopted very quickly in France for surgical operations.

Did his brother, Apolloni Pierre Préterre, adopt this technique by the end of December 1865? I think so. The memory[24] and the letter, presented in the name of Préterre, and read by Philippe Ricord[25] (1799-1889) at the meeting of the Academy of Medicine on May 29th, 1866, testifies this. Préterre recalled back in different books printed in 1866[26], or later[27], that *till these last years, nobody knew in France another method, than ether or chloroform anaesthesia to suppress pain during the extraction of teeth; but the lethal cases under the influence of these substances, even in the most skillful hands, had striken the public with horor. A new anaesthetic had to be developed. We have found in nitrous oxide gas, that we have introduced in Europe, where he was absolutely unknown as an anaesthetic before we had carried out our experiments,* and Préterre added: *We had barely made presented our experience to the Academy of Sciences and to the Academy of Medicine when the majority of the physicians and surgeons of the hospitals invited us to repeat them in front for them.*

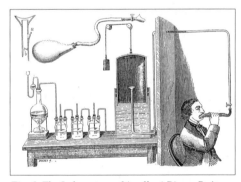

Fig. 1 The Laboratory of Apolloni Pierre Préterre A. P. Préterre: Nouvelles recherches sur le protoxyde d'azote, Paris, 1866; 10.

Several members of the Academy visited the laboratory of Préterre (Fig. 1), where the purified gas was produced by means of a tinware bell gazometer of about 400 liters, a lead, or a rubber tube, connected to the gazometer, allowed to reach the operating room. The patient inhaled the gas directly via a mouthpiece made of silver. If it was necessary to perform an extraction of a tooth at the patients home, a rubber gas bag was filled with the gas. Préterre held some filled gas bags at the disposal for colleagues who wished to utilize the properties of nitrous oxide.

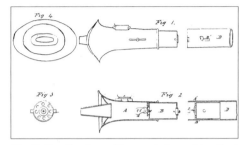

Fig. 2 Details of metallic mouthpiece of Apolloni Pierre Préterre, Drawing of his Patent N°72100

Préterres method was successful. He published a list of physicians who had watched him perform surgery, as well as the list of the operations carried in the Parisian hospitals. He was as enthusiastic as to study the technique thoroughly and take a patent, N°72100[28], on June 26th, 1866 (Fig. 2), at the same time on a new metallic mouthpiece and on a gas regulator or califactor. Like in Spragues device, Préterre located his regulator on the second or on the third washing bottle. The regulator (Fig. 3) was used to slow down or

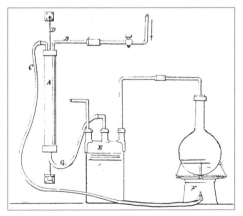

Fig. 3 The gas regulator of Apolloni Pierre Préterre, Drawing of his Patent N°72100

to speed up the admission of the lighting gas, the latter supplying the gas lamp used to regulate the release of nitrous oxide.

The mouthpiece was composed of three parts:
- the admission tap
- the inspiratory valve, whose aperture could be regulated with a key,
- the expiration valve for the exhalation of carbon dioxide gas.

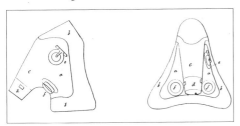

Fig. 4 Details of the Mask of Apolloni Pierre Préterre, Drawing of his Patent N°72100

On December, 3rd, 1866, an addition was made to the initial patent. The metallic mouthpiece seemed to be too stiff, and needed the help of an assistant to keep the patients lips tightly closed around the inhalation tube in many cases. Préterre constructed a mask (Fig. 4) to be adapted to different types of faces. These masks which covered mouth and nose, were composed of a main hard rubber compound, with soft rubber edges. The soft rubber was thinner than the hard part, and allowed a tight fit to the patients face. Inside the mask there were two wedge-shaped protrusions, which could be inserted between the patients teeth, to keep the jaws apart. Two valves, were usually kept closed and allowed the exhalation of the carbon dioxide, whereas the mobile valve was used for inhalation. The onset of anaesthesia occured after 30 to 40 seconds. Préterre used nitrous oxide everyday, performing dental extractions, extraction of ingroving toenails, or minor surgical acts, that did not require prolonged anaesthesia. He did not experience about unwanted side-effects. W.A.N. Cattlin[29] of Brighton supported Préterre's opinion: nitrous oxide gas was less dangerous than chloroform, but its use should be restricted to minor surgical interventions. Nitrous oxide anaesthesia was particularly valuable in dental surgery, because at that time, the only method at the dentists disposal for diminishing pain was to perform a local anaesthesia by congelation, i.e.[30] applying a small bag of fine salt and ice in front of the offended tooth, followed by another freezing mixture until its white appearance, showed a congealed condition.

The technique of Préterre was that successful that he raised many covetous glances. He said[31] that it was true for all innovations, he *saw running behind him, the thick peat of this imitators who try to take advantage of others researches, making every effort to depreciate them.* The scientific yearbook of Figuier and Henri Berthoud had already published the results of Préterre's experiments, and moreover on May 15th, 1867, Martin Lauzer[32] (1812-1897) had given an accurate description of two surgical operations performed by Préterre.

The Parmly family (Fig. 5).

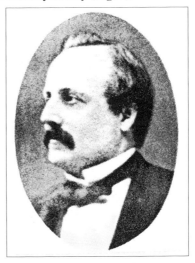

Georges Washington Parmly (1819-1892)

The Parmly family was the largest family in the United States being involved in dentistry[33]. John Parmelee and his son John settled in Guilford, Connecticut from England in 1639 and 1635, respectively. Thirteen dentists from the Parmly family out of them eleven have been very successful practitioners.

Francs; 600 liters of gas could be produced at a prize of about three francs, the nitrate of ammonia, which was the most expensive ingredient, was half a Franc per pound. Regarding the economic aspect, said Marion Sims, it was really cheaper than the best Scotch chloroform.

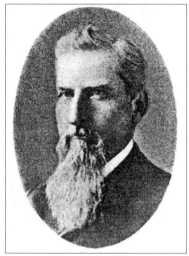

Henry Clay Parmly, (1835-1895)

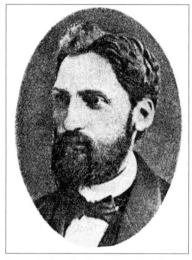

Samuel Pleasant Parmly, (1838-?)

The international prestige that the Parmly family achieved is unique in the history of dentistry. If we look at them as dentists, we are mainly talking about three persons: Georges Washington Parmly (1819-1892), who was the dentist of Alexander of Holland in 1848, Henry Clay Parmly (1835-1895), his cousin - both of them moved from Den Haag to Paris in 1863 - and Samuel Pleasant Parmly (1838-?), brother of Henry C., who lived in the United States, and who joined Georges and Henry in Paris in the same year. They built an association and opened an office on, 35, Boulevard des Capucines, Paris. Being in a similar position in Europe as Thomas Evans, they took care of famous American patients in Paris and European elite, thus it is not surprising that the Parmlys were equipped with a gazometer. According to John Crane, in those days, the costs of a complete apparatus, containing 700 liters of gas, came to 200

In 1868, Samuel Pleasant Parmly returned to the United States; Georges and Henry kept association going until 1869, when they sold the office to their cousin Levi Spear Burridge. In 1869 Georges got settled in London.
10

Jean Baptiste Rottenstein and Lond.

J. B. Rottenstein was a member of the Academy of Leopoldina Carolina and of the Odontological Society of New York. He published a treatise on galvanism in 1858 and on surgical anaesthesia in 1880[34]. There is no reference concerning Dr. Lond.

Nitrous oxide anaesthesia:
a new impetus after the Worldfair
in the year 1867.

As G. Q. Colton came to Paris at the time of the Worldfair in 1867, the method of using nitrous oxide inhalations had already been adopted broadly in France. Thomas Evans (1823-1897), a friend of Colton and his guide on this occasion, helped him to get in contact with some wealthy families in Paris. Colton had already started taking advantage of the Parisian events to give anaesthetics to British and American patients. Marion Sims[35] certifies that on December 22nd, 1867, while performing a mastectomy on a patient - Mrs. P. from St. Louis Missouri - Colton and Evans administered the nitrous oxide gas. The operation and dressing, which took sixteen minutes, was carried out with the assistance of well-known people, e.g. Baron Félix Hippolyte Larrey (1808-1895), Sir Joseph Francis Oliffe (1809-1869), Professor Charles P. Pope (1818-1870) from St. Louis, Dr. Johnston and many others. On the 28th of the same month, Colton and Evans gave the gas to Miss X. of Dublin, who had been struck down by an abdominal tumor, requiring a more extensive examination to determine, though the tumor was fibroid or cystic. She was kept under nitrous oxide anaesthesia for eight minutes and recovered promptly, even if she suffered from an organic valvular disease. In the same paper Marion Sims reports on a very interesting operation, the young American dentist John Crane administering the gas. It was performed on April, 2nd, 1868, on a woman, from Italy, where Crane kept the patient constantly under the influence of the gas for twenty minutes. Marion Sims added that he *presumes that this is the longest period of time that any one has as yet been kept under its influence*. The operation was conducted in the presence of Sir Joseph Oliffe, Dr. Dyce Duckworth from London, Dr. Schost (late of the U.S. Army), Dr. Thierry-Mieg, and Dr. Pratt.

An paper with the instructions on the application of nitrous oxide was read in front of the members of the Liverpool chemists association by the dentist, Dr. W. H. Waite[36], on November 21st, 1867. At the end of the lecture, some experiments on the anaesthetic properties of nitrous oxide were carried through. Four months later, on, March 31st, 1868, Thomas Evans performed a series of demonstrations on the use of nitrous oxide according to Colton`s method at the Dental Hospital of London, Soho Square and at the Central London Ophthalmic Hospital[37]. Most of the well-known representatives of the London dental profession, e. g. Arthur S. Underwood, Hepburn, Alfred Coleman, and other officers agreed that this anaesthetic agent undoubtedly possessed very remarkable and valuable properties. Even being very enthusiastic they concluded that this agent had to be utilized very carefully until they had obtained more experience of their own. Twelve or fifteen extractions of teeth were performed within a very short time[38], having to be afraid of hidden dangers, a lot of anxiety reigned among English physicians.

The report printed in the British Medical Journal on April 4th, 1868, p. 337, reveals that the gas administered by Evans was *prepared from ordinary coal-gas, by a process and apparatus which Colton has invented, and which Dr. Evans has modified...It (the gas) is stored in a small gazometer, and drawn off into bags. The bags are furnished with tubes, to which a tube-mouthpiece with inspiratory and expiratory valve is attached. The tube is placed between the lips, the teeth being kept apart, for the purpose of subsequent operation, by a small piece of wood, and the lips are pressed around the tube with the fingers of the operator tightly, and the nostrils are compressed.*

If that description is compared to Préterres device and mouthpiece, the modifications by Evans extremely resemble the description given by Préterre. According to Préterre`s first patent, the patient put a flattened tube between his teeth, the end of the mouthpiece being of an ovoid shape. The stiffness of the mouthpiece couldnt easily be adapted to the various forms of the jaws, and its application needed the help of an assistant, who pressed the lips of the patient to the tube. The disadvantages of this metallic mouthpiece led Préterre to develop a mask covering mouth and nose, with a protrusion inside to keep the jaws apart. Evans also used a tube inserted between the lips, and placed a small piece of wood between the teeth. Joseph T. Clover[39] (1825-1882) had noticed that the assistant of Dr. Evans emphasized that the tube did neither bend nor collapse, and was rather surprised it had not come to his mind to make use of a coil or spiral wire inside. It seems very fascitinating that Evans never saw Préterres mouthpiece or masks. Did Thomas Evans copy the latters technique? Why did he never speak of Préterres experiences? Why did'nt he publish the modifications of the device or the changing of the process?

Conclusion

An interesting statement was written by John B. Rich[40] (1811-1910), who was one of the youngest to build the first Dental College in Baltimore, and who died at the age of the one hundreds years.

We sent American dentists all over the world. Brewster was the first.

I was at Maynards in Washington when Evans came in to use his influence to get an appointment as Bearer of Despatches in Paris. Evans went to Brewster in Paris, - who was a rough operator, and filled fifty teeth in one day. Evans wife liked Paris and she convinced him that they could make more money there than in their home town Lancaster, Pa. He asked Brewster about practicing in Paris, and Brewster offered him a partnership. Evans agreed and after having negociated everything then and there on with his wife, finally bought Brewster out for $ 100,000.

Mrs. Evans was a very beautiful and diplomatic woman, and had managed to become acquainted with Prince Louis Napoleon when he was banished to in London. After returning to Paris as member of the Assembly he built his home together with the Evans family. He never forgot his friends, and the intimacy was always kept up. Evans allowed the Prince to use his bank account. Mrs. Evans introduced him to Princess Eugenie, and Dr. and Mrs. Evans were always entertained en famille at the royal palace.

Evans was a sycophant and a man worshipper. He would do anything to curry favor with somebody.

This is an unknown aspect of the eminent personality that Thomas Evans was, the dark side of a man who was 24 years old when he joined to Edward Maynard`s (1813-1891) office!

References:

[1] Wells H: Letter of Horace Wells. Lancet 1847; 266

[2] White SS: History of Dental & Oral Science in America. Philadelphia 1876; 78-82

[3] Watson J: Transactions of the American Medical Association 1848; I: 218

[4] Ellsworth PW: Nitrous oxide gas in operative surgery. Dental Cosmos 1866; VII: 444, referred to Trumann Smith. Also in: Dental Register of the West 1866; XX: 85

[5] Carnochan JM: Nitrous oxide gas in capital operations. Dental Cosmos 1866; VII: 444-445. Also in: Dental Register of the West 1866; XX: 86-88

[6] Ira M Jr: Is nitrous oxide anaesthetic? Boston Medical & Surgical Journal 1852; 435-436

[7] Bigelow HJ: Anaesthetic agents, their mode of exhibition & physiological effects. Transactions of the American Medical Association 1848; 196-214

[8] Bigelow HJ: Nitrous oxide gas for surgical purposes in 1848. Boston Medical & Surgical Journal 1868; I: 17-18

[9] Colton GQ: Nitrous oxide gaz an anaesthetic. Dental Cosmos 1864; V: 490-493

[10] Westcott A: Laughing gas. Dental Register of the West 1864; XVIII: 40-48

[11] Ring M: Dentistry - An Illustrated History. Harry N. Abrams, Mosby-Year Book. New York 1992; 231

[12] Latimer JS: Nitrous oxide in dentistry. Dental Cosmos 1863; V: 16-17

[13] The protoxide of nitrogen as an anaesthetic. Br Med J 1868; I: 508

[14] Rottenstein JB: Traité d'Anesthésie Chirurgicale. Paris 1880

[15] Sprague AW: Nitrous oxide as an anaesthetic and therapeutic. Boston Medical & Surgical Journal 1866; LXXIV: 313-315

[16] Cooper HR: The nitrous oxide gas as an anaesthetic in dental operation. Dental Cosmos 1864; V: 693-695

[17] Sims MJ: On the nitrous oxide gas as an anaesthetic. Br Med J 1868; I: 349-350

[18] Truemann WH: The history of dental journalism in the United States. Dental Cosmos 1920; LXII: 65-73

[19] Parmly BL: New light on dental history. Dental Cosmos 1920; LXII: 936-958

[20] Crane S: Obituary. Dental Cosmos 1912; LIV: 390

[21] Kingsley NW: Causes of irregularity in the development of the teeth. Dental Cosmos 1875; XVII: 168-195

[22] Four JR: Franco-American professional interrelationship in dentistry. I.C.D., Sc. Ed. Bull. 1973 VI: 2,1973

[23] Préterre AP: Propriétés physiologiques du protoxyde d'ázote appliqué aux opérations chirurgicales. Bulletin général de thérapeutique médicale & chirurgicale 1870: 160-164; 215-218

[24] Préterre AP: Nouvelles Recherches sur les Propriétés Physiologiques et Anesthésiques du Protoxyde d'Azote. Paris 1866

[25] Ricord Ph: Bulletin de l'Académie Impériale de Médecine 1865-66, Meeting 29th May 1866: 749-753, and 1866-67: 322-324

[26] Préterre AP: De l'Emploi du Protoxyde d'Azote pour Pratiquer les Opérations Chirurgicales. Paris 1866

[27] Préterre AP: Les dents, Traité pratique des Maladies de ces Organes. Paris 1889

[28] Zimmer M: Des premiers Brevets d'Invention.... Pour une Histoire du Développement de l'Anesthésie. D.E.A., E.P.H.E. Paris 1995

[29] Cattlin WAN: Nitrous oxide as an anaesthetic. Medical Times & Gazette 1868; 78

[30] Zimmer M: Therapeutic concepts of endodontic treatment in the 19th century. International Dental Journal, 1997; 47: 340-348

[31] Préterre AP: Recherches sur les Propriétés Physiques et Physiologiques du Protoxyde dAzote Liqufié. Paris 1869. Also in: L'art dentaire 1869; 42-54

[32] Martin L: Du protoxyde dazote comme agent anesthésique. Journal des connaissances médico-chirurgicales 1867; 262-264

[33] Braun PL: The greatest dental family. Dental Cosmos 1923; LXV: 251-260; 363-491

[34] Rottenstein JB:op. cit.

[35] Sims Marion J., op. cit., 349

[36] Nitrous oxide. Liverpool Royal Institution. Dental Register 1867; XXI: 527

[37] A new anaesthetic: Br Med J 1868; I: 332

[38] Anaesthesia in dentistry by protoxide of nitrogen. Br Med J 1868; I: 337-338

[39] Discussion at the Odontological Society. Br Med J 1868; I: 359-360

[40] Rich JB: Statement of Dr. John B. Rich. Dental Cosmos 1920; LXII: 958

How the French were Informed and Implemented Surgical Anaesthesia in 1846.

M. Th. Cousin, Paris, France

Information about Morton's discovery that ether would permit painless surgery came into France at least four times. Paradoxally however, only one information was followed by a trial, which besides failed.

The first event which is reported[1] is the sending of a package containing ether and a "double tubular flask" with directions for use, from W. T. G. Morton to "a young American doctor" living in Paris. This American doctor, "Morton's friend", was in Saint Louis Hospital, on december 15th 1846, the day when Doctor Antoine Jobert (de Lamballe) had to operate on a patient with an inferior lip cancerous lesion. The event was revealed by Jobert more than one month later on january 23th 1847 issue of the "Gazette des Hôpitaux civils et militaires"[1], and on february 2th 1847 at the Académie de Médecine: "I am, I think, the first surgeon in Paris who tried out ether..."[2].

The second event is reported by the surgeon Alfred Velpeau at the Académie de Médecine (on january 12th) and also at the Académie des Sciences (on january 18th). "In the middle of december", he received "Doctor Willis Fisher from Boston"[3], "a dentist"[4] who offered to try an analgesic method, the means of which was being kept secret. Velpeau refuses to use a method whose means is unknown to himself. Some days later, the secret is disclosed in a letter from "Doctor Warren from Boston"[3], his first name and details about the letter content Velpeau does not give. Again, Velpeau is reluctant, he claims he does not know how much ether may be dangerous to physiologic functions. We do not get Warren's letter content but we can suppose it is not very different from John Ware 's letter with John Collins Warren's post-sriptum, sent to Dr Forbes, editor of the English and Foreign Medical Review, and translated on january 12th in a French Gazette: "In six cases, I used this means to prevent pain in surgical procedures, with full success, and without bad consequences", signed: John C. Warren[5].

The third information comes from the chemist Charles Thomas Jackson. When he understands the Morton's trials are successful, he claims for the fatherhood of the discovery and turns towards Paris as arbitrator and especially towards the Academician Elie de Beaumont whose student he was as he learnt in Paris[6]. His first letter, dated the november 13th 1846, describes the interventions in Massachusett's General Hospital, indications, methods, results, observations, potential hazards. It is followed by a second short letter, dated the december 1st, where other anaesthesias are reported, all of them successful.

These two letters are sent together. We know that mail service came two times a month from Boston to Liverpool and from there to Le Havre, by Cunard Line (one time only in winter) and the letters were probably in the same steamer as Morton's package to Willy Fisher. Arriving to Paris the letters are deposited in Académie des Sciences by Elie de Beaumont on december 28th[3] and are kept as unsealed packages (as it was the use to take priority for an uncertain discovery). They are read only on january 18th, one week after the first Malgaigne's reports and when a number of trials have already been made in Paris. So Jackson had little influence in the development of anaesthesia in France. But the academicians had no doubt on the eminent part of Jackson in the discovery of anaesthesia, to such an extent that the Consul de France in Boston, wrote in september 1847 a letter which was read at the Academy to reestablish the actual facts[7].

To end with the news which came from America, we have to recall that Horace Wells when he was probably in Paris[8], sent letters to the Académie des Sciences[9] and to the Académie de Médecine[10] respectively to explain his part in the discovery of anaesthesia not only with nitrous oxide but also with ether, which he considered as less convenient than- and gave up for- nitrous oxide.

During may 1847, William Thomas Green Morton, in the aim to counter Jackson's claims, wrote in his turn to the Académie des Sciences[11] and in november sent his review on this question to the Académie de Médecine[12]. The two papers were recorded but nor read neither discussed. As we have just written[5] information came also by medical journals, the first to be found on jan 12th was in "Gazette des Hôpitaux civils et militaires". So informations towards French people did not miss.

I - The first trial takes place then on december 15th 1846 in St Louis Hospital and is due to Antoine Jobert (de Lamballe)[1]:

"M Jobert, on the point of making the operation, gives the patient into the American doctor's care, in order to give insensivity against pain. (The American doctor is surely the Bostonian Willy Fisher who visited Velpeau). *His way of work was so: He brought a glass globe with two tubes and a bottle containing ether. Sponge pieces were entered and the liquor of the bottle was poured into the globe. Immediately the ether caracteristic smell of ether escaped off. (...) We have said the globe had two tubes. The first was left free, in order to let air come into the globe. The second was introduced into the patient's mouth. The nostrils were left open... The patient was then recommanded to inhale strongly in order to bring air with ether vapours into the mouth, and from there into the respiratory airway. In this manner inspiration and expiration were somewhat easy, but it is conceivable that a part of unsaturated air came into the nose during inspiration and during expiration a part of expired air came into the globe and was mixed with ether vapours. The ether effects were delayed by these facts. But let us return to our patient: we can say that at the end of 18 minutes clear symptoms were not obtained. The experimentator missed of necessary materials to achieve his aim, M Jobert started his operation".*

It is to be noted
- the patient had an inferior lip lesion and so the assembling might be somewhat leaking
- Fisher's apparatus cannot be exactly similar to Morton's apparatus which had valves
- It is said that the experimentator lacked the necessary materials (manquait des objets nécessaires), probably he had an insufficient amount of ether.
- The experimentator had probably insufficient or no experience. Perhaps however, did he pull out some teeth under ether, as he said to Velpeau "he had the secret to painlessly pull out teeth"[4].

In conclusion this first anaesthesia did not work ...

II- The second trial, done in this same hospital Saint Louis, some weeks later, is due to Jean- François Malgaigne. In a later paper, Malgaigne explicitly refers to Jobert's patient`s etherization[13] (although he erroneously claims Morton himself administered ether).

On january 12th 1847 at Académie de Médecine[4], he reports his first five consecutive trials. No dating is to be found. He says his trials were started after the English and American publications had been translated in Union Médicale. (As the first surgical etherization in London by Liston on december 21st is published in the first *Lancet* issue of 1847, and no communication about ether is to be found in the *Union Médicale* before january 13th, the date of his first trial remains uncertain but surely some days only before january 12th. and perhaps even as it was the custom in these times the day itself of the communication.)

He says: *"Having no such apparatus (Morton's or Robinson's apparatus) at my disposal, I used a simple tube in which I put some amount of ether and which I introduced into one nostril, the other nostril being closed. I took care to recommend inspiration with the mouth closed and expiration with the mouth opened"*. How was exactly this assembling and how was it possible to inhale according to this rule when the patient was already fallen semi-asleep, it is the question. Malgaigne answers: *"After a short time the patients understood this little manoeuvre very well"*. In fact in his other papers[13,14] he admits the patients are not always *suited, docile or clever* to rule out their respiration.

On his five trials, he gets three full successes, one failure and an incomplete success. These observations make a great rumour, among the medical world and also among the general public. But the surgeons who attempt to repeat Malgaigne's example do not achieve any anesthesia. The assembling is probably in the cause. The other descriptions of Malgaigne's materials are not clearer than the first: *"A glass bottle with a tube on a point of its circumference and at the junction of the two inferior thirds and the superior third of its height contains several little pieces of sponge on which a certain amount of ether is poured (...). The tube must be left over the liquid level in order to let a free entrance for outer air..."*. No design is given and his *three new facts* are not very convincing. It is in these times that Jobert reports his first trial.

The constant and definitive successes occur when the Charrière's apparatus are used[15,16]. The first apparatus is made with a tube for air going down to the bottom of the bottle[15]. A second tube for ether vapours starts over the level of the sponge pieces and ends in with a mouth piece. It contains two valves for inspiration and expiration. Another apparatus is made up of metal clothes like Davis lamp to protect against fire[16].

Many successful etherizations are reported at the Académie des Sciences and the Académie de Médecine from january 25th 1847 and come from the whole country. Velpeau is from now on converted to ether administration and becomes its unfailing supporter. Jobert also from this moment does not know anymore failure.

Enthusiasmus henceforth becomes general and there is the actual beginning of the surgical anaesthesia in France.

References:

1. Gogué G: Aspiration de la vapeur d'éther. Gazette des Hôpitaux civils et militaires 1847; 9: 39-40

2. Anonyme: Compte-Rendu de l'Académie de Médecine, séance du 2 février 1847. Gazette des Hôpitaux Civils et Militaires 1847; 9: 58

3. Velpeau A: Remarques à l'occasion des précedentes communications (sur l'éther sulfurique). Séance du 18 janvier 1847, Compte-Rendu de l'Académie des Sciences 1847; 24: 76-78

4. Malgaigne JF:Emploi de l'éther. Suivi de discussion sur la communication de Malgaigne. Séance du 12 janvier 1847. Bulletin de l'Académie Royale de Médecine 1847; 12: 262-264

5. Anonyme: Gazette des Hôpitaux civils et militaires 1847; 9:19

6. Zimmer M: Des premiers brevets d'invention. Pour une histoire du développement de l'anesthésie. Mémoire de DEA, Ecole Pratique des Hautes Etudes à la Sorbonne. Paris 1995, p 22-29

7. Bulletin de l' Académie Royale de Médecine 1847;13: 7-8

8. Duncum B M: The Development of Inhalation Anaesthesia. RSM, London, 1947, p 121

9. Wells H: Extraits d'une lettre de H. Wells, chirurgien dentiste à Hartford (Connecticut). Compte-Rendus de l'Académie des Sciences 1847; 24: 373-374

10. Wells H: Effets de l'éther sulfurique. Bulletin de l'Académie de Médecine 1847; 12: 393-395

11. Correspondance: Séance du 17 mai 1847. Compte-Rendus de l'Académie des Sciences 1847; 24: 378

12. Morton W T G: Mémoire sur la découverte du nouvel emploi de l'éther sulfurique. Bulletin de l'Académie Royale de Médecine 1847; 13: 351

13. Malgaigne J F: Sur un nouveau moyen de supprimer la douleur dans les opérations chirurgicales; découvert par M. Morton de Boston. Revue Médico-Chirurgicale 1847; 1: 12-18

14. Malgaigne JF: De l'emploi des vapeurs d'éther sulfurique. Trois nouveaux faits. Gazette des Hôpitaux Civils et Militaires 1847; 9: 29 (n° du 19 janvier 1847)

15. Anonymous: Questions de l'influence de l'éther. Union Médicale 1847; 1:40

16. Anonymous: Inspirations éthérées. Nouvel appareil. Etat de la question. Gazette des Hôpitaux Civils et Militaires 1847; 9: 53

Rudolf Frey's Unfinished Legacy: History without Future

J. Rupreht, University of Ljubljana, Slovenia;
W. Erdmann, Erasmus University Rotterdam, The Netherlands

The 7th World Congress of Anaesthesiologists (WCA) at Hamburg, September 14-21, 1980, was a convenient opportunity for Prof. Rudolf Frey of Mainz (1917-1981) to gather, for a Panel, pioneers of anaesthesia from many different countries. In introduction to the booklet of Abstracts[1] he wrote: "The 7th World Congress... is an unique and perhaps last chance to bring together the pioneers of anaesthesiology". The Panel was called "Anaesthesia: Past and Future". The aim was "preparation of a booklet, provided to be edited 1981, in connection with a list of pioneers". The eight lines long sentence is rather confusing on other aims of the proposed book. A short draft of the book was promised for distribution at the WCA, but could not be traced as of 1997. Only eleven speakers were allowed 5 minutes to hold their address. The whole Panel lasted 90 minutes. Other participants were asked to have their papers read by title.

The Abstract booklet[1] of the Panel is a 57 pages long, rather attractive mess, full of shortcomings and does not leave an impression of a reliable document. On the page 4 a long list of abstracts starts at the pioneer whose name starts with letter B. First seven authors are chaotically described, addresses are incomplete and "No abstract available". In fact, majority of mentioned emeriti or pioneers provided no abstract. On the page 54 "List of Authors" mentions everyone either with an abstract or not but also some people not mentioned earlier. There are 68 names altogether on the list. All of them must have been personal friends to Prof. Frey because a multitude of pioneers from both Americas, Africa, Asia and Australia does not play a role in the show. Moreover, in some cases, mentioned persons can by no standard be regarded as either an "emeritus" or a "pioneer" when one scans their backgrounds.

Nevertheless, in the Panel booklet, Frey did invite participants to provide their curriculum vitae, list of publications, last position and address. These materials were supposed to be published by 1981.

The response to Frey's invitation must have not been all too successful which can be suspected from Frey's letter of 21 January 1981, mentioning that the Panel booklet did not represent the complete set of the "firsts". The most important part of the letter reads:

"Now we are preparing an illustrated treatise for 1981 entitled "Anaesthesia, Past and Future: with detailed careers of the initiator-developers of world anaesthesiology and a list of their most important writings, along with a statement about the pioneers' special interests and their ideas on the historical and present-day development of Anaesthesiology, resuscitation and intensive care.

You are kindly invited, to submit to my address your picture, an one page single spaced synopsis curriculum vitae and your statement on ca. 1-2 pages in typescript for this above mentioned publication at the latest by <u>1st April, 1981.</u>

Should you yourself also want to nominate another pioneer not already entered on the list, I would be grateful if you could send me the name and address, so that he can still be invited".

In the volume of "Korresppondenz, Anaesthesia: Past and Future"[2] one finds this letter, also with the deadline 1st March, 1981 and 1st July, 1981. The letter with the July deadline is dated 1st May, 1981. These repeat mailings appeared necessary when suggestions for yet more pioneers came in. It is rather embarrassing to find out how anaesthesiologists, then "in picture" failed to provide Frey with correct information about anaesthesia pioneers in their countries. Willy Dam of Copenhagen suggested that Dr. Trier Morch be included as a Danish pioneer (letter Copenhagen, March, 1981) and Dr. T. Tammisto wrote about several other Finish pioneers before him (letter of 26 March, 1981). The Canadian Dr. R.A. Gordon was surprised to find a certain name on Frey's list of pioneers, because "X" was "relatively junior, and is, in fact, almost entirely unknown in academic anaesthesia in Canada" (letter of February 2, 1981); ("X" by these authors).

Springer Publishers:
A good idea, but ...

By March 1981 a sufficient number of solicited manuscripts must have become available and the Publishers (Springer-Verlag) were approached. In a letter of 5 March 1981, Dr. J. Wieczorek, Springer-Verlag, wrote Prof. Frey that the topic was desirable. However, the Springer wished careful selection of the pioneers for the book similar to American "Who is Who in Anaesthesiology". Furthermore, quite some work was needed to make manuscripts publishable. The Publishers wondered whether a completely revised plan for the book was needed. Also, they asked directly, who else would assist Frey in making a book. Such a time consuming project was more than what Frey himself could manage, they stated bluntly. Altogether, Springer could not make the proposed book "Anaesthesia: Past and Future", as of May 1981.

On 15 March 1981, Frey sent a letter to Prof. T.C. Gray of Liverpool requesting editorial assistance and advice. "Did we forget some V.I.P.?" was another question. The book was not to be expensive but had to be "rather comprehensive". There is a letter from Prof. T.C. Gray of 21st March 1981 mentioning the draft of the title page and minor corrections on this item. On this letter, Prof. Gray kindly refused to be co-editor and offered only "co-operation of R. Janik and myself".

Materials for the Book on the Move

The whole pile of manuscripts for the book must have been sent to Liverpool shortly after March 1981, in original and not as a copy mentioned in Frey's letter to Gray (5 and 15 March 1981)[2]. Then it is quiet for a while, as far as written evidence is available. In the meanwhile, from June 1981, an intense activity towards the First International Symposium on the History of Modern Anaesthesia started from Rotterdam. Through Dr. Howatt, and directly, Prof. Gray was approached to speak about the history of The British Journal of Anaesthesia. He himself added the topic "A Tale of Two Cities"[3]. In his letter of 27th July 1981 he confirmed his participation for the May 5-8, 1982 event in Rotterdam. The second paragraph of his letter[4] reads:

"I do not think that I could possibly take any more editing work at this stage. I am afraid that I have had to tell Rudolph that I just cannot manage much help with his venture. How will your symposium tie in with his project? His collection of manuscripts is so mixed I really do not know what can be done with it. What a pity you are so far away as it would be very useful to be able to meet and have a chat".

The adressee, Dr. Rupreht of Rotterdam knew nothing of Frey's project at that time which did not make it easy to interpret Prof.

Gray's letter. Some light was thrown onto the subject by Frey's letter of 23 September, 1981, to Dr. Rupreht, in which he promised to attend the 1982-Symposium at Rotterdam[5]. Wishing to involve Professor Erdmann of Rotterdam and Dr. Rupreht to co-operate on the book "Anaesthesia: Past and Future", he mentioned also that the materials were in Liverpool with Gray for editorial work. Frey's plan was to visit Rotterdam between 17 and 22 December 1981.

In a letter of 16 December 1981 to Professor Erdmann[6] Frey asked the Rotterdam team to take over the editorial work. Dr. Rupreht could join the editorial team "according to his participation". Frey's wish became to combine his materials with those of the 1982-Rotterdam Symposium. However, he would not be in Rotterdam around Christmas 1981, but in Egypt.

Months later, following the Frey's death on 23rd December 1981, Gray wrote to Erdmann on 1st March 1982: *"I found on my desk on my return a letter from him asking him to send to you a whole pile of manuscripts which I think he sent to me in error. Whether they will be very helpful from the point of view of the new Congress is doubtful"*. In the P.S. of the same letter "I will send the manuscripts to you under separate cover as soon as I can. /TCG". On March 29th 1982 (erroneously typed 1981) Gray wrote to Dr. Rupreht accompanying letter for the two summaries and the registration form for the May Anaesthesia History Meeting[7]. He mentioned "I shall bring all the MSS with me appertaining to the Hamburg meeting".

What is all the MSS appertaining to Hamburg?

Four large volumes of manuscripts along with a catalogue of names and addresses of contributors for the planned "Anaesthesia: Past and Future" reached Rotterdam in early May 1982. The same year they were read, re-catalogized and judged unsuitable for making a book. Most contributors provided a photograph, curriculum vitae, list of publications and one or two pages of their view on the history and future of anaesthesia. Academically conscious and scientifically bred anaesthesiologist is often surprised at Frey's selection of pioneers or nestors. There is a general tendency of lesser known contributors to provide more pages of materials - much of which can often not be scientifically verified.

Sixty-eight names appeared in The Hamburg Panel booklet. The "MSS" contains records of 85 authors, albeit some incomplete. There are 7 separate letters (Table I).

Frey's planned book 15 Years on.

Apparently, authors contributed manuscripts for „Anaesthesia: Past and Future" without any second thought. very seldomly there is a remark on inability to look into the future. Concerning the past there is much repetition of standard historical information or anaesthesia lore.

Nevertheless, the biographical data may be of interest in some instances. Certainly, photographs are valuable although there is a surprising number of younger faces among the pioneers and nestors.

Of much greater interest is the psychology of the contributions, especially when set against the background of real circumstance. Not only are many contributors not historically verifiable pioneers of anaesthesia in their countries, very often they even lack insight into the local past of anaesthesia and into the history of anaesthesia in general.

The more remote we get from 1980 the more difficult it will be to make something useful of Frey's materials for "Anaesthesia: Past and Future". One might show, with the luxury of retrospect 17 years later on, that it is not possible to predict future experience.

103

Nr.	Name	Residence	Photo + or -	CV + or -	List of Publ. + or -	Pages + or -
1.	E.M. Papper	Miami, Fl.	+	-	-	4
2.	C. Parsloe	Brasil	+	+	-	12
3.	J.W. Pender	California	+	+	-	5
4.	J. Pokorny	CSSR	+	-	-	12
5.	A.M. Radwan	Cairo	+	+	+	16
6.	R. Rizzi	Italy	+	-	-	4
7.	F.W. Roberts	England	+	+	+	3
8.	J.S. Robinson	Birmingham	+	+	+	7
9.	H. Ruben	Copenhagen	+	+	+	15
10.	M. Sabathie	Bordeaux	+	+	+	4
11.	S.K. Saev	Bulgaria	+	+	+	5
12.	P. Safar	Pittsburgh	+	+	+	17
13.	O. Secher	Copenhagen	+	-	-	5
14.	N.P. Singh	India	+	+	+	13
15.	E.L. Soares	Portugal	+	+	-	6
16.	J.O.A. Sodipo	Nigeria	+	-	+	14
17.	J. Stoffregen	Mainz	-	-	-	6
18.	J. Stovner	Oslo	-	-	-	1
19.	S. Sun	Turkije	+	+	+	3
20.	M.H. Sych	Poland	+	+	-	8
21.	E.A. Stojanov	Bulgaria	+	+	-	3
22.	T. Tammisto	Helsinki	+	+	-	3
23.	A.B. Tarrow	Philadelphia	+	+	-	4
24.	E. Trier Morch	Florida	+	-	-	3
25.	S. Tupavong	Bangkok	+	+	-	3
26.	G. Vasconcelos	Mexico	+	+	-	8
27.	V. Vanievski	Leningrad	+	+	-	2
28.	D.M.E. Vermeulen-Cranch	Amsterdam	+	+	+	9
29.	H. Yamamura	Tokyo	+	+	+	5

Nr.	Name	Residence	Photo + or -	CV + or -	List of Publ. + or -	Pages + or -
30.	G.M. Wyant	Canada	+	+	+	7
31.	B.E. Abed	Damascus	+	-	-	5
32.	L. Aro	Helsinki	+	+	-	3
33.	W.G. Atherstone	South Africa	+	-	-	10
34.	L. Barth	London	+	-	-	4
35.	J.H. Birkhahn	Israel	-	-	-	1
36.	L.A. Boeré	Santpoort (NL)	-	-	-	1
37.	C. Bovay	Switzerland	+	+	-	4
38.	A. Bull	South Africa	+	+	+	4
39.	A. Bunatian	Moscow	+	+	-	5
40.	J. de Castro	Belgium	+	+	+	39
41.	M. Chayen	Tel-Aviv	+	+	-	2
42.	Woon Hyok Chung	Corea	+	+	-	4
43.	E. Ciocatto	Italy	+	boekje		
44.	S. Cuoremonos	Athene	+	+	-	4
45.	W.H. Dam	Copenhagen	-	+	-	5
46.	E. Damir	Moscow	-	-	-	1
47.	T. Darbinian	Moscow	+	-	-	4
48.	H. Wollman	Philadelphia	-	+	+	17
49.	H. Epstein	Oxford (UK)	-	-	-	1
50.	F.F. Foldes	New York	-	-	-	9
51.	R. Frey	Germany	+	+	+	4
52.	J.P. Gauthier-Lafaye	France	-	+	-	1
53.	Q.J. Gomez	Phillippijnen	+	+	+	13
54.	R.A. Gordon	Toronto	+	+	+	14
55.	T. Gorth	Sweden	+	-	-	9
56.	H. Grant Whyte	South Africa	+	+	+	5
57.	C. Grat	Liverpool	+	+	+	12
58.	M. Griffith	Montreal	-	-	-	1

Nr.	Name	Residence	Photo + or -	CV + or -	List of Publ. + or -	Pages + or -
59.	Dr. B.C. Haid	Innsbruck	+	+	+	10
60.	Prof. J. Henley	USA	+	+	-	3
61.	Prof. D. Henschler	Würzburg	-	-	-	4
62.	Roy M. Humble	Edmonton	+	+	+	10
63.	A.R. Hunter	Manchester	+	+	+?	18
64.	S. Jeretin	Saudi Arabia	+	+	-	6
65.	Prof. J. Jordanoff	Bulgaria	+	+	-	4
66.	Joseph Douglas	Sydney	+	+	+	7
67.	R. Fisher	Heidelberg	alleen foto's van Springer Verlag			
68.	W. Jurczyk	Poland	+	+	+	15
69.	H. Killian	Freiburg	+	+	-	18
70.	J. Lassner	France	+	+	-	5
71.	Z. Lett	Hong Kong	+	+	+	6
72.	G. Litarczek	Romania	+	+	-	4
73.	H.M. Livingstone	Hopkinton, Iowa	+	+	-	15
74.	I. Lund	Oslo	-	+	-	1
75.	R.R. Macintosh	Oxford	+	+	+	13
76.	A. Madjidi	Iran	+	+	+	3
77.	I. Magill	England	+	-	-	8
	opgestuurd door J. Zorab, brief bij van Zorab.						
78.	Prof. G.F. Marx	Bronx	+	+	+	18
79.	O. Mayerhofer	Wien	+	+	+	12
80.	O. Mollestad	Oslo	-	+	-	1
81.	V.D. Monterosso	?	-	+	-	2
82.	L.E. Morris	Ohio	-	+	+	16
83.	W.W. Mushin	Cardiff (UK)	+	+	+	4
84.	E. Nilsson	Lund, Sweden	+	-	-	3
85.	O. Øyen	Oslo	+	+	-	6
86.	D.H.G. Keuskamp	Rotterdam	-	+	-	4

References or Archival Materials:

1. Frey R: Abstracts. Panel "Anesthesia: Past and Future"; 7th World Congress of Anaesthesiologists, Hamburg, September 14-21, 1980. Friday 19th September 1980; 14.15-14.45 P.M. Programme & 57 pp. No bibliographical data. Archives of Anaesthesia Rotterdam, The Netherlands

2. Frey R: "Korrespondenz. Anaesthesia: Past and Future". One of the five volumes on this topic, marked: Frey II. Place: Idem Ref. 1

3. Gray TC: A tale of the two cities. In: Essays: Anaesthesia and Its History, Rupreht J. et al. (Eds.) Springer-Verlag, Heidelberg, New York, Berlin, Tokyo. 1985. pp 284-290

4. Gray TC: Letter of 27th July, 1981, to Dr. J. Rupreht. Archives of Anaesthesia, Rotterdam, The Netherlands

5. Frey R: Letter of 23 September 1981, to Dr. J. Rupreht. Idem 4

6. Frey R: Letter to Prof Dr. W. Erdmann. Idem 4

7. Gray TC: Letter of 29th March 1982 (erroneously 1981) to Dr. J. Rupreht. Idem 4

From the Beginning of Anaesthesia to the first Chair of Anaesthesia in Innsbruck (1959) – The Contribution of Bruno Haid to this Development

H. Benzer, Department of Anaesthetics, University Clinics Innsbruck, Austria

Bruno Haid was one of the pioneers of anaesthesia in Austria. I am glad that I can now introduce you to the contribution of Bruno Haid to the development of anaesthesia in Innsbruck, in Austria and in Europe.

In October 1932, the famous surgeon Prof. Burghard Breitner, assistent at Prof. Anton von Eiselsbergs clinic in Vienna, had become head of the headship of the surgical department at the University of Innsbruck. After the second world war, it was Breitners great merit having realized the significance of anaesthesiology as one of the first surgeon's in the German-speaking area. In summer 1947, American professors visited some Austrian clinics giving lectures in different cities. Prof. Stuart C. Cullen was one of the anaesthesiologists of this team. In Innsbruck he demonstrated how to perform combined anaesthesia with endotracheal intubation using muscle relaxation during thoracic surgery that was performed by the surgeon, Prof. Brunswig.

It is believed that Prof. Breitner declared that day to be a milestone in the history of surgery and anaesthesia at the medical faculty in Innsbruck. This is how everybody realized that modern anaesthesia had become a conditio sine qua non for the future development of the surgical department at the University Hospital in Innsbruck. Dr. Bruno Haid, who had been an assistant at Prof. Breitners surgical department since 1945, has been allocated to assist Prof. Cullen on this memorable day. Impressed by this anaesthetic method, Dr. Haid developed the desire to learn these new techniques.

Dr. Haid who had finished his surgical education with approbation of the sugical board in the meantime, got the opportunity to start his special education in anaesthesiology at the State University of Iowa, Medical School, under Prof. Cullens supervision with a grant. Dr. Haids education in the United States took two years. Back to Innsbruck in 1951, Dr. Haid completely supported building up a department of anaesthesiology at the Department for Surgery of the University Hopital in Innsbruck. In 1954, plans for establishing a

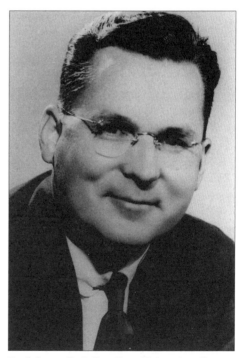

Prof. Stuart C. Cullen, State University of Iowa, Medical School

chair for anaesthesiology in Innsbruck had been made, but it seemed to be too early in spite of the existing consensus between Prof. Breitner, the surgeon, and the former minister of science.

One of the highligts in the clinical life of Bruno Haid was the 1st International Symposium for Anaesthesia and human personality in Rome in 1957. Cardiopulmonary resuscitation was a main topic at this symposium. Dr. Bruno Haid was able to discuss personally with his holiness Pope Pius 12 about ethical questions regarding this procedure.

In January 1958, a scientific meeting of the Austrian Society for Anaesthesiology took place in Innsbruck. Doz. Haid was honored in the presence the dean of the Medical Faculty, several heads of clinical departments and institutions. Among the invited speakers were Prof. Sir Robert Macintosh, head of the first chair for anaesthesiology in Europe since 1937, and head of the Nuffield chair of Anaesthesia at the University of Oxford. Sir Robert Macintosh gave a remarkable lecture about to work and to organize a department anaesthesiology in England and finally stressed the need for a department in Innsbruck. Everybody belonging to the staff, the Dean and many professors were very pleased with this idea. In 1958, the same year Professor Macintosh gave his lecture, the medical faculty applied to the Ministery for Education to establish a chair for anaesthesiology in Innsbruck.

With the ministerial approval of this application in 1959, the first independent institution in Central Europe with a chair for anaesthesiology has been established at the University of Innsbruck. Later Prof. Frey became the chair in Mainz, in Vienna Prof. Mayrhofer was appointed on the same position.

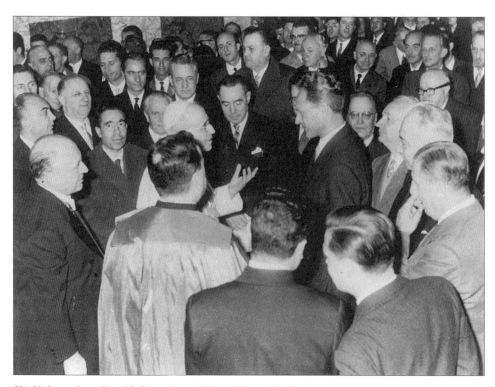

His Holiness Pope Pius 12 discussing with Prof. Bruno Haid.

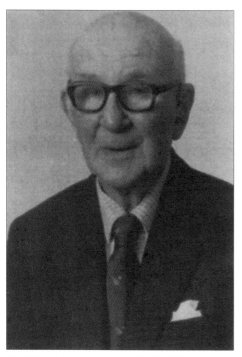

Prof. Sir Robert Macintosh, Nuffield Department of Anaesthetics, Oxford

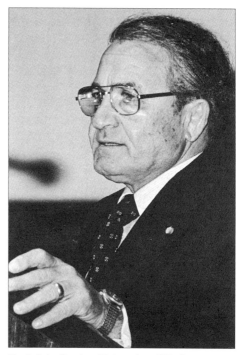

Prof. John Bonica, University of Washington, Seattle

On April 24 th, 1959, the commission at the medical faculty suggested Dr. Bruno Haid, assistent at the surgical department of the University, to be honored primo et unico loco. Other candidates where Dr. Mayrhofer, II. Surgical Clinic in Vienna, and Dr. Frey, Surgical Clinic in Heidelberg. On October 1st, 1959, Prof. Dr. Bruno Haid became chairman of the Department of Anaesthesiology in Innsbruck. One of the last highlights for Bruno Haid was the Central European Congress of Anaesthesiology that he organized in 1979.

He could speak to more than 1600 participants being the president at this conference. He spoke a few words remembering his surgical teacher Prof. Breitner, who died in 1956 and unveiled a bronze bust in memory of Prof. Breitners merits for anaesthesia. Prof. John Bonica had been the honorary speaker at this congress. On September 31st, 1985, Prof. Dr. Bruno Haid was given emeritus status after 34 years of intensive work in the field of anaesthesiology.

At that time, Bruno married his Margret and started a happy life in the Valley of Ötz in the mountains, surrounded by his friends, children and horses. He often returned to the city to visit his friends. On the occasion of the 21st Central European Congress in 1989 we celebrated the 30th anniversary of the chair for anaesthesiology in Innsbruck. The honorary membership of the Austrian Society for Anaesthesiology has been presented to Prof. Bruno Haid. Prof. Sir Robert Macintosh sent us his words of welcome for this celebration just before he died in order to remember his remarkable lecture in Innsbruck in 1958, 30 years ago.

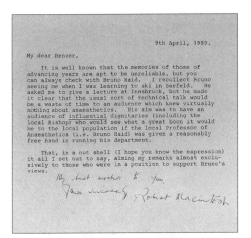

Word of welcome, sent by Prof. Sir Robert Macintosh

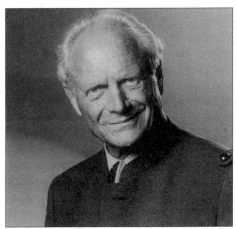

Prof. Bruno Haid

My dear Benzer,

It is well known that the memories of those of advancing years are apt to be unreliable, but you can always check with Bruno Haid. I recollect Bruno seeing me when I was learning to ski in Seefeld. He asked me to give a lecture at Innsbruck, but he made it clear that the usual sort of technical talk would be a waste of time to an audience which knew virtually nothing about anaesthetics. His aim was to have an audience of influential dignitaries (including the local Bishop) who would see what a great boon it would be to the local population if the local Professor of Anaesthetics (i.e. Bruno Haid) was given a reasonably free hand in running his department.

That, in a nut shell (I hope you know the expression) it all I set out to say, aiming my remarks almost exclusively to those who were in a position to support Brunos views.

With best wishes to you,
Yours sincerely,
Robert Macintosh

A stroke suddenly erased Bruno Haidss happyness in 1994. His dear wife Margret takes care personally, devoted to her badly handicaped and ill husband first at home, later in a sanatorium.

Bruno Haid died on Jannuary 1998.

Who was Dr. Reubens Wade?

D.J. Wilkinson,
Department of Anaesthesia,
St. Bartholomew's Hospital, London, U. K.

Introduction.

The name of Sir Ivan Magill is forever linked with Queens Hospital, Sidcup and the surgeon Sir Harold Gillies. It was in Sidcup that Magill developed his techniques of endotracheal anaesthesia with Rowbotham which were to change the practice of anaesthesia for the next 60 years. It is assumed that Gillies and Magill worked together exclusively and scant attention has been paid to other anaesthetists who worked in this hospital. One such man was Reubens Wade who perhaps initiated many of the advances that were subsequently developed and popularised by Magill.

Early life.

Reubens Wade was born on February 15th 1880, in the Lake District, the eldest son of Thomas Wade the artist.[1] He went to school in Sedburgh and then studied medicine at Christ's College Cambridge where he passed his 2nd MB in December 1902. He moved to London to complete his training at St. Bartholomew's Hospital from where he passed his Conjoint Diploma (MRCS, LRCP) in July 1906 and then subsequently obtained his MB (Cambs) in December of the same year.[2] He acted as Junior House Physician at Barts from 1906-1907 and then Senior House Physician for a further six months[3] before moving to the Great Northern Central Hospital (now the Royal Northern Hospital) in London where he remained for 3 years working as Junior and then Senior House Surgeon and then Resident Medical Officer.[4]

He then moved to Bedale in Yorkshire where he worked in general practice with a fellow Barts doctor, Dr Eddison. After 3 years in Yorkshire he moved south again to Farnham in Surrey where he presumably continued in general practice.[5]

Anaesthesia.

Reubens Wade must have been trained in anaesthetics at Barts when a medical student and it was common practice to maintain those skills in General Practice. In fact all hospital posts in anaesthesia in the UK at this time were 'Honorary' positions which meant that there was no pay and the majority of anaesthetists were forced to earn a living through general practice. The Medical Directory of 1919 lists him as an anaesthetist for the first time when his entry notes he was an anaesthetist to Queens Hospital Sidcup and was in the RAMC, but this was obviously a 'catching up' exercise as Wade had already published a paper on anaesthesia in The Lancet in 1918.[6] It is highly likely that Wade continued as an anaesthetist for all his time in general practice and then gradually 'collected' a series of honorary positions as an anaesthetist.

By 1920 he had moved back to London and was living in St. Johns Wood. The Medical Directory lists him as being Assistant Anaesthetist at St. Bartholomew's Hospital, Senior Honorary Anaesthetist at the Great Northern Central Hospital, Anaesthetist at Queens Hospital Sidcup, Late Honorary Anaesthetist at Golden Square Hospital and by

1922 he had added Demonstrator of Anaesthesia at the National Dental Hospital, Leicester Square to these.

In 1929 he was appointed a full anaesthetist to Barts where he stayed for the rest of his life. He died, following surgery at King Edward VII Hospital, Beaumont Street, London, on May 10th 1940 in his 60th year.[1] A service of remembrance was held at the church of St Bartholomew's the Less, which lies within the Hospital boundary and is the Parish Church of Barts, on June 4th 1940.

Personal details:

He married Phyllis Mary Landon in 1912 and had one son. His wife predeceased him. He was a keen oarsman as a student and rowed in his college boat. He was never a physically robust man and was profoundly deaf, a disability which in no way disadvantaged him in his chosen career. He was obviously a highly competent clinical anaesthetist but not one to 'put himself forward'. One description, from someone who was taught by him, was "a quiet, polite and a melt-into-the-background sort of chap".[7]

Anaesthesia for plastic surgery:

When Gillies first started his plastic surgery practice he worked at the Cambridge Hospital, Aldershot and he did not have a regular anaesthetist, then three Royal Army Medical Corps anaesthetists were rotated to work with him. At least one of these, Dr Reubens Wade, was to work very closely with him over the next three or four years and there appears to have been a time of 'overlap' when both Wade and Magill were together at Sidcup.

What sort of cases did Gillies work involve? These were those facial injuries which other surgeons tended to abandon as hopeless. Severe fragment and burns injuries to the head and neck produced the most horrifying injuries to the extent that during convalescence at one seaside town the Matron was requested to keep the patients indoors to prevent the local people being upset!![8] Gillies developed methods of grafting and flaps which were revolutionary for that time. He would work in close partnership with dental surgeons but the anaesthesia for such cases was very difficult.

"Surgeon and dentist were hampered by the difficulty of anaesthesia when the patients face looked like a bloody sponge. Up to 1916 they worked with open ether and chloroform. The operation would be interrupted three or four times for the surgeon to clear out the debris of blood and mucous in the pharynx and thus clear the airway. The tongue swollen with venous congestion always had to be held forward." "Gillies said that the fear of chloroform was so great that a patient warned of operation on Monday was likely to start vomiting on Saturday".[8]

Wade's contributions:

In 1916 Colonel JFW Silk visited the plastics unit at Cambridge and suggested that Wade anaesthetise these patients in a sitting up position to ameliorate the problems of blood pooling in the pharynx and causing airway obstruction. Wade adopted this technique and this was the basis of his paper in the Lancet of 1918.[6] The paper is full of understatements like "There are two main difficulties in anaesthesia for operations on the face and lower jaw, (1) maintenance of as good airway and (2) difficulty of avoiding interference with aseptic technique and field of view of the surgeon". Today's anaesthetist cannot easily imagine this type of practice without a tracheal tube or laryngeal mask airway, but most anaesthetists nowadays believe that these inventions were only to be introduced some years in the future.

Wade had five basic techniques for patients lying flat and two for those in the sitting position. For those lying flat he would use a Shipway's apparatus through which he used ether, ether/chloroform or chloroform insufflated through a Hewitt's airway via a small bent metal tube. When a sterile field was required then he would induce anaesthesia with a sterile wire frame mask and drop bottle while wearing full aseptic gown and gloves himself. For some cases he employed intratracheal warmed ether administered through a narrow bore catheter and for others a Kuhn wire re-inforced metal tube introduced into the trachea. His final technique was the use of oil/ether per rectum. These were his five techniques for those lying flat. For those in the sitting position he utilised a Shipway's apparatus or oil/ether per rectum. His paper reported the management of over 300 cases in the sitting position without any 'bad after effects or complications'.[6]

Gillies book:

In 1920 Gillies published a definitive textbook on plastic surgery based on his experiences to date. In this book was a chapter on anaesthesia written by Wade and not Magill![9] Again the book is full of mild understatements and much useful practical help, *"To begin with, the majority of plastic operations are unavoidably long."*

The use of laryngoscopes:

"For large operations upon the mouth region, intratracheal administration in some form has been adopted as a routine. Where the form of the parts permits a catheter is introduced into the trachea through a Mosher's laryngeal speculum under the guidance of vision." When Magill described his first laryngoscope the catalogue produced by A Charles King described this as a laryngeal speculum. So suddenly one is aware that the Magill straight blade laryngoscope was not the first and was just an adaptation of the Mosher scope used by Wade. Magill's paper is entitled an improved speculum for anaesthesia which it undoubtedly was but it is interesting to note it was some 6 years after Wade's description.[10]

"Administration [of the anaesthetic] by positive pressure undoubtedly relieves the patient of much of the strain of a long operation, and the ease with which pure oxygen or air can be substituted for anaesthetic through the clear airway diminishes the stress associated with cyanosis to a minimum. The difficulties consequent upon the routine adoption of these methods are easily overcome with practice. The anaesthetist must learn to depend almost solely on the respiratory movements and the pulse as his guide with rare peeps at the pupil."

Nasal tubes:

"The nasal tube:-this was described by my colleague, Captain JC Clayton in the Lancet.", Wade writes later in this same chapter. *"I always use the largest tube (size 20) which it is possible to pass down a nostril. If the tube is cut to a blunt point it will be found to pass more easily. ...Thus a clear airway is assured, always provided that the end of the tube is in its proper place just above the epiglottis, ...The mouth and pharynx are then loosely packed with gauze so as not to compress the tube."* He continues, *"One of the objections to this method is that the tube is likely to kink at the level of the ala. I have overcome this by cutting the nasal tube short at the ala, and inserting into it one end of a right-angled metal connection of the same bore as the tube."*

Here we see Magill's subsequent development of nasal intubation and the Magill endotracheal connectors set again in context of previous work.

Wade goes on to review the techniques he had described previously in his Lancet paper and adds the additional thought of premedication with 'hypodermic hyoscine' except where there is a danger of blood in the airway postoperatively. He also describes the use of rectal paraldehyde in olive oil which he found preferable to ether in oil by the same route.

Later life:

Wade continued on the staff at Barts and the Royal Northern Hospital until he died in 1940. His obituary gives further insight into the type of man he was; *"Mr Wade had the rare combination of tact and skill which makes a first-class anaesthetist. He never became flustered and carried on the most difficult work with efficient calmness. During the 20 years that the writer [Langton Hewer] knew 'Ben Wade' as he was universally and affectionately called, he cannot recall a single occasion when anyone said an unkind thing about him."*[1]

Conclusions:

The purpose of this paper is not to suggest that Sir Ivan Magill was anything but a brilliant innovator who changed the world of anaesthesia and who rightly has gained universal acclaim for his work.

It is however to suggest that, like today, there are many anaesthetists in the past like Reubens Wade who are quiet unassuming men and women who continue to provide safe anaesthesia for their patients throughout a lifetime. Often these 'unsung heroes' develop an aspect of their chosen speciality which is then 'picked up' and developed further or popularised by others.

Reubens Wade was one such 'unsung hero' except to his patients and his surgeons, who knew him well. Gillies asked him, not Magill, to contribute to his book and another surgeon, Kenneth Walker, added an addendum to his obituary which bears repetition. *"His attitude to the approaching end was typical of him. Unruffled, dispassionate and gentlemanly, he almost looked forward to it as an interesting adventure. Unruffled in death, he was unruffled in life and never during our long partnership, as surgeon and anaesthetist, have I once had to stop an operation because things had gone wrong at the other end of the table. There was something big in Wade, unexpressed in words, but implicit in his manner of living. He was the ideal anaesthetist and the ideal colleague."* Fine words indeed for a quietly efficient and innovative anaesthetist who deserves our recognition and admiration.

Acknowledgements:

I would like to thank Mr Antony F Wallace, retired Plastic Surgeon to St. Bartholomew's Hospital, for his considerable help in pointing me in some new directions and thus greatly assisting in the preparation of this paper.

References:

[1] Hewer CL: Reubens Wade, Obituary. St. Bartholomew's Hospital Journal 1939-40; 1: 174-175
[2] Register of Attendance 1902-1906. St. Bartholomew's Hospital Archives
[3] Minutes of the House Committee 1906-1907. St. Bartholomew's Hospital Archives
[4] Medical Directory 1909. 1910
[5] Medical Directory 1913. 1918
[6] Wade R: Methods of general anaesthesia in facial surgery. Lancet 1918; 1: 794-795
[7] Ellis G: Personal communication
[8] Pound R: Gillies Surgeon Extraordinary. Michael Joseph, London 1964
[9] Gillies HD. Plastic Surgery of the Face. Henry Frowde, London 1920
[10] Magill IW. Improved speculum for anaesthesia. Lancet 1926; 1: 500

Jochen Bark – a German Pioneer of modern Anesthesiology

H. Menzel
Department of Anesthesia, Municipal Hospital Bielefeld. Bielefeld, Germany

Modern German anesthesiology began half a century ago. Historically this is a short time, yet the beginnings of the specialty in Germany are already becoming obscure. We do have access to scientific publications but only rarely information on the development of the specialty in Germany is given. Jochen Bark brings to us the difficulties typical for anesthesiology in many countries where anesthesiology was a part of the department of surgery.

Most of the suggestions for improvements in anesthesia were presented orally to the chief of surgery who had the authority to accept or reject them. Barks personal notes are not available anymore. Thus, we have no written trail of the development of anesthesia in his unit and have to rely on a few meeting notes from members of the faculty. These and comments by members of his family and his associates and my own recollections from the 4 years of my tenure in his department form the basis of my presentation. Professor Dr.med. Richard Heinz Joachim Bark was known to his friends as Jochen. He was born on January 23, 1918 in Weissenborn, a small village in Thuringia where his father was a protestant parish priest. When Bark was 7 years old, his father moved the family to Gangloffsoemmern, a village north of Erfurt, where Bark started his schooling. During High School in Erfurt with a major in the humanities he also attended the conservatory of music to take piano and organ lessons. After graduation in 1937 he served the obligatory 7 months in a paramilitary organization, the Arbeitsdienst. He then started his medical education at the University of Freiburg/Br. switching to Munich later. Changing universities in midstream during medical school was common in Germany.

World War II interrupted his studies and he found himself serving in the German Navy on duty in the North Sea and the Atlantic Ocean where he saw action and sustained a penetrating chest wound with injury to his lungs, subsequently complicated by tuberculosis and bronchiectasis. He was discharged from the service and continued his medical education in Freiburg/Br. where he graduated in 1943/44, receiving his doctorate in February, 1944. Physicians were needed and the German Navy once again drafted him. He served on board and in military hospitals and was captured by the Allied on April 1, 1945, spending the rest of the war as a Prisoner of War.

In 1946 he started a three year surgical residency at the University of Freiburg/Br. under the chairmanship of Eduard Rehn, followed by a few months of otorhinolaryngology in Fritz Zoellners department. Now he was ready to practice and he accepted a position as thoracic surgeon in the Wehrawald Hospital in Todtmoos, where he had his first encounter with modern anesthesia. Spurred by his experience he decided to specialize in the field of anesthesiology and from October 1949 through March 1950 he worked at the Westminster Hospital in London and in Oxford under Sir Macintosh, the Dean of European anesthesia. When he returned to Wehrawald, his attitude towards anesthesia had changed.

He established contact with leading authorities, Hans Killian, a surgeon[1,2,3,4,5], and Hellmut Weese, a pharmacologist[3,6,7,8,9], both of whom had recognized the important role anesthesia played in modern medicine. Bark recognized that German anesthesia lagged behind the advances in the field that marked anesthesia in Great Britain and the United States. To launch an effort to advance the specialty, Bark organized the Deutsche Arbeitsgemeinschaft für Anaesthesiologie (German Study Group in Anesthesia). This important event took place in Salzburg, Austria, in 1952. At the Surgical Congress in Munich, only a year later, the Organization was named the Deutsche Gesellschaft für Anaesthesie, (German Society for Anesthesia) with Jochen Bark being the first president, serving 1953/54[10]. During his tenure Bark succeeded in having the German board of Anesthesiology established at the Deutsche Aerztetag in Lindau, thus attaining official recognition of the specialty by the organization representing the medical profession in Germany. In 1954 he organized the first Central European Congress of Anesthesiology in Munich[11].

Jochen Bark was acknowledged as a leader in the field, and in 1954 he was asked to establish a department of anesthesiology at the University of Tuebingen, preliminary as a division within the department of surgery. Only a year later Theodor Naegeli left and Hofrat Walter Dick took over the surgical chairmanship and with this the atmosphere in the department changed[22].

The new chairman was an excellent surgeon appreciating the service of the anesthesiologists, but he failed to recognize that the field needed the challenge of independence to blossom. Thus, Bark was stifled and could not expand his unit, because neither the space nor the financial resources were made available to him. His unit was soon overshaddowed by other Anesthesia Departments in Germany and Austria who could thrive under more favorable conditions. Nevertheless, Bark and his team made important contributions to anesthesia.

Bark was widely recognized as a superb teacher and lecturer[12], an outstanding clinical instructor, and a visionary in his field. Together with Johann Maurath he advocated the use of pulmonary function testing as early as 1954[14]. Calling on his background in thoracic surgery he introduced bronchoscopy and bronchography and described anesthetic methods, especially general anesthesia with artificial ventilation, for these maneuvers[15]. He was ahead of his time with the discription of preclinical rescue service, including the use of helicopters[16].

He recommended the use of battery powered cardioscopes applied directly to the chest, later realized by Helmut Kronschwitz[17]. The use of the EEG, for example during carotid endarterectomies, was advocated by Bark long before this methodology became generally accepted[18]. Relaxometry, still not generally practiced, was envisioned by Bark and an instrument introduced in 1962[19].

In 1956 Robert A. Hingson, MD, Professor of Anesthesia, Western Reserve University, School of Medicine, Cleveland/Ohio, offered Bark an appointment "as a temporary member of our Faculty, and Instructor in our teaching department, for the period December 20, 1956 through December 20, 1957".[20] This was the first offer from the USA after the War to a German anesthesiologist to give lectures on anesthesia[21].

Bark might have compared the working conditions he found in Cleveland with those in Tuebingen: both were divisions of surgery, both departments were chaired by strong surgical chiefs who recognized the importance of good clinical anesthesia services and both were not ready to grant departmental status to their division of anesthesia. The division of anesthesia at Western Reserve was not made an independent department until 1969,

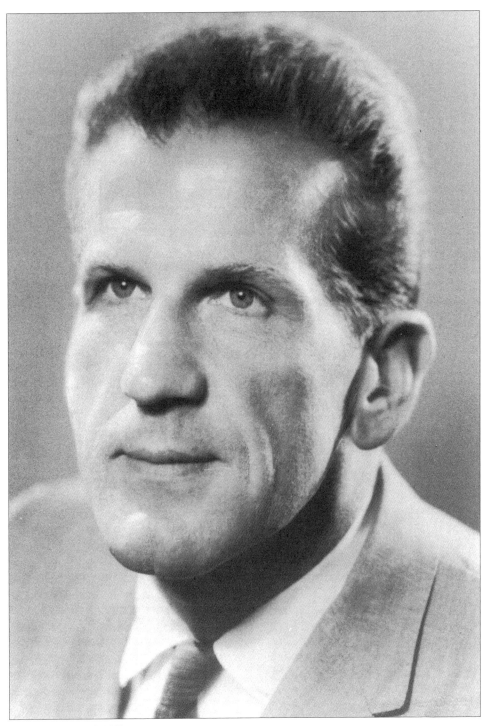

Jochen Bark (1918-1963)

when Robert A. Hingson left, while departmental status was granted to anesthesia in Tuebingen 1968, when the surgical chairman, Hofrat Walter Dick left, 5 years after Jochen Bark's death[22].

Bark was appreciated by his colleagues and, partly because of his fluency in English and French, partly because of his gracious style of chairing meetings, he moderated many a scientific session, both nationally and internationally. In 1960 he was elected vice president of the Second Congress of the World Federation of Societies of Anesthesiologists, meeting held in Toronto, Canada, under the presidency of C.R.Ritsema van Eck[23].

On the continent of Europe Bark worked closely with other leaders in the field, including Otto Mayrhofer and Bruno Haid from Austria and Georg Hossli and Werner Huegin from Switzerland.

Bark was granted only nine years of work as chief of anesthesia at the University of Tuebingen. He perished in a plane crash on April 14, 1963. His premature death cut short a promising career and the opportunity to chair one of the new departments of anesthesia at German Universities that were looking for a visionary leader in the field. Anesthesia, and particularly German anesthesia owes Jochen Bark, a charismatic visionary pioneer, not only a debt of gratitude but a place in its memory.

References:

[1] Killian H: Plan zur Neuordnung des Narkosewesens in Deutschland. Schmerz, Narkose, Anaesthesie 1941; 5:73-87

[2] Killian H: Reorganisation des Narkosewesens. Der Krankenhausarzt 1949; 9:22

[3] Killian H, Weese H: Die Narkose. Ein Lehr- und Handbuch. Thieme-Verlag, Stuttgart 1954

[4] Killian H: Fnfzig Jahre Anaesthesiologie. Ein Rckblick. Der Anaesthesist 1963; 12 (9):285ff und 12 (10):315

[5] Killian H: 40 Jahre Narkoseforschung. Verlag Dtsch. Hochschullehrer-Zeitung, Tübingen 1964

[6] Weese H: Evipan, ein neuartiges Einschlafmittel. Scharpff W: Dtsch. med. Wochenschr. 1932; 31:1205-1207

[7] Weese H: Pharmakologie des intravensen Kurznarkotikums Evipan-Natrium. Dtsch. med. Wochenschr. 1933; 2:47-48

[8] Weese H: Concerning the mechanism of anesthesia accidents in sublingual phlegmons. Anesth. and Analg 1939; 15-21

[9] Weese H, Koss F H: Über ein neues Ultrakurznarkotikum. DMW 1954; 16:601-604

[10] Bark J, Frey R: Gründungs-Protokoll und Satzung der Deutschen Gesellschaft für Anaesthesie vom 10. April 1953

[11] Bark J: Eröffnungsansprache 1. Zentraleuropäischer Anaesthesie-Kongreß, München. 24. April 1954. Der Anaesthesist 1954 ;4:137-138

[12] Bark J: Lehrbuch der Anaesthesiologie. et al: Springer-Verlag Berlin 1955

[13] Griesser G, Bark J, Mayer W: Klinische Erfahrungen in der Behandlung des schweren. Tetanus mit hohen Antitoxindosen. Langenbecks Archiv 1962; 301:455

[14] Maurath J: Lungenfunktion und Narkose - Der Anaesthesist 1954; 3:162

[15] Bark J: Bronchoscopy and bronchography under general anesthesia. Anesth & Analg 1956

[16] Bark J: Unfallrettungsdienst durch Hubschrauber. Der Anaesthesist 1960; 9:343

[17] Kronschwitz H: Direkt auf die Brustwand aufzusetzendes Kardioskop. Der Anaesthesist 1964; 13:170

[18] Bark J: Die Narkosetiefe, Untersuchungen mit dem EEG. Habilitationsschrift 1956

[19] Bark J: Kontrolle der Muskelrelaxantien. Der Anaesthesist 1962; 11:141-144

[20] Hingson R.A: Briefe an die Universität Tübingen vom November 7, 1956 und Dezember 13, 1957. Universitätsbibliothek, Tübingen

[21] Bark J: Antrag auf Freistellung an die Medizinische Fakultät der Universität Tübingen vom 26. November 1956

[22] Dietzsch F: Die Geschichte der Anaesthesie in Tübingen. Zur Entwicklung der Anaesthesie an den Tübinger Chirurgischen Kliniken im Zeitraum von 1847 bis 1968. Inaugural-Dissertation S.62, Tübingen, Med.Fakultät

[22] Griffith H.R: History of the World Federation of Anesthesiologists. Anesth & Analg 42:3:396

Robert Reynolds Macintosh – Life before Anaesthesia

A.B. Baker, Department of Anesthesiology, University of Sydney, Australia.
C. McK Holmes, Specialist Anaesthetist, Dunedin, New Zealand.

Sixty years ago in 1937 Robert Reynolds Macintosh started as Nuffield Professor of Anaesthetics in the University of Oxford, England. He was born on 17th October 1897 (100 years ago this year) in Timaru, New Zealand, as Rewi Rawhiti Macintosh). The Maori names were a tradition of the times. He spent part of his childhood in South America where his father had moved to run a newspaper following the death of his mother; (who is buried in Balclutha, New Zealand), and where he became fluent in Spanish. He returned to New Zealand to board at Waitaki Boys' High School (WBHS) in Oamaru where he had a most successful school career (Table 1)

Rewi Rawhiti Macintosh then travelled to England where he enlisted in the 2nd King's Own Scottish Boarderers later transferring to the Royal Scots Fusiliers and going briefly to France before recall to join the Royal Flying Corps (RFC) to which he had previously volunteered but been initially unsuccessful. Because of the very high casualty rate in the RFC he, along with many others, was recalled to the RFC following initial deferral.

It was at this time that Rewi Rawhiti changed his name to Robert Reynolds though this would not be confirmed legally until 1929. Robert Reynolds Macintosh undertook a course of instruction at the Central Flying School at Upavon and received his Wings on 25th April 1917 as 2/Lt R R Macintosh following a Course which on the original certificate had very carefully excluded both the words "Long" and "Short" which were the only types of courses offered. One has visions of a very abbreviated course being given as Pilots were in such very high demand at that time. One month later on 26th May 1917 on his first official sortie against the Germans he developed engine trouble soon after take-off, returned to base, obtained another aircraft (#B1685 a Nieuport 17) and attempted to regain his squadron's formation. He was unsuccessful in this and proved a lone target separated from the squadron. He was shot down by the emerging German ace Lt. Paul Strähle of Jasta 18 flying an Albatross DIII aeroplane as Strähle's 7th Victory (ultimately he achieved 14 Victories before being wounded himself in the closing stages of the war). Strähle (1893-1985), who was 4 years older than Macintosh, lived to the same age and continued to fly until very old.

Macintosh successfully crash landed his Nieuport and then promptly set it on fire so that the Germans could not obtain any information from the aircraft. This was the last successful "firing" of a landed aeroplane during World War I as the Germans had become very adept at arriving quickly at the scene of crash landings to prevent such "firing". Thereafter Robert Reynolds Macintosh was a Prisoner-of-War attempting to escape six times, two of which were relatively successful. He was initially interred in Freiburg where H E Hervey in Cage Birds (1940) reports "I spotted Mackintosh, a New Zealander, who had been with me at CFS. Mac looked worried and, on seeing me, hurriedly beckoned to me to come down......where Mac, who was waiting for me, quickly trust a small parcel into my hand

and asked me to hide it. The parcel contained an infantry compass and a small map torn from a railway carriage." (p.16) Thus right from the start Macintosh was contemplating escape. "The day after his arrival, Mac asked me to stroll around the yard, and then told me that he intended to escape from Freiburg and asked if I would join him". (p.17) This they managed to do some weeks later but the manner in which Macintosh did so is of some interest particularly with respect to later actions he would take when Professor of Anaesthetics at Oxford. Again from Hervey, "Suddenly, with the remark: "Blast this - I'm off!" Mac started to lower the rope. Craig and I held our breath, our eyes glued to the sentry, while Mac climbed out of the window, and a few seconds later, when we looked down to mark his progress, he had vanished." (p.33) The trials of waiting to see eventually had to cease and action, for better or worse, needed to occur - Mac was ever the man for that action! A few days later famished and tired but within sight of the River border which they needed to swim to safety there was " Suddenly a slight movement in the undergrowth ahead caught our eyes, and stepping from behind some bushes, a sentry, clad in the grey-green uniform of the Forest Patrol and accompanied by a large lean police dog, called on us to halt."(p.42) They were returned to Freiburg and then transferred to Zorndorf (now Sarbinowo in Poland) where other unsuccessful attempts followed, and hence a further transfer to high security Clausthal. But in Zorndorf "Mac, who had worked unceasingly at the German language, could now speak it fluently" (p.74) so was able to contemplate his most audacious attempt to escape.

"Mac told me that he and Robinson intended to jump the train shortly after it left Berlin, and asked me to get a seat in their compartment, if possible, in case they needed assistance............He was particularly anxious to jump off before getting far from Berlin, as he intended to return there, procure civilian clothes, and travel by rail to the frontier..........We were all wearing uniform, of course, but Mac had commissioned the Russian tailor at Zorndorf to line his military overcoat with a dark blue material, and this garment, turned inside out, made a passable civilian coat, which he hoped would be sufficient disguise until he reached Berlin". (p.77) The plan worked for Macintosh but not for Robinson and "We had been at Clausthal about a week, when Mac turned up with an impressive escort of German soldiers, and wearing a perfectly beautiful civilian suit". (p.81) What had transpired then unfolded "On reaching the capital, he hailed a cab and instructed the driver to take him to that quarter of the town frequented by the gay ladies of Berlin. After a drive through the city the cabman dropped him at the door of one of a row of dingy little houses in a squalid side street. A somewhat faded lady answered his knocking, and upon being admitted, Mac immediately informed her that he was a British prisoner of war, and that he needed, shelter, food and clothing. It must have been a startling revelation, but the sight of Mac's roll of German marks overcame both her patriotism and her fear of the consequences of assisting a fugitive enemy. She provided him with a meal, and then, armed with a supply of his money, went out shopping, and returned in due course with a suit and various other requirements. Having changed into his new garments, Mac bade his hostess farewell and, tucking under his arm the brown paper parcel which contained his uniform, set forth once more upon his travels". (p.82)

"In his ensuring travels Mac crossed Germany by train, but when, within a stone's throw of his destination, a peculiar circumstance resulted in his arrest..........it was then that he learnt that the fellow traveller had spotted the one weak point in his disguise - he was wearing English boots made of real leather at a time when leather was almost an unknown commodity in Germany". (p.83)

Macintosh was, despite this capture, somewhat of a hero in Clausthal. "In spite of its unsuccessful ending, this journey of Mac's was a very stout effort, particularly in view of the fact that before he was sent to Zorndorf he could speak scarcely a word of the German language". (p.83)

Following the end of the war Robert Reynolds Macintosh enrolled in Guy's Hospital Medical School graduating in 1924, trained initially as a Surgeon (FRCS Edin 1927), switched to anaesthesia, became Nuffield Professor at Oxford in 1937, and "took" the D.A Examination in 1939. In World War II he became an Air Commodore in the R.A.F and was active in experiments to design better life jackets for airmen who "ditched" into the North Sea. He was Knighted in 1955 and died on 28th August 1989 following a head injury sustained in a fall at home in Oxford.

1912	Entered WBHS as Boarder 2nd Junior Chess Championship
1913	School B Tennis Team 2nd Senior High Jump 1st in Year (1st English/Maths, 2nd Chemistry) Writing & Navy League Prizes
1914	School Cricket XI School Rugby XV (Wing Forward) School A Tennis Team #2 in School Rowing IV - 2nd to Wanganui College in N.Z. National Schools' Rowing Championships (no VIIIs at this time) Won Senior Tennis Singles Championship 1st 50yds. Senior Swimming Handicap 2nd 100yds. Senior Sprint Championship 1st Senior Long Jump Championship - setting a new record 18ft 9in (previous record set in 1908) School Debating Team
1915	Head Boy Platoon Subaltern Christian Union Leader School Librarian & Editor of School Magazine "The Waitakian" Secretary of the Camera Club School Cricket XI School Rugby XV (Wing Forward) School A Tennis Team #3 in School Rowing IV - 3rd to Christ's College and Christchurch Boys' High School in N.Z. National Schools' Rowing Championships (no VIIIs at this time) 2nd Senior Tennis Singles Championship 1st Senior Long Jump Championship - broke his own record with 19ft 3 ins School Debating Team

Reference:

Hervey HE: Cage Birds Penguin Books 287, 1960

ACKNOWLEDGEMENTS

Sir Anthony Jephcott for loan of Cage Birds.

Mr Guy Francis (step-son of Sir Robert Macintosh) for discussion and copies of personal effects of RRM.

Librarian Waitaki Boys' High School for access to school records.

Prof K Wiedermann for unravelling the new name for Zorndorf.

François Magendie: The Apostle of Pain?

C. Parsloe
Hospital Samaritano, São Paulo, SP, Brasil

François Magendie is considered the founder of experimental pharmacology. He was a vivisectionist, a precursor of modern Medicine and was vehemently against Bichats doctrine of Vitalism. His *Précis élémentaire de physiologie* published in 1816, when he was 33 years old, marked the beginning of modern physiology, later to be advanced by his follower, Claude Bernard. In his book Magendie wrote: "Facts, and facts alone are the foundations of science". Such statement ran against the discursive method commonly used at the time. In 1821 he prepared a pocket size *Formulaire sur l'emploi et la préparation de plusieurs médicaments* which became a classic. For the first time drugs were properly studied on animals. The book was translated into several languages and ran for 9 editions.

In 1821 he started and became editor of a new journal called *Journal de Physiologie Éxperimentale* which lasted 10 years and later received the additional title et de *Pathologie*. He became a member of the *Académie de Sciences de Paris* in 1824.

He visited London in 1824 performing physiological demonstrations on living animals which created much furor. He was known to be gracious and charming in private life although exhibiting a rather violent temper and combativeness in scientific matters. He was the center of the Bell-Magendie controversy over the discovery of the functions of anterior and posterior spinal nerve roots. He fully defended his priority as properly defining their separate motor and sensitive functions. He described the cerebro spinal fluid circulation and the foramen which became known by his name (apertura medialis ventriculi quarti).

In 1835 his *Leçons sur les phénomnès physiques de la vie* were published. In 1842 they were in their 4th edition consisting of 4 volumes. In this book significant and original statements were put forward such as: *Expérimentez, expérimentez, le reste viendra de soi!* and *La conviction ne nâit que de preuves.* He gave his reason for writing the book: *Mon but principal a été de contribuer à changer l'état de la Physiologie, de la ramener entièrement l'éxperience, en un mot de faire éprouver à cette belle science l'heureuse rénovation des sciences physiques.*

He was present at the *Acadmie des Sciences* Monday meeting on February 1, 1847 when Velpeau presented for the second time his excellent results with the administration of ether for surgical operations. At the same meeting Roux gave a more cautious report on the effects of ether. Magendie was then 64 years old and severely questioned the rendering of insensibility and unconsciouness with ether on moral grounds.

"For some weeks a certain number of surgeons have set themselves to experiment on man, and for the undoubdetly praiseworthy purpose - that of performing operations without pain - they intoxicate their patients to the point of reducing them, so to speak, to the state of a cadaver which one can cut and slice at will without causing suffering."

"Acting in such a way surgeons fail as to reason and morals, and may achieve dangerous consequences to public safety; thus, I decided to protest against such imprudent experiments and specially against hasty publications."

"An American dentist announced last month (sic) that breathing ether vapor caused such an insensibility that it was possible under this influence to remove a tooth painlessly, which is from time immemorial every dentists pretention, rarely achieved."

"This announcement, which perhaps was not meant to cross the Atlantic, and which probably was no more than a local advertisement, arrived in England; immediately London surgeons launched themselves upon the traces of the American artist, administered ether vapor and performed several operations equally *sans douleurs*; the news arrived in France and without a moments delay several surgeons from Hospitals in Paris hastened to immitate their overseas colleagues."

"Inebriation carried to insensibility is a deplorable state; loss of the moral sense, of the consciousness of its own existence is degrading and debasing; this state, on the other hand, can lead to a fatal end."

"As for myself, and I believe that all men of respect will think likewise, I would not for any reason allow myself to be rendered unto such a situation in which your body is handed over, in a defenceless state, to a surgeon who may be clumsy, incapable or unattentive."

"Anyone with a little courage and energy will prefer to suffer for a moment instead of being overcome by drunkness even if for a brief period."

"What will be the consequences if these experiments are carried out by uncapable, ignorant, even criminal hands (all aspects must be foreseen)? And if instead of public operations the inebriation is carried out in the intimacy of a home or in a clandestine way on women, on young persons, with perverse or guilty intentions, dont you believe that public morals and safety would be in serious danger?"

"Ether inebriation is still not well known. It should be studied not only for surgical operations but for and by itself. What are its characteristic phenomena? How do they differ from the inebriation caused by alcohol, opium, hashish, etc.? In which way does its accompanying insensibility differ from that caused by a large number of narcotic poisons? *Voilá, certes, une belle et important étude à faire!* However, this study should, like all serious studies, be carried out silently, with calm and should be of sufficient duration to lead to assured results; only then it should be applied to human beings with safety and morality."

The following paragraph, from the original, shows the intense feelings Magendie had for the haphazard introduction of ether inhalation by surgeons without prior knowledge of its hazards as well as his fear that an important discovery could be mismanaged.

Mais, si l'on continue à expérimenter sans ménagement; si on livre à la publicité, le soir même, l'expérience qu'on a faite le matin et qui n'est pas terminée, puisque peut avoir, en définitive, de funestes conséquences, on s'exposerait à compromettre un moyen qui sera peut-être utile un jour, quand il sera bien étiudié, bien connu et appliqué à propos; mais qui, au contraire, exploté comme il est aujourd'hui, pourrait prochaiment être réduit à l'une de ces prétendues découverts, à l'un de ces puffs scientifiques qui viennent périodiquement amuser la curiosité du public et satisfaire sa passion insensée pour tout ce qui est erreur et mensonge.

Velpeau protested such accusations presenting a series of arguments to which Magendie responded:

"Ether, I know, really has the attribute of such happy properties. Does it follow that it is necessary to intoxicate patients for all small operations consisting of a single stroke of the scalpel such as... opening of an abscess... ligature, excision or cauterization of hemorrhoids..."

Je n'hésite pas à répondre négativement.
"Therefore, at the moment I regard ether inhalation not only as of no use but as being formally contra-indicated in such circumstances."

"... Ether intoxication has inconvenients which seem not to have bothered surgeons.

Consider, gentlemen, is pain in the human nature, and even in the animal nature devoid of any usefulness?"

"During removal of nasal polyps blood flows abundantly into the hypopharynx and tends to get into the larynx; its contact with the glottis elicits cough and efforts to impede its entry into the trachea; but if the glottis has been rendered insensible, blood will penetrate the bronchi and suffocation may result."

Magendie was prescient, therefore, in being the first individual, upon hearing about ether unconsciousness, to warn about the unrecognized danger of aspiration into the lungs. Early in his career he had worked on the functions of the epiglottis and swallowing. Therefore, he could immediately grasp the problem which had not been mentioned by surgeons using ether without adequate knowledge.

Magendie seemed to have been taken by surprise with the news of the introduction and immediate widespread acceptance of ether inhalation for surgical operations and as a pharmacologist he decried the immediate human application without proper prior scientific knowledge and animal experimentation. He was also quite concerned with the possible moral consequences of ether inebriation, as he called it.

On the following Monday meeting, February 8th, Roux commented the letter which Magendie had written to the *Journal des Débats* in reference to such human experiments and its serious consequences.

Magendie explained the certain vivacity of his previous remarks on account of the extreme concern he had for experiments on man and stated that unfortunately he saw no reason to withdraw the essential meaning of his remarks.

He went on making statements on another type of problems.

"This type of inebriation very frequently causes dreams, which remarkably, start at the very instant the vapor is breathed. During such dreams sleep is not complete; one could even think that it does not exist."

"Without doubt ether inebriation can provoke, specially in women, erotic dreams, and even as one of them said, of complete love dreams *(rêves d'amour complet)*. Women thus inebriated have been seen to hurl themselves upon the operator, with gestures and propositions so expressive, that in this singular and novel situation, the danger is not for the patient but for the surgeon."

Such unexpected statements caused much hilarity from the Academicians interrupting temporarily the session. But, Magendie went on.

Je serait désespéré qu'on supposât que j'ai l'intention de provoquer l'hilarité; je regarde, au contraire, comme trés-graves ces conséquences de l'ivresse de l'éther. Je serait bien malhereux si ma femme, si ma fille avaient été le sujet de scènes analogues à celles dont j'ai été le temoin.

(I would be very unhappy if my wife or my daughter had been involved in scenes of this kind.)

Again Magendie was prescient in warning for the first time about the unrecognized possibilities of unforeseen dreams under such a state of ether inebriation and incomplete loss of consciousness.

To-day the rule is still followed that anesthesia should not be induced without the presence of another person, to avoid any such extraordinary or extravagant claims. Magendie was the first to express such a warning.

On the next meeting, on February 15th, Velpeau made a long pronouncement on the benefits and the dangers of ether and concluded by saying:

"...ether by preventing pain does not prevent operations from being dangerous and that the possibility of operating without suffering was not a reason to operate without necessity."

Magendie made his final comments and ended by saying:

"I do not wish to be misrepresented as the Apostle of Pain, and furthermore as resisting an useful discovery for the only reason that it was not made by me."

He never made further comments on ether at the Academy meetings.

It is remarkable that such a lucid person, who introduced experimental physiology and pharmacology, and was instrumental in the demise of Hippocratic Medicine and the Vital Force concept, failed to accept the veritable revolution in surgery caused by the discovery of ether inhalation. Perhaps his background as a vivisectionist and introducer of animal experimentation were the main factors in his abrupt and negative reaction. Some of his arguments were sound and others exaggerated but he uttered the first serious warnings as to possible complications of anesthesia which remain valid to this day. Nevertheless, the desire to abolish pain during surgery proved overwhelming and by-passed any precautions, immediately spreading the use of ether for surgical operations without any serious prior pharmacological experimentation in animals. Such experiments were a province of the physiologists like Flourens who was highly interested in the nervous system and immediately set himself to study the phenomenon.

References:

Olmsted JMD: François Magendie. Arno Press. New York 1981

Lichtenthaler C: Histoire de la Médecine. Fayard 1978

Deloyers l: François Magendie, 1783-1885. Presse Universitaires de Bruxelles 1970

Genty M: François Magendie. I Partie. Les Biographies Médicales. Revue Mensuelle Illustr. V. 9 N. 5. Mai 1935

Genty M: François Magendie. II Partie. Les Biographies Médicales. Revue Mensuelle Illustr. Volume 9, N. 6. Juin 1935

Lazorthes G et Campan L: François Magendie (1783-1855). Bull Acad Nation Md., 1984, 168. N.1-2, 105 -111. Sa'nce de 24 Janvier

Compte Rendu des Sa'nces de lAcadémie des Sciences. XXIV,

N. 5, 1er Février, 1847:134-138, 142-144

N. 6, 8 Février, 1847: 170-175

N. 7, 15 Février, 1847: 238-239

The Cushing Tradition Changes in Neuroanaesthesia within 40 Years

J. M. Horton, Cambridge, UK

Harvey Cushing was the founder of modern or twentieth century neurosurgery and his contributions are inextricably linked with the development of neuroanaesthesia. He introduced the first anaesthetic records, monitoring of blood pressure, local anaesthetic techniques for major surgery, and suggested controlled hypotension[1, 2, 3]. He also trained two of the founders of British Neurosurgery, Norman Dott of Edinburgh, Hugh Cairns of the London and Oxford, and influenced Geoffrey Jefferson of Manchester and over the years I have had the privilege of working either in departments they had founded or with neurosurgeons they had trained.[4, 5] From the standards set by Cushing neuroanaesthetists have a tradition to follow.

I wish to trace and review some of the developments in neuroanaesthesia from 1953 to 1990 from my personal experiences in London, Edinburgh, Cambridge and Hong Kong.

Although in the 1950's neuromuscular blockade and manually controlled ventilation were widely used for abdominal and thoracic surgery, it was still believed that spontaneous ventilation should be preserved for craniotomies, so that the integrity of respiration could be monitored, and it was customary to use the Magill breathing attachment, and nitrous oxide, oxygen and trichlorethylene vaporised from a Boyle bottle. The tachypnoea induced by the latter was controlled with intermittent doses of pethidine. Endotracheal intubation for neurosurgical cases at the London was accomplished with an induction dose of thiopentone, and an injection through the cricothyroid membrane of 4ml of 4% lignocaine, since Douglas Northfield did not approve of muscle relaxants (neuromuscular blockers). He did not know that I had used suxamethonium to facilitate intubation while we were in the anaesthetic room, and he was not there to see what was happening. Brain bulk was reduced by ventricular drainage and the surgeon had to be warned to hold on to the brain if there was a risk that the patient might cough.

In Edinburgh in 1960, the Department of Surgical Neurology was lead by Norman Dott who was well aware of the contributions already made by anaesthetists to neurosurgery[4]. By that time several people, the Australian, Diana Furness[6], Peter Mortimer of Bristol[7], Allan Brown of Edinburgh[8] and Andrew Hunter of Manchester[9] had realised that controlled mechanical ventilation with the use of neuromuscular blockers improved operating conditions, and so it became the practice to use controlled ventilation for all supratentorial craniotomies and spinal operations. Since positive pressure ventilation elevates the mean intrathoracic pressure[10], we tried to overcome this problem by using a negative pressure of up to 10 cm of water on the Newcastle 3 ventilator[11] and the Barnet ventilator, often by attaching the wall suction to the ventilator[12]. This practice was abandoned following adverse reports in the literature, observation of air trapping in the open chest, and that operating conditions did not seem to be improved[13, 14].

The introduction in 1960 and 1961 to the United Kingdom of the potent analgesics phenoperidine and then fentanyl lead to their use as analgesic supplements replacing pethidine, and reducing the need for inhalation agents[15]. Halothane gradually replaced trichlorethylene, but there were suspicions that it raised intracranial pressure, and it needed the late Gordon McDowall of Leeds to show us that this indeed was so.

Hyperosmolar Diuretics

In Edinburgh we used 100ml of 15% saline to control cerebral oedema, and urea when a commercial preparation became available. Both of these agents were very effective, but caused vicious skin sloughing of the skin if given extravenously or there was any extravasation. In 1961 mannitol became available, used at first in a 25% solution, but crystal formation in the bottles was such a problem that it was replaced by the 20% solution.

Elective Hypotension

I was introduced to hypotensive anaesthesia by Hale Enderby in 1951, at the Queen Victoria Hospital Plastic Surgery Unit at East Grinstead, and subsequently was always interested in its application to neurosurgery as part of a continuous search for improved and safer operating conditions for aneurysm surgery. In 1954 when at the London Hospital a friend gave me some trimetaphan given to her by a colleague in the United States, and I started to use it at the London.

By 1960, when I went to Edinburgh, Allan Brown had already evaluated and abandoned hypothermia and arteriotomy as hypotensive techniques for neurosurgery and the usual technique in the 1960's was to use trimetaphan. At that time I avoided using halothane as a supplement. In 1965 and 1966 we had an interesting time. Having visited Jack Small and Victor Campkin and their team in Birmingham, England, we did eighteen aneurysm cases, where under hypothermia, a cardiac pacemaker was inserted, tachycardia of 200 to 250 beats a minute induced, and with the fall in cardiac output the blood pressure rapidly and dramatically dropped. Such a technique was complicated, time consuming and dangerous and did not prove to be of any advantage[16,17].

In 1970 I had moved to Addenbrookes Hospital, Cambridge and at time there was renewed interest in the use of sodium nitroprusside (SNP) as a hypotensive agent. At first our pharmacy prepared it for me, and then a commercial preparation became available. I found that the tachyphylaxis and tachycardia seen with SNP unacceptable, but combined with a low concentration of halothane it provided a satisfactory and controllable level of hypotension, but this was later achieved by using isoflurane alone, with or without the aid of beta blockers. As the years have passed and neurosurgical techniques have become more sophisticated and improved, particularly with the introduction of the operating microscope, it has now been shown and is generally agreed that there is no place for elective hypotension in neurosurgery.

Brain Protection

With the growth of knowledge about intracranial pressure and cerebral blood flow and the effects of such 'physiological trespass', there had always been a search for techniques to provide 'brain protection'. Hypothermia had of course been one approach. In 1978, in Cambridge, I tried the use of high doses of thiopentone, 30mg/kg in fifty cases but found it to be of no benefit.

Head Injuries[18, 19]

In Edinburgh, Norman Dott and John Gillingham, and in Cambridge, Walpole Lewin had set up and developed specialised head injury units. Decerebrate spasms, hyperventilation and hypoxia were common observations in severe diffuse brain injuries, and it seemed that the lessons learned in the operating theatre could be applied to the patient in the ward. In 1960 we had in the head injury unit operating theatre in Ward 20 of the Edinburgh Royal Infirmary, one of the two Newcastle 3 ventilators which were available for the entire Hospital. The only other available ventilators in Edinburgh at that time were four Barnet ventilators, which belonged to Surgical Neurology at the Western General Hospital.

In 1964 after managing six serious head injuries with controlled ventilation, at the suggestion of John Gillingham, I went to the Ospedale Maggiore Hospital in Milan, to see Drs Mimmina Bozza and Marina Rossanda, who provided increased enthusiasm and inspiration for the use of the technique. They together with Emeric Gordon of Stockholm were the real pioneers of controlled ventilation and intensive care for head injuries and neurosurgery.

Air Embolism

In Edinburgh we conducted all explorations of the posterior fossa in the prone position, but in Cambridge, Walpole Lewin and his colleagues, and the Hong Kong neurosurgeons preferred the sitting position. The hazard of air embolism being well known I preferred to monitor the end-tidal CO_2, which gave adequate early warning of such an incident.

Neuroradiology

Before the introduction of the CT Scanner, the only way to outline the cerebral ventricles was by the introduction of air in to the ventricles. When this was performed by the lumbar route, lumbar air encephalography or LAEG, it was very uncomfortable for the patient. Combinations of the butyrophenones (Droperidol) and analgesics were used with some success to decrease nausea and discomfort. Ketamine, in spite of reports of increased intracranial pressure was successfully used and facilitated LAEG and then CT scans in children.

Hong Kong

The descendants of Cushing, be they anaesthetists or surgeons are now working all over the world and I have been privileged to work with many of them.

Conclusion

We have come a long way since this statement in an editorial the British Journal of Anaesthesia in 1965[2]

"However if the contribution of anaesthesia to neurosurgery is firmly established, its basis remains largely empirical. There is little precise knowledge of the numerous and interrelated ways in which anaesthetic agents influence surgical exposure of the brain. To extend this knowledge, and to participate in (initiate, even) the circumvention of those formidable anatomical and physiological obstacles which appear to bar the way to radical new progress in neurosurgery, is the challenge for the future."

Even though safer techniques and more sophisticated monitoring facilities are now available, a succesful outcome for many neurosurgical procedures will only be achieved with dedicated and meticulous attention to detail and close co-operation with surgical colleagues.[21]

References:

1. Beecher HK: The first anaesthesia records (Codman, Cushing). Surg Gynaec and Obstet 1940; 71: 689 -993

2. Cushing H: On routine determinations of arterial tension in operating room and clinic. Boston Medical and Surgical Journal 1903; 148: 250 - 256

3. Fulton JF: Harvey Cushing: A Biography. Springfield, Illinois, Charles C Thomas, 1946

4. Dott NM: Advances in Twentieth Century Neurology. Proceedings of the Royal Society of Medicine. 1971; 64 : 1051 - 1055

5. Rush C, Shaw J F: With Sharp Compassion. Norman Dott. Aberdeen University Press. 1990

6. Furness DN: Controlled respiration in neurosurgery. Br J Anaesth 1957; 29: 415

7. Mortimer PLF: Controlled respiration in neurosurgical anaesthesia. Anaesthesia 1959; 14: 205

8. Brown AS: Letter. Anaesthesia 1959; 14: 207

9. Hunter AR: Discussion on the value of controlled respiration in neurosurgery. Proceedings of the Royal Society of Medicine 1960; 53: 365

10. Opie LH, Spalding JM, Smith AC: Intrathoracic pressure during intermittent positive pressure respiration. Lancet 1961; i: 911

11. Horton JAG, Inkster JS, Pask EA: Two more respirators. Br J Anaesth. 1956; 28: 169

12. Maloney JV, Elam JO, Handford SW, Bolton GA, Eastwood DW, Brown EB, Ten Pas RH: Importance of negative pressure phase in mechanical respirators. JAMA 1953; 152: 212

13. Watson WE: Observations on physiological dead space during intermittent positive pressure respiration. Br J Anaesth 1962;34: 502

14. Galloon S, Rosen M: Trapping in the alveoli with positive-negative ventilation. Anaesthesia 1965; 20: 87

15. Brown AS, Horton JM, Macrae WR: Anaesthesia for neurosurgery. The use of haloperidol and phenoperidine with light general anaesthesia. Anaesthesia 1963;18:143 - 150

16. Brown AS, Horton JM: Elective Hypotension with Intracardiac Pacemaking in the operative management of ruptured intracranial aneurysms. Acta Anaesth Scand 1966; Supplement 23: 665

17. Gillingham FJ: Methods of circulatory arrest. In: Luyendijk W, ed Progress in Brain Research, Cerebral Circulation. Amsterdam-London-New York. Elsevier Publishing Company, 1968; 30: 367 - 376

18. Horton JM: The immediate care of head injuries. Anaesthesia 1975; 30: 212 - 218

19. Horton JM: The anaesthetist's contribution to the care of head injuries. Br J Anaesth 1976; 48: 767 -771

20. Horton JM: Current Aspects of Anaesthesia for Neurological Surgery. In: Zorab JSM ed. Lectures in Anaesthesiology. Blackwell Scientific Publications, Oxford. 1988. 2. 52 -64

21. Editorial Br J Anaesth. 1965. 37

The History of Neuroanaesthesia

I. Kiss
Department of Anaesthesiology; Alfried Krupp Hospital
Essen, Germany

The history of neuroanaesthesia starts with the history of anaesthesia in 1846. Earlier reports are of cultural interest, and I will not address them today. These last 150 years can be roughly divided into three parts. The first fifty years were dominated by trials of openly administered inhalational anaesthetics. During the second period, local anaesthesia was introduced. About the half of the operations were carried out under this technique, the others in inhalational anaesthesia, some neurosurgeons combined both. The third era started in 1957 with the general use of endotracheal intubation, muscle relaxation and controlled ventilation. From this date we can speak of *neuroanaesthesia*. The primary aim was no longer only to anaesthetize the patient and to ensure his survival of the operation, but also to find the right technique and drug.

The first neurosurgical operation under anaesthesia was probably performed in 1879 by Sir William MacEwen, a Scotsman, a pioneer of neurological surgery and anaesthesia as well[1]. The first *documented* neurosurgical operation under anaesthesia dates back to May 25, 1886 in Queens Square Hospital in London by Sir Victor Horsley[2]. He investigated already years before the effects of ether and chloroform in animals and in himself. Horsley paid special attention to the painful phases of craniotomy and administered chloroform in appropriate doses (Fig.1.) Neurosurgery underwent a boom between 1886 and 1896. More than 500 surgeons reported performing brain operations. During the following 10 years, this number dropped to below 80.

Technical advancements in the application of inhalational anaesthetics facilitated their use. Vernon Harcourt, a physical chemist, constructed for Horsley a vaporizer for chloroform, which was connected to a cylinder of compressed oxygen. Fedor Krause, the founder of German neurosurgery, used the Roth-Dräger oxygen-chloroform apparatus (1902), which permitted the application of 100% oxygen. The Ombrédanne ether inhaler was widely used in spite of the fact that the addition of oxygen or the removal of CO_2 was impossible. It could be used in patients in prone position as well.

Local anaesthesia with cocaine was first used in neurosurgery around 1900 by Kocher in Bern[3]. In 1904 procaine was introduced in clinical practice. The methode soon gained popularity. In 1917 Cushing recommended regional anaesthesia - the term comes from him - for all types of neurosurgery.

Harvey Cushing, the founder of modern neurosurgery, influenced the development of both neurosurgery and anaesthesia. In 1894, Codman and he developed charts to intraoperatively record pulse, respiration and temperature. He introduced pneumatic blood pressure measurement in the operating theatre, which he got know in Padova in 1900. He also suggested the use of continuous precordial auscultation during surgery[4].

The first anaesthetist specialised in this field was Dr. Zebulon Mennel - the father of neuroanaesthesia, as Hunter calls him - who already being an anaesthetist, was appointed to perform anaesthesia for neurosurgical operations in Queen's Square Hospital in 1911. He used a motor to drive air through an ether vaporizer and the mixture was connected to the intratracheal catheter. Mennel published his experiences very vividly[5]. At the same time, in 1911, Franz Kuhn in Kassel, Germany performed anaesthesia with intratracheal intubation for neurosurgical operations[6]. In 1935, Noel Gillespie in Oxford published his doctoral thesis entitled "Endotracheal nitrous oxide-oxygen-ether anesthesia in neurological surgery"[7]. In fact, endotracheal intubation was a very important advancement in neuroanaesthesia.

Local anaesthesia still had its proponents among the famous neurosurgeons. Olivecrona in Stockholm in 1936 operated on one of the best known Hungarian writers for an angiomatousus tumor in the posterior fossa. My Hungarian collegues sitting here all know the book by Frigyes Karinthy entitled "Travels around my cranium" in which he brilliantly described his illness, the operation under local anaesthesia in prone position and the postoperative course[8].

The new, third era of neuroanaesthesia was heralded by the works of Kety and Schmidt in the late forties. They measured cerebral blood flow and metabolism and identified the vasoconstriction of cerebral vessels following hyperventilation in humans[9].

In 1957, Diana Furness from Melbourne published a short paper in the British Journal of Anaesthesia in which she described a standard anaesthetic technique for neurosurgery[10]. This included the induction of anaesthesia with thiopentone, tracheal intubation following suxamethonium and local anaesthesia of the trachea, maintainance of anaesthesia with nitrous oxide-oxygen, muscle relaxation and controlled ventilation. Her statements still hold today.

The years to follow were filled with new developments in anaesthetic techniques.

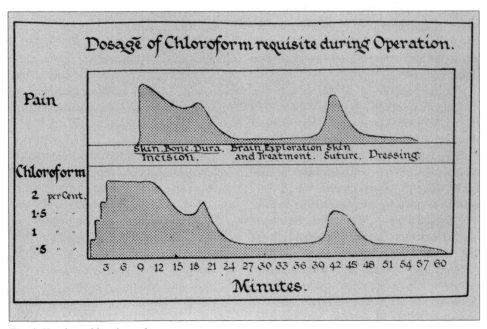

Fig. 1 Horsleys chloroform chart

Spontaneous breathing for detecting changes in respiratory patterns in posterior fossa procedures was used into the eighties. Hypothermia and circulatory arrest were introduced in cerebral vascular surgery, but were later abandoned because of high mortalitity (Fig.2.). Induced hypotension became generally done in the fifties and is still practised in aneurysma surgery. Its importance is declining since the routine use of temporary clips. In the eighties, brain protection, based on experimental works, primarly with barbiturates failed to show any significant clinical results.

Inhalational anaesthesia with halothane was for over ten years the most widely used technique of neuroanaesthesia. In 1967, Jennett and coworkers showed the detrimental effect of halothane in patients with already elevated intracranial pressure, which could not be corrected by hyperventilation[11]. Michenfelder from the Mayo Clinic, who for decades dominates neuroanaesthesia believes Jennetts opinion was based on technical failure, his patients were in fact not hyperventilated[12]. Anyway, halothane was abandoned from neuroanaesthesia. In the seventies neurolept anaesthesia became generally applied. The renaissance of inhalational anaesthesia came in the eighties with isoflurane.

The general introduction of microscopic neurosurgery in the seventies opened new fields for surgeons and inspired the development of anaesthesia. Neuroanaesthesia became a highly technical procedure. Anaesthetic managemant was generally extended into the pre- and postoperative phase of intensive care. Jennett and Teasadale from Glasgow elaborated standards for the evaluation and management of head injured patients in the seventies.

The first *Commission of Neuroanaesthesia* was founded by nine countries in Antwerp in 1960. In 1964, Hunter from Manchester published the first book on neuroanaesthesia[13]. The term Neuroanaesthesia was coined

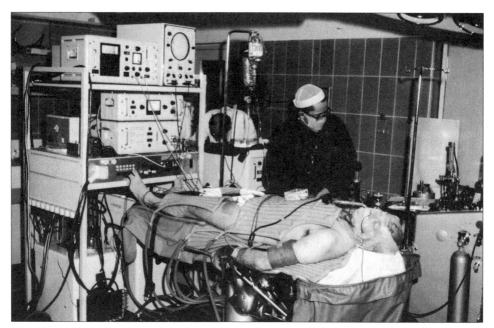

Fig. 2 Hypothermia for neurosurgical operation at Freiburg University, Germany (around 1970)

by Michenfelder in 1968. *The Journal of Neurosurgical Anesthesia* was started in the U.S. in 1989.

What is the state of art today and what is in store? Four days before the 40th anniversary of the lecture Diana Furness gave in Adalaide we cannot add much to her technique of neuroanaesthesia. Today we deepen anaesthesia with inhalational agents or opiates. There is no particular anaesthetic drug of great importance in neurosurgery. This fact was proved by Michael Todd, currently editor-in-chief of Anesthesiology. In 1993, he compared three anaesthetics for elective supratentorial craniotomy and found no difference in the short-term outcome[14].

As for the future I do not see significant changes looming in our practice. Neurosurgery itself is becoming less and less invasive, it does not inspire one to invest new anaesthetic methods. I would be pleasantly suprised if in twenty years listening to the same lecture I could hear revolutionary news about neuroanaesthesia.

References:

[1] Macewen W: Intracranial lesions. Lancet 1881; 2: 581-583

[2] Horsley V: Brain surgery. Br Med J 1886; 2:670-675

[3] Kocher TH: Hirnerschütterung, Hirndruck und chirurgische Eingriffe bei Hirnkrankheiten. Wien, Hölder 1901 p. 397

[4] Shepard DAE: Harvey Cushing and Anaesthesia. Can Anaesth Soc J 1965; 12: 431 442

[5] Mennel Z: Some difficulties which may occur in the administration of anaesthesia for some cerebral operations. Br J Anaesth 1930; 7: 52-58

[6] Kuhn F: Perorale Intubation. Berlin, Karger, 1911 pp 124-125

[7] Gillespie NA: Endotracheal nitrous oxid-oxygen-ether anaesthesia in neurological surgery. Anesth Analg 1935; 14:225-229

[8] Karinthy F: Utázs a koponyám körül. Budapest 1937

[9] Kety SS, Schmidt CF: The effect of active and passive hyperventilation on cerebral blood flow, cerebral oxygen consumption, cardiac output, and blood pressure of normal young men. J Clin Invest 1946; 25:107-119

[10] Furness D: Controlled respiration in neurosurgery. Br J Anaesth 1957; 29:415-418

[11] Jennet WB, McDowall DG, Barker J : The effect of halothane on intracranial pressure in cerebral tumors. J Neurosurg 1967; 26:270-274

[12] Michenfelder JD: The 27th Rovenstein Lecture. Neuroanaesthesia and the achievement of professional respect. Anesthesiology 1989; 70:695-701

[13] Hunter AR: Neurosurgical Anaesthesia. Blackwell, Oxford 1964

[14] Todd M, Warner D, Sokoll M. et al: A prospective comparative trial of three anesthetics for supratentorial craniotomy: Fentanyl/Propofol, Isoflurane/NO and Fentanyl/NO. Anesthesiology 1993; 78:1005-1020

The Introduction of Lidocain (Xylocain): Holger Erdtman and Nils Löfgren

M. Andreen
Department of Anaesthesie and Intensive Care
Danderyd Hospital, Danderyd, Sweden

I am going to tell you the story about the discovery of a new drug which has contributed to the development of anaesthesia in a very decisive way.

The drug is lidocain, or Xylocain, a local anaestetic, less toxic, with a longer period of action and faster onset than procain, which is the best local anaesthetic available since 1905.

I have learnt the story from my dearly appreciated teacher and close friend Torsten Gordh who introduced me to the fascinating world of anaesthesia, who plays an important role in this exiting story and whom you can see on this delightful photograph where he is preparing for an injection - maybe of Xylocain.

How did it all start? Like many other of the world's greatest discoveries it started with someone who was looking for something quite different. In fact this someone was studying the association of biochemistry and genetically inherited properties.

His name was Hand von Euler - a German chemist - and a pioneer in biochemistry, who had been working at the Stockholm University for many years. He had come to Stockholm/Sweden at the age 23 in 1896 to work with the famous Professor Svante Arrhenius. Twentythree years later he received the Nobel Prize along with Sir Arthur Harden from London, awarding their work on fermentation. It was after von Euler had been rewarded with the Nobel Prize in 1929 that he got deeply involved in chemical genetics and his research aimed at was finding answers to physiological properties based on chemistry. Among other things he focused on certain mutants of barley - in this case clorophyll-deficient plants - which seemed to be more resistant against vermin, than "normal" strains of barley. Extensive studies were undertaken and alcoholic extracts of these mutated barley plants were prepared and analyzed with V-spectroscopy. Supported by these investigations, typical absorption bands of an indol-derivative could be identified. The compound responsible for this absorption band was isolated by von Euler and co-workers in 1933.

An analysis of the chemical clements was performed so that the net formula could be determined. It was carbon 11, hydrogen 14, nitrogen 2. Based on different chemical tests it was concluded that the compound - which was called gramin - most probably was a dimentyl aminomethyl substituted indole.

Von Euler was eager to determine the exact chemical structure of this compound which he thought could be used as an agricultural insecticide.

Now another important character in this story comes into the picture. That is Holger Erdtman - a young and very clever chemist - who was given the task to synthesize gramin. From what was known about the compound (net formula, absorption characteristics) he realized that there were two, possible structures -isomeres - that could correspond to the elemental analysis of the compound. He began to synthesize one of them - realiging that the product that he had manufactured was not gramin - it was the isomer which he called isogramin. This certainly led to disappointment.

But, being a proper chemist and scientist, he tasted some of the material that he had produced. To his surprise he found that this tongue got numb, i.e. anaesthetized. That was an interesting observation that he could not ignore.

On the other hand, the job that he had been given was to synthesize gramin. Suddenly a report on a German group led by Theodore Wieland was published, since they had synthesized gramin. This surely was a scientific defeat for the Nobel Prize winner and his talented assistant, and they were not too happy having to face this fact. But Erdtman was freed from further gramin-studies and enabled to dig into the isogramin molecule and explore its remarkable qualities.

(Before we turn front the gramin story, let me just tell you that several groups of chemists had isolated the compound pretty much at the same time. Among them was a Russian group who named the alkaloid donaxin because it was isolated - not from rye - but from Arundo donax - a huge grass which had evoked their scientific interest, because it was believed that the camels in Siberia would not eat that grass.

Finally, it was shown that the clorophyll-deficient - but gramin-containing - strains of barley were not especially resistant to vermin - after all. Exit gramin!)

Erdtman now allowed himself to become totally absorbed in exploring the interesting substance that caused surface anaesthesia of the tongue when you tasted it. The only problem was that it was rather difficult to synthesize isogramin that proved to be poisonous, too. So, Erdtman thought that this dangerous quality of isogramin might even be present in the ingredients for the synthesis of isogramin, which was true, in deed. In the procedure of synthesizing isogramin an anilide was produced as a intermediate and when Erdtman tasted it his tongue got anaesthetized!

Anilides belong to a class of compounds that were much easier to manufacture and Erdtman felt that it could be promising a field to be explored.

In 1935 another important person enters the scene: Nils Loefgren - a promising young chemist working at the Chemical Institute of the university in Stockholm being very interested in the association of chemical structure and physiological effects live Erdtman. Together they synthesized 16 anilide compounds with an anaesthetizing property. But, when the substances were tested in the physiology laboratory they did not appear to be superior to procain which terminared Erdtman's interest in localey anaesthetizing anilides. He gave up looking for a local anaesthetic that could replace procain. Call their results were published in a Swedish chemical journal in 1937. Erdtman left the chemical institute of the University soon and took a position at the Royal Institution of Technology in Stockholm where he, became a very succesful professor in a few years time.

Loefgren, stayed at the institute as a lecturer and as a reseacher. He was very busy teaching, so his research had been put to rest for a while. He could not forget the captivating search for a local anaesthetic having had the opportunity to take part.

Let us review the situation concerning local anaesthetics at the time!

It all started with Carl Koller - the father of local anaesthesia - who demonstrated the anaesthetic properties of cocaine. This was reported in 1884 for the first time in Heidelberg at a Congress for ophtalmologists.

In 1905 Alfred Einhorn had managed to synthesize procain, a drug similar to cocaine, that became unsurpassed local anaesthetic for the following 40 years. Chemical and pharmaceutical industry tried to invent new anaesthetic substances, though, very few of them were useful due to toxic and irritating effects. Thus procain was finally looked upon as the ultimate local anaesthetic or as close as close could be. But it was far from ideal: it had delayed onset, a short action and shoud significant toxicity.

Obviously, Loefgren must have been aware of the fact that procain was not the answer to a surgeon's or anaesthetist's demand as a good local anaesthetic.

After a while Loefgren took up research on the anilid-compounds and their anaesthetic properties again. He systematically started to synthesize new substances with the same basic compounds, though with a new approach to the molecular structure.

All new substances in this series were given codes. One of them was called LL30 and like the rest of the newly synthesized substances it was tested for local anaesthetic properties by putting it on the tongue. If it proved to be effective it was put on a shelf for further examination. LL30 was probably put on the shelf some time in 1942.

This is when Bengt Lundqvist appears. Lundqvist was a chemist, too, but he had a different approach to testing and evaluating these substances than Loefgren. He believed that putting them on the tongue did not suffice when evaluating the anaesthetic effect. Lundqvist started to inject the new substances into his body, performing various types of nerve blocks though finger blocks seem to have been the most commonly used technique. He even performed spinal blocks- on himelf. A very dangerous business...

He was a sincere investigator and not having any experimental animals at his disposal, he played the part of a guniea pig. He was not a medical doctor and he knew nothing about nerve blocks and also very little about risks in medical practice, but he realized that they needed a more sophisticated model than the tongue testing to be able to estimate and validate the local anaesthetic properties more specifically. (He lend a textbook on regional anaesthesia from one of his friends who was a medical student and who had lend this book from one of his teachers, Dr Torsten Gordh!).

Relating to these rather heroic but systematically performed tests, Bengt Lundqvist was able to tell Nils Loefgren, that his compound LL30 was the best local anaesthetic substance that existed!

Loefgren was the elder one, he was the teacher, extremely intelligent, talented in many ways, he was a musician, an excellent lecturer, a chemical artist, very accurate but at the same time intuitive as far as his work was concerned. He became a professor -although he did not bother to keep the position very long because of heaps of tedious administrative tasks that came along with the title. He received many awards and prizes for his work on Xylocain.

Lundqvist was the younger one, he was the pupil, a shy and lonely person who loved physical challenges, he was a keen fencer and sailor. Unfortunately he died at the age of 30 from the sequelae of a head injury that he had contracted when falling down the stairs in the institute - probably under the influence of some chemical compound that he had tested on himself.

The experiment that Lundqvist performed on himself early in 1943 lead to the promising results and the conclusion made by Lundqvist. This year is the most important year in this story and I dare say the story of local anaesthesia!

If this substance was to become a pharmaceutical drug you had to investigate and define its toxicity first.

In order to do so, Loefgren turned to Leonard Goldberg, who was a Ph. D. in medical pharmacology at the Karolinska Institute and had a modern laboratory with ample resources at his disposal. He was outstanding in the field of statistical analysis of biological variation. Gladly he accepted to carry out the toxicological studies on the compound LL30. In less than fourteen days, hundreds of mice later he concluded that LL 30 was the best local anaesthetic existing surely relating it to procain. Its LD 50 was well above and its effectiveness far better that that of procain. In fact it was 3-4 times less toxic and 3 times as effective as procain and superior to it in duration as well.

Now Loefgren was convinced that LL 30 was a major hit. In May he and Lundqvist met the chief executive of the research department of the Astra company who admitted that he was interested in buying the substance.

Loefgren was worried that the news about their discovery of the new local anaesthetic and its relatively simple chemical structure would be spread. Goldberg, for instance, gare lectures on LL 30 when appointed as an associate professor of the Institute. That was on the 29th of May, ...

On the 15 th of July Loefgren and Lundqvist applied for a patent on the method for the synthesis of LL 30. In August, Loefgren and Lundqvist met member of the board of the Pharmacia company who got the licence for the drug for two weeks at the cost of 5000 Swedish crowns. They never came back to the inventors after these two weeks to complete their business. I guess, they must have regretted this...

(Instead quite unexpectedly, the science attaché of the US embassy in Stockholm invited Loefgren and Lundqvist to an informal meeting offering them US $ 25000 for this new wonder-drug. This event illustrates the turmoil their discovery raised.)

Rumours came up about several other pharmaceutical companies making different offers to Loefgren and Lundqvist in order to purchase the substance but no business was done. Until..

The Astra drug company finally bought the patent-application and the rights to market and distribute LL 30 world wide in November 1943. Loefgren and Lundqvist were guaranteed royalty of 4% on all sales and received 15000 Swedish crowns for the contract. Now Astra took over.

A method for producing the compound had to be set up. This proved to be a big problem as to the lack of raw material. (World War II) A name was chosen for the drug: Xylocain. Applications for patents in 27 different countries were delivered.

In 1945 Astra was able to produce Xylocain on a semi-large scale and clinical tests were carried out by Torsten Gordh who was the only anaesthetist in Sweden at that time working at the Karolinska Hospital. He started the tests with great enthusiasm and valuable support and assistance from a young medical student who later became his wife - Ulla Gordh. Torsten had heard rumours about this promising substance that had been synthesized at the University and he was obviously very interested in having a new local anaesthetic with better qualities than procain.

Torsten Gordh started the investigations by performing a series of blind wheal tests and the results showed that Xylocain had outstanding properties in terms of latency, duration and absence of local reactions. So he moved on to clinical studies in daily routine. More than 400 anaesthesias utilizing Xylocain, with or without adrenalin were performed and evaluated within this study. The results were excellent. This was a drug that surpassed procain in every aspect. Similar tests were carried our in dentistry leading to equally satisfying results.

Torsten presented his clinical results with Xylocain in 1947 at a meeting of the Swedish Anaesthesia Club that became the Swedish Society for Anaesthesia and Intensive Care later on. The following year Xylocain finally was registered on the 16 th of January 1948 and released on the Swedish market. Other countries were to follow soon.

The author of the first international paper to appear on Xylocain was Torsten Gordh. It was published in Anesthesia in 1949.

The year before he wrote an article on his clinical experience with Xylocain in the Swedish Medical Journal. The reason why the publications on Xylocain did not appear until 1948 and 49 respectively, resulted from the lengthy procedure to obtain the patent. Loefgren just did not want the knowledge about Xylocain to become public until he was sure that no one else could copy the molecule.

From the article in the Swedish medical journal I quote: "The introduction of a new local anaesthetic is only justified if it has advantages over already accepted. The experience hotherto show that we, in lidocaine, have gotten a drug with these qualifications. It will fulfill the classic requirements of an ideal local anaesthetic, as it has low toxicity, is non irritant to tissues, is water soluble, can be sterilized and permits storage with adrenalin. Lidocain has further, a fast and efficient effect with sufficient duration, and is, in my opinion, the most ideal of hitherto-known local anaesthetics. It is further remarkably useful in all areas, where any form of local anaesthesia can be performed".

That final remark is still valid and I dare to claim that the discovery of Loefgren and Erdtman and the investigations of Bengt Lundqvist, Leonard Goldberg and Torsten Gordh had an impact on anaesthetic practice and enabled modern anaesthesia and pain therapy to take a major step forward.

I can not help wondering what would have happened if Erdtman had synthesized gramine instead of isogramine which was his objective! Gramine is not a local anaesthetic. If you put it on the tongue nothing happens except that it tastes nasty. Would Xylocain never have been synthesized? And what about the development of regional anaesthetic techniques as valuable tools in surgical anaesthesia and in pain therapy??

Anyhow, by mistake we got Xylocain and..

The rest of the stroy you all know. Many local anaesthetics were to follow lidocain. Prilocain, mepivacain, bupivacain and all the others but it started with LL 30.

Astra has recently celebrated the 50 th anniversary of the synthesis of Xylocain by reluating this beautiful review of its history.

Development of Anaesthesiology and Intensive Therapy in Czechoslovakia after World War II

J. Pokorný, Postgraduate Medical School, Prague, Czech Republic

The beginnings of clinical anaesthesiology in the former Czechoslovakia are to be found in the early years after World War II. The father of professional anaesthesiology in the former Czechoslovak Republic was Dr. Lev Spinadel. He studied the speciality in Great Britain during the war. His teachers were Sir R. R. Macintosh, F. Bannister and S. Rowbotham. Following his return to Prague after the war, Spinadel decided not only to offer his skills and knowledge to some prominent surgeon, but also to develop anaesthesiology as a medical speciality and science.

After having been confronted by negative viewpoints of academic representatives of surgery, Dr. Spinadel was finally accepted by the Chief of the Army Medical Service who, on January 1, 1948, founded the first Department of Anaesthesiology in the country at the Central Army Hospital in Prague - with Spinadel

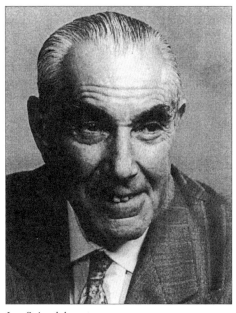

Lev Spinadel

Lev Spinadel, MD., PhD.
founder of medical speciality Anaesthesiology in Czechoslovakia
(1897-1970)

1924	graduated in medicine – Prague, Czechoslovakia
1941	residency in Anaesthesiology – United Kingdom (R. R. Macintosh, F. Bannister, S. Rowbotham)
1948-1956	Head of **First Department of Anaesthesiology in Czechoslovakia** – in the Central Army Hospital
1950	author of monograph <u>Clinical Anaesthesiology</u>
1955-1957	lecturer of anaesthesiology in the Postgraduate Medical School in Prague
1956-1970	researcher in the Czechoslovak Academy of Sciences

> **Jana Pastorová, MD., Assoc. Prof.**
> surgeon
>
> | | |
> |---|---|
> | 1949 | scholarship in anaesthesiology - Oxford, UK |
> | 1950 | text-book **General Anaesthesia**, 1st ed. |
> | 1955 | representative of Czechoslovakia on the **1st World Congress of Anaesthesiology** – Scheveningen |
> | 1958 | text-book **General Anaesthesia**, 2nd ed. |
> | 1952-1959 | Chairwoman of the **Committee for Anaesthesiology** in the Czechoslovak Surgical Society |

at its head. This department has attracted many enthusiasts who have visited it for either short or long periods of time in order to learn the principles of modern anaesthesiology.

However, in late 1940 and early 1950, there were physicians in large hospitals who, independently of Dr. Spinadel's department, devoted themselves to anaesthesiology in the framework of surgery. Dr. J. Pastorová, staff member of the 1st Surgical Clinic, was awarded a scholarship in 1949 by the Rockefeller Foundation for a 6 month study stay in Oxford and she studied anaesthesiology at the Nuffield Department of Anaesthesiology. Pastorová is the author of the first textbook on general anaesthesia, published in 1950.

She initiated courses and lectures for students and physicians and was also the representative of Czechoslovak anaesthesiology at the 1st World Congress of Anaesthesiology in 1955 at Scheveningen. Also laying the foundation at the 1st Surgical Clinic for Czechoslovak anaesthesiology was Dr. Josef Hoder, later Associate Professor and President of the Czechoslovak Society of Anaesthesiology and Resuscitation - and a pioneer of the speciality in our country.

In the early 1950s at the Clinic of Paediatric Surgery in Prague, Dr. Miloslav Drapka started professional paediatric anaesthesia and was a pioneer in this particular branch of anaesthesiology.

> **Josef Hoder, MD., PhD., Assoc. Prof.**
> (1912-1987)
>
> | | |
> |---|---|
> | 1959-1961 | Chairman **Committee for Anaesthesiology** in the Czechoslovak Surgical Society |
> | 1961-1971 | Chairman **Czechoslovak Society for Anaesthesiology** |
> | 1971-1973 | Chairman **Czechoslovak Society for Anaesthesiology and Resuscitation** |
> | 1980-1987 | Head **Clinic for Anaesthesiology and Resuscitation**, Charles University in Prague |
> | | - / - |
> | 1970 | President of the III. European Congress of Anaesthesiology in Prague |

> **Miloslav Drapka, MD.**
> (1911-)
> **founder of paediatric anaesthesia in Czech Republic**
>
> 1950s   **leading anaesthesiologist** in the Clinic for Paediatric Surgery, University Hospital Prague
> 1959-1978   Head, **Department of Anaesthesiology**, University Hospital Prague
> -/-
> 1953   introduced CPAP and PEEP into paediatric inhalation anaesthesia

At the Plzeň University Hospital, there was "the man of the hour", Dr. J. Minář, PhD. (1917-1971), who devoted himself fully to anaesthesiology from late 1940ties. He has contributed considerably to the country-wide development of modern anaesthesiology, as well as the establishment of respect among surgeons for our profession. He is also one of the three main authors/editors of the 1965 monograph, Anaesthesiology.

In 1947, orthopaedic surgeon Dr. M Hrdlica (1910-1983) began working exclusively in the field of anaesthesiology at the Brno University Hospital. His teacher of anaesthesiology was surgeon, Professor B. Hejduk, who had completed the full course in anaesthesiology in Great Britain. Dr. Hrdlica studied, developed and practised all type of modern anaesthesia. Through his expertise, he made it possible for his surgical partners to build up in Brno an internationally acknowledged cardiosurgical centre, with Prof. J. Navrátil as Head Professor.

In Slovakia, the father of anaesthesiology is Associate Professor T. Kadlic (1913-). From 1967 to 1983, he was head of the Chair and Cli-

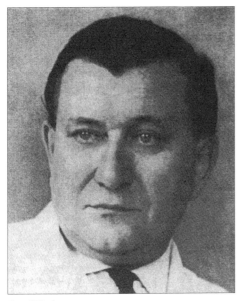

Josef Hoder

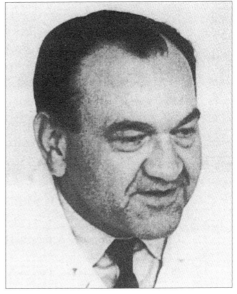

Jiri Minář

nic of Anaesthesiology and Resuscitation at the Postgraduate Medical School in Bratislava.

In early 1950, surgeons felt the urgent objective necessity to develop modern anaesthesiology and created the Committee for Anaesthesiology in 1952 as part of the Czechoslovak Surgical Society, with Pastorová as the first Chairman. This Committee concentrated the physicians' interest in developing this new branch of medicine and were successful in cooperating with the Ministry of Health. An important result of their endeavor was the incorporation in 1955 of anaesthesiology as an officially acknowledged medical speciality. Anaesthesiology was incorporated into the Chair of Surgery and Dr. L. Spinadel took over the responsibility for teaching and examinations until 1957. In 1950, Spinadel authored the first comprehensive monograph on anaesthesiology. He was succeeded by Hugo Keszler, who held the position until 1968. Keszler left Czechoslovakia after the invasion by the armies of the Warsaw Pact in August 1968. I was then nominated as Head of the Chair for Anaesthesiology and in 1972 for Anaesthesiology and Resuscitation, and held that position until the end of 1990.

In Slovakia, the second Postgraduate Medical School began activities in 1957.

Jiri Minář, MD., PhD.
(1917-1971)

late 1940s	leading **anaesthesiologist**, Surgical Clinic, University Hospital Plzeň (Pilsen)
1958	Head, **Department of Anaesthesiology**, University Hospital Plzeň (Pilsen)
- / -	
1965	monograph **Anaesthesiology**

Miloslav Hrdlica, MD.
(1910-1983)

1947	leading **anaesthesiologist,** 2nd Surgical Clinic, University Hospital Brno
1953-1966	regional **expert in anaesthesiology** for Southern Moravia
1958-1966	Head, **Department of Anaesthesiology**, University Hospital Brno
1967-1975	**Expert-Anaesthesiologist** – in University Hospital Greifswald, Germany

Tomás Kadlic, MD., Assoc. Prof.
(1913-)
pioneer of Anaesthesiology in Slovak Republic

1967-1983	Head, Chair and Clinic of Anaesthesiology, Postgraduate Medical School, Bratislava

Until 1983, the Slovak representative of anaesthesiology was T. Kadlic and his successor in Bratislava is M. Májek.

The Committee for Anaesthesiology of the Czechoslovak Surgical Society achieved independence in 1962 as the Czechoslovak Society for Anaesthesiology - in 1972 as Anaesthesiology and Resuscitation - with J. Hoder as the first President.

Due to systematic cooperation of the pioneers of anaesthesiology with the Ministry of Health, the structure and scope of anaesthesiological service has grown from individual anaesthesiologists in hospitals in late 1950s to Departments of Anaesthesiology in the 1960s and 1970s. Beginning in large hospitals in the 1970s, Departments of Anaesthesiology have, step-by-step, extended their activities to the field of intensive therapy - and ITUs have completed their structure. Such departments - Clinics of Anaesthesiology and Resuscitation in teaching hospitals - are responsible for the teaching of students and physicians. Parallel with this development, anaesthesiology was officially acknowledged in 1971 as one of twenty basic medical specialities - with primary and final degrees - and enlarged by intensive therapy with the official designation of Anaesthesiology and Resuscitation. The educational programme for full qualification requires residency for a minimum of 6.5 years.

In addition, nurses are offered the possibility of attaining a specializtion in anaesthesiology, resuscitation and intensive care. In former Czechoslovakia, anaesthesiology and resuscitation were, for a number of years, perceived by the Medical Faculties in universities as an exclusively postgraduate medical specialization. As a result, basic information was given to students for a long time by surgeons and anaesthesiologists. After 1980, a

---

Prof. Jiri Pokorny, MD., DSc., FRCA
(1924-)

1950	graduated in medicine - Charles University Prague
1956-1972	Head, **Department of Anaesthesiology** in the Central Army Hospital Prague
1972-1990	Head, **Clinic of Anaesthesiology and Resuscitation** in the University Hospital Prague-Motol
1969-1990	Head, **Chair for Anaesthesiology and Resuscitation** in the Postgraduate Medical School, Prague
since 1970s	lecturer for medical students on the Charles University
- / -	
1961	monograph **Anaesthesiological Technics**, 1st ed.
1964	monograph **Anaesthesiological Technics**, 2nd ed.
1965	monograph **Anaesthesiology**
1981	text-book **Emergency Medicine**
1989	text-book **Emergency and Disaster Medicine**
1996	book **Anaesthesiology and Resuscitation in the Czech and Slovak Republics on the Way to Professional Independence**

Professional Bodies

1952 – **Committee for Anaesthesiology** in the Czechoslovak Surgical Society, section in the Czechoslovak Medical Society J. E. Purkyně
1961 – **Czechoslovak Society for Anaesthesiology**, section in the Czechoslovak Medical Society J. E. Purkyně
1971 – **Czechoslovak Society for Anaesthesiology and Resuscitation**
1993 – **Slovak Society for Anaesthesiology and Intensive Medicine**
1994 – **Czech Society for Anaesthesiology, Resuscitation and Intensive Medicine**

Structure of Anaesthesiological Service

1948 <u>First</u> **Department of Anaesthesiology** in the Central Army Hospital in Prague
since 1957 **"Institutional Anaesthesiologist"** – Individuals in Hospitals
since 1960 **Departments of Anaesthesiology** in hospitals
since 1970 **Departments of Anaesthesiology and Resuscitation** (with ITU) in large hospitals
since 1980 **Clinics of Anaesthesiology and Resuscitation** (with ITU) in teaching hospitals

Education in Anaesthesiology and Resuscitation

A) Postgraduate Medical Schools (Prague, Bratislava)

1955 **Anaesthesiology** acknowledged medical speciality as higher specialization over: surgery, obstetrics & gynaecology, internal medicine, paediatrics
Residency Time 3 years

1971 **Anaesthesiology and Resuscitation** is basic medical speciality
Residence Time – primary degree ... 2,5 years
– final degree ... <u>4,0</u> years
total 6,5 years

B) Medical Faculties on Universities (pregraduate education)

1960s **sporadic** lectures and seminars
1980s **planned** lectures, seminars, examinations. Extension into Emergency and Disaster Medicine

new attitude was accepted and anaesthesiologists are now giving lectures to students not only in their profession, but also in the fields of emergency and disaster medicine.

Czechoslovak anaesthesiologists were busy organizing international contacts. However, these efforts were severely limited for 40 years by the conditions dictated by the Cold War. Nevertheless, landmarks of activities were the 1st Symposium of Anaesthesiology in 1965 and the III European Congress of Anaesthesiology in 1970 held in Prague, the 1977 International Congress of Anaesthesiologists in Bratislava and the 1989 International Congress on Emergency and Disaster Medicine in Piešt'any, Slovakia.

During the years of building up the speciality, 35 professional textbooks and monographs by Czech and Slovak authors were published. Since 1953, the Reference Journal of Anaesthesiology and Resuscitation, founded by L. Spinadel and J. Drábková, has been a most important link for our colleagues with the world's professional literature. Since 1990, the independent journal, fully devoted to anaesthesiology and immediate care, with J. Počta as editor-in-chief, covers the need for a professional forum.

The rapid development of anaesthesiology and resuscitology with intensive therapy has created the following challenge to medicine: give the chance everywhere to save threatened lives because the human organism is "too good to die".

The reaction to this maxim in Czechoslovakia was the concept of Differentiated Patient Care that was accepted in 1974. According to the concept, the level of medical care to be given to a patient is according to the level of threat to life and to the patient's prognosis.

There are five degrees of Differentiated Patient Care:

1. Resuscitative Care: For patients in acute failure of one or more vital functions. To be provided in Departments of Anaesthesiology and Resuscitation (Intensive Therapy).

2. Intensive Care: For patients who are seriously ill and without this care would be expected to develop failure of vital functions.

3. Standard Care: For patients who are not life-threatened.

4. Long-term and Rehabilitation Care: For patients who are expected to regain health and working activity.

5. Symptomatic Care: For patients who are close to or in a terminal state.

Another consequence of the development of anaesthesiology and resuscitation has been the ongoing creation in this country of a modern and quite effective Emergency Medical Service System and the development of Disaster Medicine.

After fifty years of development - from the most modest of beginnings with only a few enthusiasts - we can currently see a well-established medical profession with several branches (anaesthesiology and resuscitation in cardiovascular and transplant surgery, a pain clinic and Emergency and Disaster Medicine). Members of the Society of Anaesthesiology, Resuscitation and Intensive Medicine now number close to 1,300 physicians as well as hundreds of nurses and the Society is holding a strong and important position in Czech medicine.

Emergency Medical Service

District Centres of Rescue Service

Regional Centres of Rescue Service – include Air Rescue

Integrated Rescue System – includes Disaster Medicine

References:

[1] Spinadel L: Klinická anestesiologie (Clinical Anaesthesiology). Naše vojsko Prague 1950

[2] Keszler H, Minář J, Pokorný J: Anestesiologie (Anaesthesiology). SZdN Prague 1965

[3] Keszler H, Pastorová J, Jadrný J, Fencl V: Resuscitace (Resuscitation). SZdN Prague 1963

[4] Pokorný J, Bohuš O: et al. Anesteziologie a resuscitace v České a Slovenské republice na cestě k oborové samostatnosti (Anaesthesiology and Resuscitation in the Czech and Slovak Republics: Development to professional independence). PVS Prague 1996

Walter Kausch – a Pioneer in Parenteral Nutrition

K. Stinshoff, Berlin, Germany

Up to now, Walther Kausch's (1865-1928) work has rarely been discussed or appreciated and his contribution as a clinical surgeon and researcher is known to few, even in Germany. However, two American surgeons have acknowledged his achievements; Owen H. Wangensteen, a former professor of surgery at the University of Minnesota made the following comment on Kausch on 11 September 1979 in an address to the International Surgical Group in San Francisco: "It should be noted that the radical pancreatic resection for cancer has returned to the Kausch manoeuvre....it is, therefore, improper to speak of today's radical pancreaticoduodenectomy as the Whipple procedure"[1]. Wangensteen was referring to Kausch's pioneering achievement, which is still unappreciated, of carrying out the first successful partial pacreaticoduodenectomy in the world on 21 August 1909. His contributions in another sphere were referred to in Robert Elman's book "Parenteral Alimentation in Surgery"[2] on the subject of intravenous nutrition. "The idea [of parenteral intravenous nutrition] was gaining ground however, for Kausch, a German surgeon, in 1911 stated categorically that postoperative patients unable to take food by mouth or rectum urgently need nourishment and therefore must be fed artificially".

In his book, Elman describes in detail Kausch's procedures for parenteral nutrition. Before enlarging on his intravenous therapy work though, it is of interest to consider his unorthodox but impressive career. Kausch began his academic and clinical career at the

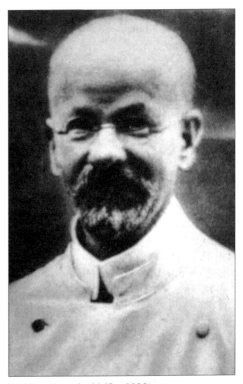

Walther Kausch (1865 – 1928)

University Hospital of Strasbourg in Alsace where he did a two year course in neurology and psychiatry. He then moved to Naunyns Medical Clinic where he went through a full course of training in internal medicine and became a lecturer in this subject. The clinic in Strasbourg was the leading diabetes research centre of his time and it was there that Oskar Minkowski (1858-1931) and Freiherr Josef von Mering (1849-1908) proved the existence of pancreatic diabetes in 1889. Here,

Kausch became a recognised expert in diabetes and remained so in his later surgical career.

In 1896, Kausch moved to the University Surgical Clinic of Breslau (Wroclaw) to work with Johannes von Mikulicz (1850-1905), who was looking for a fully trained internist for his large surgical department. Kausch was so fascinated by von Mikulicz and surgical work that he went through a complete course of surgical training, wrote a professorial thesis and was appointed Professor of Surgery in 1903. In 1906, Kausch took over the Directorship of the Auguste-Viktoria-Hospital in Berlin-Schöneberg. As already mentioned, he performed the first successful pancreaticoduodenectomy here in 1909.

Part of his success was due to his pre-operative and post-operative management. At this time he had already worked for several years on the use of highly concentrated sugar solutions for intravenous nutrition. After animal experiments with various substances, he decided on glucose as the best fuel for the body. In 1910 he had over 40 patients who had received up to 10% glucose solutions intravenously. For all patients, quantitative urine analysis, blood sugar tests and other metabolic examinations were carried out. Kausch found surprisingly small quantities of sugar in the urine. Harmful side-effects and discomfort were not observed. In his 1911 publication "On intravenous and subcutaneous nourishment with glucose", Kausch clearly favoured the intravenous application of 10% glucose solutions, and he justified this by pointing to the high tolerance of glucose by the body and the fact that he had demonstrated its almost complete assimilation. He also described how he had prepared an extremely frail patient with a carcinoma of the papilla for the necessary operation by treating him for several days with intravenous glucose infusions. In his 1912 work, he described how useful such infusions are for post-operative treatment[3].

Patients who were in a poor condition benefited especially from infusions which could provide them with 500 or more calories and 2 to 3 litres of fluid. Visible veins at the elbow or in the arm were preferred for the infusions. At the beginning of 1911, Kausch introduced a new infusion needle which he had developed. Among other features, it had a three-way tap which was a further innovation. Kausch, who compared intravenous with subcutaneous techniques - which were common at the time, was enthusiastic about intravenous feeding with glucose: "The capacity of the body to accept and utilise sugar infused intravenously or subcutaneously - i.e. into the greater circulation - in such doses and over such a long period is a surprising phenomenon and has not yet been exploited in practice". Kausch introduced intravenous therapy into everyday clinical work - at least in his own clinic. His achievements in this area are recognised in the literature. He is listed by Levenson et al[6] beside Claude Bernard (1813-1878), Albert Landerer (1854-1904), Briedl (?) and Kraus (?). As early as 1850, Bernard had treated dogs with intravenous sugar solutions, and in contrast to the findings with cane sugar, he interpreted the lack of glucose in the urine as a sign of its assimilation[3].

Landerer's great achievement in this field at the end of the 19th century, as Felix Mendel (1862-1925) described in 1908, was "to have made endovenous application of medicines common knowledge among doctors at a time when it had almost completely been forgotten"[4,7]. Intravenous therapy had almost been forgotten in the middle of the 19th century, having been replaced by subcutaneous injection and infusion as a result of the introduction of the Pravaz needle (1853) and Wood's injection needle. Mendel continued "Thus [as a result of the feasibility of subcutaneous injection] intravenous therapy was gradually forgotten, and it was hardly used for several decades".

In 1896, Briedl and Kraus experimentally treated four women patients with 200 to 300ml of a 10% sugar solution in order "to provide an understanding of the action of sugar in the human organism"[5]. After Landerer's first saline infusions in 1881, the interest of the medical world was concentrated on intravenous injections reaching a climax with Salvarsan (1909) and Neosalvarsan therapy (1911) for the treatment of syphilis. Kausch follows, in this series of research workers, with his studies on intravenous nutrition. In the German literature, Kausch's achievements were only recognised to a minimal degree. Reissigl and Fritsch mention that after the turn of the century Kausch concerned himself "...with the question of intravenous and subcutaneous nutrition with glucose..."[8]. Their subsequent sentence is about uncertainty, "... the constant changing both in the choice of the route and the choice of solutions". This uncertainty presumably refers to general attitudes towards intravenous nutrition. Kausch himself was very certain of his position on the issue: "My artificial nutrition method seems to me to be so well tested and justified by experience that I would also like to recommend it for non-surgical diseases..." For patients suffering from hysteria, with severe vomiting, for hyperemesis gravidarum, for severe gastro-intestinal catarrh and other ailments which drain the body of fluid and nutrients[3]. He regarded cholera as an almost compelling indication. But it appears that Kausch's advice went unheeded. In 1916, in his publication "Glucose infusions in cases of cholera", he almost pleaded for the procurement and use of intravenous glucose infusions for soldiers who had cholera. A year later he recommended using invert sugar as a glucose substitute for infusion purposes [invert sugar is made by boiling cane sugar with dilute acids and consists of dextrose, levulose and a small proportion of cane sugar] because it was easily assimilated by the body and was far less expensive than glucose[10].

It is clear from what has been said, that Kausch's training in internal medicine had a stimulating and integrating effect on his surgical capability and creativity. Resulting from his demonstration of their lack of toxicity and ease of assimilation in surgical patients, he was able to strongly recommend, as early as 1911, the use of infusions, for non-surgical disorders such as cholera. His achievements in this field clearly show that Kausch was a pioneer of parenteral nutrition.

References:

[1] Wangensteen O H: Mandated Celibacy in the Academic Arena. Surg Gyn Obstr. 150 (1980), 1980; 150:739-745. Reprint of an adress to the international Surgical Group, San Francisco, California, 11 September 1979

[2] Elman R: Parenteral Alimentation in Surgery. Hoeber, New York 1947, p. 11-12

[3] Bernhard C: Lecons sur les propiétés physiologiques et les altération pathologiques des liquides d'l'organisme. Paris 1859; 2:459

[4] Landerer A: Über Transfusion und Infusion. Arch klin Chir 1887; 34:807-812

[5] Briedl A, Kraus R: Über intravenöse Traubenzuckerinfusionen am Menschen. Wiener klin Wschr 1896; 9:55-58

[6] Levenson St M, Smith Hopkins B, Waldron M, Canham J F, Seifter F: Early history of parenteral nutrition. Federation Proc. 1984; 43:1399

[7] Mendel F: Der gegenwärtige Stand der intravenösen Therapie. Berl klin Wschr 1908; 19:2188

[8] Fritsch A, Reissigl H: Handbuch der Infusionstherapie und klinische Ernährung. Band 4. Einführung der Herausgeber. Karger Verlag, 1988, XIII

[9] Kausch W: Traubenzuckerinfusionen bei Cholera. Dtsch Med Wschr 1916; 15:53-54

[10] Kausch W: Die Infusion mit Invertzucker (Calorose) Dtsch Med Wschr 1917; 23:712-713

Early Reports on Deaths under Anaesthesia

C. N. Adams
Department of Anaesthesia
West Suffolk Hospital, UK

Introduction

William Morton gave the first successful public demonstration of ether anaesthesia at the Massachusetts General Hospital in Boston, United States of America on 16th October 1846. This event marked the start of modern anaesthesia. The first use outside America was by James Robinson, a dentist, on 19th December 1846 at a private house in Gower Street, London. Two days later, at University College Hospital, Robert Liston amputated the leg of Frederick Churchill under ether anaesthesia administered by William Squire. These cases established the use of inhalational anaesthesia.

It is generally accepted that Hannah Greener was the first unfortunate individual to die under anaesthesia when she received chloroform for the removal of a toenail on 28th January 1848. Her death certificate confirms chloroform anaesthesia as the cause of her demise[1]. However, in the contemporary British medical press, four earlier cases of death were reported either under or in association with anaesthesia, Thomas Herbert on 14th February 1847, Albinus Burfitt on 23rd February 1847, Ann Parkinson on 11th March 1847, and a man from Auxerre in France on 10th July 1847.

Between 1987 and 1997 in the United Kingdom, the National Confidential Enquiry into Peri-operative Death (N.C.E.P.O.D.) has examined deaths occurring during surgery and anaesthesia or in the 28 days that follow. By this standard the five deaths in 1847 and 1848 are all legitimate cases for study.

The entitlement of each of the five cases as an anaesthetic death will be considered, and the wider context of cause of death and the nature of Victorian Society discussed with reference to these individuals.

The Four Early Reports
Thomas Herbert, 14th February 1847

The first case to make the medical press in the *Provincial Medical Journal*, was that of Thomas Herbert[2,3]. The surgeon, Robert Sturley Nunn reported that he had operated on this 52 year old man on 12th February for a bladder stone. The ether had been administered by a colleague, Dr. Williams. The patient was bound to the table as was the custom, and it took eight minutes to bring the patient under the influence of the ether after which the operation was commenced. Mr. Nunn experienced some difficulty because of the state of extreme relaxation of the bladder which he noted, "seemed to fall in folds upon the forceps." The operation lasted ten minutes.

Thomas Herbert recovered consciousness, but remained in a passive state for twenty four hours after which time, "He had a severe chill, which lasted for twenty minutes." Resuscitation was administered by the house surgeon, Mr. Taylor, by giving brandy, with a equal quantity of water. That evening a state of complete prostration developed and the house surgeon sent for Mr. Nunn. continued through the night, this time with Brandy and water, arrow-root, and hot water bottles and blankets. At nine o'clock the following morning, ammonia was given.

Consultation now took place with other members of the medical staff, who agreed continuation of the treatment described, but a stimulating injection was now added. However the patient continued to decline, and he died at five o'clock.

Mr.Nunn did not consider that the death of his patient was entirely due to ether, "It is not my intention or inclination to attribute the loss of my patient wholly to the influence of the æther which was administered in this case, nor hastily to descry its use under all circumstances connected with surgical operations." He further notes that the patient did not show any signs off suffering during the operation, and makes the following observation, "Pain is doubtless our great safeguard under ordinary circumstances; but for it we should hourly be running into danger, and I am inclined to believe that pain should be considered a healthy indication, and an essential concomitant with surgical operations, and that it is amply compensated for by the effects it produces on the system as a natural incentive to reparative action."

No inquest ensued, and the house surgeon, Thomas Taylor, signed the Death Certificate[4] giving "Collapse after lithotomy" as the cause of death. We may speculate today that septicaemia was the actual cause of the patient's demise.

Albinus Burfitt, 23rd February 1847

The next case is perhaps the most disturbing, not for the insight it gives on early anaesthesia, but for what it reveals about Victorian society.

In the *London Medical Gazette* of 1847, J. Willott Eastment gives a graphic description of the case[5]. "Albin Burfitt, of Silton, aged 11 years, became entangled about 8 A.M. on 23rd of February, in the machinery of a mill, in consequence of which he sustained a very severe compound fracture of the left thigh, with great laceration of the soft parts, and a simple fracture of the right thigh. Mr. Newman, of Mere, a very able and experienced surgeon, saw the patient soon after the accident, and with the concurrence of another surgeon, Mr.Rumsey, determined on amputation of the limb as soon as the patient had recovered from the shock of the accident. I was requested to be present at the operation. Saw the case at 4 P.M., and instantly agreed in opinion, as to the necessity of an operation, with the other surgeons, who had been in constant attendance on the boy throughout the day. We did not, at this time, entertain any fears of the patient's death, either from the injuries sustained, or the intended operation. The nervous system had certainly received a great shock, but as there had been but a trifling loss of blood,- as considerable reaction had been established,-as no vital organ had apparently been injured,-as the boy was quite sensible, and had shown great fortitude and patience under his severe sufferings, we all considered there was sufficient vital force in his system to support him under the operation. The question now arose, whether the inhalation of ether should be employed? After mature consideration we determined that it should, and that we would use the apparatus we had at hand. As soon as the patient was brought under its influence, which was the case in about three or four minutes, Mr.Newman operated with his usual skill and judgement, but the patient's sufferings on making the circular incision, were so severe, that the intelligent and humane clergyman of the parish, Mr.Martin, who personally waited on the boy throughout the operation, remarked that the remedy was quite a failure. The inhalation was now employed the second time for two or three minutes, and with decided benefit, as far as the entire suspension of suffering was involved, and the operation (in which the loss of blood was most trifling) was concluded. With its conclusion our difficulties and anxiety commenced, for our patient was in such a state of exhaustion and apparent intoxication that we soon considered his life to be in danger: and our fears were but too fully realised, for in defiance of all watchful attention it was in our united power to pay, he sank in less than three hours after the operation. The state of the brain during this period was peculiarly distressing. There were alternate manifestations of excitement and depression of the sensorial powers; at one time resembling delirium, at another like approaching syncope, and again like violent intoxication, and these alternate conditions continued until the poor boy died."

Despite the fact that only eight weeks had elapsed since the introduction of ether anaesthesia into the United Kingdom, Mr.Eastment had already gained some experience with the drug by anaesthetising a Newfoundland dog for the successful removal of a schirrous tumour. In discussing the cause of death of Albinus Burfitt, he notes the partial failure of ether but concludes that death was attributed to its narcotising effects on a nervous system already depressed by extensive injuries."

The Death Certificate[6] was not issued until 12th June 1847 by the Bridport Coroner, Mr.Frampton. The cause of death is given as "By clasping with his hands a Shaft in a Mill propelled by water and having a Linen apron on his person the same was drawn around the Shaft by means wherof he received divers bruizes and fractures upon his legs and thighs." According to the Local Record Office, the archives of the case do not survive. Similar examination of the contemporary local press reveals that the incident was not apparently reported publicly.

Despite the note that the loss of blood was most trifling, the likely interpretation of the facts now is of hypovolaemia as a result of the extensive injuries.

Ann Parkinson, 11th March 1847

The case of Ann Parkinson is deserving of greater attention than has so far been afforded. Extensive coverage was given to the case by the lay press both local and national. Though she died two days after the operation, her death certificate is the first to mention anaesthesia as a cause. More importantly, for the first time medico-legal concerns were raised against her attending physicians by the Coroner. Unfortunately, the original transcripts of the Inquest do not survive Though articles are to be found in the *Times* and the *Lancet,* the primary source of both is the *Lincolnshire Chronicle*[7] of 19th March 1847.

Ann Peverill Parkinson, the daughter of Thomas Parkinson, a haymaker, had married John Parkinson, a hairdresser in Newark on 24th June 1845. They lived in Spittlegate, a suburb of Grantham which had developed as a result of the arrival of the railway. *The Lincolnshire Chronicle* explains the background to the case thus, "It appears that a respectable female, aged 21, of the name of Ann Parkinson, the wife of a hairdresser at Spittlegate, who had been married eighteen months, and had a child nine months old, had been afflicted with a tumour on the under part of her left thigh for about twelve months, which had gradually increased in size until, from its situation, it became a perpetual torment to her, as she was unable either to sit down or lie in bed with any comfort. Under these circumstances, having read of many successful operations being performed without pain under the influence of the ether vapour, she expressed a wish to her medical attendant (Mr. Robbs, of Grantham) to have the ether applied, and the tumour removed."

Surgery took place on 9th March 1847, and anaesthesia seems to have been less than satisfactory as the patient moaned and grasped her sister-in-law's hand. She is noted to have remained in a state of complete prostration post operatively and to have died two days later on the morning of the 11th March 1847.

The Inquest commenced on Saturday 13th March at the Brewer's Arms in Spittlegate. The Coroner, George Kewney made the following opening observations to the jury, "The case you are about to investigate is one of the most important that it has fallen on myself to preside over, because if it should be found after a calm and deliberate inquiry that the death of this person did result from the effect of the vapour of ether, and not from the tumour under which she was labouring, or from the operation that was necessary to remove it, it will become a question whether the person administering the ether is answerable for the consequences or whether it is unsafe or prejudicial to life to pursue the practice of administering ether, which has been introduced apparently with great success in many cases. I have every reason to believe that Mr. Robbs performed the operation with that skill he is known to possess, and no one can blame him for adopting a practice sanctioned by the highest medical authorities and which has been used in all our leading hospitals, his object being the alleviation of pain and suffering; but it will be for you to say, after a calm and dispassionate investigation, whether in doing so he has strictly adhered to the rules laid down in such cases, or whether he has been guilty of criminal negligence, inattention, or rashness in the manner in which he has treated the particular case before you. It must be remembered that credit is due to him for endeavouring to extend the advantages of a discovery apparently calculated to relieve the sufferings of humanity for it is well known that many of the greatest discoveries in medical as well as other sciences have been violently opposed on their first promulgation, of which the circulation of the blood and other equally striking instances may be mentioned; but whilst he should receive encouragement upon this view of the subject, it must never be forgotten that he was bound to bring to the case under his management the greatest care, skill, and attention of which he was master, and in no degree to exceed or go beyond the instructions laid down by competent medical authorities in similar cases. The remarks contained in a portion of the charge to the grand jury at the Central Criminal Court in a late case appear to me to be so appropriate that I cannot do better than read them. They are as follows:- 'Although it would be very hard to make a medical man amenable to a charge of manslaughter because he happened to be unsuccessful in his treatment of any particular case, yet on the other hand it was necessary for the protection of the public that persons of the medical profession should understand that if they chose to make use of dangerous and deadly ingredients they were bound to exercise the utmost care and caution in so doing. The interests of science require that there should occasionally be some departure from the beaten path prescribed by medical authority, and many important results had followed from such deviations by the alleviation of disease heretofore deemed incurable. But if dangerous experiments were attempted, the persons adopting them must be taught to keep within proper bounds, and that they must exercise the most ample caution in carrying out these experiments."

The Coroner and jury then viewed the body to allow for burial the next day. The inquest recommenced on Monday evening the 15th.

Elizabeth Leek, sister-in-law and cousin of Ann Parkinson was the first to give evidence. She testified to the tumour being evident during Mrs. Parkinson's pregnancy and how treatment in the form of poultices had been given by Mr. Bentley, a medical practitioner residing in Spittlegate. Following her confinement, the tumour continued to give problems, and so Mr. Robbs, a surgeon from Grantham was consulted. Despite puncture and application of leeches by the surgeon, the tumour continued to increase in size. The decision now appeared as to whether ether should be used. Prior to the day of surgery Mr.Robbs administered ether to Ann Parkinson by way of a trial on two separate occasions. Clearly she was aware of conversation during the administration, but resolved to have ether during her surgery.

On 9th March, the operation took place. Mr.Dibben, assisted by administering the ether using a glass jar, a pipe and a tin. Mrs.Leek stated that the deceased moaned each time she was cut, and squeezed her cousin's hand. The operation lasted fifty five minutes during which time the deceased also drank a little brandy and water. It was noted by the witness that she did not lose as much blood as expected. Following the surgery she was put to bed and it was noted that, "she never appeared to rally." The next day she took some gruel and tea, She complained of a numbness in her legs, and pain in the lower part of her back. She also said that she had felt the pain of the operation the previous day. She died quietly at twenty minutes past five the next morning, Thursday.

Inspection of the body was by William Eaton, surgeon of Grantham and Robert Shipman. They noted the wound and that surgery had been performed correctly. Post mortem examination revealed only that the heart contained less blood than usual, and the blood in general was rather more fluid than usual. It was stated that nothing in the wound or the body could be considered a sufficient cause of death. In Eaton's opinion the cause of death was the ether.

In the context of this paper, it is interesting that Wiliam Eaton's evidence now continued with a comparison of the post mortem findings in this case with those of Thomas Herbert. Particularly the congestion of the membrane of the brain which he attributed directly to ether. Robert Shipman confirmed the findings of his colleague.

Following the Coroner's summing up, the jury's verdict was, "that the deceased died from the effects of the vapour of ether, and in which no blame whatever was attached to Mr. Robbs or the gentleman who assisted him, they having the sanction of eminent men and successful cases for the use of the ether, and their object having been to confer upon the deceased the benefit so many other persons had derived from its use."

From the small clues found in the Inquest we may speculate that Ann Parkinson also died from blood loss leading to hypovolaemia. However, her Death Certificate[8] records, "Died from the effects of Ether administered for the purpose of alleviating pain during a surgical operation to remove an Osteo Sarcomatous tumour from the left thigh."

The Man from Auxerre, France, 10th July 1847

Though not reported until 1848 in the *London Medical Gazette*[9], a man died in Auxerre in France in July of 1847. The article refers to the *Gazette Médicale*[10], 4 Mars 1848, which, when translated from the original French gives the following account.

The incident happened at the Hôtel Dieu in Auxerre on 10th July 1847, in the presence of five qualified doctors, among whom some had already practised "etherisation". A 55 year old man, suffering from a cancerous tumour on his left breast dating back seven months, was etherised with the help of a Charrière device, which had already proved to work successfully. The patient who was quite strongly built and had at that point, no visible lesion resulting from his cancer, experienced a violent excitement two or three minutes into the inhaling process. The patient's chest and limbs started shaking violently. His respiratory rate accelerated, and his face blushed. Whilst trying to remove the appliance from his face, the patient was faintly speaking as if drunk.

It was decided that the process should still carry on, but that the opening of the vapour device should be widened as much as the appliance would allow, as the tap controlling the flow had only been slowly half opened.

After ten minutes (from the commencement of the inhalation), the immobility of the limbs was total, as well as the loss of sensitivity, the breathing was high and slow, but noiseless. The face muscles had stopped twitching, and the complexion had become purple red, and so had the chest. The pupils were dilated and still, turned right up.

The device was then removed, and the operation started; but the incision had at that point only produced a small quantity of black blood. When it was noticed that the face complexion had decomposed, the skin was by now totally purple, and the breathing was slow. The pulse, checked for the first time, was floppy, full, and very slow. Suddenly, it ceased to beat: all was over.

Autopsy twenty two hours after death. Each incision into the brain, lungs, heart, liver, kidneys, spleen, exhaled a very strong odour of ether. The blood in the veins was fluid, and of a deep black colour. The blood which had engulfed the while of the posterior side of the lungs was thick. The airways and the larynx were also very injected; the spleen was so sloppy on the inside, it looked like grape pith.

Hannah Greener, 28th January 1848

The death of Hannah Greener was reported in the *Gateshead Observer*, the Lancet and the *Medical Gazette*. Hannah Greener was an illegitimate child whose mother had died in childbirth. She was living with her father who had by then married Mary Rayne.

This fifteen year old girl had had her left great toenail removed successfully under ether anaesthesia in the Newcastle Infirmary on 24th October 1847. On 28th January 1848 she was operated on at Winlaton by Mr.Megginson for the right great toenail[11]. Mr.Megginson statement was as follows, "I seated her in a chair, and put about a teaspoonful of chloroform into a tablecloth, and held it to her nose. After she had drawn her breath twice, she pulled my hand down. I told her to draw her breath naturally, which she did, and in about half a minute I observed the muscles of her arm become rigid, and her breathing a little quickened, but not stertorous. I had my hand on her pulse, which was natural until the muscle became rigid. It then appeared somewhat weaker-not altered in frequency. I then told my assistant, Mr.Lloyd, to begin the operation, which he did, and took the nail off. When the semicircular incision was made, she gave a struggle or jerk, which I thought was from the chloroform not having taken sufficient effect. I did not apply any more. Her eyes were closed, and I opened them, and they remained open; her mouth was open; and her lips and face blanched. When I opened her eyes they were congested. I called for water when I saw her face blanched, and I dashed some of it on her face. It had no effect. I then gave her some brandy, a little of which she swallowed with difficulty. I then laid her down on the floor, and attempted to bleed her in the arm and jugular vein, but only obtained about a spoonful. She was dead, I believe at the time I attempted to bleed her. The last time I felt her pulse was immediately previous to the blanched appearance coming on, and when she gave the jerk. The time would not be more than three minutes from her inhaling the chloroform."

The inquest adjourned from 29th January to 1st of February to allow for a post mortem examination to be performed by Sir John Fife, surgeon of Newcastle-upon-Tyne[12]. Fife's opinion was that death had been caused by congestion of the lungs as a result of inhaling chloroform, but his subsequent testimony confirmed that he was in favour of anaesthesia. He added, "I have no hesitation in affirming that the fatal issue of this case might have occurred in the hands of the most prudent and skilful surgeon that ever lived. It sometimes happens that a person will die from the shock of the operation, within a very few minutes after, and with nothing to show the cause - merely from the shock it gives the system."

The second expert witness was Robert Mortimer Glover, a surgeon who practised as a physician in Newcastle. He confirmed the proper conduct of anaesthesia and surgery, but noted that "I consider chloroform more dangerous than ether."

The jury delivered the following verdict, "We are unanimously of opinion that the deceased, Hannah Greener, died from congestion of the lungs from the effects of chloroform, and that no blame can be attached to Mr.Meggison, surgeon, or his assistant, Mr.Lloyd."

Child Labour

The death of Albinus Burfitt highlights to us the need for the social and educational reforms that took place in the 19th and 20th Centuries. This is well illustrated by the *climbing boys*, the assistants to the sweeps who would clamber throughout the winding chimneys of the well-off in order to clean them. Charles Kingsley published *The Water Babies* in 1863 which drew attention to their plight. In 1864 an Act of Parliament was passed to stop sweeps employing children under the age of ten, and to have any assistance from children under sixteen in the actual cleaning of a chimney. By 1875 the fourth Act required sweeps to take out an annual licence, and gave the police powers to enforce the law. Liberal Governments after 1905 passed laws improving the welfare of children, for example in 1906 empowering local councils to provide school meals, and 1907 starting school medical inspections[13].

Mortality in Victorian England

Examination of the medical literature following the introduction of anaesthesia reveals many case reports of death and papers examining the causes of these events. However in the wider context of mortality, these instances are few. In the three decades that included the introduction of anaesthesia overall mortality[14] per 1000 population was 22.4 (1840's), 22.2 (1850's) and 22.5 (1860's). An example of how other causes of death were far more significant is tuberculosis. In the sixty years from 1851 to 1910 nearly four million people were recorded on their Death Certificates as having died from the disease, with one-third being in the 15 to 34 age group15. Thus tuberculosis accounted for 13% of total mortality in this period, but more importantly was responsible for over 40% of deaths amongst young adults.

150 Years of Reporting Anaesthetic Mortality

It was only nine weeks from the introduction of ether into the United Kingdom to the first report of a death, Thomas Herbert, in association with an anaesthetic. Individual case reports may be found in profusion in the literature during the ensuing fifty years. By 1848, John Snow was writing on the subject in the *London Medical Gazette*[16]. He noted from animal experimentation that chloroform killed rapidly when it pervaded to a certain extent the air that the animal was breathing. He deplored the circumstances of the few deaths reported at that stage, noting that there had been no control on the strength of the chloroform.

Reflecting on the mildness and uniformity of the action of the vapour of chloroform when more diluted, he concluded that we ought to feel confident that it is capable of being used with perfect safety, certainty and precision.

A number of authors attempted to analyse the first deaths under anaesthesia. In 1858, in a series of articles in the *Lancet,* Dr. Glover considered a wide range of aspects of inhalational anaesthesia. Included in his series are case reports of the first 21 deaths world wide. He commented then on the difficulties in giving a correct list, noting that many cases probably happened that escaped publication. Dr. Glover proposed that chloroform killed by suddenly arresting the pulmonary circulation[11]. Dr. Glover's interest in the subject may have been as a result of his being called as an expert witness in the Inquest of Hannah Greener.

The controversy over the safety of chloroform continued well into the twentieth century. Perhaps the most interesting chapter in this story were the two Hyderabad Chloroform Commissions in 1888 and 1889. Edward Lawrie, a doctor in the Indian Medical Service attempted to settle the issue for the first time in 1888. The other Commissioners were Surgeon, Patrick Hehir, and two colleagues Drs Kelly and Charmarette[17]. Experimentation took place on 128 pariah dogs and their conclusion was that, "Chloroform can be given to dogs by inhalation with perfect safety, and without any fear of accidental death if only the respiration-and nothing but the respiration-is carefully attended to throughout."

However after publication of these conclusions, the Editor of the *Lancet* was sceptical suggesting that the results were at variance with the experience in Europe. Undaunted, Laurie persuaded the Nizam of Hyderabad to fund a second Commission in 1889, this time with the Commissioners included Dr. Thomas Lauder Brunton, nominated by the *Lancet,* Surgeon-Major Gerald Bomford, and Dr. Rustomji Hakim, as well as the original members of the first commission. This time the 490 animal included dogs, horses, monkeys, goats, cats and rabbits. The conclusion agreed with the first Commission, "The administrator should be guided as to the effect entirely by the respiration. Chloroform may be given in any case requiring an operation with perfect ease an absolute safety as to do good without the risk of evil." However, this conclusion was still not universally accepted by the establishment.

In 1912, the American Medical Association banned the use of chloroform, though by then the drug was little used in the United States. Chloroform continued in use for many years in the United Kingdom.

Organised mortality reporting continues to this day in the United Kingdom with the work of such studies as the triennial Confidential Enquiry into Maternal Mortality, and the National Confidential Enquiry into Perioperative Death.

Discussion

It took only two months from the introduction of anaesthesia into the United Kingdom, until the first reports of death in association with the technique appeared. The deaths of Thomas Herbert and Albinus Burfitt, occurred after anaesthesia and were not recorded as having been caused by anaesthesia on their Death Certificates.

The case of Ann Parkinson is more important as for the first time, anaesthesia was recorded on her Death Certificate as the cause. Also, for the first time the Coroner, George Kewney, raised the possibility of a surgeon and anaesthetist being guilty of a crime whilst in pursuit of their profession. This contention in the Coroner's introduction was not, however, proven.

With the benefit of hindsight, the case of Thomas Herbert may now be attributed to septicaemia following instrumentation of the bladder. However, in the cases of Albinus Burfitt and Ann Parkinson, blood loss leading to hypovolaemia would make anaesthesia a contributing factor to their deaths in an age when fluid resuscitation was not comprehended.

There is insufficient corroboration to confirm the case in Auxerre as the first death during anaesthesia especially as reporting was so late, indeed coming after that of Hannah Greener. However, this case does appear worthy of further investigation.

Whilst the medical press did debate death and anaesthesia, the lay press did not seem to devote the same attention. Similarly, examination of *Hansard* and the Parliamentary Papers of the time did not reveal a single item on death and anaesthesia until 1854 when Sir John Hall cautioned against it use in the battlefield during the Crimean War. This is perhaps not surprising given the other important causes of death such as tuberculosis.

The case of Albinus Burfitt gives an insight into the cruel nature of Victorian Society where child labour was accepted.

References:

1. Death Certificate. Hannah Greener. Quarter, June 1848; District, Gateshead; 24: p 119

2. Nunn RS: Operation for lithotomy performed under the influence of æther: Death. Provincial Medical Journal 1847, p 134

3. Nunn RS: Fatal effects of ether vapour in a case of lithotomy. London Medical Gazette 1847; 39: 414-5

4. Death Certificate. Thomas Herbert. Quarter, March 1847; District, Colchester; 12: p 50

5. Eastment JW: Another case of the fatal effects of ether in operations. London Medical Gazette 1847; 39: 631-3

6. Death Certificate. Albinus Burfitt. Quarter June 1847; District, Mere; 8: p 303

7. Anonymous. Death from inhaling the vapour of ether. Lincolnshire Chronicle 19 March 1847; p 6 Cols 1 & 2

8. Death Certificate. Ann Parkinson. Quarter March 1847; District Grantham; 14: p 349

9. Anon. Therapeutics. Death from the inhalation of ether vapour. London Medical Gazette 1848. 41: p 432

10. M.R: Mort rapidement causée par l'inhalation d'éther. Gazette Médicale 4 Mars 1848; 13: p 170

11. Glover RM: Report on anæsthesia and anæsthetic agents, No. II. *Lancet* 1858: p393-4

12. Legal Medicine. Fatal application of chloroform. Edinburgh Medical and Surgical Journal 1848. 69: p498-502

13. Hill CP: British Economic and Social History 1700 - 1982. 1985 Edward Arnold p 186-7.

14. Anon. The recent English death rate. Br. Med. J. 1883 (i): p263

15. Woods R and Woodward J (eds.) Urban Disease and Mortality in nineteenth-century England. 1984 Batsford Academic and Educational London, New York, p83

16. Snow J: Narcotism by the inhalation of vapours. London Medical Gazette 1848; 42: p 614-9

17. Ramachari A & Patwari A. Edward Lawrie and the Hyderabad Chloroform Commissioners.. In: Boulton TB & Atkinson Rs. (eds.) The History of Anaesthesia. Proceedings of the Second International Symposium on the History of Anaesthesia; July 1987, London: Royal Society of Medicine, 1989; p236 - 240

Death under Anaesthesia in the Middle East

M.S.M. Takrouri*
Department of Anaesthesia
Medical College, King Saud University, Riyadh, KSA
* This paper was presented by R. Westhorpe, Australia

Abstract

It is well established that the first anaesthetic used in the Middle East for the purpose of initiating surgical anaesthesia was chloroform, and it was mentioned in the surgical book of George Post professor of surgery at Syrian Protestant College of Beirut (1873).: "a man came to St. John Hospital with a dislocated shoulder of three months. He was given chloroform and it was reduced".

In that context it would be a good assumption that death under chloroform should be researched. In his book Post indicated the possibility of death from chloroform if anaesthesia went too deep. He described five stages of anaesthesia: Excitement, drowsiness, sedation, anaesthesia and deep sleep. Then he goes on to say "If anaesthesia is not stopped there is fear of death by asphycia".

By the year 1895 death under chloroform was reported. Dr. Spiridon Abourousse attacked the use of chloroform and described it as risky: Anaesthesia with this substance is very frightful... Ether is preferable. He cited a case of cardiac arrest which took place at the Greek Orthodox Hospital where a young man was 'killed' by chloroform, had he not died in that particular hour, he would still be alive. He described the management of this case as follow: "They tried their best to resuscitate him from the deep sleep he was in, when all their attempts were of no avail and death was definite, they run away; one mounted on his horse, and the surgeon hide in a neighboring house until a cart reached him wherein he vanished from sight."

Introduction

The introduction of inhalational anaesthesia 1846 by Morton of Boston using ether was followed by the introduction of chloroform by Simpson of Edinburgh, the new discovery traveled to all the corners of the planet in no time. The use of the new agent in the surgical anaesthesia brought to the human race the most amazing blessings. Soon the zenith was refrained when death was attributed mainly to agents used in anaesthesia. In the Middle East the first recorded anaesthesia was the record of Dr. G. Post in his book on surgery. Post was a professor of surgery at Syrian Protestant College of Beirut (1873). He wrote: "a man came to St. John Hospital with a dislocated shoulder of three months. He was given chloroform and it was reduced"[1]. It seem that ether may have been used but never documented, and it is presumed that chloroform was the major inhalational agent used for the purpose of alleviating the pain of surgical procedures. So evidently it would be logical to look into chloroform mortality.[1,2]

Where, When, Why, Who and its consequences

In the medical books and journals in Arabic language, in the era of chloroform and ether, we can trace the discussion of chloroform risk and the potential lethal situation which may follow what it was termed poisoning. Obviously there were concern about the inherited toxicity of chloroform which may have followed the vogue of comparing the merits

167

of chloroform versus ether and the never ending debate about which is better and which can depress the ventilation or the circulation first. This was the case in Great Britain. By the year 1875 in Beirut comparisons were being drawn between the effects of ether and chloroform on the same logic: ether stops respiration before circulation... chloroform stops the heart before respiration. There were what we all know about the investigation of death under chloroform in what termed Hayderabad chloroform Commissions 1888-1889. However, chloroform continued to be used in the Middle East. Death following its usage was discussed in literature by the year 1895. As editorials in the journal Altabib. By the year 1899. Dr. Spiridon Abourousse wrote two articles in the journal Almashrik where he discuss the risk of chloroform, and the first death under the effect of chloroform and later on he mentioned some current statistics about its mortality as compared to ether.

The account of the death under chloroform came in the first article entitled the danger of chloroform (Anaesthesia). The author narrated end described the cardiac arrest of a patient who was in the Greek Orthodox Hospital. He made an inflamed account of the story: A young man in his eighteen, was hit by a bullet from a pistol. It hit him in his thigh. He was then admitted to the hospital for treatment, After more than a month, a surgeon decided that he should have his leg been amputated. So he solicited the help of a young doctor to give chloroform (yuokalfira). The surgeon holding his knife waiting for the patient to sleep. In fact the patient only took few breath from the air impregnated with chloroform, and he stopped breathing. His movement stopped and his sensation abolished, he slept but for ever. The doctors were surprised from this terrible situation, and they tried their best to resuscitate and revive the patient but without success. When they felt certain of his death they flee the place and ran away, one mounted his horse, and the surgeon went hiding to neighboring house until a cart reached him wherein he vanished from sight.[3,4,5,6,7,8]

The author continue in his article to describe the aftermath of the incident and the logic al explanation of his death:

1. The story did not die out. All Beirut was vibrating the echo, the local government sent a committee to study this case and to investigate the cause of death, looking into the previous condition of the patient, his illness and the amount of chloroform were used. He did not know the result of this investigation.

2. His opinion in regard the cause of death is the chloroform poisoning, and if this patient did not receive this agent then he could have been alive. He also thought that the attitude of the surgeon was not proper to decide for surgery where another experienced surgeon denied the surgery because of the weak state of the patient which could not permit him to tolerate the shock of the chloroform. He thought that the patient died from "syncope" which means fainting and cardiac arrest, due to the shock chloroform can cause to the cardiac nervous supplies, and due to vasoconstriction which cause a high resistance to the heart so it can not pump the blood to the periphery. He stated then that the major mistake of the surgeon (and all surgeons of Syria for that matter) and his assistant is not to use ether instead of chloroform. ether which is used alone by the majority of the surgeon of Lyon in France, Boston in America and Berlin in Germany.

In his second article he drew a clinical comparison between ether and chloroform, ending his article with some convincing statistics:

Conclusion

The first reported death under anaesthesia in the Middle East surprisingly is due to chloroform

Where?: It was in the Greek Orthodox Hospital in Beirut.

When?: It was in the year 1899.

Why?: The patient was exhausted after gunshot wound in the thigh spending a month in the hospital then the surgeon decided for amputation. The patient was so ill so when he was anaesthetized by chloroform, His heart stopped.

Who?: A nameless eighteen years old young man.

The sequences: Local government investigation into the cause of death, more awareness of the chloroform lethal dangers, and a vigorous call to return to ether, and later on to use less harmful local analgesics.

References:

[1] Haddad Fuad Salim (personal communication) 1997

[2] Post G. Almisbah Alwaddah Fi Sinaat Aljarrah (Arabic) 1873

[3] Editorial: Death under chloroform, Altabib 2:37:1875

[4] Editorial: The real cause of death under chloroform, Altabib 9:161;1897

[5] Editorial: Death of child under chloroform, Altabib 16;290;1904

[6] Abourousse S: Danger of chloroform. Almashrik 2;775-777;1899

[7] Comparison between chloroform and ether. Almashrik S:875-879;1899

[8] Haddad Fuad Salim: History of anaesthesia in Lebanon; Middle East J Anaesth 6:5; 241-280; 1982

Early Reports on Death under Anaesthesia in German Speaking Countries

H. Petermann[1] und M. Goerig[2]
[1] Department of Anaesthesiology, University Erlangen-Nuremberg, Germany
[2] Department of Anaesthesiology, University Hospital Eppendorf, Hamburg, Germany

Soon after the introduction of sulfuric ether for surgical procedures without pain, the first cases with fatal complications were reported. The data we got until now shall answer the question whether the death of the patients was caused by anesthesia or by other influences.

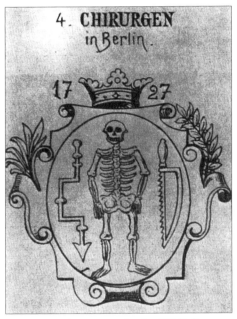

Badge of the Surgeons in Berlin (1733). From: W. Block: Der Arzt und der Tod. 1966. S. 137.

The Situation in 1847

Normally in 1847 people died either because of an accident of any kind of disease at home. Whoever could afford avoided going to a hospital. Death in hospitasl was common - just the opposite of todays's situation.

This can be explained by the fact that the hospitals did not have much capacity. In Erlangen with more than 10 thousand inhabitants, they only had about 25 beds (internal and surgical) for patients. In times before anti- and asepsis there was also a high risk to get an infection in the clinic. Hospitalbrand (hospital gangrene) or Flecktyphus (typhoid fever) brought death to a lot of people although they had survived the operation or the treatment.

As the badge of the society of surgeons in Berlin shows (Fig. 1), death must have been part of a doctors daily life. Founded in 1772 they used a skeleton in their emblem representing anatomy as well as death.

The Beginnings of Modern Anaesthesia in 1846

William T. Morton (1819-1868) and Charles T. Jackson (1805-1880) first demonstrated in public on October 16th, 1846, that sulfuric ether could be used for anaesthesia at the Massachusetts General Hospital in Boston. Hermann Demme (1802-1867), Johann F. Heyfelder (1798-1869), Franz C. Rothmund (1801-1891) as well as the dentist Heinrich E. Weickert (?) and Carl F. E. Obenaus (?) were pioneers in German speaking countries regarding the application of ether in order to perform painless surgery. Early reports on this new agent showed great enthusiasm, but quite soon complications of this procedure were observed.

The Early Reports about Fatal Complications

A few months after the introduction of ether for narcosis the first cases of fatal complications were published.

"Wenn man die Berichte über die Aetherwirkung in geschichtlicher Reihe verfolgt, so fällt es auf, dass die Jacksonsche Entdeckung in dem Grade, als sie sich vom Lande ihrer Geburt entfernte, auffallender Weise immer mehr an ihrer Wunderkraft zu verlieren schien. In Boston, wo sie das Licht der Welt erblickt, und in New York wirkte der Aether nur wunder, und Fälle, in denen er die Aerzte im Stiche gelassen oder zu strenden Nebenerscheinungen Anlass gegeben hätte, waren groe Seltenheiten. In England aber schon wuchs die Zahl der Individuen, welche den Zauberwirkungen des Aethers hartnckigen Widerstand leisten konnten; zahlreicher noch wurden die Ausnahmefälle in Frankreich, Belgien, der Schweiz und Deutschland." (2, p.103)

With increasing distance from the place, where it was discovered, the application of ether lost a lot of its amazing effects. If you are far away from the United Stated you get more reports about disturbances caused by the application of ether.

In his essay about "Sulfuric Ether and its New Applications" Alexander Bauer mentioned a list of nine contra-indications ending with: *„Jedenfalls lasse sichs Jeder zur Warnung dienen, das zur Mode gewordenen Mittel ferner nicht zu geringfügigen Zwecken zu missbrauchen!"* (1, p.38) This was a warning for everybody not to use this agent for trivial cases. Although he described a lot of complications Bauer did not mention a single patient dying due to the inhalation of ether.

Dieffenbach wrote in "Der Aether gegen den Schmerz" (1847): *If one takes into account, over a large number of patients, all the small disadvantages bound with etherization, the sum total of illness is found to be raised, so that out of a thousand etherized and a thousand unetherized cases a few more deaths occur among the former than among the latter.* (5, p.139)

The first articles about fatal complications after inhaling ether were published about two cases, that have occurred in Great Britain and were well-known in German speaking countries at that time. The case reports of Mrs. Parkinson and of Mr. H. were printed in several periodicals reviewing Lancet or other English periodicals. In the case of Mrs. Robinson the article in Lancet closes with: *"At the conclusion of the case, Mr. Robbs stated that he fully concurred in the verdict, as he had no doubt whatever that the ether alone was the cause of death, and it was a duty he owed to the public to say so. The verdict was then signed, and the inquiry terminated."* (8, p.342)

Mr. Roger Nunn, surgeon in the second case with fatal consequences stated at the end: *"I trust the publication of this unsuccessful case may lead to the publicity of many others which have occurred, so that the profession may not be led away by the erroneous supposition that the prevention of pain is so vital a desideratum in operative surgery."* (8, p.343)

The fatal case of Mrs. Parkinson was discussed in detail in a review article in the "Rheinische Monatsschrift" 1847 titled "Tod durch Einathmen des Aetherdampfes": *Death because of inhalation of ether vapor. - The application of the vapor of ether is spreading very fast and has now come to a state, in which the following unhappy case has to be reported, so much the more that his case will lead to a lot of considerable practical advice.* (13, p.324ff.)

In "Notizen aus der Heilkunde" 1847 the case report was analyzed again in an article entitled "About Etherization and the Death of Mrs. Parkinson caused by it." *The opinion about etherization and its effects, that were caused by the reports about the death of Mrs.*

die Kosten der Untersuchung und Bescheidung zu tragen.

München, den 27. Februar 1847.

Königl. Regierung von Oberbayern, Kammer der Finanzen.

In Abwesenheit des kgl. Präsidenten:

Schilcher, Director.

Aschenbrier, Director.

Heydolph, Secr.

ad Nrum. 9,761.

An sämmtliche Polizeibehörden und Physikate von Oberbayern.

(Die Anwendung des Schwefeläthers betr.)

Im Namen Seiner Majestät des Königs von Bayern.

Die Anwendung des Schwefeläthers bei vorzunehmenden Operationen ist in der jüngsten Zeit so häufig geworden, daß offenbar auch ganz unberufene Personen hievon bei den unbedeutendsten Gelegenheiten Gebrauch machen zu dürfen glaubten. Nachdem aber hierüber noch keineswegs ganz sichere Erfahrungen bestehen, am wenigsten aber ausgemittelt ist, ob nicht hievon nachtheilige Folgen für die Gesundheit und das Leben entstehen, im Gegentheile mehrern Ansichten zu Folge mitunter bedenkliche Erscheinungen bei dessen Gebrauche hervorgetreten sind, so sieht sich die unterfertigte Stelle veranlaßt, zu verfügen, daß die Anwendung des Schwefeläthers bei Vornahme chirurgischer Operationen von nun an nur unter der Aufsicht und Leitung practischer Aerzte vorgenommen werden dürfe, keineswegs aber von dem untergeordneten wundärztlichen Personale allein.

(30 *)

Die practischen Aerzte werden sich zur Aufgabe machen, allenfalls vorhandene körperliche Leiden und krankhafte Anlagen, welche eine solche Einathmung nicht vertragen, vorerst genau zu würdigen, und sind verbunden, ihre deßhalb gemachten Erfahrungen von Monat zu Monat unter genauer Berücksichtigung der einzelnen Fälle den vorgesetzten Physikaten anzuzeigen, um diese in den Stand zu setzen, an die königl. Regierung hierüber Bericht zu erstatten.

München, den 28. Februar 1847.

Königl. Regierung von Oberbayern, Kammer des Innern.

In Abwesenheit des kgl. Präsidenten:

Schilcher, Director.

Dubois.

ad Nrum. 9,172.

An sämmtliche Districts-Polizei-Behörden von Oberbayern.

(Die Aufgreifung einer blödsinnigen Weibsperson in Nürnberg betr.)

Im Namen Seiner Majestät des Königs von Bayern.

Nach einer Mittheilung der königl. Regierung von Mittelfranken, Kammer des Innern, vom 23. v. Mts. ist die Inhaltliche der Ausschreibung vom 13. December v.Js. (Intelligenzblatt Seite 2056) zu Nürnberg aufgegriffene blödsinnige Weibsperson nunmehr ausgemittelt, weßhalb dieser Ausschreibung keine weitere Folge zu geben ist.

München, den 3. März 1847.

Königl. Regierung von Oberbayern, Kammer des Innern.

In Abwesenheit des kgl. Regierungs-Präsidenten:

Schilcher, Director.

Dubois, Secr.

Decree of February 1847. From: Intelligenzblatt für Oberbayern. 1847. Sp. 437f.

Parkinson, must be adjusted. (11, Sp.195)

German articles about Mrs. Robinson's case were repeatedly reported, but all of them published the jury's decision. So ether was responsible for this death. Three other cases with fatal consequences under the influence of ether were also published. Two of them occurred in Paris and one in Madrid.

It is remarkable that most of the German publications only reported about cases without any omplications.

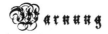

Title-page B. Kopezky.

The First Deaths under Anesthesia

First notes about fatal complications, as far as we know, were given in the middle of the year 1847. Reports reviewing eight cases reported deaths after inhaling ether, four of occured in Vienna, two in Ansbach, one in Erlangen and another one in Munich.

In his booklet Benedikt Kopezky stated: *There is no lack of reports of an unfortunate development of the disease after operation, that was followed by death. It may be difficult to prove in all cases that the inhalation of ether is fully or partly responsible for the death. But in all cases the state of insensibility lasted very long or the patient did not regain awareness.* (7, p.19)

And later on: *Warren already wrote in one of his letters to Forbes in London about the difficulties to take the decision the application of such an agent like ether. There might be aspects we just do not know right now or complications we are not aware of.* (7, p.28)

In their essays Benedikt Kopezky and Franz Schuh (1805-1865) described the four cases of death after the application of ether in Vienna.

Case 1	Vienna
Sex:	unknown
Age:	unknown
Anamnesis:	very poor general state of health
Diagnosis:	Tumor albus genu
Therapy:	Amputation of femur
Death:	6. postop. day
Cause:	Pneumonia or aspiration followed by sepsis

In this case the patient's death probably was caused by the pre-existing and long lasting diseases. This means he died due to a septic-toxic cardiac failure.

Case 2	Vienna
Sex:	female
Age:	unknown
Anamnesis:	unknown
Diagnosis:	Traumatic contusion of hand, elbow and foot
Therapy:	Amputation of upper arm
Death:	5. postop. day
Cause:	Sepsis caused by injury of foot

The reason for death of this patient was the untreated injury of the foot. An early therapy might have avoided this death.

Case 3	Vienna
Sex:	male

Age:	? (young)
Anamnesis:	unknown
Diagnosis:	Hydrocele
Therapy:	Herniotomy
Death:	13. postop. day
Cause:	Hospital gangrene (Hospitalbrand)

Hospital gangrene was a typical complication in 1847 after surgical interventions. Patients that had survived the surgical operations often died because of this infection.

Case 4	Vienna
Sex:	female
Age:	26 yrs.
Anamnesis:	very poor general state of health
Diagnosis:	Tumor albus genu
Therapy:	Amputation of femur
Death:	4. postop. day
Cause:	Sepsis or hospital gangrene (Hospitalbrand)

This young women died because of an infection. This case is comparable to case 2.

Schuh wrote about these cases: *I myself was enthusiastic about the application of ether vapor. But I convinced myself that this has an unfortunate or bad influence on the development of disease after operation.* (14, p.36f)

As far as we can comment on this Schuh made the inhalation of the vapor of ether responsible for deaths of patients, but they probably would have also died even without narcosis.

Two other reports were given by Heidenreich, a professor of surgery and ophthalmology in Erlangen with Heyfelder, in the „Medicinisches Correspondenzblatt".

Case 5	Ansbach
Sex:	female
Age:	60 yrs.
Anamnesis:	good general state of health
Diagnosis:	Scirrhus ulceration of left mamma
Therapy:	Amputation of left mamma
Death:	24. postop. day
Cause:	Pneunomia

The pneunomia could have been caused by respiratory embarrassment due to pain.

Case 6	Ansbach
Sex:	female
Age:	53 yrs.
Anamnesis:	good general state of health
Diagnosis:	Inguinal hernia
Therapy:	Herniotomy
Death:	9 hours (!) postop.
Cause:	Aspiration, Gangrene of the intestine

Although Heidenreich denied it, the cause of death was probably gangrene of the intestine because of the hernia. Another reason could have been aspiration during narcosis. But according to the given information this seems very unlikely.

Case 7	Erlangen
Sex:	female
Age:	? (young)
Anamnesis:	unknown
Diagnosis:	Ovarian atrophy
Therapy:	Ovariectomy
Death:	? postop.
Cause:	Circulatory breakdown

An intensive loss of blood was responsible for the circulatory breakdown.

This case is an example for an intraoperative complication with fatal consequences Most of them just happened and were never reported as „death under the influence of ether". On the other hand they do not differ from the six cases reported before. The question, whether ether is responsible for this death of the patient can not be answered.

To get more information about fatal complications after the application of sulfuric ether for operations without pain, one has to look at all cases with death of the patient in one clinic.

Sulfuric ether was not only applied before surgical operations, it was also used for the treatment of tetanus. In most cases, that were reported in periodicals, its use helped the patient to get through the state of tetanus and afterwards they recovered well.

Case 8	Munich
Sex:	male
Age:	73 yrs.
Anamnesis:	good general state of health
Diagnosis:	Hypermia medull. spinal. - Tetanus traumaticus
Therapy:	Inhalation of sulfuric ether
Death:	3. days post inhalationem
Cause:	Respiratory paralysis

A fatal complication was reported by Meinel in his dissertation titled „A Case of Etherization with Fatal Complications by Tetanus traumaticus". Maybe the death of the patient was not only caused by his disease but also by his age of 73 years.

Kopezky wrote: *Because of all our experiences the vapor of ether cannot be regarded as an innocent or harmless agent. It has to be applied with thoughtfulness and skilled caution, and it is careless to use it just for pleasure.* (7, p.27)

According to the known facts we summarize the above reported 8 cases:
1. Case No. 1 and 6 are the only ones, where the cause of death was related to the surgical operation.
2. The pre-existings conditions might be responsible for the fatal end in all cases.
3. The use of inhalation agents causes insufficiency of the immunological response with great probability of infection (nosokomial infection).
4. The purity of the inhalation agent is not known in any of those cases.

It can be presumed that the fatal complications might not have been avoided in any of those cases. All in all, it can neither be proved nor denied that the inhalations of ether had been the reason for the death of those patients.

Other typical complications due to ether narcosis at that time were too long lasting insensibility, disturbances of the mind for a few hours up to several days, problems with heart and respiration after surgery.

Kopezky recommended to overcome the complications in his booklet: *As helpful counter-measures we have right now, if the ether narcosis lasts too long or is too deep:*
 - *inhaling of fresh air or pure oxygen*
 - *sprinkling cold water on face, neck and breast*
 - *shaking the patient lightly*
 - *low dose of a pretty good vine* (7, p.40)

The Consequences of these Facts

As shown in a drawing, sulfuric ether might also have been used for affair of honor, abolition of physical pain or just for amusement. Application for surgical operations without pain was a convenient use. (plate 3)

Most of the German speaking areas were in 1847 were part of a confederation called „Deutscher Bund" which consisted of up to 34 sovereign states. The kingdom of Bavaria was one of them and shall be taken as an example, whether abuse or the death of a patient lead to further steps being taken regarding the

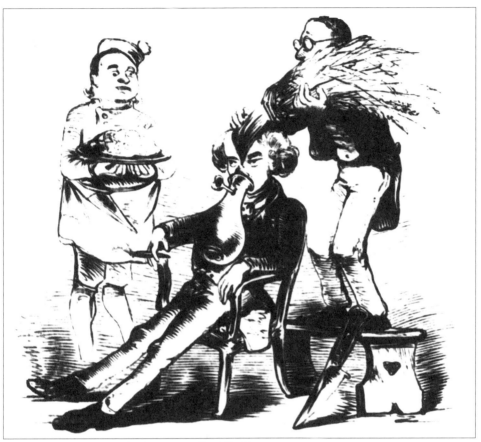

Caricature "Application of Ether Against Stupidity."
From: Illustrierte Zeitung, Leipzig. Bd. 8 (1847), S. 189.

matter. One of the first publications about the new agent sulfuric ether and its use was publsihed in the "Allgemeine Zeitung Augsburg", on January 10th, 1847. Only nine days later, the ministry of internal affairs advised Heyfelder in Erlangen to carry out some experiments on ether narcosis (6).

At the same time Rothmund in Munich started his trial and both, Rothmund as well as Heyfelder published their results in March 1847. As soon as February 26th 1847, the government of Oberbayern published the first "Verordnung die Anwendung von Schwefelaether betr.", titled *Decree concerning the application of sulfuric ether King* Ludwig I.

enacted a law on the use of sulfuric ether on June 6th, 1847. In Saxonia, Hannover, Vienna (Austria) and Poland similar instructions were given, too.

All those decrees contained the same instructions:

- It is only academic doctors allowed to use sulfuric ether.
- All other medical staff like dentists, midwives, travelling healers is prohibited to use the drug.

In Poland the following additional order was put to the above mentioned: *In every case the doctor wants to administer ether, he has to consider two other doctors.* (7, p.42)

177

Obviously these instructions resulted from the abuse of ether by medical laymen and so-called "Etherfrolics" and its lethal complications, since it was a doctors major task to turn away danger for body and soul *("Gefahr für Leib und Leben abzuwenden.")*

Soon after the introduction of chloroform in January 1848 there was already enacted a law regulating its use. There is no obvious reason for this, since Rapp wrote in 1850: *In former publications I wrote that there is no case of death known in German speaking countries. But now I have to report myself a case of sudden death after inhaling chloroform.* (12, p.157f.)

At the end of his booklet Kopezky wrote: *"Wahrscheinlich wird die zu oft, selbst in geringeren Graden producirte Aetherbetaeubung zu demselben traurigen Ende fuehren, wohin der leidenschaftliche Wein- oder Branntweintrinker geraeth, zum Saeuferwahnsinn (Delirium tremens potatorum). - Producing insensibility by inhaling the vapor of ether willprobably lead toa similar bad condition as followed by drinking vine and brandy with passion, the horrors (Delirium tremens potatorum)".* (7, p.43)

References:

1. Bauer A: Ueber Schwefelaether und seine neueste Anwendung, mit einem Anhange ueber die in den öffentlichen Anstalten Prags gewonnenen Resultate. Prag 1847

2. Bergson J: Die medicinische Anwendung der Aether-Daempfe in Bezug auf Physiologie, operative Chirurgie, Nervenpathologie, Psychiatrie, Geburtshlfe, Zahn- und Thierheilkunde, historisch und kritisch beleuchtet. Berlin 1847

3. Bericht ueber die fuenfundzwanzigste Versammlung der Gesellschaft Deutscher Naturforscher und Aerzte in Aachen 1847. Aachen 1849

4. Dieffenbach J F: Der Aether gegen den Schmerz. Berlin 1847

5. Duncum B: The Development of Inhalation Anaesthesia. London 1947

6. Intelligenzblatt für Mittelfranken. Ansbach 1847

7. Kopezky B: Warnungen vor den schaedlichen Wirkungen der Aether-Einathmung nebst einer Vergleichung mit den Narkosen durch Weingeist, Opium, Tabak und Coca. Wien 1847

8. Lancet. 1847; Jg.2

9. Medicinisches Correspondenzblatt der bayerischen Ärzte. Erlangen 1847

10. Meinel C: Ein Fall von Aetherisation mit lethalem Ausgang bei Tetanus traumaticus. Muenchen 1847

11. Notizen aus dem Gebiete der Natur- und Heilkunde. 1847 ; 2, Bd.3.

12. Rapp J: Ploetzlicher Tod nach Anwendung des Chloroforms durch Inhalation. In: Deutsche Klinik. 1850 ; 15 : 157f

13. Rheinische Monatsschrift für praktische Aerzte. 1847; Jg.1

14. Schuh F: Einige warnende Worte gegen die zu allgemeine Anwendung der Schwefelaetherdaempfe. In: Zeitschrift der k.k. Gesellschaft der Aerzte zu Wien1847; Jg.4

Early Mortality from General Anesthesia

D. K. Cope
University of Pittsburgh,
Pain Evaluation and Treatment Institute, Pittsburgh, USA

Edmund Andrews, a midwestern surgeon and medical educator, was a little known innovator in anesthesia practice who conducted the first outcome study of general anesthesia morbidity in over 200,00 surgical cases conducted during the first twenty five years after the introduction of surgical ether and chloroform.

Early Record-Keeping

In the 1860's during the American Civil War, massive battlefield casualties, the spread of infectious diseases like measles and erysipelas, and the overcrowding of military prisons often taxed the resources of both armies to provide adequate medical care. One Union surgeon, Dr. Edmund Andrews (Fig. 1), in spite of his heavy daily workload, was frustrated by his inability to follow his patients from his initial care in the field hospitals through their post-operative treatment in hospital boats or general hospitals. In fact, most physicians at this time were unable to ascertain the outcome of their patients' treatment. Dr. Andrews was exceptional among surgeons of the time in his efforts in carefully collecting data from each of his patients that he treated in the field. Within a few months after caring for the wounded in the battles fought near Vicksburg, Mississippi he published a report in the *Chicago Medical Examiner* entitled "Complete record of the surgery of the battles fought near Vicksburg, December 27, 28, 29 and 30, 1862," in which he methodically reviewed the outcomes of hundreds of his patients. In addition to the completeness of his records, he carefully categorized all of his surgical cases by regiment, injury, operation, anaesthetic technique and included follow-up reports on each patient varying in time from days, to in some cases, over a month. In his article, he contended that without adequate record-keeping "...the enormous statistics of almost all our great battles have been lost to the profession, and the vast and costly experience of so much blood and death have been rendered worthless for the

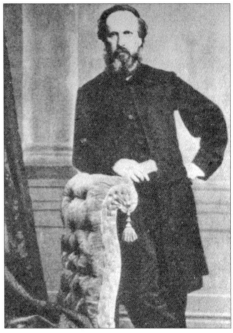

Fig.2: Dr. Edmund Andrews at the time of the Civil War

settlement of the many questions in practical surgery."[1]

This lack of outcome data not only affected the individual surgeon but the state of medical practice as well. "It is a painful fact, that after these battles the results of the various operations and injuries remained entirely unknown to the original operators, and they gained almost nothing by their experience, except the skill of hand acquired in their manipulations."[1] After presenting his detailed tables and supporting text he concluded with the comment: "...it is peculiarly gratifying to me that at length we are able to bring the maxims of military surgery to the corrective test of a large collection of facts, obtained on the western fields."[1]

Observations from Reviewing Cases

Practical conclusions that he drew from this data included the observation that most gun shot injuries were sustained on the right side of the body as the skirmishers delivered their fire from behind the right side of the trees where they stood while sheltering their left sides. Another pertinent clinical observation Dr. Andrews made was that contrary to external appearances, a gun shot wound entering a limb anteriorly generally caused hundreds of shattered pieces of bone and was more likely to require amputation than a shot traveling in a posterior to anterior direction in which case splinters were driven outward with less resultant injury. He noted that often a posterior wound "was so hideous, that it is not uncommon for the inexperienced operator to be moved by it to cut off the better limb and save the worse."[1] These lessons he applied after the war in his popular lecture series in Chicago in which he shot cadavers and dissected the damaged areas for medical students. Fortuitously, Edmund Andrews also became interested in comparing the effectiveness and risk of death from chloroform and ether general anesthesia and this is where our story begins.

Personal History of Edmund Andrews

First of all, who was Edmund Andrews? He was, born in Putney, Vermont in the United States of America on April 22, 1824, and was descended from a long line of Congregational ministers who originally settled in Hartford, Connecticut in 1640.[2] His older brother was a pioneer medical missionary to Hawaii where to this day the ABC Company (A for Andrews) is a flourishing diversified corporate conglomerate. As a result of his own effort and his mother's teaching, Edmund Andrews matriculated as a sophomore at the University of Michigan when it first opened in Ann Arbor in 1846[3], the year of the first public demonstration of ether anesthesia. In addition to premedical studies he worked his way through college by teaching vocal music and directing a church choir, while still finding time to serve as the president of his college's literary society[4]: On graduation he spent a year observing medical practice in the office of Dr. Zena Pitcher, who later became the tenth president of the American Medical Association.

During this time he supported himself by teaching school and working as the University of Michigan's Superintendent of Grounds and Buildings.[5] Edmund Andrews then entered the first class of the University of Michigan's medical department, where he attended class working his way through school via his appointment as Demonstrator of Anatomy with the responsibility of obtaining all necessary cadavers for the school. After receiving his medical degree in 1852 he stayed at the University for two years as a Professor of Comparative Anatomy before accepting the position of Lecturer on Comparative Anatomy at Rush Medical College in

Chicago, Illinois, where he again had the responsibility of obtaining anatomic subjects.[6] He became a noted teacher and lecturer and in 1859 a founding member of the Chicago Medical College, which later became Northwestern University.[4]

During his early medical practice years in Chicago he demonstrated his eclectic interests and bustling personality by his innovative contributions in such diverse arenas as a geology, natural science, medical education, poetry, music, church organ design and building. He also contributed important new techniques to the medical specialties of urology, military surgery, orthopedics and colon-rectal surgery.[7] After the outbreak of the War Between the States in 1861, he served on the staffs of both General Sherman and General Grant at Shiloh, Corinth and Vicksburg. He refused several promotions to Union Army Headquarters to remain in the field treating wounded soldiers.[4] He was the first Civil War surgeon to keep records of the sick and wounded doing such a thorough job that his system was eventually adopted by the United States Surgeon-General's office.

Nitrous Oxide-Oxygen Anesthesia

During this time, in addition to his Vicksburg outcome study, published in 1863, Dr. Andrews carefully recorded the type of anesthetic used for each of his surgical cases. He decided that he favored nitrous oxide over ether or chloroform anesthesia because of its rapid induction, early recovery and minimal post-anesthesia distress that he observed in his patients. However he also noticed the rapid onset of asphyxia with nitrous oxide anesthesia. After mulling the problem over, he decided to try adding free oxygen to improve the safety of nitrous oxide. Fortunately for Edmund Andrews, he was unaware that Dr. Benjamin W. Richardson of England, a pupil of Dr. John Snow, and at that time the greatest living authority on all matters of anesthesia, had already decided that mixing oxygen with nitrous oxide was "unsafe" and "not successful." This widely disseminated opinion was sufficient to deter all other investigators from experimentation with oxygen enrichment of nitrous oxide anesthesia except the practical Dr. Andrews, who continued his experimentation.

Thus, three years after the ending of the Union and Confederate hostilities in 1868, Dr. Andrews published another paper entitled "The Oxygen Mixture, a New Anesthetic Combination." In this paper he described nitrous oxide and oxygen anesthesia in five preliminary experiments on rats followed by a description of the administration of nitrous oxide and oxygen to four of his patients. "Every surgeon who has seen the prompt and pleasant anaesthetic action of the nitrous oxide gas, so much used by dentists, has wished that in some way it might be made available in general surgery. The patient usually goes under the influence in 30 to 40 seconds, and wakes with equal promptness, without vomiting or other unpleasant symptoms, all of which is in striking contrast with the slowness, the nausea, and the discomforts of chloroform and ether. There have been, however, great obstacles to the use of the gas, owing to its evanescent action. The oxygen contained in it is in a state of chemical combination, so that it is not available for oxygenation of the blood; hence if any attempt is made to continue its action, the patient becomes purple in the face, showing all the signs of asphyxia; subsultus tendinum then supervenes, and shortly after he almost ceases to breathe, and, if allowed nothing but pure nitrous oxide, would doubtless die in a few minutes. I have for some time been experimenting, to see whether by the addition of free oxygen to the nitrous oxide, a mixture would not be obtained, by which a patient might be anaesthetized for an indefinite period without danger of asphyxia, and thus render gas available for the most prolonged operations of surgery."[8] In addition, in this same set of experiments Dr. Andrews describes the first attempt at carbon dioxide absorption in a closed anesthesia delivery system by the use of lime water spray. It was not until ten years later, on November 11, 1878 at the French Academy of Sciences that Paul Bert reported the successful amputation of a dog's leg under nitrous oxide-oxygen anesthesia. His anesthetic rendered a dog insensible with muscle relaxation prior to surgery and resulted in the demonstration of the safety of nitrous oxide-oxygen anesthesia to a wide audience.

Anesthesia Case Reports

Throughout his practice, Edmund Andrews kept record books of over 10,000 surgical cases with detailed histories and outcomes of each patient. These were maintained at the hospital, at his home, his office and even on occasion in the dispensary. He assigned numbers to each case to avoid duplication and he carefully bound the cases in sequence. Later he cross-referenced cases of the same type or in the same patient. An example of a case study in which he compared different general anesthetics in the same patient is illustrated by Case 6064. His report reads: "Mixed gas anesthesia, pure gas anesthesia, sulfur ether anesthesia in the same patient. October 3, 1868, Mrs. Beber very anxious temperament ingrowing toe nail. Two months ago I took sulpha ether for operation on left foot for the nail. Got to sleep slowly felt no pain. Six months ago - took pure nitrous oxide for extraction went to sleep in about a minute, felt no pain, face blue, was wild a long time after waking and felt uncomfortable several days. Today took gas mixed with oxygen for extirpation of other nail. Anesthetized in minutes, no blueness of lips. Kept inhaling 3 minutes from beginning. Wakes up wild after three minutes more. Continuous wild 15 minutes, but recovered quicker and with more comfort than from pure nit (sic) ox gas."[9]

First Outcome Study of the Morbidity Of General Anesthesia

Beginning in 1867, Edmund Andrews began systematically investigating the morbidity of general anesthesia. Although contemporaries of his such as Drs. M. M. Perrin and Lallemand of France had deemed a comparison of anesthetic mortality an impossibility Dr. Andrews persisted. In the introduction to his study he stated: "other surgeons seem to have been equally hopeless of success in this matter, so that our best works on anaesthesia are often perfectly silent, on the important point of the relative dangers of the different articles. Yet this is the very thing on which the surgeon most needs light, at the present time. It is well known that chloroform is by far the most convenient article for use, and, therefore, always to be preferred, if equally safe; but if it is materially more dangerous than ether, the conscientious surgeon will choose the latter, for the sake of the safety of his patient. This is, therefore, a question of tremendous magnitude, possibly involving thousands of lives in its decision, hence the surgical profession will not quietly acquiesce in the opinion that its solution is impossible."[10] Certainly Dr. Andrews could not ever have been said to quietly acquiesce in the face of difficulty. He solicited data from the U.S. Government, large teaching hospitals, and searched the British and European literature. In addition, he obtained data regarding nitrous oxide general anesthesia from dental practices. His methods were described as follows: "In obtaining these facts, my method of procedure was, take from

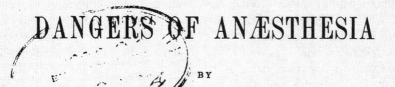

Fig. 2: Title page from "Relative Dangers of Anaes-thesia by chloroform and ether, from statistics of 209,893 cases", the first large outcome study of the morbidity of general anesthesia[10]

the records of each hospital (where reliable records existed), the number of anaesthesias and the number of resulting deaths. Reports of deaths, not accompanied with the number of anaesthesias, and reports of anaesthesias, not stating the number of deaths, are rigidly rejected. Where reliable records did not exist, I obtained, by personal consultation with the house surgeons, a careful statement of the annual number of anaesthesias, based on the known average frequency per week, and carried this estimate over any period, during which the same offers could certify positively as to the number of deaths..... In deciding what deaths were really caused by the anaesthetics, I have generally followed the opinion of the officers reporting them; but where this could not be obtained, I have adopted the principle, that for a death to be fairly attributed to the anaesthetic, it must be immediate, or nearly so, and there must be no other probable cause present. These rules exclude a great number of deaths, vaguely reported as due to chloroform and ether. Thus, out of 21 reported to the Surgeon-General of the U.S. Army, as caused by chloroform, only seven were found fairly attributable to that agent. It is not possible to keep absolutely clear of all errors, on this point, but I think I have obtained a close approximation to the truth; and as I have pursued exactly the same course with ether as with chloroform, the errors, if any exist, must be fairly distributed on both sides of the question, and the results of the comparison of the two anaesthetics cannot vary much from mathematical verity."[10]

Since the information about the morbidity and mortality of ether or chloroform general anesthesia during first twenty five years after its introduction is almost wholly anecdotal it is interesting to examine the correspondence he received from large hospitals in response to his queries. Surgeons from the Alms-House section of Philadelphia Hospital responded that both ether and chloroform were administered by four attending surgeons: one who used "all together chloroform" which he even gave successfully to an 8 day old patient; "two surgeons who gave primarily ether; and a fourth surgeon who uses more ether than chloroform."[11] Also in Philadelphia at the Pennsylvania Hospital "sulphuric ether is used in this institution in all operative cases requiring an anesthetic to the almost entire exclusion of all others" without any known deaths.[12]

Dr. Cheever at the City Hospital in Boston (Fig. 3) understood Andrews' methodology immediately and was able to calculate the death rate from ether anesthesia in 8760 cases over 5 years.[13] Also from Boston, Dr. Hodges from the Massachusetts General Hospital wrote that "two patients were killed by chloroform....by Dr. J.C. Warren when that anesthetic was first introduced, and since those cases, which occurred on the same day, nothing but ether has been used."[14] In another response from the Massachusetts General Hospital Dr. Elliott Richardson, a resident surgeon in 1869, commented on his own interest in deaths from anesthesia and his preliminary attempts to "score" or "tally" the use of ether anesthesia. However since it was given so frequently and "so absolutely safe is it considered" his attempts at documentation were discontinued. He claimed that "students, nurses, and even patients administer it [ether] with perfect safety without any particular watching of pulse or any anxiety about respiration, the sponge being removed only when snoring becomes marked."[15]

On July 3, 1869 the U.S. Government, Surgeon General responded in a typical bureaucratic fashion by referring Dr. Andrews to a government form, circular No. 6 SGO page 87.16 After asking for a more specific response, Edmund Andrews was sent another letter which again directed him to the same printed circular with the explanation: "in reply I would say, that the inquiry you make, if I comprehend it, would involve the

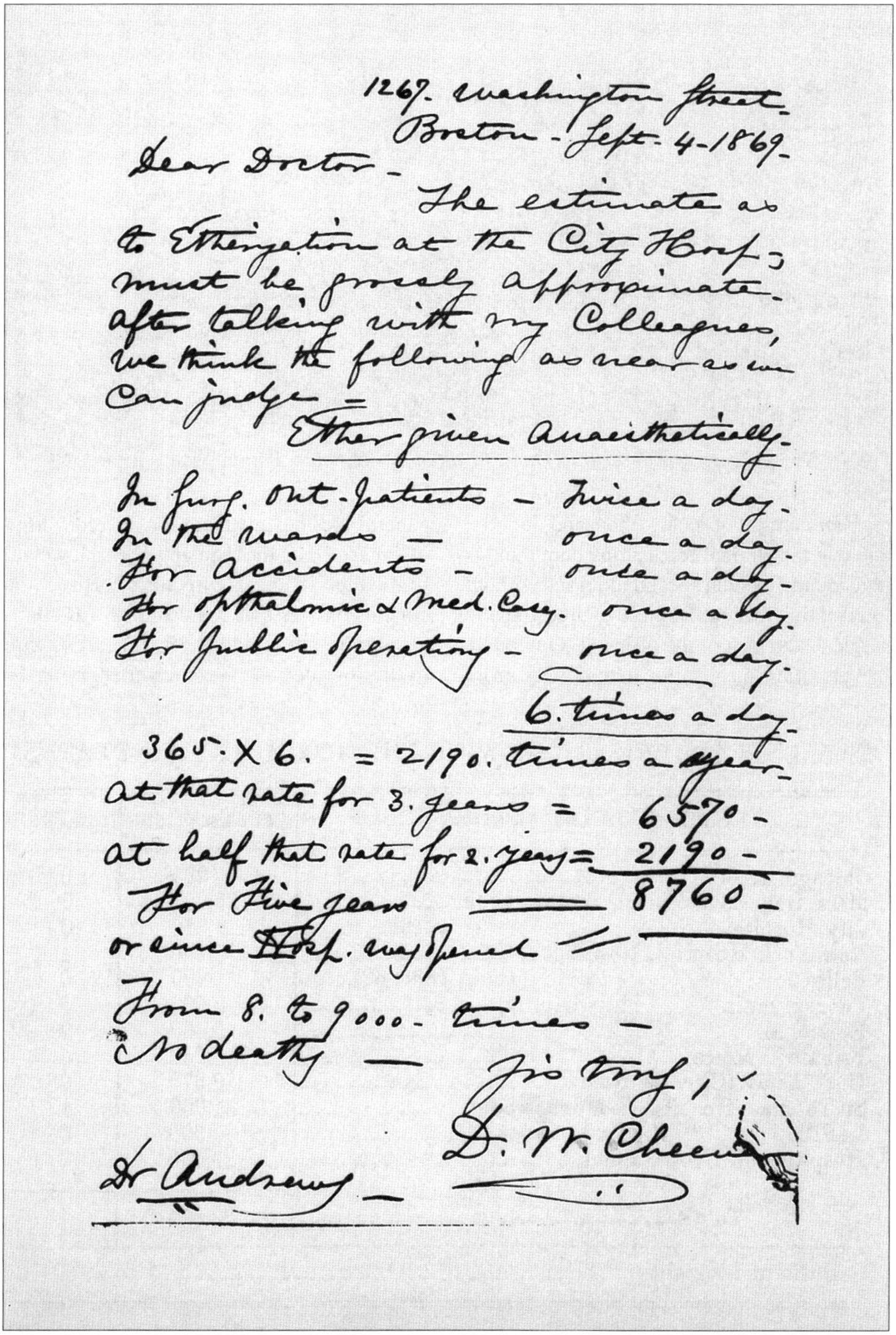

1267. Washington Street –
Boston – Sept. 4 – 1869 –

Dear Doctor –

The estimate as to Etherization at the City Hosp. must be grossly approximate. After talking with my Colleagues, we think the following as near as we can judge –

Ether given Anaesthetically –

In Surg. Out-Patients — Twice a day.
In the Wards — once a day.
For Accidents — once a day.
For Opthalmic & Med. Cases. once a day.
For Public Operations — once a day.
                              6. times a day.

365 x 6. = 2190. times a year.
At that rate for 3. years = 6570 –
At half that rate for 2. years = 2190 –
For Five years   8760 –
or since Hosp. was opened

From 8. to 9000. times –
No deaths —   Yrs truly,
                    D. W. Cheever

Dr Andrews –

Fig. 3: Personal correspondence from Dr. W. Cheever, City Hospital, Boston, September 4, 1869

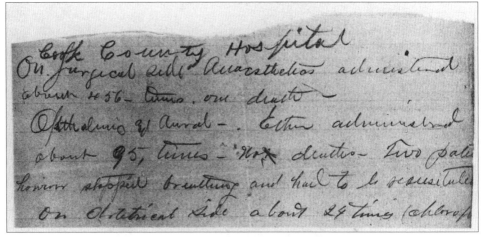

Fig. 4: Personal correspondence from Dr. W. Cheever, City Hospital, Boston, September 4, 1869

re-examination of many thousand reports, and that the clerical force at my command is inadequate for such special inquiries without interrupting the regular work of digesting the surgical statistics of the office."[17] Obviously the importance of surgical morbidity from general anesthesia was not considered worthy of "interrupting the regular work". However, from this medical director's office, the conclusion was that "chloroform was administered in not less than 80,000 cases" with twenty-one deaths.[17] Yet even after giving the

TABLE OF ETHERIZATIONS WITH THE ACCOMPANYING DEATHS.		
Sources of Information.	Etherizations.	Deaths.
Chicago Records,	895	0
Mass. General Hospital, Boston, about	25,000	0
City Hospital, " "	8,760	0
New York Hospital, New York,	5,100	1
Bellevue " " (about 1868–69),	600	0
Pennsylvania " Philadelphia,	2,500	0
Episcopal " "	3,432	0
Private Practice, "	250	0
U. S. Army (Circular No. 6.),	6,978	0
St. Thomas' Hospital, London, about	1,000	1
LaPitie " Paris, about	300	0
Hospitals of Lyons, about	38,000	2
Totals,	92,815	4
Ratio of Mortality,	1 to 23,204	

Fig. 5: Table of "Etherizations" and rates of mortality from Dr. Andrew's published outcome study[10]

requested statistics, the answering government official, George A. Otis, protests with the comment: "it is simply impossible for me to interrupt my own inquiries to enter upon investigations involving much labor and the employment of numerous clerical assistants. On so large a subject as that to which you refer, it would be necessary to consult many thousand reports."[17] It is interesting to note the degree of bureaucratic inertia present one hundred and thirty years ago.

In contrast the response from Cook County Hospital in Chicago, known to this day as a hospital with many indigent patients and large caseloads, appeared to be very simple and direct as it appears to have been quickly jotted down without wasted energy on a scrap of paper (Fig. 4): "on surgical side anaesthetics administered about 456 times - one death. Ophthalmic and aural ether administered about 95 times - no deaths. Two patients however stopped breathing and had to be resuscitated. On obstetrical side about 24 times chloroform."[18]

Dr. Andrews published his compiled findings, three years later in 1870 in the

TABLE OF CHLOROFORMIZATIONS, WITH THE ACCOMPANYING DEATHS.

Sources of Information.	Chloroformizations.	Deaths.
Chicago (Hospital and private records),	6,726	5
Bellevue Hospital, N. Y. (about 1867–8),	600	1
Charity " "	1,460	2
Private practice of a Surgeon in Phila., about	1,000	0
U. S. Army Records (Circular No. 6),	13,956	7
Royal Infirmary, Liverpool,	2,000	2
Workhouse Hospital, "	1,800	0
Southern " "	2,000	1
Northern " "	950	0
Charing Cross " London,	800	1
Middlesex " "	600	0
Royal Ophthalmic Hospital, London,	2,808	1
Guy's Hospital (Eye Department),"	3,224	0
" " (Surg. Department)"	11,500	3
* University Hospital, "	18,250	4
Dreadnaught " "	1,400	1
London " "	13,000	3
St. George's " "	8,000	2
Westminster " "	3,120	1
St. Thomas' " "	3,746	2
Other London Hospitals,	9,826	3
La Pitie, Paris,	312	2
K. K. Allg. Krankenhaus, Vienna,	10,000	2
Totals,	117,078	43
Ratio of Mortality,	1 to 2723	

Fig. 6: Table of "Chloroformazations" and ratio of mortality from Dr. Andrew's publication[10]

Chicago Medical Examiner. The mortality data for general ether anesthesia, derived from 92,815 cases in 12 hospitals, was 1 death per 23,204 cases (Fig. 5). This contrasts with the chloroform morbidity calculated from 117,078 cases at 23 hospitals which was calculated to be 1 death per 2723 cases (Fig. 6). Mixed chloroform and ether anesthesia resulted in 11,176 reported cases with 2 anesthetic deaths for a rate of 1 death per 5588 cases.[10]

However, when compared to the mortality of ether and chloroform general anesthesia the statistics for nitrous oxide anesthesia obtained by the Colton Dental Association showed nitrous oxide to be quite safe with no reported deaths occurring in 75,000 cases. To the American data, Dr. Andrews added reports from the English and European literature showing the relative safety of chloroform, ether and even bichloride of methylene. His concluding table, seen in Fig. 7, demonstrates the overwhelming safety of nitrous oxide general anesthesia followed by ether anesthesia in 1870.10

Conclusion

In the 1860's, a commonly held belief was that one anesthetic agent was superior to all others and therefore should be given to all patients. Therefore a continuing debate was carried on across the Atlantic regarding the safety of ether versus chloroform anesthesia, with anecdotal information and a gamut of opinion ranging from the position that all anesthesia was dangerous and experimental, to the position that many more lives were saved by surgery and anesthesia than lost. The problems of under-reporting and the rarity of an anesthetic death in a single practitioner's lifetime contributed to the frustration of conducting outcome studies. Another study during this time was undertaken by French physicians in Lyons in 1859 in which chloroform morbidity was estimated as one death in 6,000 patients. However the authors balanced their findings with the conclusion that an unknown number of lives were indeed saved by chloroform anesthesia.[19]

In 1858 John Snow analyzed 50 deaths associated with the administration of chloroform concluding that "cardiac syncope" and not pure anesthetic effect was the cause of death.[20] Twenty years later, the Hyderabad Commission reports, which were published beginning in 1890, stated that the principle cause of anesthesia death was overdosage.[21]

Finally, if we summarize the whole matter, it seems that the various anæsthetics have the following rates of mortality:—

Sul. Ether,	1 death to 23,204 administrations.
Chloroform,	1 " " 2,723 "
Mixed Chloroform and Ether,	1 " " 5,588 "
Bichloride of Methylene,	1 " " 7,000 "
Nitrous Oxide,	No death in 75,000 "

CHICAGO, No. 6, 16TH. ST.
April 5, 1870.

Fig. 7: Summary table of the rates of mortality from the various anaesthetics[10]

Andrew's study, occurring in time between these two investigations, was exceptional in that he contrasted different anesthetic agents, including even mixtures of agents, to compute a relative danger from each anesthetic. He presumed that in a series as large as his, risks pertaining to particular patients, surgeons or institutions and errors made by approximating cases, would be true across all of the anesthesia groups that were examined.

Clearly this early outcome study has many shortcomings, not the least of which is the approximate nature of the calculations of the number of anesthetics and anesthesia-related deaths. Another significant confounding factor is the bias in favor of nitrous oxide which was administered in dental procedures which presumably are shorter and have less risk of mortality than the general surgery performed in sicker patients. Another important factor not considered in Dr. Andrew's study were the sociological factors present at the time. Extremely ill, poor, or desperate patients were more likely to be hospitalized in the 1860's as compared to the less sick or more prosperous patients who usually received medical care and anesthesia at home. Thus reports from hospitals did not reflect the entire general population undergoing surgery. However the collection of such a large number of cases from so many different institutions so early after the introduction of general anesthesia is a very important contribution from Dr. Andrews study.

For a medical educator with a very busy professional and personal life, Dr. Edmund Andrews (Fig. 8) pursued the question of anesthesia safety to a remarkable degree for a surgeon of his time or any other time. It is interesting to contemplate what the indefatigable Dr. Andrews might have done with the modern statistical techniques of meta-analysis and the assistance of current computer technology. In his investigation of the oxygen enrichment of nitrous oxide, CO_2 absorption in the anesthesia circuit, careful record keeping and comparative outcome studies the remarkable Edmund Andrews stands ahead of his time as a paragon of practical Midwestern common sense and energetic determination.

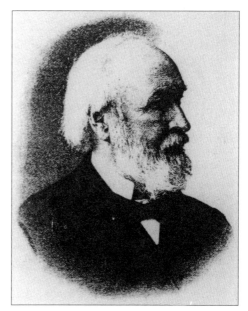

Fig. 8: Dr. Edmund Andrews from: Chicago Medical Record, 1904; 26:112

Acknowledgments

The author acknowledges the courtesy of Dr. William K. Beatty, retired Professor of Medical Bibliography, Northwestern Medical School, Chicago, for his suggestions; the Northwestern University Medical Library Historical Education for making the Edmund Andrews Surgical Case Books available; Patrick Sim of the Wood Library-Museum for his help; and Doug Bacon for his encouragement in presenting this data for publication.

References:

1. Andrews E: Complete record of the surgery of the battles fought near Vicksburg, December 27, 28, 29 and 30, 1862. The Chicago Medical Examiner 1863; 4:12-58
2. McArthur SW: Edmund Andrews, 1892-1941. Proceedings of the Institute of Medicine of Chicago 1942; 14:90
3. Quine WE: Edmund Andrews. Surg Gyn and Obstetrics 1922; 42:323
4. Arey LB: Northwestern University Medical School 1859-1979. [2nd ed.] Evanston, Ill., Northwestern University, 1979, p 429
5. Chicago Medical Society: History of Medicine and Surgery and Physicians and Surgeons of Chicago. Chicago, Biographical Publishing Corp., 1922, p 65
6. Sperry FM: A group of distinguished physicians and surgeons of Chicago. Chicago, JH Beers, 1904, p 53
7. Beatty WK: Edmund Andrews surgeon, inventor and record-keeper. Proceedings of the Institute of Medicine of Chicago 1985; 38:59-69
8. Andrews E: The oxygen mixture, a new anaesthetic combination. Chicago Medical Examiner 1868; 9:656-661
9. Andrews E: Case Reports, 1857-1903, 26 vols. Case 6064. Housed in the Historical Collection, Northwestern University Medical Library, Chicago, Illinois
10. Andrews E: The relative dangers of anaesthesia by chloroform and ether - statistics of 209,893 cases. Chicago Medical Examiner 1870; 11:257-266
11. Andrews E: Case reports, 1857-1903, 26 vols. Housed in the historical collection, Northwestern University Medical Library. Personal correspondence, July 20, 1869
12. Andrews E: Case reports, 1857-1903, 26 vols. Housed in the historical collection, Northwestern University Medical Library. Personal correspondence, July 25, 1869
13. Andrews E: Case reports, 1857-1903, 26 vols. Housed in the historical collection, Northwestern University Medical Library. Personal correspondence, September 4, 1869
14. Andrews E: Case reports, 1857-1903, 26 vols. Housed in the historical collection, Northwestern University Medical Library. Personal correspondence, July 12, 1869
15. Andrews E: Case reports, 1857-1903, 26 vols. Housed in the historical collection, Northwestern University Medical Library. Personal correspondence, June 25, 1869
16. Andrews E: Case reports, 1857-1903, 26 vols. Housed in the historical collection, Northwestern University Medical Library. Personal correspondence, July 3, 1869
17. Andrews E: Case reports, 1857-1903, 26 vols. Housed in the historical collection, Northwestern University Medical Library. Personal correspondence, July 12, 1869
18. Andrews E: Case reports, 1857-1903, 26 vols. Housed in the historical collection, Northwestern University Medical Library. Personal correspondence, 1869
19. Editorial: Ether and chloroform compared as anaesthetics. Boston Med Surg J 1859; 61- 129
20. Snow J. On Chloroform and Other Anaesthetics: Their Action and Administration. London, John Churchill, 1858
21. The Hyderabad Chloroform Commissions. Lancet 1890; 1:149, 1:921, 1:486; 1:1140, 1:1389

Early Reports on Death under Anesthesia in the XIXth Century in Spain

A. Franco, J. C. Diz,
Servicio de Anestesiología, Reanimación
Hospital General de Galicia, Clinico Universitario, Spain

During the second half of last century, chloroform was almost the sole anesthetic used in Spain, since it replaced ether in December 1847. In general terms, the use of chloroform was very cautious in Spain, and it seemed that surgeons were afraid of such a powerful agent, and with little resources for counteracting its undesirable actions. Certainly, these were some of the reasons that explain that in many operations performed in Spain the surgeons used very small doses of chloroform, with a technique they called „incomplete anesthesia". They often said that it was preferable a superficial anesthesia to an irreversible tragedy. In Spain there were even many operations without any kind of anesthesia. Sometimes the surgeon did not want to have any anesthetic accident, but in other cases the patient himself rejected anesthesia, and there were also operations in which the surgeon was unable to anesthetize the patient[1].

Many surgeons maintained passionately this way of operating without anesthesia or in very superficial stages of anesthesia, and they stated that this was the reason of the very low incidence of anesthetic deaths in Spain, and even many surgeons believed that the incidence in Spain was lower than in other countries. There were many statistics published in Spain in the XIXth century in which anesthetic mortality was almost zero, and some authors stated that in Madrid there was not any case of anesthetic death in the final twenty years of XIXth century[2]. However, the reality was quite different, and in this paper we will show some well documented cases of anesthetic mortality published Spain.

In one of the very first clinical administrations of sulfuric ether in Spain, in the Hospital General in Madrid, the surgeon Antonio Saez administered liquid ether per rectum twice to a 50 years old patient the day before the operation, and inhalatory ether during the operation, in which he extirpated a giant breast tumor[3]. The anesthesia was incomplete, and the patient died soon after the operation, without recovering the conscience completely. In Spain nobody attributed this death to anesthesia, but John Snow in 1858 described this case as a possible anesthetic death, although he admitted that he did not have enough information[4].

Dr. Antonio Mendoza, on February 16, 1847, in Barcelona, amputated a leg under ether anesthesia, and the patient died a few hours after the operation. Dr. Mendoza attributed this death to ether, explaining that there was an overdose, since the patient did not recover the conscience[5-6].

A very famous accident occurred in Madrid, on March 24, 1849, when a 12 years old boy died suddenly in the *Hospitales Generales* de Madrid during an induction with chloroform[7]. Snow also described this case in his classical book of 1858[4].

There were several cases of death after inhalation of chloroform in the Military Hospital of Madrid, in the second half of last century. In 1849, a soldier with hydrophobia died after chloroform administration for the treatment of seizures[8]. In 1859, another soldier died during chloroform inhalations used for the treatment of traumatic tetanus. Later, in 1875, there were two cases of chloroformic death, one due to „prolonged action of chloroform", and the other to „syncope" at the end of the operation[9].

A man died suddenly during the induction of anesthesia with chloroform in the *Hospital de la Princesa*, in Madrid in 1884, due to „congestive eclampsia". The necropsy showed ingurtigation of cerebral vessels[10].

In Barcelona, between 1880 and 1900 we could record seven deaths attributed to anesthesia, according to statistics of that date[11]. In Madrid, in 20.000 operations, there were ten cases of anesthetic death, according to a publication of 1910[12].

We could also find in Spanish medical journals many cases of postoperatory death, attributed to shock or collapse, without describing the exact cause, but they were not related to anesthetics[13-17].

The main problem we find when we try to make an analysis of these cases is the definition of „anesthetic death", since not every death under the effects of anesthetics is a death caused by anesthesia. In general terms, most surgeons of the period we studied consider only as anesthetic deaths those occurred during the operation, and in many cases they were related to cardiac or respiratory syncope, or „congestive eclampsia". But they seldom included as anesthetic deaths those which happened in the few hours or days after the operation, although in many instances these deaths were really caused by anesthesia.

In Spain, at the end of XIXth century, there was a development of the techniques of abdominal surgery, and the operations were longer and more aggressive. There was also an increase in the problems with chloroform anesthesia, and this was one of the reasons that explain why chloroform was gradually substituted for ether or combined ether-chloroform techniques, as these were safer for abdominal surgery. In this period several surgeons published statistics with a very high postoperative mortality, attributed to shock or collapse, but no related to anesthesia[13,16]. Some surgeons of the beginning of this century imputed to chloroform the high morbidity and mortality during surgery, and they were of the opinion that there were important differences among surgeons of the same hospital. Some of them believed that the incidence of anesthetic deaths and postoperative collapse was higher in the slower surgeons, and in those that discontinued the operation with explanations to the students. But for many, the real cause of the supposed low anesthetic mortality in Spain was that many surgeons did not publish the real number of deaths, and they assumed that mortality was, at least, twice as much as they said[18].

In summary, in Spain, as in many other countries during the XIXth century, there were many anesthetic deaths. Certainly, the real number of cases is higher than the number published in the journals. In many instances the surgeons hid the cases of deaths they had, and this makes very difficult to do an accurate estimation of the problem. Most surgeons considered as anesthetic deaths only those which occurred during the operation, but they did not relate to anesthesia those happening in the postoperative period. With the analysis of the cases we have found and of other publications we estimate that the overall mortality attributed to anesthesia in Spain was around 1 each 2.500 operations in the second half of XIXth century, a number very far from the optimistic estimations of many of our surgeons.

References

[1] Franco A, Cortés J, Vidal MI, et al.: "Historia de la anestesia clorofórmica en España 1847-1927. Una aproximación a su morbimortalidad." Act. anest. reanim. 1993, 3: 188-222

[2] San Martín A: "La insuflación nasofaríngea en la anestesia general, la calefacción de los operados y actitudes operatorias." Rev. Med. Cir. Pract. 1905, 66: 5-21.

[3] Roel F.G: "Tumor escirroso enquistado de la mama derecha que pesó trece libras (de á 16 onzas) y un cuarterón." La Facultad, 1847, 10: 155-157

[4] Snow J: "On Chloroform and other Anesthetics; their Action and Administration." John Churchill, London, 1858

[5] Anonymous: "Efectos de la inhalación del éter en un caso de amputación de la pierna, practicada en el hospital de Santa Cruz de Barcelona por el Sr. Mendoza." La Facultad, 1847, 2: 155

[6] Hervás J: "La anestesia en Cataluña. Historia y evolución." Tesis Doctoral, Barcelona, 1986

[7] Anonymous: "Muerte por el cloroformo." La Union, 1849, 82, 165

[8] Anonymous: "Varias mordeduras causadas por un perro: cauterización poco tiempo después. Hidrofobia a los 48 días; uso del cloroformo. Muerte." Gaceta Medica (Madrid), 1849, 153: 67-68

[9] Anonymous: "Hospital Militar de Madrid (Cuadro estadístico)." Gaceta de Sanidad Militar, 1875, 1: 222-223

[10] Anonymous: "Muerte por el cloroformo." IV y V ejercicios, Instituto Rubio de Madrid, 1884-1885

[11] Recasens S: "Ventajas del éter sobre el cloroformo como anestésico general." Tipo-Litografía de Balmas, Barcelona, 1897

[12] Faure S: "Anestésicos por Inhalación." Tesis Doctoral, Madrid, 1910

[13] Pombo L: "Memoria estadística de las operaciones verificadas en el quirófano de la Facultad de Medicina." Imp. Asilo Huérfanos, Madrid, 1895

[14] Pintado M: "Reseña de las contraindicaciones del cloroformo." Rev. Med. (Santiago), 1848, 1/7: 129-135

[15] Magaz J: "Inconvenientes graves del uso de las inhalaciones clorofórmicas: medio de evitarlas." Rev. Med. (Santiago), 1848, 1: 236-240

[16] Arpal F: "Estadística operatoria." Tip. Mariano Sala, Zaragoza, 1899

[17] González Olivares J: "Una víctima más por el cloroformo." Rev. Cienc. Med. (Santiago), 1856, 4: 121-128

[18] Guedea L: "Anestesia local." Anales de la real Academia de Medicina, Madrid, 1911

An early Chloroform Death in Berlin.

B. Panning*, H.-G. Klös, S. Piepenbrock*
* Medizinische Hochschule Hannover
Department of Anaesthesiology, Germany

At the Fourth International Symposium of the History of Anaesthesia in Hamburg a small bronze sculpture was presented in the exhibition in the Kunsthalle[4]. This work of art (Fig.1) is connected with an early use of chloroform in the Zoological Garden of Berlin. A short description of this event is given in the text of the catalogue[4]. Details will be described later. The story was presented several times in the literature[1, 2, 3, 8, 9, 10, 11].

A new and completely different version was published 1994 in the memorial book on the occasion of the 150th anniversary of the zoological garden of Berlin[6]. This report is presented here. It is based on the personal knowledge of the retired director of the zoo Dr. Heinz-Georg Klös who obtained his information from the late director Dr. Heck. Dr. Heck had private connections with the surgeon and artist Prof. Carl Ludwig Schleich who knew the story from his father Carl Schleich. C. Schleich was a contemporary of the bear anaesthetic. As a friend of the famous Albrecht von Graefe, Carl Schleich should have had a relatively objective view of the events[13].

According to the "Klös-Schleich-version", which is how we want to call this variant[6], a cataract operation on a bear was to be performed on May 12th, 1851. A zookeeper Mr. Lütgens tied the bear, and then a physician, Dr. Krieger, administered chloroform to the animal. The operation could not take place because the bear could not be anaesthetized adequately. The reason for this may have been the lack of a sufficient amount of chloroform. It was reported that only 1.5 ounces of chloroform had been available.

It seems that this event soon became known in the town and the topic was widely discussed among the citizens. The town-peoples' imagination may have induced another variation; and this is the tenor of the other descriptions: Johann Lucas Schönlein (1793-1864) from Bamberg, medical professor in Berlin from 1839 till 1859, was interested in the use of the new anaesthetic substance chloroform. He was permitted by King Friedrich Wilhelm IV from Prussia to use an animal of the zoo for a "clinical trial". A cataract operation was to be performed on a bear. This opportunity was chosen to gain experiences with chloroform before using it on human beings. The operation was performed successfully but the bear did not awake after the anaesthesia. The King of Prussia found this event so interesting that he induced the famous animal-sculptor Albert Wolff to create the bronze as a memory of the event (Fig. 1). This approximately 40 cm high sculpture consists of 6 animals dressed as human beings. In the middle is a bear sitting on a chair, surrounded by 5 other animals with human faces. On the right side of the bear is an ape and a fox, on the left side an owl and a young bear. Behind the bear a goat. A part of these animals allegorized famous doctors of Berlin who in the phantasy of the citizens were told to have been involved in the experiment. The ape represented the surgeon and ophthalmologist Prof. Dr. Joh. Christian Jüngken. The owl stands for the neurologist Prof. Dr. Moritz Romberg. The goat

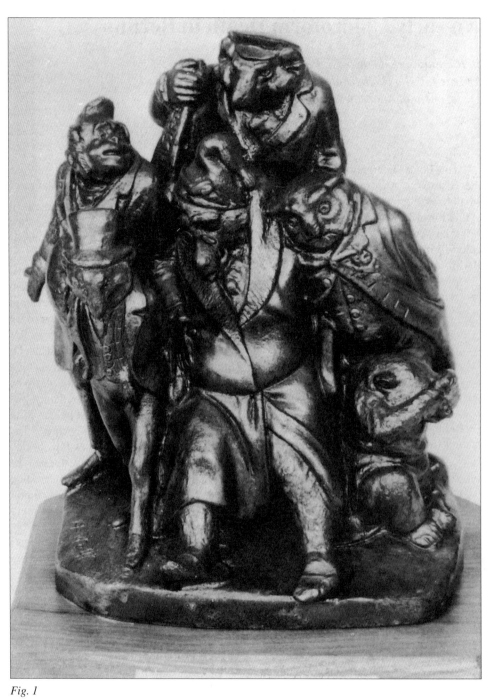

Fig. 1

symbolizes the above mentioned Prof. Schönlein. This goat holds a bag with the lettering "chloroform" in his right hand. So he was certainly seen as the "anaesthetist". The fox is an allusion to the sculptor Wolff. Only for the young bear no allusion could be found. A competition for the best poem to the sculpture was induced. The young Paul Heyse who 1910 became a winner of the Nobel-prize for literature won the prize, a copy of the bronze with the following poem:

"Der Bär ist nun ein toter Mann

das Chloroform ist schuld daran.

Ein ärztliches Kollegium

ging mit dem Vieh zu menschlich um.

Das Füchslein greint,

das Böcklein flennt,

der Wolf setzt ihm dies Monument."

A translation of these verses can be found in a paper of Ebstein[1]

A dead man is the bear I fear.

The reason well this chloroform here.

A consultation of medical men

Treated too humanly the animal then.

The foxlet grins, little bear will lament,

The wolf erects this monument.

As mentioned above several references can be found in the literature. The eldest one originates from C. T. Jackson. 1851 he gave a short note in his description of anaesthesia in animals which appeared 1852[5]. The first sentence reads: "In Berlin, chloroform was administered to a bear without due admixture of air and it killed him". 1915 the German engineer Feldhaus included the tale in a collection of short scetches[2]. 1921 Holländer used the story for a short paragraph in a book on caricature and satire in medicine. In this book a picture of the animal group can be found[8]. 1923 Ebstein took up the tale in his account on Schönlein[1]. 1946 Frankel retold it in his paper "on the introduction of general anaesthesia in Germany"[3]. Frankel was an urologist from Berlin who emigrated to Manila 1933. 1952 a Dr. F. W. R. gave a short summary of the bear-anaesthetic in the Ciba-Journal[9]. According to the medical historian Prof. Schadewald from Düsseldorf the initials belong to Dr. F. W. Rieppel from Basel who was an employee of the Ciba-company[12]. 1965 an article of Reuter appeared in a regional medical journal in Berlin which narrated the event once more[10]. All these references assumed that the bear was operated on and did not recover from the anaesthetic and did not take the "Klös-Schleich-version" into consideration.

It seems difficult to find out the truth today. One way of discussing this question may be looking at the date of the event. The Klös-Schleich-version states May 12, 1851[6]. The inscription at the base of the bronze, which was exhibited in the Kunsthalle in Hamburg, presents the year 1847[4]. This date seems unlikely but not impossible because chloroform was first introduced on November 14th, 1847. The reference from Jackson[5] suggests the year 1851 as the latest date. Feldhaus[2] and also Robinson[11] names 1852. The other references do not give an explicit date.

A recently discovered detail may give further support to the "Klös-Schleich-version". Prof. Schadewald found the plaster form of the bronze. This is in the possession of a Dr. Krieger in Düsseldorf[7, 12]. He inherited the cast form from his grandfather who lived from the beginning till the last third of the 19th century in Berlin. This grandfather was a medical officer of the Prussian government[7]. As it is stated above in the "Klös-Schleich-version" Dr. Krieger was the physician involved[6]. Research in old newspapers of Berlin is in progress in order to find out whether this assumption can be supported.

References:

[1] Ebstein E: Anecdotes about Schönlein. Medical life 30 (1923) 463-465

[2] Feldhaus FM: Modernste Kriegswaffen – alte Erfindungen. Abel und Müller, Leipzig 1915.

[3] Frankel WK: The introduction of general anesthesia in Germany. J. Hist. Med. 1946; 10: 612–617

[4] Goerig M: Anaesthetic Equipment in the History of German Anaesthesia. Catalogue of the exhibition held at the Museum für Kunst und Gewerbe, Hamburg from 23 April to 4 Mai 1997. Catalogue. Edrs.: J.Schulte am Esch, M. Goerig. Dräger, Lübeck 1997

[5] Jackson CT: Etherization of Animals and of Man. Trans. Am. Inst. City of N. Y. for 1851, Albany, 167-173, 1852 Reprinted in: S. B. Nuland: The origins of Anesthesia. The classics of medicine library, Birmingham, 1983

[6] Klös H-G, H Frädrich, U Klös: Die Arche Noah an der Spree, FAB-Verlag, Berlin 1994, p.p. 58–59

[7] Krieger R: Personal communication, 1994

[8] Holländer E: Die Karikatur und Satire in der Medizin. Enke, Stuttgart 1921

[9] Rieppel FW: Der chloroformierte Bär. Ciba-Zeitschrift 1952; 11: 4808

[10] Reuter H: Wilhelm Wolff: Karikatur auf die erste Chloroformnarkose in Berlin. Bln Med 1965; 16: 363

[11] Robinson V: Victory over pain, Schuman. New York 1946, p.p. 231–233

[12] Schadewald H: Personal communication, 1996

[13] Schleich CL: Besonnte Vergangenheit, p.p.49-51. Rowohlt, Berlin 1922; p.p. 49–51

Gurlt's Report "Zur Narkotisirungs-Statistik" in 1897 - an Early Contribution to Quality Assurance in Anaesthesia

W. Röse, Department of Anaesthesiology and Critical Care Medicine
Otto-von-Guericke-University, Magdeburg, Germany

Numerous contemporary medical scientific publications consider aspects of quality assurance, quality measurement and quality management. In this context it seems sometimes neglected or forgotten that problems of quality in connection with medical treatment were recognized, documented, discussed and published already 100 years ago. One example for this is the initiative of the German Society for Surgery in 1890 to start a multicenter study on surgical anaesthesia. This project was headed by the surgeon Ernst Julius Gurlt (1825-1899) (Fig. 1) from Berlin. He reported on the occasion of the annual congresses of the German Surgeons in 1891, 1892, 1893, 1894, 1895 and 1897[1-6] on the basis of a questionnaire, answered by the majority of the leading German surgeons and by some German speaking surgeons from abroad.

The nine items of this questionnaire were
1. Observation period for the report
2. Anaesthetics (chloroform, ether, mixtures etc.)
   and the frequency of their application
3. Manufacturer of the anaesthetics
4. Application devices for the anaesthetics
5. Duration of exceptional long lasting anaesthetic procedures (1 hour and more)
6. Consumption of anaesthetics per minute, or as average for each anaesthesia, or
   maximal need for very long lasting anaesthesia procedures
7. Number of patients, to whom morphine or other pharmaceutics were injected before anaesthesia-induction
8. Glucose and/or protein determination in the urine
9. Complications during and after anaesthesia:
   a. asphyxia (treatment, tracheostomy etc.)
   b. deaths (causes, obduction results)
   c. postanaesthetic complications following chloroform and ether anaesthesia
      (collapse, pulmonary oedema, bronchitis, fatal and non-fatal pneumonia)

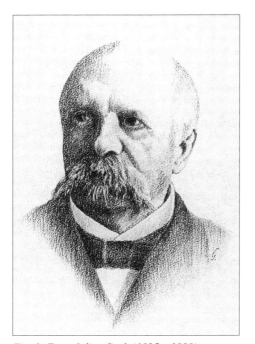

Fig. 1: Ernst Julius Gurlt (1825 – 1899)

On April 24, 1897, Gurlt gave his sixth (and last) report to the participants of the German congress of surgery in Berlin. (Fig. 2) This report summarizes the results of the questionnaires for the two periods 1895-1896, 1896-1897 respectively, because in 1896 no report had been presented.

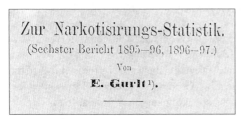

Fig. 2: Title of Gurlt's sixth report on anaesthesia statistics

Gurlt reviewed 92 answers given by authors from surgical departments in Germany. 12 came from Austria, Russia, Sweden and Serbia.

Additionally Gurlt repeats the data of the proceeding years, so that a survey from 1890 to 1897 can be demonstrated. (Fig. 3)

Referring to these data with a total number of 330 429 anaesthetized cases and 136 anaesthesia-related deaths Gurlt calculates a mortality rate of 1:2429. This number is much better during and after anaesthesia with ether, with a combination of chloroform and ether, with Billroth-mixture and with bromethyl. The highest mortality rates resulted from anaesthesia with pental and last but not least in connection with chloroform. Although chloroform has had the same unfavourable results in the years before it was in 1895/96 as well as in 1896/97 the anaesthetic of first choice in most surgical departments.

Gurlt's comment is concentrated on less than two pages. Repeatedly he refers to the former 5 publications and to some of the 36 original reports, printed on 40 extra pages as appendix to the sixth report.

Extracts of some of these very comprehensive and detailed reports may find the

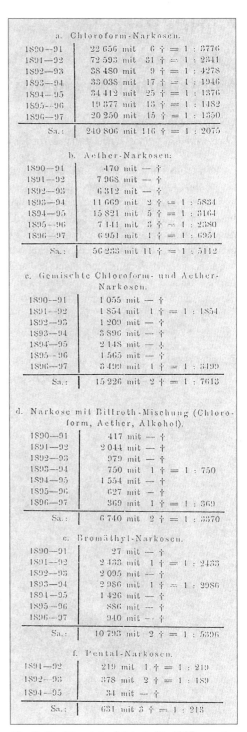

Fig. 3: Gurlt's original data in his 1897 report

interest of the contemporary reader. The numbers correspond to those of the questionnaire.

Appendix 1:

Charité-Hospital Berlin (von Bardeleben up to 1895, from 1896 KÖNIG)

1. March 1895 - March 1896
2. 666 chloroform-anaesthesia-procedures
3. Manufacturer: Merck company, Darmstadt
4. Esmarch mask
   24 cases with Junker or Kappeler apparatus
5. 83 cases 60 - 90 min (average chloroform consumption 34,5 ml)
   44 cases 90 - 120 min (average chloroform consumption 59,4 ml)
   20 cases 120 - 150 min (average chloroform consumption 70,0 ml)
6. Overall chloroform consumption:
   22 ml/case
   0,57 ml/minute of anaesthesia
   Tendency to decreased consumption following more carefully administered drop-method:
   0,57 ml/minute in 1896 versus 0,71 ml/minute in 1894.
7. Principle morphin premedication with exception of children
8. no comment
9. Extraordinary excitation in
   18 patients
   Vomiting during anaesthesia in
   8 patients
   Intermittent pulselessness in
   9 patients
   Asphyxia (6 of them severe) in
   10 patients

"Traction of the tongue, pressing down the epiglottis and cardiac massage were successful in all cases to overcome the live threatening situation."

Description of an anaesthesia-related death after 6 ml chloroform in a 36 years old man scheduled for the reposition of a fractured leg. Unsuccessful reanimation trials for 60 minutes including external cardiac massage. The Charité-report ends with the sentences: "Finally it should be mentioned, that in this year experiments with compressed oxygen (produced in the ELKAN factory) were undertaken to investigate, whether the postanaesthetic recovery could be shortened by inhalation of 100 % oxygen. In 20 chloroform-respectively ether-anaesthetized patients a significant success of oxygen on recovery could not be detected."

Appendix 4 (extract):

University Königsberg (Braun, von Eiselsberg, i.V. Stetter)

In this report the use of the Kappeler apparatus is described with special consideration of a metall insufflation catheter - to administer the chloroform-air-mixture via nose or mouth for operations at the head.

Appendix 5 (extract):

University Tübingen (Bruns)

In this surgical department the application of ether predominates (485 cases with ether, 152 with chloroform, 155 with bromethyl). Bruns reports: "In numerous cases general anaesthesia was replaced by local anaesthesia with ether anaestheticus or ethyl chlorid, but especially by the Schleich infiltration method."

Appendix 6 (extract):

University Heidelberg (Czerny)

Among 1670 operations in ambulant cases only 103 had general anaesthesia. The majority of the patients were locally anaesthetized with Cocain. The results were very good without any example of intoxication symptoms.

Appendix 30 (extract):

Hamburg-Eppendorf-Hospital (Kümmell and Sick)

Chloroform anaesthesia: 1371 cases
Chloroform anaesthesia deaths: 3

"Case report III: very fat 29 years old brewer with 36 hours existing incarcerated inguinal hernia. Because of suspected pericarditis and alcoholism the herniotomy is started using the Schleich local anaesthesia method. This procedure proves insufficient. Now 0,01 Morphin is injected, Cognac given, than Chloroform administered; very heavy excitation, frequent awakening during anaesthesia. After 40 minutes anaesthesia with consumption of 75 ml Chloroform at the end of the operation, when the skin was sutured, cessation of breathing, followed by pulselessness. Unsuccessful reanimation trials.

Obduction: Pleuritis adhaesiva, obliteratio pericardii totalis, degeneratio adiposa myocardii et hepatis."

Gurlts 1897 report including the added detailed answers to the questionnaire in many respects reflects the situation of anaesthesia quality at the end of the 19th century in Germany with

- very simple equipment
- unexperienced, non-specialised personnel
- lack of intra- as well as postoperative monitoring
- minimal or missing documentation.

On the other hand the reporting surgeons give a very realistic picture on the situation in the different hospitals, and Gurlt has to be congratulated to have added again so many appendices to his annual report given by some of the most respected heads of surgical departments of his time.

Compared with the 5 former reports a tendency to the administration of local anaesthetics can not be overlooked in 1897. But there are only few remarks concerning the advantages of the Schleich infiltration method and no data on complications or deaths. The main statement refers to the enormous number of more than 300.000 anaesthetized cases reported in 7 years with special consideration of fatal and also non-fatal complications.

Gurlt may have been disappointed to see in 1896/1897 again the big number of chloroform anaesthesia cases and chloroform-associated complications. It is very unclear, why the contemporary physicians did not trust in the impressive statistical data demonstrating the advantages of ether as well as of different combined inhalational anaesthesia techniques.

One reason against broader ether administration may have been an increasing number of reported ether-related post-anaesthetic complications such as bronchitis or pneumonia. These mainly non-fatal complication were only casuistically documented.

Severe chloroform-related complications with cessation of breathing and circulation obliged the surgeons to improve the measures and methods of reanimation. The recommendation of external cardiac compression by Maass in 1892 in cases of chloroform-syncope is one example for this intention.[7] Also in the 1896/97 report there are several references to artificial breathing and circulation, intravenous infusion, electric phrenic stimulation and pharmacologic stimulation of the circulation.

Summarizing it can be stated that Ernst Julius Gurlt was an early pacemaker of quality assurance in anaesthesia. There was no seventh report on anaesthesia statistics. Gurlt died on January, 18, 1899.

References:

[1] Gurlt E: Zur Narkotisirungs-Statistik (Erster Bericht 1890-1891), Verh.Dtsch.Ges.Chir. 1891; 20: 46-65

[2] Gurlt E: Zur Narkotisirungs-Statistik (Zweiter Bericht 1891-1892), Verh.Dtsch.Ges.Chir. 1892; 21: 308-366

[3] Gurlt E: Zur Narkotisirungs-Statistik (Dritter Bericht 1892-1893), Verh.Dtsch.Ges.Chir. 1893; 22: 8-45

[4] Gurlt E: Zur Narkotisirungs-Statistik (Vierter Bericht 1893-1894), Verh.Dtsch.Ges.Chir. 1894; 23: 11-62

[5] Gurlt E: Zur Narkotisirungs-Statistik (Fünfter Bericht 1894-1895), Verh.Dtsch.Ges.Chir. 1895; 24: 460-537

[6] Gurlt E: Zur Narkotisirungs-Statistik (Sechster Bericht 1895-1896, 1896-1897), Verh.Dtsch.Ges.Chir. 1897; 26: 202-248

[7] Maass F: Die Methode der Wiederbelebung beim Herztod nach Chloroformeinathmung Berlin.Klin.Wschr. 1892; 29: 265

The Circulatory Risks of Anaesthesia in Leiden before 1930.

M. van Wijhe
University Hospital, Groningen, The Netherlands

Introduction

The problems associated with the effects of anaesthesia on the circulatory system can be divided into two main categories: 1. sudden failure of the heart at the beginning of the procedure, and 2. slow, progressive failure of the circulation in the course of the procedure. The terminology used by different authors before 1930 being confusing, the different interpretations and resulting treatments will be presented, as found in original theatre books and lectures of the Leiden University Hospital. The degree to which physiological and pharmacological knowledge was integrated into clinical practice will become apparent.

Examples

The annual reports of the operations performed in the surgical department from 1875 onward were reviewed with regard to circulatory problems. Of the 146 patients operated upon in 1879-1880, 20 died peri-operatively, 6 in a state of "collapse". In 1883 a 38 year old man had an operation on his hand, a quarter of an hour after induction he suddenly became cyanosed and died. In 1889 a patient was reported to be in a "collapsed" state due to abdominal obstruction. He was given subcutaneous ether injections. Right hemicolectomy with colostomy lasting three hours was done under chloroform anaesthesia. Post-operatively he was given more ether injections and champagne to drink. The next day he complained of terrible thirst, he also vomited, for which he was given morphine powders, port wine, eggs, and clear soup. All went well however, he went home after four months with a closed colostomy. In 1891 a 5 year old girl died after bilateral correction of congenital hip joint luxation was attempted. A few hours after the operations she was sweating, vomiting, and had a thready pulse. Desperate, her surgeons gave her 1/8 litre of physiologic saline solution subcutaneously and intravenously in "the vein that accompanies the radial artery". The postmortem examination showed all the signs of blood loss. In the ensueing years several more such cases were described, operations with major blood loss, post-operative signs of serious fluid depletion, death and anemia at postmortem. Infusion of intravenous normal saline, up to 750 ml., was done when the signs became serious. From 1916 onward haemoglobin was measured in operation patients using the Sahli method[1].

Terminology

The terminology used between 1850 and 1930 to describe what we now call "shock" is different from that of today, and differed between authors. John Snow defined the cardiac complications of anesthesia as being due to: (1) cardiac syncope, primary heart failure, or (2) anaemic syncope, a lack of blood returning to the heart[2]. van Iterson, the Leiden professor of surgery between 1878 and 1901, used the term "collapse" when a patient had the signs of a rapid and weak pulse, clamminess, sweating, lowered consciousness, extreme thirst and nausea. Collapse was thought to have a nervous cause. Hammes, the author of the first authoritative dutch textbook on anaesthesia, also used "collapse" in this sense. "Syncope" he reserved for signs of acute or subacute cardiac failure[3]. van Itallie, a pharmacologist who reviewed anaesthetic drugs in 1928, defined syncope to be of the "reflex" and the "toxic" kind; as did the German surgeon Sauerbruch[4,5]. The table shows the relationship between the different terms.

Author	Ventricular fibrillation	myocardial depression	vagal	haemorrhage
Snow 1858	cardiac syncope		anemic syncope	
van Iterson 1899	reflex syncope	"too deep"	collapse	→ shock
Hammes 1908	syncope		collapse	
van Itallie 1928	reflex syncope	toxic syncope	surgical shock	
Sauerbruch 1933	"fruhsyncope"	overdosis	reflex death	collapse → shock

Treatment

The treatment of the circulatory problems during and after anaesthesia varied from doing nothing to strong stimulation of the heart with various cardiotonics. Hammes' opinion exemplifies the former: *"... thirst after lengthy chloroform anaesthetics can be very troublesome. A light, even anaesthetic gives the best postoperative results; ether with lack of air causes more problems than when air can be freely drawn in. Treatment consists of rest, and no food or drink. If the thirst becomes very agonizing, the mouth can be wetted with cold water or an ice-cube. Some vinegar on a swab held under the nose is a good remedy for postoperative nausea. If the patient has been operated upon in the morning, he is usually capable of drinking water, diluted milk, light soup or weak tea. Wine or champagne seem irrational to me, but are generally well taken. That beverages such as strong coffee are recommended is a mystery to me. Thus, in normal cases treatment is unnecessary. It is more a matter of leaving well enough alone. There are however cases where the most troublesome symptom, vomiting, lasts too long and becomes an agony. Then we also like to have the illusion of doing some thing. Ice-cubes, sips of warm water, strong coffee with or without bicarbonate of soda, champagne, warm towels on the stomach area, and stomach lavage have all been recommended and are worth trying. I think "qui bene suggerit, bene curat". Hypodermoclysis, by the way, by dilution and more rapid excretion of the toxins, could also be successful."*

Risk evaluation took place pre-operatively: if a patient had signs of heart disease and could not hold his breath for at least twenty seconds, he was considered unfit for operation.

Acute cardiac problems were treated with various cardiotonics, mostly stimulating drugs. Common were: camphorated spirits, hexetone, ether, digalene, caffeine, adrenaline, lobeline, strychnine, morfine, and atropine. Resuscitation and artificial ventilation ensued if necessary.

Cardiac syncope

The slow development of insight in the mechanism of acute anaesthetic death under chloroform anaesthesia demonstrates how slowly discoveries in basic science percolate into clinical practice. In Leiden, Willem Einthoven developed the string galvanometer, with which it became possible to register the electric activity of the heart from 1906 onward. An achievement for which he received the 1924 Nobel prize. Goodman Levy wrote his observation concerning the mechanism of ventricular fibrillation due to the interaction of the influences of chloroform and catecholamines on the myocardium in 1914. Yet an official government publication on anaesthetic drugs by the Leiden pharmacologist van Itallie in 1928 did not elucidate the mechanism of acute chloroform death. In practice ether was the anaesthetic of choice in adults in Leiden, until Zaaijer introduced nitrous oxide in 1923.

Anemic syncope

In the beginning of the period studied, shock, or anemic syncope as it was called was treated with drugs considered to be cardiac stimulants, such as digitalene, caffeine or camphorated oil. Visser investigated the effectiveness of these drugs in 1908, concluding that only digitaline had some effect[6]. The others were continued to be used for many years however.

During the whole period studied blood pressure was not measured to monitor its' changes, as the surgeons felt it could cause unrest in the operating theatre, something much to be avoided. As reports in the international literature on the use of normal saline and Bayliss' (acacia gum) solution in surgery and resuscitation of the wounded increased especially after the First World War, evidence of its' cautious use can be found in the operation report books.

Conclusion

In conclusion the application of new medical developments in surgery in the Leiden University Hospital in the late 19th and early 20th century was typical for continental Europe. The importance of the physiologic backgrounds of acute cardiac catastrophe and of excessive blood loss took decennia to understand and implement into clinical practice.

References:

[1] van Wijhe M: From Stupefaction to Narcosis. Dissertation Leiden, 1991
[2] Snow J: On Chloroform and other Anaesthetics. London, 1858
[3] Hammes T: Leerboek der Narcose. Amsterdam, 1919
[4] van Itallie ea: Narcotica. Leiden, 1928
[5] Sauerbruch F, Schmieden V: Chirurgische Operationslehre I: Leipzig, Barth, 1933
[6] Visser MJ: Aether of Chloroform? Dissertation Amsterdam, 1908

The Lahey Explosion

G. L. Zeitlin,
Brigham and Women's Hospital, Boston, Massachusetts, U.S.A.

Although cyclopropane was introduced into clinical practice in the early 1930's there was initially very little serious research into preventing explosions.

It took an explosion in a particular hospital, in a department of surgery headed by a unique man, to stimulate much-needed investigations. A young woman was killed by a cyclopropane explosion on the morning of October 31 1938 in Operating Theatre Number 2, at the New England Baptist Hospital in Boston.

This paper describes the remarkable and unusual response to this tragedy by the head of the Lahey Clinic, Dr. Frank Lahey, and outlines some of the many ramifications of his response.

Frank Lahey was born in Haverhill, Massachusetts in 1880 and attended Harvard Medical School. When America entered the war in 1917 he became a Major in the Army Medical Corps and was appointed Chief of Surgery at an evacuation hospital in France for wounded American soldiers. After the war he opened an office at 638 Beacon Street in Boston. The first two associates he chose were Dr. Sara Jordan, a gatroenterologist and Dr. Lincoln Sise, an anesthesiologist. These would appear very shrewd and logical choices for an abdominal surgeon. His selection of a physician anesthesiologist foreshadows his later and intense interest in the development of professional anesthesia specialists.

He was so successful that by 1924 his was the third largest private clinic in the U.S.A. with patients coming from all over the East Coast and Canada. Later the Clinic attracted patients from all over the world including Sir Anthony Eden, future Prime Minister of the United Kingdom.

But on that morning in 1938, a much more humble patient undergoing breast surgery, became the victim of an explosion. Her name was Mary Lahiff; she was 44 years old and worked as a secretary at a fuel supply company in Cambridge. Dr. Urban Eversole who was giving anesthesia in the adjacent operating room described what happened when interviewed some years later.

"The operation was just about over when we heard the bang in the next room. I immediately turned my patient over to the anesthesia resident and went into the adjoining room. I examined the patient. She seemed alright. An immediate bronchoscopy was performed, but in doing so a pharyngeal tear was missed. She developed emphysema clear down to her knees and died about 18 hours later". We also know from another description that a tracheostomy was performed. I have been unable to find any evidence that ventilatory support was provided, other than supplemental oxygen.

An autopsy was reported by the Boston Medical Examiner. Mary Lahiff died of what we would now term massive lung contusions and mediastinal emphysema. She is buried in the Cambridge Catholic Cemetery among other deceased relatives. She and William Morton, in the adjacent Mount Auburn Cemetery, sleep quietly about 500 yards apart.

Dr. Eversole continues: "Dr. Lahey, with his usual alacrity called a meeting of representative experts from throughout New England and the country."

But the very first action Lahey took was to issue what we now would call a press release. In essence it is a detailed description of what happened that fateful morning. This is also a remarkable action. In 1938 the feeling of invulnerabilty on the part of the medical profession and the awe in which it was held by the public led to virtually complete supression of medical error and adverse outcome.

Dr. Lahey asked one of the younger anesthesiologists, Dr. Phil Woodbridge to coordinate a meeting of experts. This led to intense activity by a number of people and their findings were presented just 12 weeks later.

The meeting was held at the Lahey Clinic on the evening of January 23 1939. A copy of the printed report of that meeting has recently come to light. It is 24 pages long; The meeting ran very late that bitter winter night. Because of this only a few of the highlights are presented here.

In Dr. Lahey's opening statement we read: "The room in which the explosion occurred was immediately locked up. We telephoned Dr. Karl Connell, the manufacturer of the apparatus and he immediately started for Boston from New York and made an investigation of the accident and the apparatus."

Lahey continued:

I felt it particularly incumbent on me as an individual to have a frank discussion of the situation in an open meeting; also I feel keenly the obligation to the lady who was the victim of this catastrophe and to the members of her family.

I have said to the anesthetists that they are somewhat sheltered from criticism, while I represent the outpost against which surges all the undiluted criticism which may come up as a result of this. This must be discussed both from the point of view of logic and sentiment. I have hoped that there might take place (tonight) an expression of opinion regarding the wisdom of continuing the use of cyclopropane, oxygen, ether and ethylene, OR of discontinuing the use of explosive anesthetics".

Dr. Connell's report was read by Dr. Woodbridge and is summarized thus:

1. The gas mixture was 18% cyclopropane in oxygen.
2. The explosion took place at the patient's end of the circuit. This was deduced from damage to the valves.
3. There was sufficient humidity - a wet bulb hygrometer showed relative humidity of 65% 15 minutes after the explosion.
4. The operating room floor was conductive and the drag chains were in use.
5. The interior of the tubing was quite moist 8 hours after the explosion. The external conductive wires on the tubing had been disrupted and therefore could not be tested.

Connell continued:

"The police method of reconstructing the crime was instituted by mock operation. One observation stood out, namely that anyone with rubber soled shoes sitting on the anesthetist's stool on arising suddenly developed a charge of static so high as to jam the electroscopic voltmeter at its maximum reading."

Lahey had also invited J. Warren Horton, Professor of Biological Engineering at M.I.T. to study the situation.

Prof. Horton confirmed many of Connell's observations. He found that NONE of the following was an absolute guarantee against the collection of significant electrostatic charges. That is to say he was able to measure substantial voltages in these and many other circumstances.

1. A relative humidity as high as 65%.
2. The then current practice of a wire running from the machine along the tubing to the face mask.

3. A person wearing crepe soled shoes and cotton clothes, as had Miss Edgar the nurse anesthetist who gave Mary Lahiff the anesthetic.

He concluded that the only certain safeguard against these possibilities was to interconnect the patient, the anaesthetist, the gas machine and the operating table to bring them all to the same potential.

Prof. Hoyt Hottel, Prof of Chemical Engineering from M.I.T. had in the intervening weeks experimentally defined the limits of explosibility of all the commonly used anesthetic vapours and gases in both air and oxygen. This had been done by Waters and others when the gas first entered clinical use. That night he gave a dramatic live demonstration for the audience.

Also during those three months Dr. Woodbridge had surveyed 100 leading anesthesiologists in the U.S.A. in attempt to gauge the frequency of explosions and also their opinions. His results were published later in the Journal of the American Medical Association.

Many others present also spoke; here are just two examples:

Dr. George MacIver from the Worcester Hospital: "I am interested in this subject as an executive. I am glad to hear what I have tonight and my fears have subsided. My feeling is that if the clinical men wish to resume the use of cyclopropane I would be willing and ready to agree with them".

Dr. William Brickley, Medical Examiner of Boston: "In 6000 deaths from unnatural causes I have seen no explosion from cyclopropane and only two deaths from syncope while under the influence of cyclopropane. I would feel that it is not a burning question (sic) in regard to a great number of accidents."

Although this seemed to be the end of the matter it was, as Winston Churchill said in another context, the end of the beginning. Examples of research resulting from this one fatal explosion include:

1. Further extensive research by Horton to find the limits of explosibility of complex gas mixtures;
2. The development of the Intercoupler by Horton.
3. The development of codes of behaviour in the operating room to prevent explosions.
4. The development of practical and routine testing for conductivity.

This paper contends that a single fatal cyclopropane explosion at the Lahey Clinic in 1938 and the vigorous response of its founder led to the greatest outburst of preventative research and activity from the time of its introduction in 1931 to its ultimate dis-0,appearance from clinical practice in the West in January 1996.

The Woolley and Roe Case - 1: The Anaesthetist's Thoughts

J. R. Maltby
Foothills Hospital, Calgary, Canada

Chesterfield is an iron mining and engineering town with a population of 80,000, about 20 km south of the much larger city of Sheffield. The year 1997 marks the 50th anniversary of one of the best known British medicolegal trials of the 20th century. The plaintiffs were Albert Woolley and Cecil Roe who had spinal anaesthesia on the same day at Chesterfield Royal Hospital and both suffered permanent spinal cord damage.

The patients

Woolley and Roe were on the same operating list at Chesterfield Royal Hospital on Monday, October 13, 1947. They each received spinal anaesthesia using 10 ml of light nupercaine 1/1500.[1] Roe, age 45 years, was first on the list and had a semilunar cartilage removed from his knee. Next came an emergency patient who was very ill from intestinal obstruction and died on the fifth postoperative day from peritonitis and bronchopneumonia. He also had light nupercaine spinal. Whether he had spinal cord damage is unclear, although Dr. Malcolm Graham, the anaesthetist, and the Roe family believe that he did. Woolley, age 56 years, had repair of a hydrocoele the same afternoon.

The postoperative courses of Woolley and Roe were similar, although Roe was always more severely affected than Woolley. The day after surgery both men had developed acute myelopathy involving the roots of the cauda equina and the lower spinal cord where the concentration of the injected solution would have been greatest.[2] The presenting features were flaccid paralysis of the legs, and anaesthesia of the lower abdominal wall, legs and perianal region with incontinence of urine and faeces. The symptoms progressed to painful spastic paraparesis after some initial improvement. There was never any clinical evidence of meningitis or meningism but the similarity of the conditions of both men strongly suggested a common aetiology.

In February 1948 Woolley improved for about a month when he was able to walk with the aid of two sticks and had partial control of micturition but a month later his walking

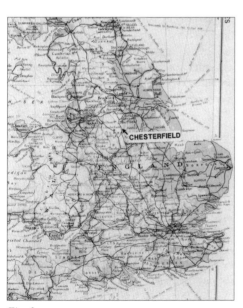

Fig. 1

deteriorated again. By May 1950 Roe was suffering from such severe flexor and adductor spasms that his legs and buttocks had to be tied down, even when he was lying prone. A myelogram showed arachnoiditis at L1 upwards and complete occlusion below L1. At laminectomy, a large arachnoidal cyst was found on the right side and posteriorly under the laminae of T10-11. It was thick walled and contained yellowish fluid under tension which was released. Below the level of the cyst, the conus medullaris and roots of cauda equina were enclosed in a dense mass of arachnoidal adhesions. The whole contents of the dural sheath had been converted into a solid mass of fibrous tissue with scarcely any identifiable neural elements. The spasms were much less severe for about three months and then increased again. Attempts to control them were made by injections of intrathecal alcohol and surgical division of nerves and muscles.

Both men survived for several years in a severely disabled condition. Roe had no sensation below the lower chest and no control over his bowel function. He had spastic tremors in both legs which were so violent that they threw him out of his chair or out of bed. He could wash, shave and feed himself but could not turn over or sit up without assistance from his wife or from a chain fitted over his bed. Before he became paraplegic he worked as a farm labourer, grew all his own vegetables and flowers, did his own house decorating and family shoe repairs. Woolley's disabilities were similar. He was no longer able to work, keep his own garden or pursue his hobby of pigeon racing.

The anaesthetist

Dr. James Malcolm Graham was born in Holmewood near Chesterfield where his father was the village doctor.[3] He graduated in medicine from Sheffield University in 1939, then joined his father's practice to help out because the assistant had joined the armed forces. He expected to be 'called up' himself but was never allowed to go because there was no one to look after the practice. The following year, having given 20 anaesthetics as a medical student, he was asked to give anaesthetics on Tuesday afternoons at Chesterfield Royal Hospital, the surgeon giving his own spinals in the morning - a practice that was not uncommon in 1940. Graham agreed, but claimed he was terrified every Tuesday because he knew he lacked training and experience. After a time he became interested, started reading and passed the Diploma in Anaesthesia (DA) on his first attempt in 1945. He also attended a one-week course at the Department of Anaesthetics in Oxford. While he was there, he saw a prototype of the Macintosh laryngoscope and ordered one before they were commercially available. He was therefore one of the first anaesthetists in England to own one.

Spinal anaesthesia

Spinal anaesthetics were common in 1947, particularly in a mining area such as Chesterfield where many men had respiratory problems and the commonest general anaesthetic was ether. Graham estimated that probably 40% of his anaesthetics in 1947 were spinals.

For many years after the introduction of spinal anaesthesia in 1898,[4] little attention was paid to sterilizing the external surface of ampoules of local anaesthetics. In 1942 Hewer and Garrod[5] drew attention to the fact that ampoules with gummed labels, as were used in the Woolley and Roe case, could be contaminated. Storing ampoules in antiseptic solutions was widely practised, although Hewer and Garrod favoured formaldehyde vapour. If this was not available, they recommended that the ampoule should be regarded as frankly septic, held in a sterile towel or gauze, its neck etherized and nicked with a sterile file, and the solution drawn into a syringe without the needle touching the neck of the ampoule. In 1951, four years after the Chesterfield tragedy, Macintosh condemned the storing of ampoules in antiseptic solutions and recommended sterilization by autoclaving.[5]

The senior anaesthetist in Chesterfield Royal Hospital, Dr. Pooler, was aware of the risk of infection if the spinal needle touching the unsterilized surface of the ampoule. Ciba, the manufacturers of nupercaine, recommended against autoclaving so Pooler and Graham agreed that immersion in phenol would be a sensible alternative. At the time the ampoule was to be used, it was taken out of the phenol with forceps, washed in sterile water, the top filed off using a sterile file, and the local anaesthetic aspirated into a sterilized glass syringe.

The anaesthetics

Roe was the first patient on the morning list for removal of his left semilunar cartilage. He received premedication of omnopon 20 mg and scopolamine 0.4 mg one hour preoperatively. He received spinal anaesthesia in the left lateral position, 10 ml light nupercaine 1/1500 at the first attempt. During the operation, he complained of headache and felt a burning sensation in his knee when the surgery began. He also had pain in his spine and head which continued for the remainder of the day when he returned to the ward.

The second patient, unnamed, was extremely ill with intestinal obstruction. His spinal anaesthetic appeared to be satisfactory but he remained very ill and died five days later.

Woolley was anaesthetized the same afternoon. He also received spinal anaesthesia, 10 ml light nupercaine 1/1500. He was turned prone for seven minutes, then turned supine for radical cure of a right hydrocoele. He did not complain of pain or headache and returned to a different ward from that of Roe.

The following day it was apparent that both patients had suffered major neurological damage, Roe worse than Woolley, that was to cripple both men for the remainder of their lives. Graham had administered all three anaesthetics and had used a new ampoule for each of the three patients.

The ampoules

The 20 ml glass ampoules containing light nupercaine 1/1500 were manufactured by Messrs. Ciba Ltd. and arrived at the hospital in packages of 12. The hospital routine was for the theatre sister to place the ampoules, each with its gummed label, in a jar containing 1/20 phenol, coloured blue, for 12 hours, during which the labels soaked off. The now unlabelled ampoules were then transferred to a jar containing 1/40 phenol, coloured pink. The pink dye had no other purpose than to identify the antiseptic solution as phenol. When the anaesthetist removed an ampoule from the phenol solution, he held it to the light to check for possible cracks before using it.

Woolley and Roe versus Ministry of Health and Others

Writs alleging negligence were issued in 1949 against the Ministry of Health as Trustees of the hospital, Graham the anaesthetist, and Messrs. Ciba Ltd., the manufacturers of the drug. The trial lasted for 11 days in 1953. The plaintiffs alleged either direct injury by the spinal needle, introduction or failure to prevent the introduction of infective organisms, or injection of carbolic acid (phenol) which had entered the ampoule in circumstances which Graham should have prevented or detected. They made similar allegations against the hospital and, against both, pleaded res ipsa loquitur. The allegation against Ciba, that the injuries were caused by the contents of the ampoule, was withdrawn soon after commencement of the trial.

After hearing evidence from Graham and experts in neurology and anaesthesia, the judge accepted Professor Macintosh's theory that the damage was caused by phenol that had leaked into the ampoules through cracks that were invisible to the naked eye. During the trial, Macintosh recommended autoclaving everything, but agreed that this method was not in widespread use in 1947 and that anaesthetists were not generally aware that disinfectants could seep through invisible cracks.

In his summing up, the judge commented that Graham had given his evidence "in a very careful and forthright manner, and having heard him describe and demonstrate the method of examination to which he subjected the ampoules before aspiration, I find it extremely difficult to believe that he could in the case of two successive patients have missed a visibly cracked ampoule." He therefore found that the plaintiffs' claims failed both against the hospital and against Graham.

The Appeal was dismissed by the unanimous judgments of three Lords. In spite of their terrible disabilities, neither Woolley nor Roe received any compensation.

Interview with Dr. Graham 1983

In 1964-65 I was a general practitioner in Chesterfield and met Graham without knowing of his involvement in the Woolley and Roe case. During my anaesthesia training in Sheffield 1967-69 I never gave, saw or heard of a spinal anaesthetic being given in the Sheffield hospitals. The consultant anaesthetists did not accept the phenol theory and since neither they nor anyone else had a credible alternative explanation, they were not prepared to take any risks. Having moved to Canada where spinals were common, my interest in the case grew and, in 1983, I visited Graham in Chesterfield. We reviewed various explanations of what could have caused the tragedies and he was clear and forthright on the following points.

Wrong drug

Impossible. There were no other ampoules of similar size or shape in the hospital. The pharmacy and operating theatre were searched for other 20 ml ampoules and none were found.

'Invisibe cracks' in ampoules

Impossible under normal conditions. Graham said that he and Pooler did "all sorts of experiments banging these things about. And we couldn't crack one. We could smash them, but we couldn't crack them."

In court he was given ampoules to look at and was asked, "Would you see that crack?" He said he could eventually find the crack, but would not have seen it in the ordinary visual check. The 'invisible' cracks were thermal cracks. He knew, because 'people' had talked that these were not accidental but had been made by touching the glass with a hot wire in a laboratory.

Intrathecal phenol

Not believable. Graham never accepted that the clinical condition of Woolley and Roe was due to intrathecal phenol. He also said that the neurologists at the trial[1] categorically denied this possibility, "This is not due to phenol. It cannot be. It would not produce this sort of syndrome."

Contamination of needles and/or syringes

Believable and possible. Graham was certain that there must have been a common cause. How else could the same thing happen three times in one day? - assuming the third patient between Roe and Woolley was also affected. But what was that cause? If the correct drug was given and the cracked ampoule with phenol leakage theory was wrong, it must have been due to some form of contamination of either the needles and/or syringes.

On the day that the spinal anaesthetics were given, the theatre sister was ill with violent headaches and vomiting and went off duty at lunch time. In fact she had a pituitary tumour that was later successfully removed. Was it possible that, because she was unwell, she had not supervised the preparation and sterilization of the needles and syringes to the usual standard? Without being able to identify the contaminant, Graham was sure that 'something' had been contaminated in 'some way'.

The human and humane side of Cecil Roe and Dr. Graham

Three years after the trial, the assistant matron of Chesterfield Royal Hospital came to Dr. Graham to tell him that Mr. Roe was being admitted for terminal care. Graham's natural reaction was that he would try to avoid meeting him. A few days later she came again and said Roe would like to see him. Although Graham was not comfortable because of possible unpleasantness, he went to Roe's bed. The conversation went as follows:

Graham: "Good morning, Mr. Roe. How are you?"

Roe: "I am not very well, Doctor."

Graham: "I know that, and I am very sorry."

Roe: "I wanted to see you because I wanted to tell you how sorry I am for all that trouble I've caused you. I did not want to bring the case at all, it was the union."

Graham: "Mr. Roe, they were quite right. You came in here for a simple operation and you finished up with your legs paralyzed. But, I would like you to know, to this day I do not know what went wrong. I can promise you that it was not that we, somebody gave the wrong thing to you by mistake. We just do not know."

Roe: "Oh, well, thank you very much for telling me, Doctor."

Graham's final comment on Roe was, "What a marvelous chap. To send and say 'I am sorry for the trouble I have caused you.'"

Final solution?

In 1990, seven years after this discussion and more than forty years after the tragedy, a possible explanation was suggested[6]. Before use, needles and syringes were sterilized in a boiling water sterilizer that was descaled each weekend with an acid liquid. Contamination of the needles and syringes could have occurred if the sterilizer had not been properly rinsed after descaling. If this is the final solution, it would explain why other sporadic cases of post-spinal paraplegia occurred in that era, and why such cases disappeared when autoclaving became standard and, later, disposable needles and syringes became available.

References:

[1] Cope RW: The Woolley and Roe case. Woolley and Roe versus Ministry of Health and Others. Anaesthesia 1954; 9: 249-270

[2] Hutter CDD: The Woolley and Roe case. A reassessment. Anaesthesia 1990; 45: 859-864

[3] Graham JM, Maltby JR: The Woolley and Roe Case. (Audiotaped discussion: copy and transcript at Association of Anaesthetists of Great Britain and Ireland, 9 Bedford Square, London, WC1B 3RA, England)

[4] Corning JL: Spinal anaesthesia and local medication of the cord. New York Medical Journal 1885; 42: 483-485

[5] Hewer CL, Garrod LP. Meningitis after spinal analgesia. Br Med J 1942; 1: 306

[6] Macintosh RR: Lumbar Puncture and Spinal Analgesia. Edinburgh: Livingstone 1951

The Woolley and Roe Case - 11: an Explanation

C. Hutter
City Hospital Nottingham UK

Professor Maltby has just described the background details of Albert Woolley and Cecil Roe's spinal anaesthetics, otherwise known as the Woolley and Roe case. In the 1950s[1] this case had a devastating effect on the practice of spinal anaesthesia in the UK and abroad. The fundamental problem was that there was no satisfactory explanation for Woolley and Roe's paraplegia, nor in fact for other clinically similar cases. There were many reports, but two well known papers discussing this problem came from the USA[2,3] ..... Professor Nickolas Greene and Foster Kennedy. Britain was not the only country where serious neurological problems were being seen after spinal anaesthesia.

At the Woolley and Roe trial in 1953[4], because of the clinical similarities between Woolley and Roe and these cases abroad, the neurologists giving evidence as expert witnesses expressed the opinion, and I believe correctly, that the post-spinal paralyses suffered by Woolley and Roe and these other similar cases were all caused by the same unknown agent.

The only plausible conclusion was that the correct spinal solution had been given, but that it had been contaminated. When I investigated this problem, I asked when did the contaminant get in? Not how and not why, but when, and this very simple question was the vital step that led me to the answer.

I next spoke to Cecil Roe's son and daughter-in-law. This is Cecil Roe himself in a wheelchair (see figure), and I expect, for many of you, this is the first time that you have seen someone in a wheelchair as a direct consequence of receiving a spinal anaesthetic. Cecil Roe lived in a small coal-mining community called Tibshelf in central England in Derbyshire. Just consider what sort of advertisement he must have provided for spinal anaesthesia in the 1940s and 50s, being pushed around these streets in a wheelchair.

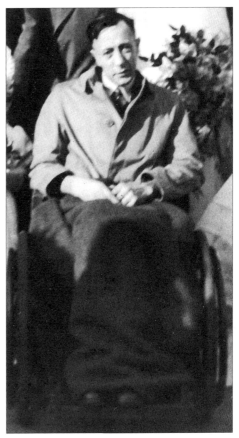

Cecil Roe

With the help of new information from Cecil Roe's family, I concluded that contamination happened when the needles and syringes were boiled in the water boiling sterilizer[5]. The only contaminant I could identify was the acidic descaler - two possibilities are phosphoric acid and sulphurous acid. The pathological changes in Cecil Roe's spinal cord were those of chronic adhesive arachnoiditis. These are fully consistent with the known toxicology of acid poisoning.

I concluded that the most likely sequence of events was that the hospital staff failed to wash the acid descaler from out of the water boiler after descaling, and that Woolley and Roe were paralyzed because their spinal needles were boiled in acid which then contaminated the spinal needles and syringes. I also concluded that this was the most likely explanation for the cases described by Greene and Foster Kennedy where the symptoms were similar to Woolley and Roe.

The first report of paralysis after spinal anaesthesia is attributed to König[6], although there may be an earlier report in the Belgian literature[7]. Water boilers had been in use for almost 20 years by the time König reported his case, König's patient had a similar clinical picture to Woolley & Roe, and at postmortem, the pathology was compatible with early arachnoiditis. Thus it is possible that König's patient had also been injured by acid. The problem of acid is still with us in the form of spinal anaesthetic solutions with low pH, and these can be associated with arachnoiditis[8].

It is forgotten that these water boilers remained in intermittent use in English hospitals up till at least the late 1960s. Surveys of complications after spinal anaesthesia which quote work carried out when these water boilers could still have been used, does not therefore give a fully reliable assessment of the safety of spinal anaesthesia as practiced today.

This leads us to an important medico-legal point. When the cause of these early neurological problems was not known, it was very easy to blame any post-operative neurological disability on the spinal or epidural anaesthetic, which unfortunately continues to this day. Now that we have a good explanation for these early problems such as Woolley and Roe, we can credibly argue that spinal anaesthesia is not the cause of post-operative neurological disability unless there is good evidence.

These water boilers remain in use today in developing countries and, as a result of this historical reassessment, we can now draw attention to all the attendant risks.

Finally, from this review, we see that the answer to the very long-standing enigma of the Woolley & Roe case was obvious and simple. Perhaps it is because the answer was too simple that it was overlooked for so long. Should we now look at other long-standing and seemingly insoluble medical problems and ask whether, if history repeats itself, the right approach to the problem will also produce an obvious and simple explanation?

References:

[1] Morgan M: The Woolley and Roe Case. Anaesthesia 1995; 50:162

[2] Greene N M: Neurological sequelae of spinal anesthesia. Anesthesiology 1961; 22: 682-698

[3] Kennedy F, Effron A S, Perry G: The grave spinal cord paralyses caused by spinal anesthesia. Surgery Gynecology and Obstetrics 1950; 91: 385-398

[4] Cope R W: The Woolley and Roe Case. Woolley and Roe versus Ministry of Health and Others. Anaesthesia 1954; 9: 249-270

[5] Hutter C D D: The Woolley and Roe Case. A Reassessment. Anaesthesia 1990; 45: 859-864

[6] Konig F: Bleibende Rückenmarkslähmung nach Lumbalanästhesie. Münch Med Wschr 1906; 53: 1112-1113

[7] Dandois R: Accidents cerebro-spineaux, tardifs et prolongés après cocainisation de la moèlle. Journale de Chirurgie et Annales de Societé Belge de Chirurgie 1901; 1: 282

[8] Reisner L S, Hochman B N, Plumer M H: Persistent neurologic deficit and adhesive arachnoiditis following intrathecal 2-chloroprocaine injection. Anesthesia and Analgesia 1980; 59: 452-454

Karl E. Hammerschmidt
Scientist, Humanist and Pioneer of Anaesthesia

W.F. List, A. Kernbauer
Department of Anaesthesiology Graz, University Clinics Graz, Austria

Karl Eduard Hammerschmidt was born in Vienna on June 12th, 1801. (Fig. 1) His father was a civil servant. At the age of 17 years, after finishing highschool, he started philosophical studies at the University of Vienna in 1818/19. In the year 1819-20 he began to study law and finished receiving a doctoral degree in January 1826. Besides law he also took lectures in natural science. In the beginning of 1830 he probably conducted medical scientific studies without proven graduation. In historical books we find hints that Dr. Hammerschmidt started final examinations for obtaining the degree of a Doctor of Surgery in 1853, although no examination and graduation protocols could be found. In an official document of the Interior Ministry about "dubious persons" Hammerschmidt's name is found as a Doctor of Law and a Doctor of Medicine. But this document has not proven reliable regarding other cases.

Dr. Hammerschmidt published a considerable number of entomological and other scientific papers and was accepted in the Kaiserlich-Leopoldinische Akademie of Scientists in Bonn in acknowledgement of his scientific contributions. His papers on the etherization of humans were published between February 1847 and March 1848, he especially emphasized his cooperation with the dentist Dr. Josef Weiger. He was also a distinguished entomological collector, his shell collection was awarded a scientific price. He furthermore helped to arrange the entomological collections of the archdukes Albrecht, Karl-Ferdinand and Wilhelm.

After 1835 he became co-editor of an agricultural journal besides his entomological interests, in 1838 he became its sole editor. From 1840 Dr. Hammerschmidt got into increasing and permanent problems with the censors of his journal. Highly regarded people tried to intervene but this did not improve the situation. In his agricultural journal he criticized the construction of a monument for the Emperor Franz. Frustration caused the political system and the limitation of free speech accumulated in Dr. Hammerschmidt that made him switch to the revolutionary side in 1848. He became a vehement opponent of the goverment. One year later he

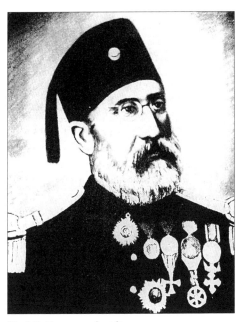

Karl E. Hammerschmidt

was sentenced to 12 years in contumatium in his absence for his active participation in the Revolution of 1848. Only a few of the prisoners survived this ordeal.

Dr. Hammerschmidt fled to Hungary after the suppression of the revolution. In 1849 he arrived in Istanbul. The Habsburg Monarchy asked for the exchange of all refugees involved in the revolution of 1848, the Ottoman Subleme Porte denied. Dr. Hammerschmidt did not go to the custodial camp for refugees in Aleppo in 1850 as ordered but worked as a doctor in the Gülhane Hospital in Istanbul and later on in Damaskus also as well being a doctor in a hospital. A personal inquiry was made from the Austrian internuntius to the Ottoman foreign secretary Ali Pascha on behalf of Dr. Hammerschmidt without result, finally returned to Istanbul and became Professor at the Medical Faculty for Geology, Mineralogy and Zoology.

Dr. Hammerschmidt participated in the International Conference for the foundation of the Red Cross, and the Red Crescent in Geneva in 1860. He was the decisive delegate of the Ottoman Empire. He converted to Islam faith and called himself Abullah Bey. He also became colonel in the Turkish army during the Crimean war. He received the gold medal for scientist and other awards from the Habsburg Monarchy in 1869. The Turkish Goverment also honored him at the occasion of the 100th year of the foundation of the Red Crescent with a stamp in 1968. Highly respected he died in 1874 in Istanbul. His scientific work was published in Vienna between 1834 and 1848 covering a wide range of topics like the American pigeon, the Mexican butterfly, oxyuris, mushrooms in Austria, fossils and mineralogical questions; in 3 publication between 1847 and 1848 he critically discussed the miserable situation of animals used for medical experiments.

His first report on the etherization of humans appeared on February 19th, 1847 and gave information about the healthy individuals and himself as well as a description of the first 50 patients under anaesthesia. He summarized his results as follows:

1. Human power cannot inhibit but delay the onset of ether narcosis
2. Interindividual differences could be found regarding the period of time needed to achieve a sufficient degree of anaesthesia.
3. Individuals who have been etherized desire further anaesthesia.
4. Of all senses hearing fades last and returns first.

In a statistical overview on 1560 etherizations carried out between January and July 1847, Dr. Hammerschmidt comments on the usefulness and harmlessness of ether. He performed 300 etherizations on himself, 600 etherizations on healthy individuals and about 200 etherizations on animals without any surgical intervention with the help of the dentist Dr. Joseph Weiger. Based on this he was able to distinguish between five stages of ether narcosis, findings that could be supported by the results of John Snow and Arthur Guedel that have been published by the end of 1847 and 1920, respectively. John Snow was able to achieve an even deeper level of anaesthesia in animals.

Hammerschmidt also suggested a protocol which he used for his statistics including date, number, kind of operation, apparatus used, duration of inhalation, duration of sleep, age, sex and body composition. All in all Hammerschmidt states 4500 operations under ether and chloroform anaesthesia in the first year after introduction. He thought ether to be superior to chloroform as an anaesthetic, since Weiger and Hammerschmidt found that chloroform reduces the quality of physical and psychic life wereas ether increases it. Bleeding during and after operations was less under chloroform anaesthesia as compared to ether.

Ether narcosis was introduced in Austria on January 22 nd, 1847 being performed on dogs. Only a few days later, on January 27th, 1847, a minor surgical procedure was carried out on a patient by Ernst Krackowiczer - the assistant of Professor Franz Schuh who was the head of the second Department of Surgery at the University of Vienna and had conducted the above mentioned trial on dogs. The next day the first official amputation of a femur could be demonstrated under the influence of ether at the same place. It took only one more day until Professor von Watmann, of the First Department of Surgery dared to resect a lower jaw under repeatedly continued ether inhalation. This is believed to have been a major surgical intervention at that time. Hammerschmidt started applying ether on end of January, Weiger on February 1st, while the first operation under ether narcosis in Graz was performed on February 2nd under the supervision of the surgeon Anton Hinterthür.

Professor James Simpson from Edinburgh published data on fifty anaesthesias carried out using chloroform on November 10 th, 1847. Here he stressed the advantages of chloroform over ether, to name a few : faster onset of action, smaller quantities of narcotic are required, more pleasant smell, easy to handle, especialy while on transport, no need for an apparatus for its administration. A month later, on December 8th, 1847, an article was published in a newspaper called "Wiener Zuschauer" on the administration of chloroform by the famous dentist Weiger. In Graz the first chloroform anaesthesia was performed by Professor J. N. Kömm on December 16th, 1847. Josef Weiger published his book in 1850 covering 21.000 etherizations. He again stresses his findings concerning the advantages of ether over chloroform even after having conducted 350 anaesthesias with chloroform. Weiger mentions his scientific cooperation with K. E. Hammerschmidt and others. In 1892 Julius Gurlt published an overview of 100.000 anaesthesias where he proved that a lethal outcome was 4 times more likely when using chloroform as compared to ether.

Hammerschmidt was the first person to recognize that hearing fades quite late in the process of anaesthesia, a problem we are still facing.

Karl Eduard Hammerschmidt was a scientist, recognized problems and facts concerning anaesthesia very early.He was able to give relevant scientific statements and suggestions by observing the events during narcosis. A protocol for each anaesthesia performed documenting respiratory and pulse rate was first suggested by E. A. Codman in Boston 1894. Other hemodynamic parameters were not taken until the 20th century.

K. E. Hammerschmidt and J. Weiger performed hundreds of anaesthesias on themselves using ether and chloroform. Hammerschmidt emphasizes that people having undergone narcosis once, share the desire for further anaesthesias. We conclude that these persons, especially both above mentioned doctors might have been addicted to chloroform and ether due to their work on these drugs.

First Surgical Anaesthesia in the Czech Countries

J. Pokorný, Postgraduate Medical School
Prague, Czech Republic

In the 19th century, the Czech Countries, known as the Kingdom of Bohemia, were an important cultural and economic part of the former Austrian Empire.

The report of the discovery of "a new method of rendering patients insensitive to the pain of surgical operation" - Morton's ether anaesthesia - came from Boston to Europe, starting in the United Kingdom in December 1846. In London on December 21, Robert Liston had performed, for the first time, the painless amputation of the thigh of a butler named Frederick Churchill. The ether anaesthesia was administered by William Squibb. As reported in V. Robinson's excellent 1946 book on the history of anaesthesia, *Victory over Pain*, in the first weeks of 1847, the news had been disseminated throughout Europe via newspapers and messengers.

Unfortunately, there is no verifiable information as to how this important news came to Prague. We know for certain, however, that in the oldest Prague hospital - the Hospital of Merciful Brothers founded in 1350 - a Brother-surgeon, Coelestin Opitz (1810-1866), had tested sulphuric ether on animals - rabbits and dogs - in January 1847. Because of his experiments, Opitz is regarded as the "patron" of Czech experimental pathologists. By February 6, he had anaesthetized, without operation, several healthy human volunteers. On February 7, 1847, 113 days after Morton's famous demonstration in Massachusetts General Hospital in Boston, Opitz administered inhalation ether anaesthesia to several patients. Some had tooth extractions and one underwent the "excision of a large ulcer". The surgeon was Dr. Hofmeister. In the following days, ether anaesthesia was applied for more extensive and serious surgical operations - with great success.

By the mid-nineteenth century, the Prague Hospital of Merciful Brothers was such an acknowledged medical institution that the Medical Faculty of Charles University sent medical students there for seminars, study stays and education. In the 1840s, the Surgical Clinic of the University Hospital was headed by a prominent surgeon, Professor Franz Pitha. Quite soon after the success of Opitz and Dr. Hofmeister, Professor Pitha had introduced ether anaesthesia in his clinic. Because Pitha was cautious and reserved about the first reports of anaesthesia (as were some of his colleagues) he awaited Opitz' results. Because of this, however, he lost the priority.

In the first comprehensive report on the introduction of ether anaesthesia in Prague and

Ether Anaesthesia

16. 10. 1846	–	Boston, USA	**Morton**	**Warren**
21. 12. 1846	–	London, UK	**Squibb**	Liston
21. 1. 1847	–	Vienna, Austria	?	Schuh
7. 2. 1847	–	**Prague**	**Opitz**	**Hofmeister**
9. 2. 1847	–	Olomouc	**Heller**	?

the Kingdom of Bohemia, the author Professor J. Halla (1814-1887) wrote that Opitz had administered ether to 186 patients by April 20, 1847; Pitha immediately began the regular use of anaesthesia in his clinic; the use of anaesthesia was quickly introduced in many hospitals outside of Prague. Interestingly enough, in the Moravian city of Olomouc, Dr. J. S. Heller successfully administered ether anaesthesia on February 9, 1847, just 2 days after Opitz. It is a shame that we have no knowledge of the method used by Opitz and Heller. We can only suppose that a glass instrument was used similar to the one used by Morton.

Frank Coelestin Opitz was born in 1810 in Heřmánkovice-Hermsdorf, a small village in Eastern Bohemia. His parents were poor farmers. At the age of 20, wishing to begin medical studies, he entered the Order of Merciful Brothers of St. John as a candidate for full membership. After three years, he obtained full membership in the Order and achieved the qualification of "practicing surgeon". When he was 37, he convinced the physician-surgeon Dr. Hofmeister that ether could be applied as an anaesthetic for surgery. In 1848, Opitz left Prague for Brno, where he completed his philosophical and then medical studies. In 1851, he graduated in Vienna. He was nominated as Provincial for the Order in Bohemia and Moravia in 1859 and died in Vienna in 1866. (Fig. 1)

German newspaper reports on anaesthesia and its expansion in Europe in the first months after its discovery have been successfully collected in a book by L. Brandt and G. Fehr, *A Discovery in Surgery (Eine Entdeckung in der Chirurgie)*. One can see the efforts of

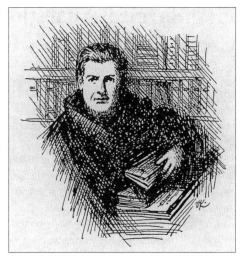

Fig. 1: Coelestin Opitz (1810-1866)

many to be acknowledged as the first to have introduced ether anaesthesia in their country. This fact reflects not only the high ambition of our past colleagues, but also the unmeasurable significance of anaesthesia for suffering patients as well as for surgeons who were stressed by the element of torture that was inherent in their work.

I am in full agreement with the German surgeon-historian J. Thorwald, who stated that the history of surgery as a medical science began on October 16, 1846 - the day of the discovery of surgical anaesthesia.

The story of Opitz has charmingly been described in a novel by Professor V. V. Tošovský, the renowned Czech pediatric surgeon. An English version, edited in cooperation with his Canadian colleague, R. Zachary, under the title Pain? No!, has been published in Australia and is available worldwide in English-speaking countries.

References:

[1] Brandt L, Fehr G: Eine Entdeckung in der Chirurgie (A Discovery in Surgery). Wiesbaden 1996
[2] Pokorný J, Bohuš O: et al. Anesteziologie a resuscitace v České a Slovenské republice na cestě k oborové samostatnosti (Anaesthesiology and Resuscitation in the Czech and Slovak Republics - Development to Professional Independence). PVS Praha 1996
[3] Thorwald J: Die Geschichte der Chirurgie (The History of Surgery). Steingruben-Verlag G.m.b.H., Stuttgart 1965

The first Anaesthesia with Ether at Lisbon, Portugal

A. F. Espinheira, Lisbon, Portugal

The Royal Hospital of St. Joseph today known as St. Josephs Hospital was the first place where anaesthesia was tested for surgical procedures in Portugal. The application of ether, as a general anaesthetic for surgery took place at the Royal Hospital of St. Joseph in Lisbon Portugal on July 20th 1847. The patient (J.L.) was a young officer of the Portuguese Army. An artillery projectile had destroyed his left foot and a third of his left leg was amputated without anaesthesia the 1st of May, 1847. An infection developed in the remaining part of the leg showing purulent spots and gangrene. The general condition was bad and it was necessary to interfere by carrying out another surgical operation.

This second operation took place on July, 20th 1847, i.e., 81 days later. The report on this second operation contained the following note : Patient has been previously etherized before. It is really extraordinary the registration of this operation and He reason that made me present this communication. The etherization was performed using the pneumatic system with Walters equipment. The pneumatic theory was based on the discovery of new gases, including oxygen for treatment of respiratory diseases.

From the Bulletin of Anesthesia History Volume15, Number 2 April, 1997: Humphry Davy`s small circle of Bristol friends: Pneumatical/Pneumatic/Pneumatology: adj. noun, moved by the wind; relative to the wind;consisting of spirit or wind. A branch of mechanics, that considers the doctrine of air, or laws according to which that fluid is condensed, or gravities. In the schools, the doctrine of spiritual substances, Gods, angels, and the souls of men. The doctrine of spiritual existence. (Reid). - Dr. Johnson, Dictionary. (Stafford, Body Criticism, p.417). This technique is used at Thomas Beddoes Medical Pneumatic Institution in Clifton near Bristol, England.

In the dictionary of Medicine and Surgery written by P. H. Nysten, and published in Paris in 1885, one can read on page 760: Equipment to be used with certain gases for the treatment of lung diseases. In the functioning of this type of equipment the airs coming out from the lungs, do not enter the recipient containing the gas. Source of the exhalation valve.

The equipment used at Lisbon was a little more sophisticated than others. It was made of a bell shaped glass or any other container stuck on a circular base with two holes: one for inhaling the gas and the other for its way out with a tube for the patient to breath through the mouth. The ether was poured in small container placed under a bell shaped glass. Forty minutes the ether had evaporated, the patient remained awake with a slight cough, restless, moved and took the buccal out of his mouth. The glasses were replaced by sponges soaked with ether, andafter one and a half hour the patient was asleep, finally while the surgical procedure itself took eighteen minutes only.

12.00 p.m.
- 12.45 p.m.: Beginning of etherization, pulse 80.
- 12.49 p.m.: Pulse 120, hot skin.
- 12.53 p.m.: Pulse 100, cough, very hilarious laughter.
- 12.58 p.m.: Temperature, back to normal, aware of evironment, pulse 100.

1.00 p.m.
- 1.03 p.m.: Normal sensitivity, same condition.
- 1.06 p.m.: Pulse 92, some sleepiness, cries.
- 1.09 p.m.: Feels drows.
- 1.14 p.m.: Pulse 104, normalsensitivity. Because he is not allowed to speak he writes clearly down what he wants to express.
- 1.27 p.m.: He becomes restless, moves and takes off the buckle from his mouth. The ether has completely evaporated, the patient is awake. Time spent 42 minutes, the ether is renewed replacing the bottles by sponges soaked in ether in a similar process to the one used by Morton.
- 1.32 p.m.: He fells drunk and hilarious.
- 1.35 p.m.: It shows that he is drunk.
- 1.40 p.m.: Pulse 108, less restless.

2.00 p.m.: More restless and the patient says I feel as if I had drank a few glasses of Porto wine.
- 2.20 p.m.: Patient calm and breathes normal.
- 2.35 p.m.: The operation is done with complete insensitivity of the patient. Time spent during second period : 63 minutes. Total time of anaesthesia : 105 minutes
Time spent for surgery: 18 minutes
Final comment :

This explains the disappointment of the whole team involved in this operation, although the surgeon was one of the best at that time Doctor J. Theotnio da Silva Chief Ward Surgeon. Pretty soon this equipment was replaced by Open Mascara that really made history. One would say: I am going to do an Open Mascara, instead of I am going to perform an anaesthesia .

Chloroform Anaesthesia in the Practice of Military Surgery in 1849 in Hungary

M. Terekes
Department of Anaesthesia and Intensive Therapy, Medical University of Pecs, Hungary

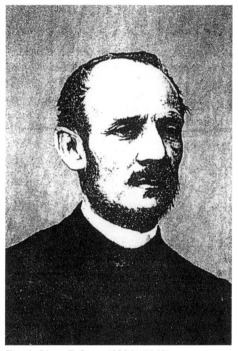

Fig. 1. János Balassa (1814 - 1868)

The introduction of ether anaesthesia by Morton at the Massachusetts General Hospital on 16th October 1846 was a turning point of the history in medicine. The great discovery of inhalational anaesthesia spread world-wide very fast and within six months ether anaesthesia was applied in many countries in all over the world including Hungary too.

Dr. János Balassa, Professor of Surgery of the Medical School of Pest applied ether surgical anaesthesia first in Hungary on 11th February, 1847 after having seen and studied the ether inhalation technique at the University Department of Surgery in Vienna (Fig.1). Very soon after the first successful use of ether narcosis during surgery ether inhalation was introduced in many hospitals of Hungary. The Hungarian pioneers of surgical anaesthesia were the following excellent physicians: Flór, Markusovszky, Brunner, Halász, Schöpf, Arányi, Ábrahám Pattantyús, Paár, Sághy, Szathmáry and Kraft who administered ether successfully for surgical intervention of adults and children too.

Rosenfeld published the first book of anaesthesiology in Hungarian entitled "The effect of the vapour of aether sulfuricus particularly from the surgeons` point of view" in 1847 (Fig. 2). His book was published in German too. The effect of ether, the clinical feature of narcosis and technique of administration were described. The application of different instruments used for ether inhalation are explained and illustrated in his book too (Fig.3).

Professor James Simpson introduced chloroform anaesthesia in November, 1847 in Edinburgh. The advantage of chloroform that was said to be more potent more comfortable to inhale and it was so much easier to give. Chloroform anaesthesia was very popular at this time particularly in Scotland.

Dr. Sándor Lumnitzer (1821-1892), well known Hungarian surgeon studied clinical surgery in Berlin in 1847 and he described the inhalational anaesthesia in his report (Fig. 4). Dr. Lumnitzer received medical diploma in Pest and he was an excellent surgeon

THE EFFECT
OF VAPOUR OF AETHER
SULFURICUM

PARTICULARLY FROM
THE SURGEONS' POINT OF VIEW

BASED ON EXPERIENCE

AND SCIENTIFICALLY ELUCIDATED

WRITTEN BY

DR. JÓZSEF ROSENFELD
PRACTITIONER PHYSICIAN

PEST
THE PROPERTY OF HECKENAST GUSZTÁV
1847

KÉNÉGÉNYGŐZ

HATÁSA,

KÜLÖNÖSEN SEBORVOSI TEKINTETBŐL;

TAPASZTALATI ADATOKRA ÉPITVE

S TUDOMÁNYOSAN FELVILÁGOSITVA.

IRTA

ROSENFELD JÓZSEF,

ORVOSTUDOR, SZÜLÉSZ-MESTER, A' KIR. MAGYAR EGYETEMI ORVOSKAR, A BUDAPESTI KIR. ORVOSEGYESÜLET, S A KIR. MAGYAR TERMÉSZETTUDOMÁNYI TÁRSULAT RENDES TAGA; A HONI IZRAELITÁK KÖZÖTT MAGYAR NYELVET TERJESZTŐ PESTI EGYLETNEK E. I. MÁSOD-ELNÖKE, GYAKORLÓ ORVOS PESTEN.

EGY KÖRE METSZETT TÁBLÁVAL.

PEST.

HECKENAST GUSZTÁV TULAJDONA.

1847.

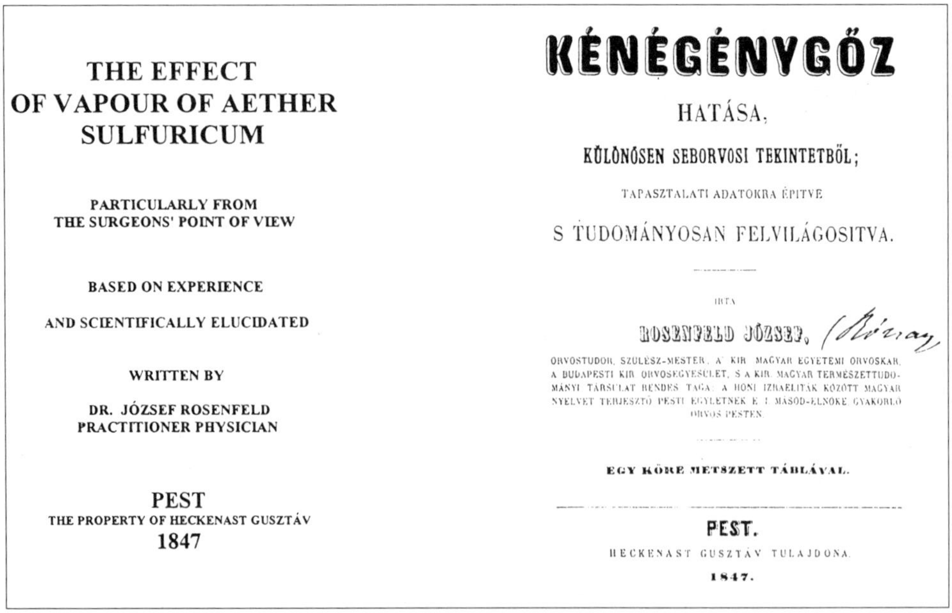

Fig. 2 The first book of anaesthesia by J. Rosenfeld published in Hungarian in 1847

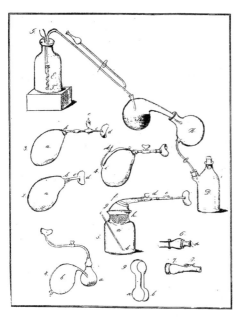

Fig. 3 Laboratory instruments for the production of ether and the anaesthetic equipment for the inhalation of ether vapour used in 1847. Illustration from the book of Rosenfeld, 1847

practising at the Department of Balassa. During his study of surgery he had experience with inhalational anaesthesia in Vienna, London, Zurich and Paris.

1848 was the year of the volcanic disruption of revolutions in Hungary and in many other countries in Europe. During the War of Liberty many casualties required surgery in Hungary.

Dr. S. Lumnitzer joined the Army and he became an excellent military surgeon and he was appointed Army Staff Chief Medical Officer of the Hungarian revolutionary troops. He was a highly appreciated and brilliant surgeon and the attending personal physician of A. Görgey, the famous colonel of the Army. Dr. Lumnitzer moved with the troops to the Northern Warfare of the War of the Liberty.

He made notes and brief medical records in his diary during this time of the War. In 1848-49 military surgeons performed surgical interventions under chloroform

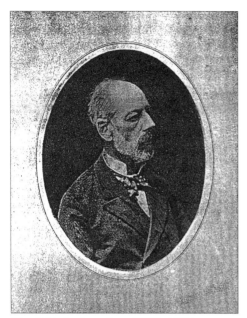

Fig. 4 Sándor Lumnitzer (1821 -1892)

the arm of an injured was performed under chloroform anaesthesia. The place of the quartering of the troops and army hospital can clearly be identified with the name of the towns mentioned.

The following notes give the documentary evidence of the application of chloroform in case of surgery of wounded during the 1848 Liberty War in Hungary (Fig. 5):

"Schlacht bei Kremnitz... Abzug nach Neusohl und Schlacht bei Schemnitz - Görgei bei Zsarnóc ...Einquartierung in Neusohl Horváth's Spitaler...Eine Amputation in Neusohl mit Chloroform...Geheilt... eine zweite...Arm...(non legible words)...mit Chloroform...in Radva..."

"Battle at Kremnitz...moving to Neusohl and battle at Schemnitz...Görgei at Zsarnóc...quartering in Neusohl...Hospitals of Horváth...amputation with chloroform in Neusohl...- recovered... a second (amputation) ...arm with chloroform...in Radva."

inhalational anaesthesia during the War of Liberty in Hungary.

The following fragments of his notes in German clearly showed that amputation of

Hungarian physicians together with many other European doctors basically changed medical care of patients with the introduction

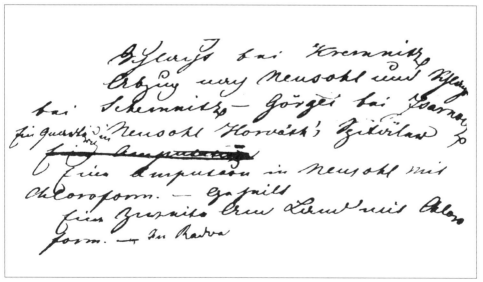

Fig. 5 Copy of the notes from the diary of Sándor Lumnitzer. Document of the first use of chloroform anaesthesia In the military surgery In Hungary in 1849.

of inhalational anaesthesia. That was the Revolution of Medicine too opening a new way of development of surgery providing a painless surgical medical care for the patients in every country.

Rosenfeld cited the saying of Seneca in his book on ether anaesthesia which is really an essential point of the achievement of human being in medicine:

"Multa jam nobis miracula revelavit natura, et plura adhuc revelabit, et ubi sunt limites? quis hoc mortalium possit decidere."

(The original Diary of Dr. S. Lumnitzer was the property of late Professor J. Szentágothai, Budapest, Hungary, and the copy of the document is published with his personal permission.)

References:

Hügin W: Anaesthesia, discovery progress breakthroughs. Editones Roche, Basel 1989

Balassa J: De Juvene Medico. Thesis, Pest 1838

Rosenfeld A: „The Effect of the Vapour of Aether Sulfuricus Particularly from the Surgeons` Point of View". Pest 1847 (in Hungarian)

Hõgyes E : Emlékkönyv a Budapesti Királyi Magyar Tudomány Egyetem orvosi karának múltjáról és jelenéről. (Almanch, the History of the Medical Faculty of the Budapest Royal University). Magyar Orvosi Könyvkiadó Társulat, Budapest 1896 (in Hungarian)

Korbuly Gy :The history of ether narcosis in Hungary". Orvosi Hetilap 1937; 37 : 924 (in Hungarian)

Antal J: Lumnitzer Sándor. Magyar Nemzet 1979;10. August (in Hungarian)

The Role of the "Societas Medicorum Germanicorum Parisiensis" for the Spread of Anaesthesia in Europe

M. Goerig,
Department of Anaesthesiology, University Hospital Hamburg, Germany
C. Nemes*,
Department of Anaesthesiology, Municipal Hospital Pfaffenhofen, Pfaffenhofen, Germany
A. Straimer*,
Department of Anaesthesiology, Municipal Hospital Pfaffenhofen, Pfaffenhofen, Germany

Hardly any other medical achievement spread as fast as ether anaesthesia, a technique important and indispensible to the development of modern surgery[3]. After the discovery of the anaesthetic properties of sulfuric ether by the American physician and chemist Charles Thomas Jackson (1805-1880), the dentist Thomas Green Morton (1819-1868) from Boston on September 30th, 1846 managed to conduct a painless tooth extraction employing ether anesthesia. He then asked the head of the department of surgery at Massachusetts General Hospital John Collins Warren (1756-1856) for permission to demonstrate his technique during major surgical procedures[25]. On October 16th, 1846 critically watched by a large audience, he successfully performed an ether anaesthesia. Since then this date has been regarded as the beginning of modern anaesthesia. Throughout the German speaking nations the news about the successful application of vaporous ether and the possibility of painless surgery was mainly covered by the daily press – a phenomenon that was observed in the United States[29].

Apparently Aloys Martin (1818-1891), a member of the "Society of German Physicians in Paris" played an underrated part in the spread of the knowledge about the anaesthetic properties of sulfuric ether across the German speaking nations[24]. The following text gives information on Martin's biography and deals with the history of the mostly unknown "Societas medicorum Germanicorum Parisiensis" as well as some of its most important members.

The news about the first successful ether anaesthesia reaches Europe

It is common knowledge that the information about the first successful ether anaesthesia was published by the surgeon Henry Jacob Bigelow (1818-1890) who at that time worked at the Massachusettts General Hospital. His contribution to the Boston Medical and Surgical Journal, later the New England Journal of Medicine was called "Insensibility during surgical operations, produced by inhalation"[6]. The news was carried to his friend Francis Boote (1792–1863) from Liverpool, England, by the "Acadia", a steam boat of Cunard Line and arrived there on December 15th, 1846. After receiving this information, he immediately informed the English press and the surgeon Robert Liston (1794–1847)[27]. Only three days later Boote proleeded to perform a tooth extraction under ether anaesthesia in Liston's presence on 19th of December. Deeply impressed by the new method on 21st of December Liston carried out an amputation of the lower leg while the patient was inhaling sulfuric ether. The news about this occurence quickly spread all over England[5].

The first use of ether on the continent

It is still to be definitely revealed how the news about the anaesthetic properties of ether reached the Continent. But very likely Edward Warren (?) (not related to the surgeon Warren of Massachusetts General Hospital) whom Morton employed as his legal advisor concerning patents, took the information to Paris. He had also crossed the Atlantic on board the "Acadia" and reached the city 19th or 20th of December, 1846[6]. There he met the physician F.W. Fisher (?), an old aquaintance from Boston, who worked at the same hospital as Joseph Jobert de Lamballe (1799–1867). Only one day after Liston in London, on December 22nd, they performed the first ether anaesthesia on the Continent at the hospital "St. Louis". They continued to carry out successful etherizations the following days[27].

The surgeon Joseph François Malgaigne (1806–1865) was among the first to successfully etherize a person in front of an audience at the "Académie de Médicine" on January 12th in 1847. That very day his colleagues Philibert Joseph Roux (1780-1854) at the "Hotel Dieu", and Armand Louis Marie Velpeau (1795-1867) at the "Charité" of Paris tried to do the same, but failed. That was why they stated that further experiments were futile and dangerous[6]. They were supported by the famous physiologist François Magendi (1783–1855) who also primarily opposed the idea of an ether anaesthesia. On top of that he doubted it was ethical to cause people to fall unconscious by inhalation[4].

But a few days later Malgaigne performed another etherization in front of the members of the academy and Velpeau who had been among those opposing the use of the new technique had to confess his misjudgement of the situation and said: "Je doutais, il y a huit jours, mais aujourd'hui je n'hésite pas à dire que c'est la est une grande chose, une découverte capitale et destinée à un immense avenir"[29].

Etherization on its way to become a common technique

Many contemporary articles, documents and letters prove that there were several more successful ether anaesthesias in various hospitals during the following days and rapidly spread the news about the prodigious new technique[6]. Among the people reporting on these incidents was the Danish physician Emil Theodor Pauli (1814–1874). He mentioned a series of self-experiments performed by the members of the "Society of German Physicians in Paris" – among them Aloys Martin from Munich[1, 27].

Aloys Martin – some biographic data

Aloys Martin (Fig. 1) was born in Bamberg in 1818 and studied medicine in Munich, Vienna and Berlin. He found employment as practitioner at the "Münchner Poliklinik" and kept the position with the except of several short interludes until 1854. Aside from his demanding duties as general practitioner he

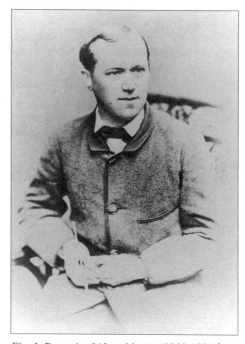

Fig. 1 Portrait of Aloys Martin (1818-1891)[8]

became involved in pharmacological studies and gained the doctoral degree by publishing the article "Über Urokinin und einige andere Farbstoffe im Menschenharne" ("About urokinin and other coloring substances of humane urine")[12,13]. After passing the Bavarian state exam, Martin decided to continue his studies and moved first to Vienna and then to Paris. Shortly afterwards the first news from Boston concerning successful sulfuric ether anaesthesias reached France[15].

In the early summer of 1847 he went back to Munich and published his comprehensive monograph "Zur Physiologie und Pharmakodynamik des Aetherismus" ("About the physiology and pharmacodynamics of etherism")[16]. This publication brought him the "venia legendi" of the Ludwig Maximilians University of Munich and possibly was the first treatise in the world dealing with anaesthesiology and helping its author to achieve the professoral title[24].

When scientific interest turned to the new inhalational agent "chloroform" in 1848, Martin began his own studies about its anaesthetic properties and published his results together with his friend Ludwig Binswanger (1820-1880) in their well-respected monograph "Das Chloroform in seinen Wirkungen auf Menschen und Thiere" (Chloroform and its effect on humans and animals)[17]. He then continued to publish articles about the pharmacological properties of ether and of other narcotics such as different forms of chlorinated ether and nitrous oxide[12].

When in 1848 an epidemic cholera stroke the northern part of Germany, the Bavarian government sent Martin to the cities of Magdeburg, Stettin, Braunschweig and Berlin in order to study the situation and report on his work regularly[12]. In Berlin he met Rudolf Virchow (1821-1902) who at that time was working as prosector at the Institute of Pathology of the University in Berlin and did postmortem examinations of cholera victims. Because of his merits in science, Martin was made private lecturer in 1848 and "Honorary professor" (a term bestowed to professors who are not head of a department and are paid for doing lectures etc.) in 1860. From 1876 on he was working as professor at the Ludwig Maximilians University in Munich. Apart from his clinician career he worked as chief editor and kept on writing for papers like the "Bayrisches Aerztliches Intelligenzblatt" and others until 1869. When Martin died as highly respected physician in Munich on January 10th, 1891, he was praised for publishing articles on ether anaesthesia in the "Augsburger Allgemeine Zeitung"[12]. But his important role concerning spreading of the use of sulfuric ether throughout the German speaking nations was not mentioned. Only a few years ago this was revealed by some Spanish authors[7].

Paris – "The Mecca" of medicine

In order to learn about the latest achievements in medicine, Martin went to Paris in early summer of 1847. There he met a lot of German colleagues and many others from different nations sharing the same objectives. At that time Paris for decades had attained holding a leading position in medical science. It had taken over this role from the "First Medical School of Vienna" due to the Revolution of 1789[21].

From all over the world physicians poured into the city of Paris that was called "the Mecca of medicine"[11]. They wanted to take part in lectures and demonstrations by famous doctors and become familiar with the latest discoveries in medical practice taught at hospitals, clinics and private practices. It is interesting that two of those arriving at Paris from the United States were to become directly involved in the historic discovery of ether anaesthesia at the Massachusetts General Hospital: one was the surgeon John

Collins Warren (1778-1856) who was to perform the famous first operation under ether anaesthesia, the other was Jacob Bigelow (1818–1890) who was part of the audience at that time and afterwards began reporting on the new successful method of painless surgical procedures to various audiences among them the "Boston Society of Medical Improvement"[30]. Among those from Germany was Johann Friedrich Dieffenbach (1792-1847) who performed one of the first ether anaesthesias in Germany in Berlin and only some weeks later published a monograph on this new technique that was to become widely spread. Another German pioneer of ether application was the surgeon Johann Ferdinand Heyfelder (1798-1869) from Erlangen who some years later lived in Paris for a longer period of time[10]. Afterwards he kept on preferring French medical journals to others, a fact demonstrating his strong attachment to the French medical community. One of these magazines was the "Révue Médico-Chirurgicale de Paris" which was edited by Malgaigne and featured an article on the anaesthetic properties of sulfuric ether. It was read by Heyfelder on January 21st of 1847 and lead him to undertake his own experiments. It is also worth mentioning that Heyfelder like Martin was interested in cholera and like him travelled to regions struck by the epidemic[24].

1830-1831 – The Society of German Medical Practitioners in Paris

It was probably in the winter of 1830/1831 that several German physicians thought about establishing a "Vereinigung Deutscher Heilkundiger ("Society of German Medical Practitioners"). The majority of these were doctors who had been working in Paris for several years and wanted to support those colleagues, coming to Paris, who did not speak French[21]. Others stayed only for a few months and many of them saw to the wounded of the riots of July 1830. In addition they attended the lectures of famous surgeons like Guillaume Dupuytren (1777–1835), Jaques Lisfranc (1790–1847) or Philip Roux (1780–1854) or watched the experiments of outstanding physiologists like François Magendi (1783–1855)[20].

In order to get to know each other and to talk about interesting cases they agreed to come together every week at the "Palais Royal" and usually continued their sessions at a restaurant called "Richefeu" which offered a comfortable atmosphere for further discussions. But this society was never formally established and fell apart a few years later. That is the reason, why there is no further information on the first Society of German Medical Practitioners, a fact that was regretted already a few years later[19].

1844 – the "Society of German Physicians in Paris" established

In 1844 there was another attempt to establish a "Society of German Physicians in Paris" (Fig. 2). After preliminary discussions several physicians who had been working in Paris for longer period agreed to found a new society with its own statutes. The idea behind this association mainly was to intensify the national cohesion of the members and on the other hand to persue scientific objectives. In order to support scientific work, a library was set up. By purchasing literature and through generous donations it grew remarkably fast. German medical journals according to the statutes were acquired with the intention to spread the latest German scientific findings throughout France[21].

The unstable political situation in Paris between 1846 and 1848 influenced the social life of this particular association as well, so that, temporarily, meetings were held less regularly[19]. With the cessation of public unrest the members tried to revive their society. They gave the society strict statutes and defined

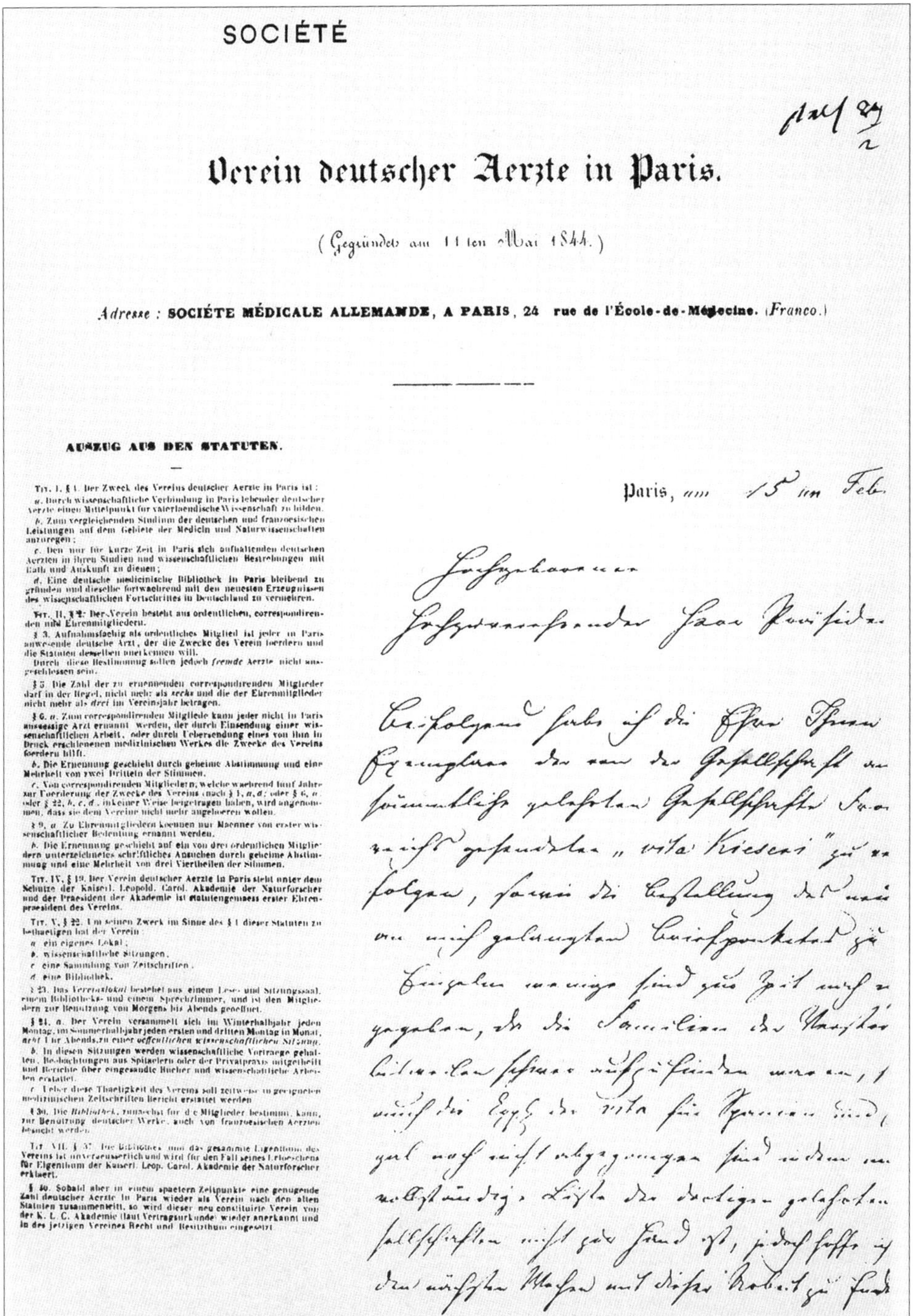

SOCIÉTÉ

Verein deutscher Aerzte in Paris.

(Gegründet am 11ten Mai 1844.)

Adresse : **SOCIÉTÉ MÉDICALE ALLEMANDE, A PARIS, 24 rue de l'École-de-Médecine.** (*Franco.*)

AUSZUG AUS DEN STATUTEN.

Tit. I. § 1. Der Zweck des Vereins deutscher Aerzte in Paris ist :

a. Durch wissenschaftliche Verbindung in Paris lebender deutscher Aerzte einen Mittelpunkt für vaterlaendische Wissenschaft zu bilden.

b. Zum vergleichenden Studium der deutschen und franzoesischen Leistungen auf dem Gebiete der Medicin und Naturwissenschaften anzuregen ;

c. Den nur für kurze Zeit in Paris sich aufhaltenden deutschen Aerzten in ihren Studien und wissenschaftlichen Bestrebungen mit Rath und Auskunft zu dienen ;

d. Eine deutsche medicinische Bibliothek in Paris bleibend zu gründen und dieselbe fortwaehrend mit den neuesten Erzeugnissen des wissenschaftlichen Fortschrittes in Deutschland zu vermehren.

Tit. II, § 2. Der Verein besteht aus ordentlichen, correspondirenden und Ehrenmitgliedern.

§ 3. Aufnahmsfaehig als ordentliches Mitglied ist jeder in Paris anwesende deutsche Arzt, der die Zwecke des Verein foerdern und die Statuten desselben anerkennen will.

Durch diese Bestimmung sollen jedoch *fremde* Aerzte nicht ausgeschlossen sein.

§ 5. Die Zahl der zu ernennenden correspondirenden Mitglieder darf in der Regel, nicht mehr als *sechs* und die der Ehrenmitglieder nicht mehr als *drei* im Vereinsjahr betragen.

§ 6. *a.* Zum correspondirenden Mitgliede kann jeder nicht in Paris ansaessige Arzt ernannt werden, der durch Einsendung einer wissenschaftlichen Arbeit, oder durch Uebersendung eines von ihm in Druck erschienenen medizinischen Werkes die Zwecke des Vereins foerdern hilft.

b. Die Ernennung geschieht durch geheime Abstimmung und eine Mehrheit von zwei Dritteln der Stimmen.

c. Von correspondirenden Mitgliedern, welche waehrend fünf Jahre zur Foerderung der Zwecke des Vereins (nach § 1, *a*, *d*; oder § 6, *a*, oder § 22, *b*, *c*, *d*.) in keiner Weise beigetragen haben, wird angenommen, dass sie dem Vereine nicht mehr angehoeren wollen.

§ 9, *a.* Zu Ehrenmitgliedern koennen nur Maenner von erster wissenschaftlicher Bedeutung ernannt werden.

b. Die Ernennung geschieht auf ein von drei ordentlichen Mitgliedern unterzeichnetes schriftliches Ansuchen durch geheime Abstimmung und eine Mehrheit von drei Viertheilen der Stimmen.

Tit. IV, § 19. Der Verein deutscher Aerzte in Paris steht unter dem Schutze der Kaiserl. Leopold. Carol. Akademie der Naturforscher und der Praesident der Akademie ist statutengemaess erster Ehrenpraesident des Vereins.

Tit. V, § 22. Um seinen Zweck im Sinne des § 1 dieser Statuten zu bethaetigen hat der Verein :

a ein eigenes Lokal ;

b. wissenschaftliche Sitzungen,

c eine Sammlung von Zeitschriften,

d. eine Bibliothek.

§ 23. Das *Vereinslokal* bestehet aus einem Lese- und Sitzungssaal, einem Bibliotheks- und einem Sprechzimmer, und ist den Mitgliedern zur Benutzung von Morgens bis Abends geoeffnet.

§ 24. *a.* Der Verein versammelt sich im Winterhalbjahr jeden Montag, im Sommerhalbjahr jeden ersten und dritten Montag in Monat, *acht* Uhr Abends, zu einer *oeffentlichen wissenschaftlichen Sitzung.*

b. In diesen Sitzungen werden wissenschaftliche Vortraege gehalten, Beobachtungen aus Spitaelern oder der Privatpraxis mitgetheilt und Berichte über eingesandte Bücher und wissenschaftliche Arbeiten erstattet.

c. Ueber diese Thaetigkeit des Vereins soll zeitweise in geeigneten medizinischen Zeitschriften Bericht erstattet werden.

§ 30. Die *Bibliothek*, zunaechst für die Mitglieder bestimmt, kann, zur Benutzung deutscher Werke, auch von franzoesischen Aerzten besucht werden.

Tit. VII. § 37. Die Bibliothek und das gesammte Eigenthum des Vereins ist unveraeusserlich und wird für den Fall seines Erloeschens für Eigenthum der Kaiserl. Leop. Carol. Akademie der Naturforscher erklaert.

§ 40. Sobald aber in einem spaetern Zeitpunkte eine genugende Zahl deutscher Aerzte in Paris wieder als Verein nach den alten Statuten zusammentritt, so wird dieser neu constituirte Verein von der K. L. C. Akademie (laut Vertragsurkunde) wieder anerkannt und in des jetzigen Vereines Recht und Besitzthum eingesetzt.

Paris, am 15 ten Feb.

Fig. 2 Official letter head of "Société Verein deutscher Aerzte in Paris"; please note on the left some extracts of the society's statutes[8] themselves as: "Sociable and scientific association of German physicians". The fact that among other things – there were again "scientific evenings", is a proof that they succeeded. The meetings, which were all taken down, were primarily held at the rue Hautefeuille on Saturday evenings at 8 p.m[20,22]. It was in 1849, that the members agreed to share their rooms and library with "the Association of English Physicians" which had also existed for several years[19]. But lack of space caused them to split up again just a year later and to meet regularly at spacious rooms rented especially for this purpose.

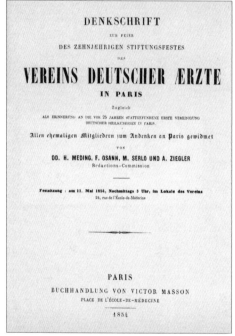

Fig. 3 Cover page of a publication of the Society in 1854[19]

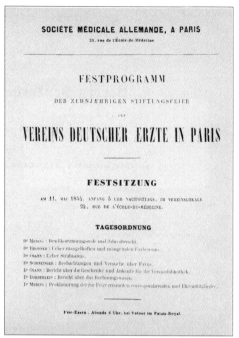

Fig. 4 "A Festprogramm" on the occasion of the 10ths anniversary of the Society's foundation in 1854[19]

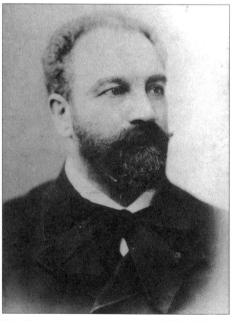

Fig. 5 Jean Baptiste Rottenstein (1832-1897), the Society's last librarian[8]

1853 – Association of the "Society of German Physicians in Paris" with the "Leopoldina" of Halle

In 1852 the members decided to co-operate more closely with the "Leopoldinisch-Carolinischen Akademie" of Halle. This

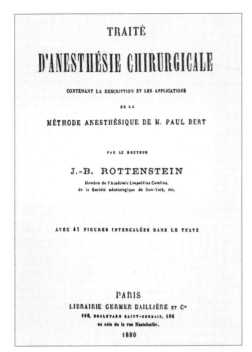

Fig. 7 Cover page of the well-known textbook of anaesthesia, which was written by Jean Baptiste Rottenstein in 1880[8]

society was highly esteemed and had already been in existence for 200 years[20]. Hence, representatives sentatives of both associations signed, after legal questions regarding the contract had been settled, a "Treaty of Protection", which was called as "affiliation" in Breslau on June 28th of 1853[19]. With this step the "Association of German Physicians in Paris" became a subsidiary of the "Leopoldina". At the same time they revised their statutes again and defined their main interest as: "To represent German science in France". On the other hand the objectives of the "Leopoldina" gained weight as well. Thus, for example, the society's possessions and the outstanding library were to become the property of the "Kaiserlich-Leopoldino-Carolinischen Aka-demie der Naturforscher" ("Imperial Leopoldinisch-Carolinische Aca-demy of Natural Scientists") in case the association in Paris broke up. And it's because of this agreement that many documents of medical history and the associations publications still exist[9,28].

1881 – The inglorious end of the "Society of German Physicians in Paris"

Because of the war between Germany and France (1870 till 1871) the activities of the society, which had not been lively throughout the 1860ies, were even more reduced. The library was given into the custody of Wülfing Luer (1803–1883), a manufacturer of instruments and member of the society[9]. That it did not become part of the "Leopoldina's" possession was due to the fact that the association of German physicians was never officially closed down. Moreover, those members who had the authority to do so, had left Paris and lived somewhere else in France or had returned to Germany or sought refuge somewhere abroad[28]. Thus the library stayed with Luer for five years and was handled over to commissioner when the house was sold in 1876. He also tried to transfer the library to the "Leopoldina".

The society´s last librarian, Jean Baptiste Rottenstein (1832–1897), born in Frankfurt and one of the most influential dentists of Paris, finally was entrusted with the transfer of the library. He was an early protagonist of nitrous oxide anaesthesia involving the pressurized chamber developed by Paul Bert (1833–1886). Presumably about 1880 Rottenstein, who had promoted the use of "electric anesthesia" and the generous use of ethyl chloride spray, also published a well-known and frequently cited textbook in anesthesia (Fig. 7).

The club's library

The Society had the protocols taken down at the weekly meetings as well as their members's scientific works published in the highly regarded – French medical journal – "Gazette Hébdomadaire de Médicine et de Chirurgie" and separately printed for members. They received their issues "free of charge and did not have to pay for the postal delivery as far as Leipzig"[19]. Since the French magazine mentioned above was read by many German physicians and most of the bigger libraries had subscribed the journal as well, the members publications were widely read.

Political newspapers were not to be subscribed by the society's library. The only paper exempt from this statue was the liberal "Augsburger Allgemeine Zeitung", because, "it featured a scientific supplement"[19]. But in the end it is not possible to find out today why it was the "Augsburger Allgemeine Zeitung" exclusively. Anyway, it was preferred by many Germans living in Paris, since it was the most widely published liberal paper in a nation that consisted of many small states[23]. Moreover the Pfalz then was a part of Bavaria, a fact that encouraged communication with the French capital, because letters could reach Augsburg by courier within three days[24].

Members of the "Society of German Physicians in Paris"

Over the decades so many medical celebrities from Germany and other countries have joined up with the club, that it is impossible to mention them all in this article[19,21] (Fig. 8). Many famous members were later bestowed with an honorary membership, quite a few of them were surgeons, who demonstrably were among the first to use ether anaesthesia in the German speaking nations: Viktor von Bruns (1823–1883), Bernhardt von Langenbeck (1810–1883), Franz Christoph von Rothmund (1801–1891), Georg Friedrich Stromeyer (1804–1876), and Kajetan Textor (1782–1860). Furthermore people like the physiologist David Gruby (1810–1898) and Eduard Friedrich Pflueger (1829–1910) were among the honorary members. Other famous personalities were the pathologist Rudolf Virchow (1821–1901) or the internist Reinhold Wunderlich (1815–1877). Last but not least Alexander von Humboldt (1759–1859) and Justus Freiherr von Liebig (1803–1873) were among the club`s members for many years. Among the corresponding members were the neurologist Pierre Paul Broca (1824–1880) and his colleague Jean Martin Charcot (1825–1893), the pediatrician Theodor Escherisch (1857–1911), the hygienist Max von Pettenkofer (1818–1901) and the opthalmologist Robert Ritter von Welz (1814–1878). More names mentioned in the club's archives were Adam Hammer (1818–1878), Friedrich von Esmarch (1823–1908), Albrecht von Graefe (1828–1870), Oskar Liebreich (1839–1908), Nepomuk Nussbaum (1829–1890) and Carl Thiersch (1822–1895). Their names are connected to many important developments regarding anaesthesia during the second half of the 19th century[19].

Aloys Martin and his correspondence with the "Augsburger Allgemeine Zeitung" in spring 1847

Finally, taking into account the historical facts concerning the "Society of German P≠hysicians in Paris" described above, the frequent reports on ether anaesthesia by the Physician Aloys Martin from Munich, are worth mentioning. He published them in the "Augsburger Allgemeine Zeitung" which was well regarded and read nearly everywhere in the German speaking nations[23]. His periodical articles, altogether more than twenty pages, were printed from the 10th January 1847 on. During this short period of time Martin wrote a total of ten press reports-which all dealt with the use of sulfuric ether. Thus, he became one of the important chroniclers of the first ether anaesthesias on the Continent. Obviously he had recognized the

Mitglieder-Verzeichniss

DES VEREINS DEUTSCHER ÆRZTE IN PARIS

Nach der Eintrittszeit aufgestellt.

ORDENTLICHE MITGLIEDER

1844

Am 11. Mai : OM : Dr ** Stromeyer, Hannover.—Dr**Szokalsky, Warschau.—Dr ** Kolb, Augsburg. — * Dr Feldmann, München. — * Dr Otterburg, Landau. Juni.-October : Dr Schlund, Mannheim. — Dr Pigné, Limoges. — Dr ** Sichel, Frankfurt. — Dr ** Mandl, Pesth. — ** Dr Schuster, Celle. — Dr Danyau, Paris. — Dr Kuhn, Strasburg. — Dr * Blanche, Passy. — Dr Davis, Kindenheim, Rh. Bayern. — Dr Macarthy, Paris. — D. Clancy, Irland.
AOM : DD. Weber, Kiel.—H. Balser, Giessen.—Liman, Berlin.—D. Bunsen, Altona.—G. Keiler, Dresden. — Vesenmeyer, Ulm. — Türk, Wien. — Erhardt, Heidelberg. — Thygesen , Kiel.—Unna, Hamburg.—Herzfelder, Würzburg.—Hillebrand, Gratz.—Schumacher, Achsen. — Ewerbeck, Dantzig. — Hagen, Velden. — Baumert, Berlin. — Füllkruss†, Leipzig. — Millies, Leipzig. — Stumpf†, Berlin. — Petersen †, Landau. — Günther, Braunschweig. — Brandes. Celle. — Tiemann, Biefeld. — Rabus, Bayreuth. — Doyer, Amsterdam. — Schenck, ... — Wieniawsky, Petersburg. — Valentiner, Holstein. — Claus, Limburg. — Wedl, Wien. — Buhl, Kempten. — Merbach, Dresden, Anger, Carlsbad. — Esterle, Padua. — Fraschina, Tessin. — Cahen, ... Joos I, Schaffhausen. — Müller, Celle.— Helbert, Hamburg.

1845

OM : DDr Oliffe, Edimburg. — Vogt (Giessen), Neufchatel. — Pappenheim, Breslau.— Schiff, Frankfurt. — Belin,Paris. — Fleury, Mayence.
Januar : AOM : ** DDr Gerlach, Baiern.— ** Lebert, Berlin.— Hoelder, Stuttgard.— Schrader, Wolfenbüttel. — Rousseau, Paris. — Proell, Wien. — Bassow, Moskau. — Ross, Holstein. Februar : Beck, Freiburg.—Prieger, Kreutznach.—Kraft, Hamburg.—Frey, Basel.—* Finelius, Preussen.—Schrader,

---

Anmerkung. — OM. bedeutet : Ordentliche Mitglieder, AOM. Ausserordentliche Mitglieder eine Trennung die in den nur ersten Jahren bestand.

Diejenigen Herren welche beim Abgang oder spæter zu correspondirenden Mitgliedern erwæhlt wurden, sind mit einem *, die Ehrenmitglieder mit zwei ** ausgezeichnet.

Die ungleiche Handschrift der verschiedene Secretære mœge etwaige Irrthümer entschuldigen, die trotz aller Sorgfalt sich eingeschlichen haben kœnnten.

Die Todesfælle waren bei der Entfernung oft schwer, bisweilen nicht zu ermitteln; dies gilt in noch ausgedehnterem Maasstabe von den Ortsverænderungen der Mitglieder. Man bittet deshalb um Nachsicht.

Mitglieder welche den Verein zweimal besuchten sind beim jedesmaligen Eintritt aufgeführt.

Die Red. Commission.

Fig. 8 Copy of the list of members of the Society, about 1854[20]

importance of a detailed description of the historical facts and therefore had reported on the "History and spreading of etherism" in the pharmacological magazine "Repetitorium für die Pharmacie" as early as 1847[15].

It is through this article that he probably became the first to record the "history of surgical anaesthesia". Presumably he was inspired by the well-known quarrel between Horace Wells (1815-1848), Charles Thomas Jackson (1805-1880) and William Thomas Green Morton (1819-1868) about the question who was the first to employ ether anaesthesia, a question that even had become subject for discussion at the "Académie Français" of Paris[6]. And since he had regularly taken part in the meetings of January 1847, which dealt with the not yet understood properties of the new agent, he also witnessed these debates. There he personally got known Wells, who had come to Paris in March of 1847 to defend his own position regarding this controversy. Because of Martin's detailed descriptions people in Germany could read about Well`s opinion a few days later. Moreover, Martin reported on the unsuccess-ful attempts of etherization by French scientists and described the findings about the pharmacodynamics of sulfuric ether published by Velpeau, Gruby and Flourens[3].

The self-experiments of club members

His detailed reports includes descriptions of numerous self-experiments regarding etherization that he and serveral members took part in[1,29]. The fact that people had repeatedly failed to successfully anaesthetize a patient made many physicians demand to first find out more about the effects of ether inhalation in animal models. Additionally there were people who called for self-experiments in order to find out more about the substance's properties.

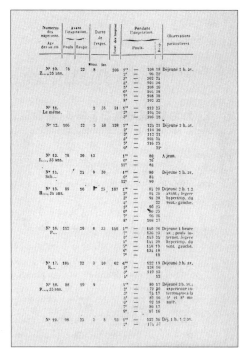

Fig. 9 Schedule of some results during the self-experiments of members of the Society[1]

It is probably true that the members of the "Society of German Physicians in Paris" were the first scientists ever to perform extensive self-experiments to ascertain more facts about the effect of ether inhalation[4]. According to a contemporary author, they, agreed "to create separate committees, one, conducting the experiments, the other commenting on cases already published". Young physicians between 24 and 37 years of age tested the effects of inhaled ether on themselves "at a room temperature of 16 to 18 degrees of Celsius" just after they had had their "morning coffee". They registered possible changes in respiration, heart-rate and sensitivity to pain and noted them using special charts[1]. They first published their findings in the "Gazette Médicale de Paris" (Fig. 9). Later many magazines of the German speaking nations printed those articles[2,29] (Fig. 10).

It is because of the fact that Martin published so many articles on the topic, that

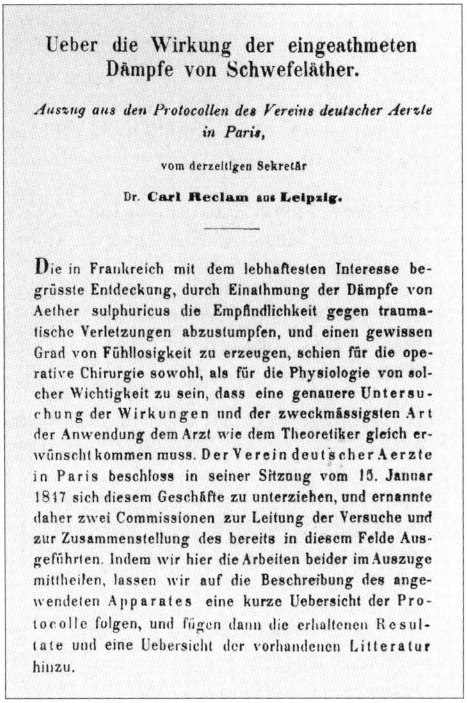

Ueber die Wirkung der eingeathmeten Dämpfe von Schwefeläther.

Auszug aus den Protocollen des Vereins deutscher Aerzte in Paris,

vom derzeitigen Sekretär

Dr. **Carl Reclam aus Leipzig.**

Die in Frankreich mit dem lebhaftesten Interesse begrüsste Entdeckung, durch Einathmung der Dämpfe von Aether sulphuricus die Empfindlichkeit gegen traumatische Verletzungen abzustumpfen, und einen gewissen Grad von Fühllosigkeit zu erzeugen, schien für die operative Chirurgie sowohl, als für die Physiologie von solcher Wichtigkeit zu sein, dass eine genauere Untersuchung der Wirkungen und der zweckmässigsten Art der Anwendung dem Arzt wie dem Theoretiker gleich erwünscht kommen muss. Der Verein deutscher Aerzte in Paris beschloss in seiner Sitzung vom 15. Januar 1847 sich diesem Geschäfte zu unterziehen, und ernannte daher zwei Commissionen zur Leitung der Versuche und zur Zusammenstellung des bereits in diesem Felde Ausgeführten. Indem wir hier die Arbeiten beider im Auszuge mittheilen, lassen wir auf die Beschreibung des angewendeten Apparates eine kurze Uebersicht der Protocolle folgen, und fügen dann die erhaltenen Resultate und eine Uebersicht der vorhandenen Litteratur hinzu.

Fig. 10 Cover page of a publication in which the self-experiments were described in detail[8]

the anaesthetic properties of ether were made known all over the German – speaking nations[23,29]. It is noteworthy that, at that time, due to the existence of the "K. u. K." Monarchy of Austria, the use of German language was common in many countries like today's Czech Republic, Hungary and northern Italy. Thus, first Martin's reports reached Augsburg by carriage via major cities like Strassbourg and Karlsruhe, "at noon, three days after they had been posted". Since papers were the most important source of information for many people, his articles were accepted and published and supplemented by comments. We can understand, how the news was spread so fast to places where the "Augsburger Allgemeine Zeitung" was sold. Because the sensational news about the properties of ether had appeared in the newspapers, the technique became such common knowledge, that items on the subject could hardly be found in non-medical journals after early summer of 1847. In spite of this the issue is still featured in today's medical magazines[3].

References:

[1] Anonymous: Recherches et expériences sur l'inhalation de l'éther sulfurique; Communiqués par la Société des Médicins Allemands à Paris. Gazette Médicale de Paris 1847; 6:101-104

[2] Anonymous: Vermischtes-Ueber die Einatmung des Aetherdunstes, Aetherrausch, Aetherschlaf, als Betäubungsmittel bei chirurgischen Operationen. Zschr f ges Medicin 1847; 35: 425-439

[3] Brandt L, Fehr G: Eine Entdeckung in der Chirurgie. Abbott GmbH, Wissenschaftliche Verlagsabteilung, Wiesbaden 1996

[4] Elkeles B: Der moralische Diskurs über das medizinische Menschenexperiment im 19. Jahrhundert. Fischer, Stuttgart-Jena-New York 1996

[5] Ellis RH: Introduction of ether anaesthesia in Great Britain. Anaesthesia 1976; 31:766-777

6. Fischer H: Zur Frühgeschichte der Inhalationsnarkose 1846/47. Gesnerus 1947; 4: 150-166

7. Franco A, Cortés J, Vidal M I, Rabanal S: Erste Abhandlung über Ätheranästhesie in Deutschland aus dem Jahre 1847. Anaesthesist 1993; 42: 51

8. Goerig M: Collection Goerig, Hamburg

9. Gruhlich O: Geschichte der Bibliothek und Naturaliensammlung der Kaiserlich Leopoldinisch-Carolinischen Deutschen Akademie der Naturforscher. Blochmann & Sohn Dresden

10. Hintzenstern, U v, Schwarz W: Frühe Erlanger Beiträge zur Theorie und Praxis der Äther – und Chloroformnarkose. Anaesthesist 1996; 45: 131-139

11. Jones RM: American doctors and the Parisian medical world 1830-1840. Bull Hist Med 1973; XLVII: 40-65 and 177-204

12. Ling H: Nachruf: Dr. Aloys Martin. Beilage Allg Zeitung, Nr. 220:10. August, 1891; Beilags-Nr. 184, S. 6-8

13. Martin A: Ueber Urokranin und einige andere Farbenstoffe im Menschenharne. München 1845

14. Martin A: Über die durch Schwefelaether bewirkte Narkose als Mittel, chirurgische Operationen schmerzlos zu machen. Teil 1, 1847; Beilage Nr. 21, S. 163-164, Augsburger Allgemeine Zeitung

15. Martin A: Geschichte der Entdeckung und Ausbreitung des Aetherismus. Repertorium für die Pharmacie 1847; 96:351-387

16. Martin A: Zur Physiologie und Pharmakodynamik des Aetherismus. Inauguraldissertation Universität München. Franz, München 1847

17. Martin A, Binswanger L: Das Chloroform in seinen Wirkungen auf Menschen und Thiere. Brockhaus, Leipzig 1848

18. Martin A: Das Civil-Medicinalwesen im Königreich Bayern. München 1883/1884

19. Meding HL: Fest-Bericht der zehnjährigen Stifungsfeier des Vereins deutscher Aerzte in Paris. Paris, Leipzig und Bonn. In den Buchhandlungen der Herren Victor Masson, Michelsen (Goetze & Mierisch) und Eduard Weber, Breslau 1854

20. Meding A, Martin A: Recueil de travaux lus à la Société Médicale Allemande de Paris. Victor Masson, Paris 1856

21. Mettenheim: Zur Geschichte der Societas medicorum Germanicorum Parisiensis. Med Welt 1942; 4: 91-92

22. Nees von Esenbeck, Th: Paris Médical, Vade-Mecum des Médecins Étrangers. Paris 1852

23. Nemes C: Aloys Martins Pariser Berichte an die Augsburger Allgemeine Zeitung (1847) – eine Spurensicherung. Anaesthesist 1994, Suppl 1, S 77

24. Nemes C: Aloys Martin – Wegbereiter der chirurgischen Anästhesie in Deutschland. Anaesthesist 1994; 43:330-331

25. Petermann H: 16. Oktober 1846 – Wendepunkt in der Chirurgie. S 47-55. In: Petermann H (Hrsg) Der schöne Traum, daß der Schmerz von uns genommen, ist zur Wirklichkeit geworden. Lengenfelder, Erlangen 1997

26. Rothe CG: Zur 50 jährigen Gedächtnisfeier der Entdeckung der Aethernarkose. Münch Med Wochenschr 1896; 41: 980-983

27. Secher O: The introduction of ether anaesthesia in the Nordic Countries. Acta Anaesthesiol Scand 1985; 29: 2-10

28. Ule W: Geschichte der Kaiserlich Leopoldinisch-Carolinischen Deutschen Akademie der Naturforscher während der Jahre 1852-1887 mit einem Rückblick auf die frühere Zeit ihres Bestehens. Blochmann und Sohn, Dresden 1897

29. Walser H: Zur Einführung der Äthernarkose im deutschsprachigen Sprachgebiet im Jahre 1847. H R Sauerländer & Co, Aarau 1957

30. Wolff H: Zum 200. Geburtstag von Johann Friedrich Dieffenbach. Zbl f Chir 1992; 11: 238-243

Some Remarks Regarding the First Etherization in Germany

U.v.Hintzenstern
Department of Anaesthesiology, Municipal Hospital Forchheim, Germany
W. Schwarz, H. Petermann
Department of Anaesthesiology, University of Erlangen-Nuremberg, Germany

The era of modern anaesthesia in Germany began on January 24th, 1847. It was supposed for a long time that, on this day, Johann Ferdinand Heyfelder (1798 - 1869), professor and chairman of the department of surgery and ophthalmology of the University of Erlangen, was the first to anaesthetize a patient with sulphuric ether in Germany[5].

The patient was the 26-year-old Shoemak-er's journeyman, Michael Gegner. Heyfelder characterized him as "pale, shrunken and not strong, suffering for a long time from a voluminous cold abscess on his left buttock". First he inhaled the ether via his mouth with closed nostrils. After 3 minutes Heyfelder interrupted the administration because of a fit of coughing. Then the glass tube of the inhal-er was put in the right nostril and the inhalations were continued. Three and a half minutes later mydriasis was observed, another one and a half minutes later bradycardia occurred. Another two minutes later, the heart rate went up again. Five minutes later the patient collapsed, two more minutes later sensation was very much reduced but the patient remained conscious. Due to another coughing fit, inhalation had to be interrupted for two minutes and then continued via the left nostril. During the following three minutes the pulse was only vaguely palpable, inhalation was tried via mouth again. A new violent coughing fit forced cessation of the procedure without incision of the cold abscess. The following day, Heyfelder succeeded in performing surgery on the same patient under ether despite repeated interruptions due to coughing fits. The patient did not feel any pain and said that he had dreamed during the operation. Therefore, the new drug was recognized to be effective[4].

Heyfelder himself was convinced that with this case, he had been the first in Germany to administer etherization for a surgical operation. He mentioned this in a chapter on the history of ether inhalation in his book entitled "The experiments with sulphuric ether"[4]. This monograph, published in March 1847, represents one of the first complete treatises on sulphuric ether in German literature. The late Ole Secher, who made a reprint of Heyfelder's book in 1987, believed in Heyfelder's priority[13]. He therefore wrote in his epilogue to the reprint: "Heyfelder has been busy. The first patient was anaesthetized on January 24th. If it was a competition of being the first to use ether for anaesthesia in Germany, Heyfelder would have won it, but the others were very close: ... v. Rothmund in Munich on January the 25th, ... and ... v. Bruns on the 26th or 27th of January in Tübingen".

What was the motivation for Heyfelder to get involved in etherization? In the preface of his book *The experiments with sulphuric ether*, Heyfelder reported that he learnt about *Malgaigne's* experiments with sulphuric ether by reading articles in the January issue of the *Revue medico-chirurgicale de Paris* and *Gazette medicale de Paris* of January 16th. He continued that because of the good results of his first etherizations he had within a short time - in his words - "a lot of material" to study the action of sulphuric ether during application.

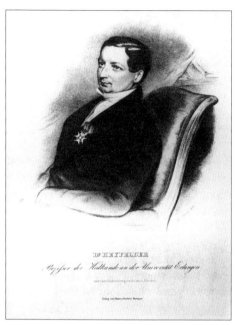

Johann Ferdinand Heyfelder (1798 - 1869). From the portrait collection of the Library of the University of Erlangen.

Perhaps Heyfelder's success was not due only to himself, as he would have people believe. Recently, the authors found an interesting article dated from February 17th, 1847, in the *Königlich Bayerisches Intelligenz-Blatt für Mittelfranken* (in English: Royal Bavarian Official Gazette for Mid-Franconia, which is the region Erlangen belongs to)[7]. Under the heading *In the Name of his Majesty the King*, there is an order dated February 13th, 1847, to refer surgical patients to the surgical department of the University Hospital of Erlangen to get more experience regarding etherization. A ministerial order of January the 19th that Heyfelder should administer ether was also referred to in this article. That means that the royal government of Mid-Franconia had officially ordered Heyfelder's activity regarding etherization.

Meanwhile, in the state archives at Nuremberg, the authors have found a letter of Heyfelder's hand dated from March 21st, 1847, which Heyfelder sent to the Royal Bavarian Government of Mid-Franconia together with a copy of his book "The experiments with sulphuric ether"[1]. In an obsequious manner - as was usual in those days - he wrote that he had undertaken his experiments with sulphuric ether following the above mentioned ministerial order of January 19th, 1847. Additionally, he asked the royal government to draw the doctors' attention to his book by means of the *Official Gazette for Mid-Franconia* and to renew the order to send surgical patients to his clinic so that he could continue with his experiments on sulphuric ether and start with experiments with salt ether. An order according to Heyfelder's requests, dated March 29th, 1847, was published in the *Royal Bavarian Official Gazette for Mid-Franconia* in the issue of April 5th, 1847[7].

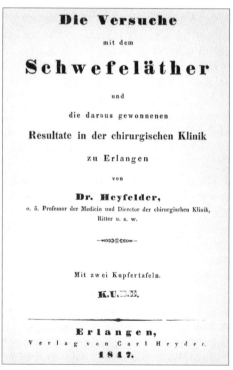

Frontispiece of Heyfelder's book The experiments with sulphuric ether, published in 1847.

Recently, in her medical dissertation[2], Fehr published an interesting article from the *Königlich privilegirte Berlinische Zeitung* (later *Vossische Zeitung*) of January 28th, 1847[8]. Therein, a painless tooth-extraction under etherization was reported performed by two physicians, Weickert und Obenaus on January 24th, 1847, at Leipzig. During the operation the patient was intoxicated but not completely unconscious. The patient did not notice the extraction of the molar tooth but became aware of the pain only a few moments later. Heinrich Eduard Weickert und Carl Friedrich Eduard Obenaus worked at that time as assistants at the royal clinical institute of the Jakobsspital at Leipzig. This article on the *first successful* etherization in Germany was reprinted in a few newspapers (e.g. *Kölnische Zeitung* of February 5th, 1847). Another short reference to that event is given in a small monograph on the history of etherization published by Aloys Martin (1818 - 1891) in 1847[9]. However, until now, no written comment of Weickert and Obenaus themselves could be found regarding the administration of ether on January 24th, 1847, or on further anaesthesiological work. Due to that, their achievement presumably did not become well-known or quickly fell into oblivion whereas Heyfelder became well-known by publishing two books and several articles referring to his numerous experiments with ether and chloroform. In his book on the administration of sulphuric ether, published in 1847, even C. E. Hering, a dentist who practiced in Leipzig, pointed to Heyfelder as the first who tried experiments with etherization in Germany (misdated as February 1st, 1847). He did not, however, mention the pioneering work of Weickert and Obenaus at all[3].

In our opinion, it makes no sense to discuss a priority claim of who was the first in Germany to administer ether. All these so-called *first* experiments were performed within a few days or hours. Should a difference be made between the first etherization for a tooth extraction or a surgical operation? Or does the honour of the first etherization go to the physician von Rothmund who first tried to etherize a patient in Munich on January 22nd, 1847? This experiment was reported by the clinical assistant of von Rothmund in the

Königlich Bayerisches Intelligenz-Blatt für Mittelfranken from April 5, 1847, p. 173

introduction to his dissertation of 1847 entitled *The Sulphuric Ether. Composition, Action and Application*[10]. Von Rothmund did not publish his experiment because it was not at all successful.

Additionally one has to consider another interesting aspect. There was not a political unit called "Germany" in 1847 but a confederacy of a lot of sovereign states called "Deutscher Bund" ("German Federation"). So it might be more relevant to look at all German-speaking countries. Considering this aspect, Hermann Askan Demme (1802 - 1867) from Bern, Switzerland, who operated on three surgical patients under ether narcosis on January 23rd, 1847, was the very first to perform a success-ful etherization in this region[6, 11, 12, 14].

Regarding the question of the "first etherization in Germany", the authors would prefer to state the following:

The very first public etherization was administerd by William Thomas Green Morton (1809 - 1868) on October 16th, 1846, at Massachusetts General Hospital in Boston, USA, and - about three months later - there were several physicians who performed "their" *first* etherizations in German-speaking countries more or less at the same time in January 1847.

References:

[1] Acten der Koeniglich Bayerischen Regierung von Mittelfranken Kammer des Innern. Schriften im Fach der Menschen und Thier-Heilkunde 1831-1878. Staatsarchiv Nürnberg, Rcp. 270/II, no. 396

[2] Fehr G: Eine Entdeckung in der Chirurgie. Diss. med Mainz (published as: Brandt L, Fehr G (1996) Eine Entdeckung in der Chirurgie. Wissenschaftliche Verlagsabteilung Abbott GmbH, Wiesbaden (1994)

[3] Hering CE: Die Schwefeläther-Frage nach eigner Erfahrung und nach den neuesten Forschungen beleuchtet. Verlag von Robert Friese, Leipzig, 1847

[4] Heyfelder JF: Die Versuche mit dem Schwefeläther und die daraus gewonnenen Resultate in der chirurgischen Klinik zu Erlangen. Heyder, Erlangen, 1847

[5] Hintzenstern U v, Schwarz W: Frühe Erlanger Beiträge zur Theorie und Praxis der Äther- und Chloroformnarkose. Teil 1. Heyfelders klinische Versuche mit Äther und Chloroform. Anaesthesist 1847; 45:131-139

[6] Intelligenzblatt für die Stadt Bern 14, no. 21 from January 25, 1847

[7] Königlich Bayerisches Intelligenz-Blatt für Mittelfranken from February 17 and April 5, 1847

[8] Königlich privilegirte Berlinische Zeitung no. 23 from January 28, 1847

[9] Martin A: Geschichte der Entdeckung und Ausbreitung des Aetherismus. Report Pharm 96 (=2. Reihe, vol 46): 351-387, 1847

[10] Merck WCh: Der Schwefeläther in seiner Bereitung, Wirkung und Anwendung. Diss med München 1847

[11] Pasch T, Mörgeli C: (eds) 150 Jahre Anästhesie (exhibition catalogue) . Wissenschaftliche Verlagsabteilung Abbott GmbH, Wiesbaden 1997

[10] Schwarz W: Die Entwicklung der Anästhesie des deutschen Sprachraums im 19. Jahrhundert. Therapeutische Umschau 1991; 48: 360-364

[13] Secher O: Johann Ferdinand Heyfelder (epilogue to the reprint of Heyfelder's book of 1847 [4]), Janssenpharma A/S, Birkerod, 1987 p 3

[14] Walser H: Zur Einführung der Äthernarkose im deutschen Sprachgebiet im Jahre 1847. Diss med Zürich. Sauerländer, Aarau 1957

We thank Lynne Lörler very much for her critical proof reading of our manuscript.

"Der schöne Traum, dass der Schmerz von uns genommen, ist zur Wirklichkeit geworden."

German Publications on Ether and Chloroform Anaesthesia in 1847.

H. Petermann
Department of Anaesthesiology, University Erlangen-Nuremberg, Germany

"The beautiful dream, that pain is taken from us, has come true." This is the first sentence in Johann Friedrich Dieffenbach's publication about "Ether against pain" in 1847 (Fig. 1).

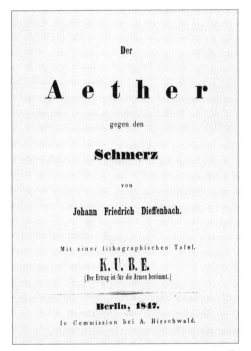

Fig. 1: Title-page J. F. Dieffenbach (1792-1847)

The first year ether narcosis was introduced in German speaking countries, a lot of publications were made.

This is a short abstract about the literature in the first year 1847.

The book "Struwelpeter" was published in the forties of the 19th century which was retitled by Mark Twain as "Slovenly Peter or Happy Tales and Funny Pictures" in 1891. The news about painless surgery sounded like "happy tales" and were sometimes illustrated with "funny pictures."

Informations about ether narcosis and its effects in 1847 were published as:

1. monographs
2. articles in periodicals
3. reports in newspapers
4. scientific publications (dissertations)

1. Monographs

In German speaking countries 19 different monographs on ether narcosis could be traced as shown in the table. Regarding the authors of these publications it is quite astonishing that they were not necessarily the first who administered ether in the region they worked in. Hermann Berend (1809-1873) in Berlin and the dentists Heinrich Weikert (?) and Carl F. E. Obenaus (?) for example in Leipzig probably were the first physicians to etherize patients in the above mentioned cities – obviously they do not show up in the list. Another interesting fact that should be mentioned is, that Conrad Schenk (?) wrote his monograph for the public. I would also like to refer that Joseph Rapp (?) and his colleague both were family doctors.

Books Published on Ether Narcosis in 1847

1. Bauer, Alexander: Ueber Schwefeläther und seine neueste Anwendung, mit einem Anhange, über die in den öffentlichen Anstalten Prags gewonnenen Resultate. Prag 1847. 55 S
2. Bergson, Joseph: Die medicinische Anwendung der Aetherdämpfe in Bezug auf Physiologie, operative Chirurgie, Nervenpathologie, Psychiatrie, Geburtshülfe, Zahn- und Thierheilkunde. Berlin 1847. 133 S
3. Bibra, Ernst von und Harless, Emil: Die Wirkungen des Schwefeläthers in chemischer und physiologischer Beziehung. Erlangen 1847. 190 S
4. Dieffenbach, Johann Friedrich: Der Aether gegen den Schmerz. Berlin 1847. 228 S
5. Grenser, Waldemar Ludwig: Über Aether-Einathmungen während der Geburt. Leipzig 1847
6. Hammer, Adam: Die Anwendung des Schwefeläthers im Allgemeinen und insbesondere bei Geburten. Mannheim 1847. 32 S
7. Hering, Carl E.: Die Schwefelätherfrage nach eigner Erfahrung und nach den neuesten Forschungen beleuchtet. Leipzig 1847. 90 S
8. Heyfelder, Johann Ferdinand: Die Versuche mit dem Schwefeläther und die daraus gewonnen Resultate in der chirurgischen Klinik zu Erlangen. Erlangen 1847
9. Jenni, Jakob J.: Erfahrungen über die Wirkungen der eingeathmeten Schwefelätherdämpfe im menschlichen Organismus. Zürich 1847. 71 S
10. Kopezky, Benedikt: Warnungen vor den schädlichen Wirkungen der Aether-Einathmung nebst einer Vergleichung mit den Narkosen durch Weingeist, Opium, Tabak und Coca. Wien 1847
11. Kronser, Victor Nicolaus: Der Schwefeläther. seine chemische Bereitung, Eigenschaft und Anwendung, nebst ausführlichem Berichte der ersten und interessantesten damit gemachten Versuche bei Operationen und verschiedenen Krankheitsfällen, so wie deren Verlauf und Nachbehandlung. Wien 1847. 72 S
12. Martin, Aloys: Geschichte der Entdeckung und Ausbreitung des Aetherismus. München 1847. 39 S
13. Nathan, Elias: Ueber Aether-Rausch (Phrenopathia aetherea), mit besonderer Rücksicht auf die jüngsten Erfahrungen in England und Frankreich. Hamburg 1847. 50 S
14. Rapp, Joseph Anton und Wieser, : Erfahrungen über Einathmungen der Schwefelätherdämpfe, gemacht und mitgetheilt von den praktischen Aerzten. Bamberg 1847. 20 S
15. Rosenfeld, Josef: Die Schwefeläther-Dämpfe und ihre Wirksamkeit, vorzüglich in Bezug auf operative Chirurgie. Pest (Ungarn) 1847. 63 S
16. Schenk, Conrad: Die Einathmung der Schwefelätherdünste zur Verhütung und Tilgung von Schmerzen. Eine Schrift für Aerzte und Nichtaerzte. Quedlinburg 1847. (populär) 45 S
17. Schlesinger, Joseph: Die Einathmung der Schwefel-Äthers in ihren Wirkungen auf Menschen und Thiere, besonders als ein Mittel bei chirurgischen Operationen den Schmerz zu umgehen. Leipzig 1847. 48 S
18. Siebold, Eduard Caspar Jacob von: Ueber die Anwendung der Schwefel-Aether-Dämpfe in der Geburtshülfe. Göttingen 1847. 27 S
19. Welz, Robert von: Die Einathmung der Aetherdämpfe in ihrer verschiedenen Wirkungsweise mit praktischer Anleitung für jene, welche dieses Mittel in Gebrauch ziehen. Nach eigenen Erfahrungen bearbeitet. Würzburg 1847. 24 S

German Medical Periodical Published in 1847

1. Allgemeine medicinische Central-Zeitung. Berlin. Jahrgang 16 (1847)
2. Allgemeine Zeitung für Militär-Aerzte. 1847
3. Archiv für die gesammte Medicin. Jena. Bd.8 (1847)
4. Archiv für physiologische Heilkunde. Stuttgart. Jahrgang 6 (1847)
5. Archiv für physiologische Medizin. 1847
6. Casp. Wochenschrift. 1847, 19
7. Hannoversche Annalen für die gesammte Heilkunde. Hannover. 1847, N.F. 7,1, 2
8. Harless Zeitschrift. Bd.4 (1847)
9. Heidelberger medizinische Annalen. 1847
10. Journal für Chirurgie und Augenheilkunde. Bd.7 (1847)
11. Journal für Kinderkrankheiten. Erlangen. Jahrgang 6 (1847)
12. Medicinische Zeitung. Hg. von dem Vereine für Heilkunde in Preußen. Jahrgang 16 (1847)
13. Medizinisches Correspondenzblatt Bayerischer Aerzte. Erlangen. 1847
14. Medizinisches Correspondenz-Blatt des würtembergischen Ärztlichen Vereins. Stuttgart Bd.17 (1847)
15. Neue medicinisch-chirurgische Zeitung. München. Jahrgang 5 (1847), Bd.1-4
16. Neue Zeitschrift für Geburtskunde. Berlin. Bd.22. 1847
17. Notizen aus dem Gebiete der Natur- und Heilkunde. Weimar. 3. Reihe, Jg.2 (1847)
18. Oesterreichische medizinische Wochenschrift. Wien. Jahrgang 7 (1847)
19. Oesterreichisches medizinisches Jahrbuch. Wien. 1847
20. Repertorium für die Pharmazie. Nürnberg. 2. Reihe (1847), Bd.45-46
21. Rheinische Monatsschrift für praktische Aerzte. Köln. Jahrgang 1 (1847)
22. Schweizerische Zeitschrift für Medicin, Chirurgie und Geburtshülfe. Jg.5 (1846), Jahrgang 6 (1847)
23. Vierteljahresschrift für praktische Heilkunde. Prag. 1847
24. Zeitschrift des Norddeutschen Chirurgen-Vereins für Medicin, Chirurgie und Geburtshülfe. Magdeburg. Jahrgang 1 (1847)
25. Zeitschrift für physiologische Heilkunde. 1847
26. Zeitschrift für rationelle Medizin. Heidelberg. Jahrgang 6 (1847)
27. Zeitschrift der k.k. Gesellschaft der Aerzte zu Wien. Redigirt von Karl Haller. Wien. Jahrgang 4 (1847)
28. Zeitschrift für die gesammte Medicin. Hamburg. Bd.34 (1847)

An analysis of the content of these monographs shows the following result:

In General about Application of Ether	12
Obstetrics	3
Dentistry	1
Physiology	1
History	1
Popular	1

Johann Friedrich Dieffenbach (1792-1847) in Berlin, Franz Christoph Rothmund (1801-1891) in Munich. Quite a few of the doctors were members of the "Verein Deutscher Aerzte in Paris", among them: Viktor von Bruns (1823-1883, Tübingen), Robert Ritter von Welz (1814-1879, Würzburg) and Adam Hammer (1818-1878, Mannheim). All the other authors, that were not named till now, were in touch with persons listed above.

Topics in the Periodicals (11 out of 28)

Bez.	ACZ	APH	JfK	MZ	MCB	MCW	NNH	NMC	ÖMW	RM	RP
Σ	56	3	4	8	7	10	44	36	19	7	5
General	2	3	4	7	4	9	6	2	5	4	3
History	-	-	-	-	-	-	-	-	1	-	2
Obstetrics	-	-	-	-	1	-	2	-	-	1	-
Physiology	-	-	-	-	-	-	1	-	-	-	-
Forensic	-	-	-	-	2	-	3	-	1	1	-
Animal	-	-	-	-	-	1	2	-	-	1	-
Internal	-	-	-	-	-	-	2	1	1	-	-
Reviews	12	-	-	1	-	-	-	11	11	-	-
Various	42	-	-	-	-	-	28	22	-	-	-

ACZ - Allgemeine medizinische Central-Zeitung
APH - Archiv für physiologische Heilkunde
JfK - Journal für Kinderkrankheiten
MZ - Medicinische Zeitung
MCB - Medicinisches Correspondenzblatt Bayerischer Aerzte
MCW - Medicinisches Correspondenz-Blatt des württembergischen Aerztlichen Vereins
NNH - Notizen aus dem Gebiete der Natur- und Heilkunde
NMC - Neue medicnisch-chirurgische Zeitung
ÖMW - Österreichische medizinische Wochenschrift
RM - Rheinische Monatsschrift für praktisches Aerzte
RP - Repertorium für die Pharmacie

If we look at the number of publications the question about the authors knowing each other arises. This can partly be answered considering that Cajetan Textor (1782-1860), professor for surgery and ophthalmology in Würzburg taught some of the physicians who were pioneers in administering ether like Hermann Demme (1802-1867) in Bern,

2. Periodicals

In 1847 a great number of articles and notes has been published in different periodicals. The list includes 28 periodicals and I am not sure, whether there are still more. The authors of the above mentioned monographs and their co-workers contributed to periodicals and – insome cases – to newspapers, mainly describing the effects of etherization on patients suffering from different medical problems.

Considering the topics, that were published in the different periodicals, I did an evaluation on eleven of them out of twenty eight:

Reports about the above mentioned topics were not only published in medical journals, but also in the so-called "Familienzeitschriften" (periodicals for the whole family).

The drawing here describes the effects of sulfuric ether pre- and postaperatively. Another one describes the application against stupidity and infidelity.

Punch suggested the application of ether to the members of the parliament in order to shorten their discussions. (Allgemeine Zeitung, Augsburg).

Punch empfiehlt den Schwefeläther im Parlament anzuwenden, so daß gewisse unliebe Maßregeln angenommen, oder auch Parteien zu Kochfleisch verhackt werden können, ohne daß es den Mitgliedern wehe thue. Noch besser wär' es jedes Mitglied mit einer Aetherblase zu versehen, für den Fall, daß einer der vielen langweiligen Gesellen im Haus eine Rede hielte.[1]

3. Newspapers

One or more newspaper were published in every city. Since education kept spreading more and more the number of newspapers was increasing. To name a few of them:

Nürnberger Kurier, Mittelfränkische Zeitung, Deutsche Allgemeine Zeitung, Königlich Priviligierte Berlinische Zeitung, Kölnische Zeitung, Illustrirte Zeitung (Fig. 2 a, b).

The newspapers being distributed all over – even to Paris – was the Allgemeine Zeitung, Augsburg.

---

1. **Dissertations on Ether in 1847**

   1. Barschall, Leopold: De casu quodam Anaesthesi dimidatae accedit excursus physiologico-pathologicus. Königsberg, Diss. med. 1847

   2. Bromberger, Theodor: De aetheris Sulphurici vaporibus. Berlin, Diss. med. 1847

   3. Diesterweg, Julius: De aetheris sulfurici in organismum per vias respiratorias inducti efficacitate. Berlin, Diss..med. 1847

   4. Jablonski, C.F.: Abhandlung über die Wirkungen der Schwefelätherdämpfe. Bern, Diss. med. 1847

   5. London, Ludwig: De aethere sulfurico. Berlin, Diss. med. 1847

   6. Martin, Aloys: Zur Physiologie und Pharmakologie des Aetherismus. München, Inaug.abh. pro facultate legendi 1847 (Fig. 3)

   7. Meinel, Carl August: Ein Fall von Aetherisation mit lethalem Ausgang bei Tetanus traumaticus. München, Diss.med. 1847

   8. Merck, Wolfgang Christoph: Der Schwefeläther in seiner Bereitung, Wirkung und Anwendung. München, Diss. med. 1847

   9. Nolten, Wilhelm: De usu aetheris vaporum obstetricio, adiectis observationisbus de chloroformi effectu. Bonn, Diss. med. 1847

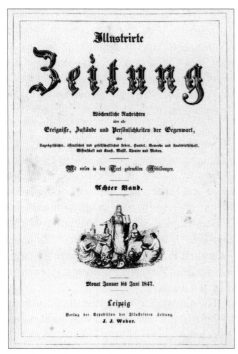

Fig. 2 a: Title-page Illustrierte Zeitung, Leipzig

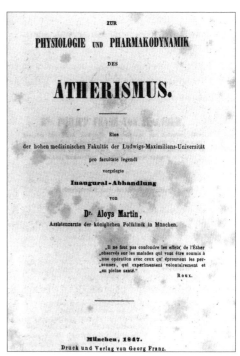

Fig. 3: Title-page A. Martin (1818-1891)

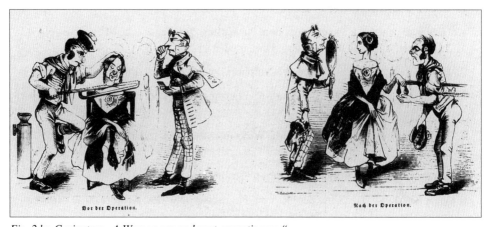

Fig. 2 b: Caricature „A Woman pre and post operationem."
From: Illustrierte Zeitung, Leipzig. Bd.8 (1847), P. 189

This was the paper with the first note about ether narcosis being published on January 10th 1847, being followed by a lot of short notes, that mostly described how the new method worked. 11 more articles were published, most of them written by Aloys Martin (1818-1891), a surgeon from Munich, who was in Paris at that time and member of the "Verein Deutscher Aerzte in Paris". The Allgemeine Zeitung was famous for its scientific section where the reports on ether and - later - on chloroform were published.

	1)L.B.	2)Th.B.	3)C.J.	4)C.J.	5)L.L.	6)A.M.	7)C.M.	8)W.M.	9)W.N.
Case Description	X						X		
History		X	X	X	X	X		X	X
Physiology		X		X	X	X		X	
Animal		X	X	X	X	X		X	
Effects		X		X	X	X		X	
Application		X	X	X		X		X	
Surgery		X		X	X			X	
Obstetrics				X				X	X
Apparatus				X				X	

4. Dissertations

The most renowned universities at that time were: Jena, Göttingen and Tübingen. As the knowledge about the application of ether spread they also started using sulfuric ether. Interestingly no medical dissertations on sulphuric ether or its use had been published at either of these universities.

This was the paper with the first note about ether narcosis being published on January 10th 1847, being followed by a lot of short notes, that mostly described how the new method worked. 11 more articles were published, most of them written by Aloys Martin (1818-1891), a surgeon from Munich, who was in Paris at that time and member of the "Verein Deutscher Aerzte in Paris". The Allgemeine Zeitung was famous for its scientific section where the reports on ether and - later - on chloroform were published.

4. Dissertations

The most renowned universities at that time were: Jena, Göttingen and Tübingen. As the knowledge about the application of ether spread they also started using sulfuric ether. Interestingly no medical dissertations on sulphuric ether or its use had been published at either of these universities.Nine thesis on ether or chloroform narcosis were written in 1847. As you can see in the list above, three of them were published in Berlin, one in Bonn, one in Berlin, one in Königsberg and one in Munich. Five of these medical dissertations were written in Latin. The contents are comparable to those of today and are shown in the table. Perhaps for all of these the last sentence of the dissertation of L. Barschall might be the programme: "Die Hypothese, ein interimistischer Gedanke, ist immer besser als Gedankenlosigkeit."

Who were these publications written for?

Most of the monographs, dissertations and articles in medical periodicals were written for doctors and other medical staff to spread the news. The surgeons wanted to inform their colleagues about their experiences with the inhalation of ether and chloroform. They wrote about their problems, but also described apparatus they used. This was in order to publish "Brauchbares und Nützliches".[2]

The general public got its informations by newspapers. The "Allgemeine Zeitung, Augsburg", had a scientific section where medical persons could gain informations on ether, e.g. concerning the activities in Paris or ether application in obstetrics. People at that time were interested in medical topics, especially in unusual or exceptional things. If these topics concerned their own life, they were even more important. Medical topics were quite popular at that time anyway, since a lot of regulations for the medical professions came up and because of the cholera epidemic. Telegraphy was just beeing invented and helped to spread news rapidly to the big cities.

What about the number of publications?

In 1847 there were a lot of German speaking countries, that were united in the 'Deutschen Bund'. But all of these states still kept their sovereignity. The most important ones were the kingdoms of Prussia, Bavaria, Hannover, Saxony and the 'House of Austria'. This is the reason why most of the articles were only published for the people within one state. Out of the above mentioned monographs three were published in Austria, two in Prussia, five in Bavaria, four in Saxony and at a time one in Baden, Hamburg and Switzerland. On the other hand, if there were notes given about other men also using ether, one can see the way how news spread. Not every article or monograph was read in all states of the 'Deutschen Bund'. For example the monograph of Bibra and Harless got book reviews from August to December, but was also not noted in some periodicals. On the given premises publications could not easily spread wide. Communication ways like streets and railways or modern transfer devices were not yet available or in bad condition. Because of these reasons the great number of monographs and reports in periodicals was obviously written to spread the "Great News" on operations without pain within one state.

In 1847 there was another publication titled "Schwefeläther" (Sulfuric Ether), written by August Heinrich Hoffmann von Fallersleben (1798-1874) and a collection of 27 songs. In a letter to a friend he wrote: *"Da ich mit Zensur nirgend politische Lieder damals drucken lassen konnte, so versuchte ich es ohne Zensur. Mein Freund Hoff (in Mannheim) scheute den Teufel nicht, noch weniger die Polizei. Damit die Sache doch nicht so leicht ausgekundschaftet würde und auch noch später den Reiz der Neuheit behielte, hatten wir 1847 in 1857 verwandelt!"*[3]

This note shows that the topic "Schwefeläther" (Sulfuric Ether) was quite common in 1847 and nobody thought about political songs better with this topic. A. H. Hoffmann von Fallersleben is better known as the author of the German National Hymn known and songs for children like "Alle Vöglein sind schon da, Ein Männlein steht im Walde."

The topics (sulfuric) ether and chloroform narcosis and their effects on human beings and animals were of common interest in 1847 as can be supported and proved by the number of publications.

References:

[1] Allgemeine Zeitung, Augsburg. 1847; 17: p 130
[2] Bauer A: Ueber Schwefeläther und seine neueste Anwendung. Prag 1847, p 3
[3] Benzmann H: Hoffmann von Fallersleben Ausgewählte Werke in vier Bänden. Band 2, Leipzig 1905, p 193

Robert Ritter von Welz (1814-1878) and the First Experiences with Ether Anaesthesia in Würzburg

Ch. Weißer
Department of Surgery, University of Würzburg,
Institute for the History of Medicine, University of Würzburg, Würzburg, Germany

Even being only a student, Robert Ritter von Welz turned his scientific interest on the influence of drugs on the human body. After learning from the newspapers that ether anaesthesia had been performed in Germany in January and February 1847, Welz started experiments on the effect of ether on anaesthesia following the advices of, Cajetan von Textor, professor of surgery. For the administration of ether, he constructed a special vaporizer (which he dedicated to the Bavarian King Ludwig I.), differing from the contemporary ones.

Robert Ritter von Welz was born on December 15th 1814 at Kelheim/Danube being the son of a judge. After his father's death the family went to Würzburg in 1828, where von Welz studied medicine between 1833 and 1838. In 1841 he graduated with a doctoral thesis about a subject of medical history, titled 'Des Asklepiades von Bithynien Gesundheitsvorschriften'; then he became fellow at the Juliusspital from 1842-1847 and also worked as a general practitioner at Würzburg. In 1849 he submitted his thesis 'De pulmonum collapsu, qui fit thorace aperto' and became a Privatdozent. In 1854 he decided to concentrate on ophthalmology only. To ensure better care of his patients he founded an eye-clinic with private means in 1857. In the same year he became professor extraordinary. In 1866 he was appointed first professor ordinary of ophthalmology at the Würzburg University. He died on November 11th, 1878 in Würzburg.

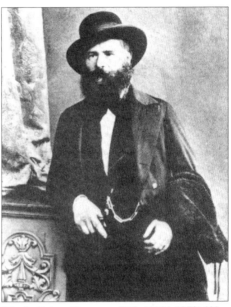

Fig. 1: Robert Ritter von Welz (1814-1878) [3]

Ether Anaesthesia in Würzburg

After physicians in Germany learned about anaesthesia through articles published in the daily press, e. g. on January 1st, 1847 in the Deutsche Allgemeine Zeitung (Leipzig), on January 10th in the Augsburger Allgemeine Zeitung, and on January 22nd in the Kölnische Zeitung, experiments and first applications in patients were performed at many locations (Tab. 1).

The path of information about ether came to Würzburg is not known. Textor however suggested von Welz to study the effects of ether on anaesthesia. Von Welz started his investigations with experiments on himself

Jan 23 1847	H. A. Demme	Bern/Switzerland
Jan 24 1847	H. E. Wickert/C. F. E. Obenaus	Leipzig
Jan 24 1847	J. H. Heyfelder	Erlangen (unsuccessful)
Jan 25 1847	F. Ch. v. Rothmund	Munich
Jan 25 1847	F. Schuh	Vienna/Austria
Jan 1847	V. v. Bruns	Tübingen
Feb 03 1847	**R. v. Welz**	**Würzburg**
Feb 1847	G. F. L. Stromeyer	Freiburg
Feb 06 1847	F. Pitha	Prague
Feb 06 1847	H. W. Berend	Berlin

Tab. 1: Chronology of ether anaesthesia in German speaking countries

or other proband and on February 1847 the first ether anaesthesia at the Juliusspital at Würzburg was carried through.

Welz published his experimental studies and his first results in a small monograph of 30 pages (Fig. 2) published on May 1st, 1847: The small monograph neither gives the exact date of the first performance of ether anaesthesia in Würzburg (the date of February 3rd 1847 for the first Würzburg ether anaesthesia is published by Cajetan v. Textor in the Neue Würzburger Zeitung of August 25th, 1847) nor the precise number of anaesthesias performed until the date of publication. But 28 major operations within 3 months (e. g. eye enucleations, tonsillectomies, tumor extirpations, tenotomies, amputations, cauterizations), and many other smaller procedures (e.g. abscesses, tooth extractions, atheromas etc.) were performed which suggest a quantity of about 100 ether anaesthesias during this period. In the beginning of July Textor testifies 80 major operations for von Welz's ether inhaler.

Summarizing his experience with ether anaesthesia, von Welz reported, that the duration of the operations performed reached up to half an hour, that the onset of anaesthesia

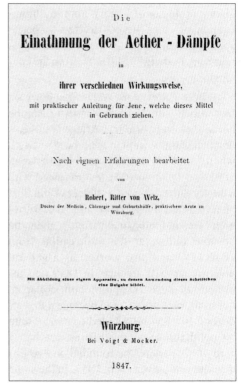

Fig. 2: Title-page of von Welz's paper of 1847

was quick, that analgesia was certain, and no complications were observed (no death, no cardiac or respiratory depression).

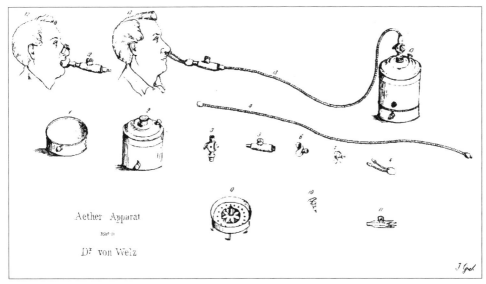

Fig. 3: von Welz's ether inhaler [6]: 1 water container; 2 vaporizing chamber; 3 tap; 4 flexible tube; 5 valve device; 6 mouth-piece; 7 nose clamp; 8 nose-piece; 9 grate inside vaporizing chamber; 10 three-way-tap; 11 valve device; 12 inhaler in use with mouth-piece and nose clamp; 13 inhaler in use with nose-piece and mouth closed.

von Welz's Ether Inhaler

For generating and administering the ether vapor, von Welz constructed his own inhaler (Fig. 3) which was built by Franz Sebastian Gerster (1789-1871) from Würzburg.

The main part of Welz's ether inhaler is the vaporizing chamber (2): it is a tin can with two openings for the access of air, one at the bottom and one on the top, that can be closed alternately. A grate for sponge or cotton saturated with ether is located inside the vaporizing chamber (9) with a central air-tube. A three-way-tap (3) with a lateral opening for air access, adjustable in the positions air only, air-ether-mix, and ether only, allows to mix air to the ether vapor which arises from the ether-sponge in the can. A flexible tube (4) connects the three-way-tap of the vaporizing chamber with the valve piece and a mouth- (6) or nose-piece (8). The valve device (5; Fig. 4) which is made of horn with an inspiration valve inside and an exspiration valve outside permits the flow of ether vapour in one direction only. A container (1) filled with warm water, could be put beneath the ether-can to hasten vaporization of ether.

von Welz's ether inhaler shows some peculiarities:

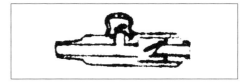

Fig. 4: Valve piece of von Welz's inhaler

1. The quantity of ether vapor getting to the patient can be regulated in multiple ways. The three-way-tap enables to change the concentration of ether in 3 steps: air only, air-ether mixture, or ether vapor only. Additional flow of air can be allowed through the closeable top opening of the vaporizing chamber.

2. Inhaling the ether vapor nasally (the way of inhaling suggested by von Welz) is more comfortable than orally, since the nose does not have to be closed with a nose clamp, and

breathing through both nostrils is much more comfortable than breathing through only one nostril, which is compulsory when using other inhalers.

3. The vaporization of the ether can be accelerated by warm water.

4. The dead space of Welz's inhaler is very small resulting from a close arrangement of the valve device and the nose- or mouth-piece.

Technique of Ether Anaesthesia by von Welz

100 cc of sponge or cotton is saturated with about 1 fl. oz. ether and put on the grate. Then the three-way-tap and the elastic tube are connected with the vaporizing chamber and the patient's mouth- or nose-piece in the air only position. When the patient is familiar with the kind of breathing through the apparatus, the concentration of the ether can be increased gradually by means of the three-way-tap and the additional air opening on top of the ether-can. As soon as the onset of anaesthesia (on the average within 6-15 minutes), the water-can filled with hot water can be put beneath the vaporizing chamber in order to speed up vaporization. Respiration can be observed by connecting a small whistle with the exspiratory valve or the inspiration opening in the vaporizing chamber. Refill of ether is possible through the top opening of the can without disconnecting the inhaler from the patient. 1-2 fl. oz. of ether is sufficient for most of the patients and surgical procedures.

Importance of von Welz's Inhaler

von Welz's ether inhaler has been used exclusively for ether anaesthesia at the Würzburg Juliusspital since April 1847. The contemporary professors of the Würzburg Medical Faculty Marcus, Rinecker, and Textor attest a secure, fast and comfortable anaesthesia performed with Welz's inhaler, in particular breathing through both nostrils is most pleasant.

In a letter dated July 22nd 1847, von Welz dedicated his inhaler to the Bavarian King Ludwig I. The Ministry of the Interior requested Professor F. Ch. v. Rothmund of Munich who had conducted the first ether anaesthesia at Munich 9 days before von Welz to examine the inhaler. The Ministry of the Interior recommended the inhaler to all Bavarian hospitals and practicians after learning that even von Rothmund was pleased.

The further employment of von Welz's inhaler is not evident: no mail order sending lists of the producer of the apparatus, no records of other users are available. Regarding the ministerial recommendation we can assume that von Welz's inhaler must have been spread widely at least for some years.

References:

1. Baar H: Zur Entwicklung der Anaesthesiologie an der Universität Würzburg. In: Baumgart P. [Hrsg.], Vierhundert Jahre Universität Würzburg. Eine Festschrift. Neustadt/Aisch 1982, p 951-956

2. Brandt L: Fehr G: Eine Entdeckung in der Chirurgie. Die ersten Monate der modernen Anästhesie im Spiegel der deutschsprachigen Tagespresse. Wiesbaden 1996

3. Sperling M: Die Entwicklung der medizinischen Fächer an der Julius-Maximilians-Universität Würzburg. In: Baumgart P [Hrsg], Vierhundert Jahre Universität Würzburg. Eine Festschrift. Neustadt/Aisch 1982, p 811-826

3. Stauber R: Robert Ritter von Welz 1814-1878. Med Diss Würzburg 1983

4. Sticker G: Entwicklungsgeschichte der medizinischen Fakultät an der Alma Mater Julia. In: Buchner M [Hrsg] : Aus der Vergangenheit der Universität Würzburg. Festschrift zum 350jährigen Bestehen der Universität. Berlin 1932, p 383-799

5. Textor C v: Äthernarkose im Juliusspitale zu Würzburg. Neue Würzburger Zeitung vom 25.8.1847

6. Welz R v: Die Einathmung der Aether-Dämpfe in ihrer verschiednen Wirkungsweise, mit praktischer Anleitung für Jene, welche dieses Mittel in Gebrauch ziehen. Würzburg 1847

7. Wirth M: Das Leben und Wirken des Chirurgen Cajetan von Textor. Med Diss Würzburg 1980

Was the Rausch-Narkose born in Hamburg?

R. J. Defalque, (*), B. Panning, (**), A. J. Wright, (*)
(*) Department of Anesthesia, UAB School of Medicine, Birmingham, Alabama, USA 35233
(**) Anaesthesieabteilung, Medizinische Hochschule, Hannover, Germany

Introduction

From 1900 through 1945 German surgeons frequently did minor surgery in debilitated patients with an anesthetic technique called Rausch-Narkose. Narkose in German means general anesthesia, Rausch means a brief state of intoxication or ecstasy produced by a drug, as alcohol.

P. Sudeck and Aether-Narkose

In 1901 Paul Sudeck,[1] of Hamburg, coined the name Aether-Narkose for a brief analgesic and amnesic state produced by inhaling a few breaths of ether poured on an open mask under the surgeon's repeated suggestion, that no pain would be felt. This allowed minor surgery for a few minutes in debilitated or ambulatory patients. In 1911 D. Kulenkampff[2] adopted Sudeck's name and technique for ethyl chloride.

Aether- and Aethylchloride-Narkose were popular in Germany and Central Europe[3] until 1945. German military surgeons for mass casualties in WW1 and WW2 extensively used it.[4]

Foreign surgeons visiting Germany from 1910 through 1930 brought back the techniques and its German name to the U.S. (Kelly; Collier; Coughlin; Gwathmey) and Great Britain (Ellis; Wilkie).

Was Sudeck the Original Discoverer of the Rausch-Narkose?

Sudeck postulated in his first paper[1] that he probably was not the first to have used the technique and after reviewing the literature he confirmed his suspicion in subsequent articles.

Indeed both the name "Rausch" and the use of an anesthetic's first analgesic stage to do surgery had been known long before Sudeck:

A. Carl Thiersch in 1888[5,6] had called Rausch the initial stage of excitement produced by chloroform and morphine. However, he does not seem to have made clinical use of it.

B. John H. Packard, an eminent Philadelphia surgeon, reported using a technique identical to Sudeck's in 1866.[7] He called it "primary anesthesia" or "first insensitivity". Ivanovich Pirogoff, in St. Petersburg, also used light ether analgesia in 1890.

In fact the use of inhalation anesthetics for conscious analgesia had long preceded Packard. In 1847-1848, James Young Simpson, John Snow, and E. W. Murphy in Great Britain used chloroform (and occasionally ether) inhalations for the relief of labor pain (narcose a la reine). Later on, chloroform analgesia was also tried in Great Britain by A. E. Sansom (1865), and in Germany by Sabarth (1866) and Bloch ("primäre Narkose") in 1900.

Misuse of the Rausch Concept

Sudeck's and Kulenkampff's Rausch-Narkose were well defined, specific methods of administration. However, the name Rausch-Narkose soon became applied to any rapid and brief general anesthesia for minor surgery, even when deep anesthetic planes were reached, as with ethylchloride or even with intravenous evipan.[8] Sudeck bitterly deplored this misuse of his technique.

Modern Versions of the Rausch

Shortly after the disappearance of the Rausch-Narkose in 1945 the concept of conscious analgesia was resurrected with the use of trichloroethylene and methoxyflurane in obstetrics and (less) minor surgery. Those agents were extensively used from 1950 through 1980, often with special inhalers; Tecota, Cyprane, Emotril, Minnit, etc. ...

Analgesia of Emergence

The analgesic stage during emergence from deep anesthesia has occasionally been used for surgery; J. Snow (1847-1848), Dastre's "anesthesie de retour", Kronacker's "koupierte Narkose" in 1905. The most recent and interesting example is J. F. Artusio's "ether analgesia" used for cardiac surgery (1955).[9] Analgesia of emergence of course lacks the advantages of safety and speed of analgesia of induction.

Conclusion

Although he was not the creator of the name or of the technique of the Rausch-Narkose, P. Sudeck extensively pioneered and promoted the technique. One is thus justified to call him the "Father of the Rausch-Narkose" and Hamburg its cradle.

References:

[1] Sudeck P: Das Operieren im ersten Aetherrausch. Dtsch Med Wschr 1901; 27: 102-103

[2] Kulenkampff D: Über die Verwendung des Stadium analgeticum der Aethylchloridnarkose. Beitr Klin Chir 1911; 73: 384-419

[3] Hirsch M: Der Aetherrausch. F. Deuticke, Leipzig & Wien, 1907

[4] Kafer H: Feldchirurgie. Steinkopff, Dresden, 1944: 170-171

[5] Dietze GM: Über Inhalationsanalgesie. Inaug. Dissert. B. Georgi, Leipzig 1905

[6] Brunn V M: Die Allgemeinnarkose. Enke, Stuttgart, p. 1913: 271-290

[7] Packard JH: Verbal communication on the subject of ether. Am J Med Sci 1966; NS 51: 154-156

[8] Killian H: Narkose zu operativen Zwecken. Springer, Berlin 1934; p. 154-155

[9] Artusio JF: Ether analgesia during major surgery. JAMA 1955; 57: 33-36

The Historical Development of Anaesthesia during the Times of the Austro-Hungarian Monarchy until the Decade after the First World War

H. Eiblmayr, Department of Anaestesia and Intensive Care, Landesfrauenklinik oÖ, Linz, Austria

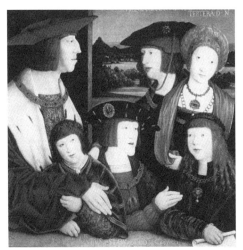

Fig. 1 Kaiser Maximilian, his wife Maria von Burgund; son Philip, grandchildren Ferdinand, Karl; Ludwig of Hungary, son of King Wladislaw of Bohemia and Hungery. (Brigitte Hamman: "Die Habsburger" - ein biographisches Lexikon. Verlag Ueberreutter 1988, p 384)

The history of the time I would like to relate to you spans four centuries. The Austro-Hungarian Monarchy developed the idea of arranged marriages to expand the empire. Following the death of his son Philip in 1506 Kaiser Maximilian I arranged partners for his three grandchildren to expand the political influence of the "Haus Habsburg" in Europe.

The first picture shows Kaiser Maximilian (Fig.1), his son Philip and daughter Margarete and the three grandchildren Ferdinand, Karl and Maria. Maria married Ludwig, the son of Wladislaw, King of Bohemia and Hungary in Vienna; Ferdinand married his beloved "Jagellonic princess" Anna, a daughter of King Wladislav in 1521 in Linz. Five years later, when King Ludwig died at the battle of Mohacs/Hungary, this couple had to take the vindication for the widened empire as Monarchs.

When Karl retired as the Roman-German Kaiser in 1556, the Roman-German Curia elected his brother Ferdinand was his successor in 1558.

At the beginning of the 18th century, the time when Kaiser Karl VI - the father of Kaiserin Maria Theresia - the power of the Austro-Hungarian Monarchy reached its climax; the motto "bella gerant alii, tu felix Austria nube" was weakened by wars all over Europe. The extraordinary fresh attempt to unite Europe failed on account of developing nationalism, racism and unsolved social problems. The two world wars ended the Austro-Hungarian Monarchy and dictatory politics.

Let us try to follow the tracks of anaesthesia in Austria and its development from the Middle Ages to the visions of a new age! Natural science was influenced by the dictatorship of Scholasticism in Europe for approximately two hundred years; the traditional alleviation of pain by drugs - handed down by cultures around the Mediterranean - was not accepted by the Roman Catholic Church, who considered the suffering of Jesus Christ to have been ideal.

In the 16th century Humanism influenced science and arts more and more; the philosophy of nature and human being created a new

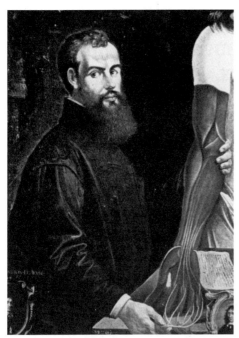

Fig. 2 Portrait of Andreas Vesal, performed by Poncet after a portrait in "Fabrica", (17th century). (Delmas André: Geschichte der Anatomie in "Sternstunden der Anatomie", Verlag Andreas & Andreas, Wien 1984, p 27)

view of life. At this time Paracelsus and Andreas Vesalius were outstanding people in science within the Habsburg Territories; their novelty in medicine was protected by authorities in politics and they used their medical knowledge as a defense against Catholic Inquisition. Vesal (Fig. 2) - an anatomist and the residing physician to Kaiser Karl V. intubated a dog by tracheostomy to observe lung function.

Paracelsus (Fig.3a,3b), famous for his knowledge in alchemy and holistic medicine, used sulphuric ether named "sweet Vitriol" in the therapeutic management of epilepsy and for painful surgery. Nevertheless he was familiar with drugs like Papaver somniferum, hyoscyamus, conium maculatum and mandrake - in the shape of a hypnotic sponge to be applied into the nose, a hypnotic drink or an alcoholic solution of drugs; there was no way, that the effect to be foreseen, it varied from hardly any reaction to life-threatening consequences. Born in Eisenach, Switzerland in 1493, he came to Villach (Austria) as a child with his father Wilhelm Bombast von Hohenheim; his father worked as a physician, the son began his education and initial studies in medicine and alchemy there. It seems that he was a scholar in Bologna and Vienna and completed his medical diploma in Ferrara - noteably twenty years before (1501) Kopernikus studied medicine at this university, which was one of the most famous ones at that time. In times of profitable wars Switzerland, tried to obtain imperial influence in Europe but denied Warfare after the composition with France at Marignano in 1515.

Paracelsus travelled all over Europe as a surgeon in the service of various military commanders; he returned to Villach after a great deal of scientific writings (in ordinary German instead of high styled Latin) and a troublesome time as a professor in Basel.

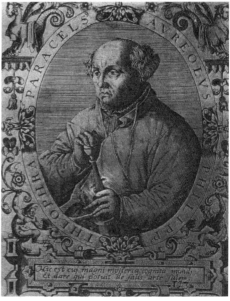

Fig. 3a Portrait of "Aureolus Philippus Theophrastus Paracelsus"

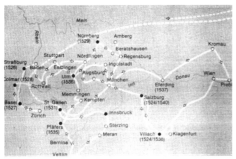

Fig. 3 Paracelsus's travels through Europe
(Strebel J., Vol. I St. Gallen 1944, p 284-302)

Theophrastus Bombastus von Hohenheim - known as "Paracelsus" - died in Salzburg and was buried at St. Sebastian in September 1541. His attempt to propagate the entirely of holistic medicine was overcome at this time by the new philosophy of a real and commensurable world without mysticism which was founded by Descartes.

At the beginning of the last century when "war cry" around the "Haus Habsburg" paused for a while, natural and technical science which had begun to alter the world in the 18th century, sent out a spark to medicine in Austria; the "Second Medical School of Vienna" related to natural science instead of natural philosophy and to scholarly mediation in German language at patients bedside instead of the usual teaching "ex cathedra" in Latin.

The History of Anaesthesia, eds. R. S. Atkinson & T. B. Boulton

Dates on which various European cities were attributed earliest known anaesthesias

1846	Dumfries, Scotland	19 December	William Scott (1820-87)
	London, England	19 December	Francis Boott (1792-1863)—J. Robinson (1813-1861)
	London, England	21 December	Robert Liston (1794-1847)
	Paris, France	22 December	A. J. Jobert de Lamballe (1799-1867)
1847	Bern, Switzerland	23 January	Hermann A. Demme (1802-67)
	Erlangen, Germany	24 January	J. F. Heyfelder (1798-1869)
●	Vienna, Austria	25 January	F. Schuh (1805-65)
	Munich, Germany	25 January	F. Chr. v. Rothmund (1801-1891)
	Riga, Latvia	c. 25 January	B.F. Baerens (?)
●	Timișoara, Austria	5 February	Musil & Siesa (?)
	Prague, Czechoslovakia	6 February	Joseph Halla (1814-87)
	Berlin, Germany	6 February	H. W. Berend (1807-73)
	Stockholm, Sweden	c. 6 February	E. G. Palmgren (1910-55)
●	Krakow, Austria	6 February	L. Bierkowski (1801-1860)
	Moscow, Russia	7 February	Fedor Inozemcev (1802-1860)
	Gothenburg, Sweden	11 February	C. Dickson (1814-1902)
	St Petersburg (Leningrad), Russia	14 February	Nikolaj I. Pirogoff (1810-81)
	Madrid, Spain	14 February	Diego de Argumosa y Obregón (1792-1865)
	Warsaw, Russia	15 February	L. Koehler (1799-1871)
	Copenhagen, Denmark	20 February	Søren Eskildsen Larsen (1802-90)
●	Ljubljana, Austria	24 February	L. Nathan (?)
	Christiania (Oslo), Norway	4 March	Christen Heiberg (1799-1872)
	The Hague, The Netherlands	5 March	A. T. C. Schoevers (?)
	Helsingfors (Helsinki), Finland	8 March	L. H. Törnroth (1796-1864)
●	Zadar, Austria	13 March	I. Bettini (?)
	Lisbon, Portugal	12 April	Gomes B. A. (?)

Countries following the name of a city denote political dependence in 1847.

Fig. 4 Dates on which various European cities were attributed earliest known anaesthesia.
(The History of Anaesthesia. RS Atkinson & Boulton TB(ed), Alden Press Oxford 1987, p 84)

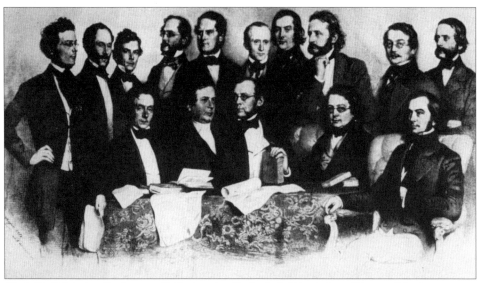

Fig.5 Medizinisches Professoren-Collegium der Hochschule Wien (after a lithograph by August Prinzhofer 1853). Please note the surgeon Franz Schuh who is the first in the line sitting from left (Lesky E: Meilensteine der Wiener Medizin Wilhelm Maudrich 1981, p 94)

In 1872 medical education developed finally into an "academic" - the surgical profession, protected by law after 6 years education with a barber surgeon and one year travelling throughout Europe to visit other barber surgeries, finally disappeared from the "royal trade regulations". I think it is of interest, that army doctors received a complete medical education as physicians and surgeons at the military hospital "Josephinum" in Vienna since the year 1785. At the middle of the 19th century the heroic and painful times in surgery came to an end; Anaesthesia, antisepsis and asepsis formed the base for modern surgery. Until that time mortality associated with surgery was - statistically verified - more than 90 %. Today the 16th of October 1846 is celebrated as "Ether Day", the birth of modern Anaesthesia. William T. G. Morton demonstrated at the Boston Massachusets General Hospital ether anaesthesia for the painless ligation of a large vascular malformation in the neck performed by Prof. Dr. John Collins Warren. The successful message on this event, announced by Prof. Dr. Henry Jacob Bigelow in the "Boston Medical and Surgical Journal" spread all over to Europe ....

Six weeks later the London medical paper "The Lancet" published this good news, political papers in European capitals followed soon after. 24 years earlier Henry Hill Hickman had brought his experiments with nitrous oxide and sulphuric ether to the attention of his medical colleagues at the "Royal Society" in London and the "Académie Francaise" in Paris; his progress against pain was brusquely refused as immoral as pain was seen as "God`s will".

Nitrous oxide and sulphuric ether were used for popular festivities, spectacles and among students.

European cities to which the earliest known anaesthesias were attributed. (Fig. 4)

The tabluation on this slide demonstrates, how swiftly the new method of "Etherization" spread across Europe. As "History of

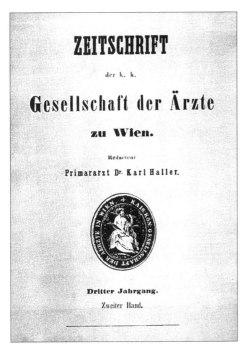

Fig. 6 Cover page of the journal in which Franz Schuh reported his expiriences with ether anaesthesia

Anaesthesia" does not exist in Austria, I tried to follow the alleged places of note in the Austro-Hungarian Monarchy. The empire comprised 17 Crown Lands in 1847. There were 9 faculties of medicine in the 14 universities and another 5 "Lycees" (specialised medical high schools) which provided medical education. Seventy years later we find 11 faculties of medicine in 12 Crown Lands. Ether anaesthesias was not applied in University hospitals only but also in high school nursing houses and small hospitals.

The University of Vienna was founded in 1365; the "New University" was the greatest in the Danube-Monarchy in the middle of the 19th century. Sixteen university professors, 12 "academic" university lecturers and 14 assistants were employed as doctors and teachers.

A pioneer in anaesthesia Prof. Franz Schuh (Fig.5) belonged to the innovating team of the "IInd Medical School of Vienna". He was born in 1804 in Scheibbs, lower Austria. His father was "Turnergeselle" - that meant a sacristan and musician for sacred music. Franz Schuh attended grammar school at the monasteries of Admont, Seitenstetten and Kremsmünster where he could finance his education and board by being a choir boy. He studied medicine in Vienna and obtained a scholarship for two years in 1831 at the "Institute of Surgery at Vienna General Hospital", which was founded in 1807. He became Chief Surgeon at this hospital in 1837 and was awarded University lecture professor in 1841; he presided a Clinic for surgery at the university, but remained primary surgeon of the G. H. and lived in the hospital because of this reason. He died in 1865 - probably due to a septic infection, as he neglected antisepsis as he was convinced of "miasma", a hostile air current which ensued wound infection. He had no confidence in disinfection with chlorinated water, which had been carried out by Prof. Semmelweis in Obstetrics since the fourties. In January 1847 Schuh published his conclusions on ether anaesthesia (Fig. 6) for 21 surgical procedures following animal trials. He used the tool constructed by Mr. Heller: an ox bladder (made of ox bowel) filled with ether, a mouth piece with a damper and a metal oral mask which fitted to the mouth tightly.

Even today this objective report can be considered fascinating as the stages of the development of anaesthesia are delineated! On the other hand he assumed, that ether could influence blood compounds and alter wound healing; he reported on the first death due to ether anaesthesia. Nonetheless the resection of a jawbone, which became necrotic after chewing on phosphorous matches, performed by the famous Prof. Wattmann under ether anaesthesia by Prof. Franz Schuh on the 29th of January 1847, was a big medical sensation worldwide!

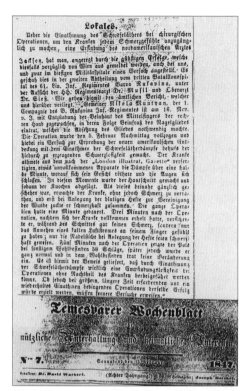

Fig. 7 Cover page of „Temesvarer Wochenblatt", in which a detailed report the successful use of ether for pain relief was published on February 13th, 1847

It is notable, that there are no known attempts of pain reduction in obstetrics in university hospitals - neither in Vienna nor in the medical "stronghold" Berlin; in smaller hospitals, for example "the Royal House for parturients" in Vienna it was usually carried out. Dr. Eduard Mikisch performed 7 gynaecological operations in 1847. The obstetricians there were aware of the tocolytic influence of the sulphuric ether. On the 1st of February 1847 one man had the opportunity to benefit from the new painless surgery for the amputation of his lower leg in the hospital for prisoners in Vienna; even the "District Hospital" in Wieden and the Children's Hospital at "Schottenfeld" (both in Vienna) applied ether anaesthesia for surgery early in this year. Besides surgery, ether was used in dentistry, in the therapy of epilepsy, as an enema in cases of kidney, biliary or gut colic as a result of lead poisoning and as inhalation therapy in cases of pulmonary disease.

Only in ophthalmology ether could not be instituted as it caused irritation of the conjunctiva.

Prague - the most famous and venerable university in Europe, dated back to the year 1348 and owned only one medical faculty in 1847. By 1917, there were two medical faculties at three universities.

Prague was regarded as "the Mecca" in medicine! In February 1847 eighty foreign guests went there to observe major diagnostic and surgical procedures under ether anaesthesia. Friar Coelestin Opitz demonstrated analgesia administered to patients of Franz Hofmeister, chief surgeon of a hospitaller cloister. Opitz is regarded as the patron of "experimental pathologists" in Czechia, as he performed many experiments on animals

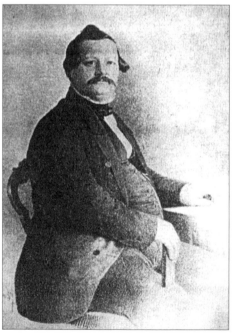

Fig. 8 Anton Hinterthür (1815-1860), the first "anaesthetist" in Graz

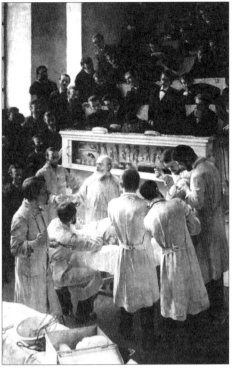

Fig. 9 Anton von Eiselsberg, Theodor Billroth`s "anaesthetist"; painting by A. F. Seligmann (standing upright in the first row) 1890. (Lesky E : Meilensteine der Wiener Medizin. Wilhelm Maudrich 1981, p 104)

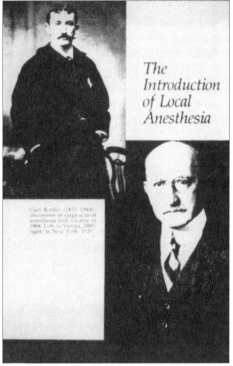

Fig. 10 Carl Koller (1857-1944) - discoverer of local anesthesia with cocaine in 1884. (Wood-Library-Museum of Anesthesiology 1984)

(rabbits and dogs) and healthy human volunteers using ether. Prof. Franz Pitha, head of the Surgical Clinic of the University in the 1840's, introduced ether anaesthesia there; Joseph Halla, director of the outpatients department and noted medical historian must be mentioned as a pioneer in diagnostic medicine using ether anaesthesia.

Temesvar did not have a university at that time.

But the "Temesvarer Wochenblatt" (Fig.7) (entertainment and information on about local events) dated Saturday, 13th February 1847 describes in detail, that the soldier Nicola Muntyan came to the military hospital for the amputation of a gangrenous middle finger of his right hand on the 5th of February 1847. He stated not to have felt any pain during the intervention, only noticing the feeling of a cold current of air on his finger at the end of the procedure. The medical officer Dr. Matthias Musil provided anaesthesia by "etherisation". Krakow - the "Jagellonia University", one of the first schools of that type in central and northern Europe, founded in 1364, based its teaching on medical and legal sciences from the first day of its existence.

Reviewing the History of Anaesthesia, edited in 1987 by Richard S. Atkinson and Thomas B. Bolton, (Royal Society of Medicine, London and Boston), we find a report on an operation of an inguinal hernia and abscess incision carried out by Prof. Ludwig Bierkowski in 1847 in Krakau, using ether anaesthesia. A colleague of his in Warsaw, Alexander Le Brun, applied chloroform for many surgical procedures; in 1858 some anaesthesia related deaths were recorded there.

In my search of the history of medicine I used the annual reports documented in the "KK Hof- und Staatshandbuch", including names and numbers of the teaching personal

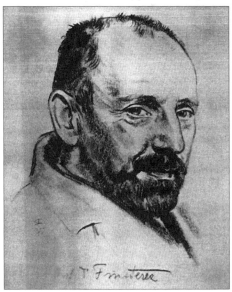

Fig. 11 Hans Finsterer (1877-1955) (Lesky Erna: Meilensteine der Wiener Medizin. Wilhelm Maudrich 1981, p 121)

attending the schools in the empire. Sometimes it is nevertheless difficult to follow the development as there were no issues between 1848 and 1854 - a period of revolution throughout Europe.

Leopold Nathan resided in Laibach as a honorary Doctor of surgery and teacher of obstetrics; he applied anaesthesia, but I was unable to find any more information on his work. Dr. Bettini seems to have practised as a doctor in Zara (Zadar), but I could find neither his name nor any other remarks in the previously mentioned KK annual reports. Within the Crown Lands there were two more notable Universities in 1847, namely Graz and Innsbruck. The University of Graz was founded in 1585; in 1847 it had seven professors and three to five assistant lecturers. At the General Hospital at Paulus Tower the royal and honorable Prof. Johan Nepomuk Kömm - chief surgeon and teacher of obstetrics was also able to attend patients from the neighbouring duchy Krain too, as he was familiar with the "Windisch" language. He and Anton Hinterthür (Fig. 8), who obtained his medical education at the famous Surgeon's High School in Vienna, were both named as protagonists in painless surgical medicine. The University of Innsbruck was built in 1677; there existed a minor medical faculty with four professors and three assistant lecturers in 1847. I do not known any information about the first experiments with ether anaesthesia there.

Dated the 10th of October 1847 the Royal Court Chancellary declared that ether should only be used by physicians, who had been educated in anaesthesiology to avoid misuse by laymen or insufficiently qualified medical staff. At the end of 1847 chloroform anaesthesia was introduced in the clinic of Prof. Schuh and was appreciated for its rapid onset without troublesome induction. The next supporter of anaesthesia was Prof. Theodor Billroth (Fig.9) who is said to be the Austrian revenge for the lost battle at Königgrätz, as he was born the son of a Prussian protestant pastor on the Rügen peninsula in 1829. After his surgical studies with Prof. Langenbeck in Berlin, he went to Zürich in 1860, seven years later he came to the University of Vienna. By the time of his death, at the age of 65 he had earned honors not only in paving the way for gastric surgery, he was also engaged in social politics and cultural life and was a famous teacher and scientist in surgery. At his clinic phenol was introduced in wound disinfection on the advice of Sir Joseph Lister. At that time the so called "ACE - mixture", an alcoholic solution of ether and chloroform was introduced to anaesthesiology; in the Austro-Hungarian Crown Lands it was known as the "Billroth-mixture" and was used until the end of the first decade of the new century.

To escape from the feared "surgical shock" at the beginning of surgical intervention, Morphine was injected pre-operatively; Friedrich Wilhelm Sertürner, a pharmacist in Paderborn- Germany - had already crystallized the pure drug from Opium in 1806! Alkaloid chemistry, invented in Germany, developed as a new revolution in anaesthesiology. Albert Niemann extracted pure Cocaine out of various coca plants and published his scientific findings in his dissertation in Göttingen in 1860. In Vienna Sigmund Freud wanted to help morphine addicts and tried the new drug, which failed as it led to cocainism instead of morphinism.

Influenced by the findings of his friend, Carl Koller (Fig.10) experimented with cocaine in ophthalmology; his successful results were presented at the Congress in Ophthalmology on September 15th,1884 in Heidelberg by Dr.Josef Brettauer, a colleague from Triest, who recognized the fundamental importance of this work. Carl Koller himself was too poor to attend the scientific meeting there. The scientific paper and the demonstration were enthusiastically acclaimed not only by participants at the congress but also at home in Vienna, when Koller was invited to the Medical Society of Vienna on the 17th of October 1884. In no time the news spread over the "Old" and the "New World". Koller incited his friend Jelinek, employed at the laryngological clinic, led by Prof. von Schrötter, to attempt cocainisation of the mucous membrane of the larynx; the next step to spread local anaesthesia had been taken.

William Halsted, Paul Reclus, Carl Ludwig Schleich, Maximilian Oberst, Heinrich Braun and August Bier are all subsequent well-known protagonists for local anaesthesia in other countries; Austrian medicine was

Beiheft zur „Medizinischen Klinik". 1908. Heft 11.
Redigiert von Professor Dr. E. Abderhalden, Berlin.

Die Lokalanaesthesie
in der Hand des praktischen Arztes.

Von

Dr. Most,
Dirig. Arzte der chirurgischen Abt. des St. Georg-Krankenhauses in Breslau.

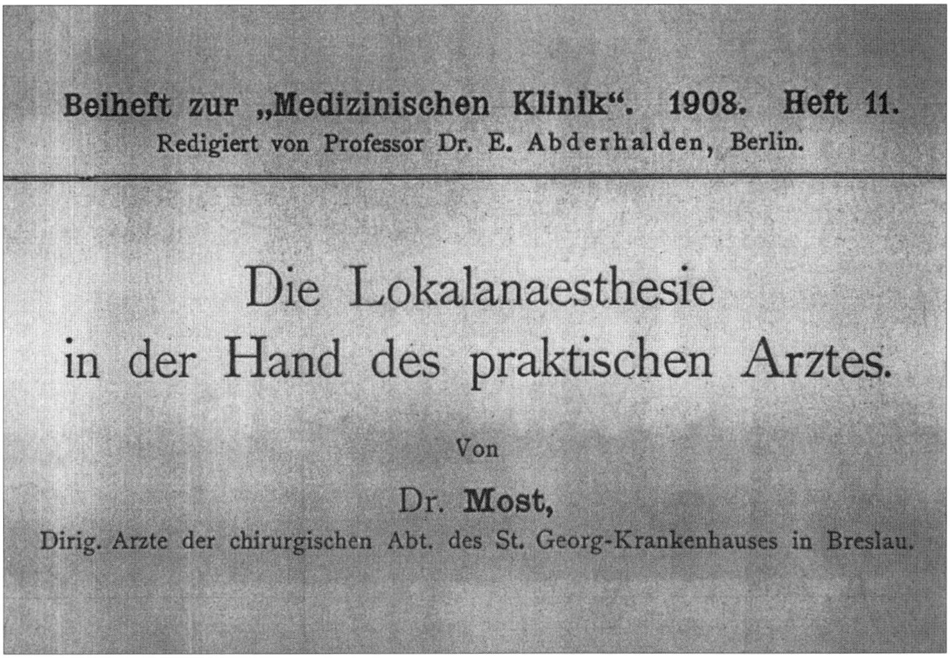

Fig. 12 Cover page of a publication of Most : "Local anaesthesia in the hand of the practitioner"

influenced by them. Carl Koller was exiled from Vienna and eventually Europe in 1886, as antisemitic propagation gradually spread over Europe by the end of the 19th century. Many famous scientists, musicians and authors who had been educated in Austrian schools and whose families had lived in the Austro-Hungarian Monarchy for many generations followed him.

Let us think about another remarkable man in anaesthesiology, whose proven methods in surgery and local anaesthesia influenced many generations of physicians in many parts of the world until the middle of this century; his name is Prof. Hans Finsterer (Fig. 11). Born in 1877 the son of a cottager in Weng, a small village in Upper Austria, he had undergone education at school and studies in medicine by strenuous efforts! As a surgeon he became a scholar at Julius von Hochenegg. A few years later he was chosen primary surgeon in the GH Vienna - being the last one to reside there, as this hospital developed exclusively as a University Hospital in 1951. Finsterer developed mesenteric, splanchnic, paravertebral and parasacral anaesthesia. His colleague Carl Landsteiner demonstrated the new method of major gastrointestinal interventions under regional anaesthesia in New York, Chicago and San Francisco in 1923. On top of that Carl Landsteiner began his well known research on ABO incompatibility in Vienna in 1901.

It was very informative for me how the knowledge about local anaesthesia spread abroad to physicians, who normally performed operations at the patient`s home or in the their own house, which was much quite usual as compared sending the patient to the hospital. Dr. Most, leading surgeon at the St. Georg Hospital in Breslau, published his empiric knowledge in a Supplement to Medical Clinics in 1908 (Fig. 12). Besides the well-known application of cocaine he was familiar with the use of Novocain®, manufactured by the German chemists Alfred Einhorn and Uhlefelder at the Merck laboratories in 1906; it was the first sterilizable local anaesthetic. He combined it with Suprarenin, whose property as a vaso-constrictor he used to extend the duration of anaesthesia and in order to avoid the toxic effect of the drug. In his paper one can find, that the color manufacturer "Hoechst" brought into commerce Novocain-Suprarenin tablets in tubes; they consistend of 125 mg Novocaine und 160 µg Suprarenin and had to be dissolved in physiologic saline. In addition one could use non-sterilizable cocaine-powder, which was mixed with water as a 1 - 10 % solution. One of the instructions ran thus: "Pravaz-syringes , which are cleaned in a cooked soda solution must be rinsed with sterile water prior to use, to prevent skin necrosis following infiltration" ....

The turn of the century was clouded in many ways: exuberant nationalism and growing racism besides many unsolved social problems in the numb politics of the monarchy led to the emigration of many gifted men and women, prior to World War I. Among them were the Foregger brothers from Tyrol, who joined a medical instruments company in the America. Richard von Foregger is renowned as one of the pioneers in the construction of anaesthetic systems. Due to the economic crisis in the shrunken empire after the lost war no further innovations in anaesthesia were invented until the fifties, when specialisation in this field began. The "Austrian Association of Anaesthetists" was the first to be founded in Europe in 1952 after World War II; it was followed by Switzerland in 1953 and Germany in 1954. Very soon the three associations organized two annual meetings and constructed up the Central European Society for Anaesthesiology.

Coming to the end of my paper, I would like to present an impression on anaesthesia in the past, anaesthesia and intensive care in the present time and a vision of the future.

References:

Vacha B: Die Habsburger; Styria 1993

Hamann B: Die Habsburger - ein bibliographisches Lexikon 1988

Simany T: Er schuf das Reich - Ferdinand von Habsburg; Amalthea 1987

Illustrierte Geschichte der Medizin, Wiener Verlag 1984

Braun L: Paracelsus, Alchimist - Chemiker, Erneuerer der Heilkunde; SV international-Schweizer Verlagshaus Zürich 1988

Meier P: Paracelsus - Arzt und Prophet; Amman Verlag 1993

Bigelow H J : Insensibility during Surgical Operations; The History of Anaesthesiology. Wood-Library-Museum of Anaesthesiology 1972

Guggenberger E: Der Zunftbrief der Bader und Wundärzte 1774; Oberösterreichische Ärztechronik 1962

Atkinson RS and Boulton Th B: The History of Anaesthesia 1989

Stiebitz R: Franz Schuh, ein Chirurg aus Niederösterreich; aus "Kunst des Heilens", Katalog zur Ausstellung in der Kartause Gaming NÖ 1991

Schuh F: Erfahrungen über die Wirkungen der eingeathmeten Schwefeläther-Dämpfe bei chirurgischen Operationen.

Mikschick Ed: Primararzt: Erfahrungen über die Wirkung der Äthereinathmungen bei chirurgischen Operationen

Haller K: Beitrag zur Würdigung der Äther-Einathmung während der Vornahme chirurgischer Operationen; nach Beobachtungen im k.k.n.ö. Provinzial-Strafhaus-Spital

Seifert, k. k.: Versuche über Äthereinathmungen an Thieren, mitgeteilt in der allgemeinen Versammlung am 17. Februar 1847

Zeitschrift der k. k. Gesellschaft der Ärzte zu Wien. Dritter Jahrgang, zweiter Band. Verlag Kaulfuss Witwe, Prandel & Comp. , Wien 1847, p 344 - 387

"Hof- und Staatshandbuch des österreichischen Kaiserthums": k. k. Hof- und Staats-Aerarial-Druckerey 1847, 1848, 1854-1918

Tochowicz L: Outline of the History of the Cracow School of Medicine 1364-1918; Reprinted from the Jubilee Edition of Medical academy in Cracow 1962

Karger-Decker B: Besiegter Schmerz - Geschichte der Narkose und der Lokalanästhesie; Koehler & Amelang; Leipzig 1984

Lesky E: Meilensteine der Wiener Medizin; Wilhelm Maudrich, Wien-München-Bern 1981

Bárány R und Kraft Fr: Die Symptomatologie der Billroth-Mischungsnarkose; Zeitschrift für Heilkunde Jahrgang 1905; Wilhelm Braumüller, k. und k. Hof- und Universitäts-Buchhändler, Wien und Leipzig 1905

Skopec M: Zur Entdeckung der Lokalanästhesie durch Carl Koller (1884) und ein kurzer Überblick über die moderne Anästhesiologie in Österreich; Institut für Geschichte der Medizin derUniversität Wien, 1987

Koller-Becker H: Carl Koller and Cocaine. The History of Anaesthesia - the Introduction of Local Anaesthesia; Wood Library-Museum of Anesthesiology 1984

Guggenberger Ed: Dr. Hans Finsterer; Oberösterreichische Ärztechronik 1962. Most Dr., dirig. Arzt der chirurgischen Abt. des St. Georg-Krankenhauses in Breslau: Die Lokalanaesthesie in der Hand des praktischen Arztes. Aus : Beihefte zur Medizinischen Klinik 1908; 11 :293-316

Intraoperative Anaesthesia and Analgesia in the Middle Ages and in Early Modern Times

Ch. Maier
Pain Clinic of the Department of Anaesthesiology and Surgical Intensive Care, Christian-Albrechts- Unversität Kiel, Germany

The commonly known date of birth of intraoperative anaesthesia is the 16th of October 1846, the day when Morton demonstrated the efficiency of ether narcosis in public for the first time. The American surgeon Bigelow had the idea of the following inscription on Morton's tombstone: "Before whom in all time surgery was agony". This sentence was true for the last 300 years before 1846, but for the times before I would like to put a question mark. As I will prove with the following, there have been means of intraoperative pain alleviation - some of which were obviously sufficient - even in mediaeval and early modern times. I would like to illustrate their effectiveness in the light of contemporary reports and portrayals in fine arts. In the end the question has to be discussed why this early knowledge had fallen into oblivion.

From the 16th to the early 19th century before 1846 we find plenty of evidence which vividly depicts the excruciating pain of patients during various operations. "Nothing was available to prevent their torment, nothing was effective to soothe them. They had to be operated fast, and the feature esteemed highest in a surgeon was his nimble work with the knife" the French surgeon Ollier wrote in his memories in 1893 (translated from[2]). There are many detailed illustrations, for example in the famous book from the German surgeon Frabricius von Hilden (1560-1634). Descriptions regarding bonding as the only means to immobilize the patient can be found in all modern-time surgical standard publications, like those by Garingeot from France or Lorenz Heister from Germany. Heister refers to at least one possible option of postoperative pain therapy by applying phytogenic opioids, for example an extract from the seeds of white poppy. But, as we know, there is no reference to intraoperative anaesthesia neither in his publications nor others like e.g. Fabricius von Hilden, Jacque Boulier or Ambroise Paré. The incapability to ease intraoperative pain adequately - which is admitted to by all authors - seems to justify the inscription on Morton's gravestone.

If we take a few steps back into the Middle Ages, we find pictures in the illustrations of different surgical, almost indifferently patients undergoing procedures like amputations and femoral herniotomies which is contradictory to statesments made above. One example is the wood-engraving of the book on von Gersstorf dated 1517[9]. It should be emphasized at this point that we are not dealing with sources written in Latin but with publications written by practising surgeons in their native, - at times - colloquial language. Partly, surgeons like Hans von Gerssdorf did not even hold the rank of a scholar. This seems to be important evidence of real medical day-to-day routine. Why should a non-scholar, who is not committed to scholastic tradition give a concrete description if he did not have any experience with it himself: Hans von Gersstorf, a so-called „war surgeon", is known to have gained extensive experience with amputations in patients with St. Antonius fever, induced by ergotamin intoxikation. He is often cited as an example of a mediaeval physician who knew about the possibilities of intraoperative analgesia by tradition, without applying this ancient knowledge himself[4,17]. In his book "The Miracle Doctor"[9] relating to the above cited illustration he states :

"A lot is said and wisdom is collected as to how draughts which make (you) sleep should be administered ...I let it be. I have never applied it or seen it being administered...I have never used it, because I know great harm can come from it. I am going to write about something which is a little better than a draught administered to the body then."

Obviously, he is suggesting inhalational instead of oral application by a piece of cloth, soaked with a special liquid, to achieve analgesia and then describes the formula of a so-called sleeping sponge in detail. His description of the contents of this sleeping sponge is based primarily on a recipe of his important idol, the French surgeon Guy de Chaliac (1300-1368 approximately). Guy de Chaliac himself, was not able to refer to own experience, but had taken over his recipe from one of his predecessors Arnoldus von Villanova. In his „Parables of Medical Art", he wrote :

"To put a patient to sleep which is deep enough that you can operate and he is not aware of it, almost as if he was dead, you have to take opium, mandrake root and hendane in equal shares and blend everything with water. If a patient requires amputation you have to soak a piece of cloth with this liquid, apply it to forehead and nose of the patient. To wake him up again, you soak the cloth with very strong vinegar." (cited from[16])

He described the technique for general anaesthesia and also how to reverse the effects of the analgetic drugs. In mediaeval times, i.e. 6th to 15th century), a large number of prescriptions existed referring the same combinations of substances[7,8,10,11,16]. The following prescription from the Antidotarium Bamberg (cited from[11]) in the 9th century is well-known. It is the oldest one passed on to future generations in German-speaking countries describing a recipe for a "hypnoticon adiutorium, id est somificum conveniens his qui chirurgiam operantur aut sectiones ut dolore non sentiant soporati..". The same inscription could be found on the label of a sleeping sponge from the Codex Kopenhagen in the 11th century: "Ypnoticon, id est somificum conveniens his qui chirurgia curantur ut sectionem doloris soporati non sentiant". The drugs in both prescriptions are identical (Fig.1).

Both recipes refer to hypnotics explicitly, i.e achieve intraoperative analgesia, thus anaesthesia ('so that a patient who needs surgery can sleep and will not have to suffer from pain during his sleep'). All compositions have in common, that they recommend a combination of opiates with various solanaceae. Hence, we are not talking about narcotics, as we find them described by Paracelsus. He used only opioids without any psychotropic co-medication and used his forumala to induce sleep only in insomnia patients, not for surgery[12]. The

Fig. 1: **Mediaeval prescriptions** (Unc(us) is equal to 1/12 pound or 30,5 gram)

Antidotarium Bamberg (9th century)		Codex Kopenhagen (11th century)	
Recipit		Recipit	
opio tevaicu	unc. II	Opium thebaicum	unc. II
mandragoris sucus ex foliis	unc. VII	mandragore sucum ex folies expressum	unc. VII
cicute his viridis sucus		cicute herbe sucum viridis	
iusquami sucu	unc. III		

Fig. 2: Content of Paper somniferum (sleeping poppy)

Occurence:	wild: Cyprus, Greece, Asia; today everywhere	
Content of morphine:	poppy juice (lacrima papaveris)	9-15%
	poppy seed	0,003-0,006%
	poppy head (mellow)	less
	greed	0,3-0,04%
Other relevante components:	narcotine, codein, narceiine, papaverine and more than 18 other alkaloids	

combination of opiates and solanaceae in the Middle Ages is nothing new at all. It was already specified by Galen and Diuscorides[13]. The contribution during the Middle Ages is the development and modification of the sleeping sponge. One of the first known German recipes for a sleeping sponge for narcosis was composed by Heinrich von Pfolspeunt (1460). In his book "Buch der Bündt-Erznei" he wrote: "nim saffte vom swartzen mohen.. den findestu in der apoteken, den heys man opium, und den safft von pulsenßamen, und den safft von alrawen bletter... nim den safft von thalm krawth" (cited from[11]).

Which substances is it all about? First of all, it is opium extracted from the Sleeping poppy. Depending on whether we are dealing with the white or the black form, this poppy has a high concentration of morphine[3,5]. By means of specific extraction of substances obviously one was able to modify the depth of sleep and anaesthesia (Fig.2)

The second substance - which is referred to in the ancient prescriptions in particular - is the mandrake. This plant is not native in northern and western Europe. It belongs to the family of solanaceae. It is related to the belladonna or „deadly nightshade", to Hendane and thorn-apple. All of these plants contain hyoscamine, atropine and scopolamine as medically relevant alkaloids (Fig 3). These substances have a stimulating effect in lower dosages, however, in a higher dose they can give rise to hallucinations. With an increasing dose they induce sleep, but also epileptic seizures and eventually even fatal central respiratory depression[5,6,10,11,13,18].

Mandrake has been known for different effects since biblical times. It served as a narcotic drug, as an aphrodisiac, but also as a medical preparation. In the Middle Ages it was available in Europe from travelling merchants. According to police reports of those days, these preparations were often forgery[13]. These difficulties in logistics explain that one can find references to other solanaceae in Northern European prescriptions.

Examples of this are the recipes of the German surgeon Heinrich von Fulspoint dated 1460, and so called sleeping or "doll" draughts in other German references, i.e. Hieronymus von Brynschwieg. Also, as cited above, Heinrich von Fulspoint described the usefulness of the sleeping sponge and he replaced mandrake by native plants containing alkaloids, like other North and West European authors. In his opinion the main advantage of this sponge was, that it allowed to reactivate an already prepared plant extract immediately before an operation by plunging it into warm water (see below the same description in the novel of Bocchaccio). In a very detailed manner he depicts how to reverse narcosis by means of a cone made of

Fig. 3: Mandragora officinarum (mandrake)

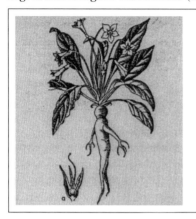

Family of Solanaceae (night dead shadows) related with
   Belladonna, henbane and thorn-apple

Occurence
   Italy, Greece and parts of Asia,
   but not in Western or Nothern Europe

medicaly important alkaloids
l-Hyoscyamin	0,3-0,4%
d/l-Hyoscyamin (atropine)	0,3%
l-Scopolamin	?%

cotton wool soaked in vinegar and fennel seeds which is then introduced into the nose. He emphasizes that the cone should not be too large, in order for the patient still being able to braethe through his nose.

There is also a Middle English prescription (about 1328 A.C.) for sleeping potions with a albel saying "For to make a drank that iz cald dwale to make a man sleepe while man brenne hym": " Tak III sponful of the galle of abarow swine..., III sponfull of hemlok jus,and III sponfull of the wylde neep, III sponful of lectuce, and III sponful of pope (poppy), and III sponful of hennebane... and medle al hem to geder ...and do ther of III sponful to apotel of good wine...and lete him, that schal be ycouren,... make him dryngke ther, of til he falle asleep, and thou moyst savely corye hym and when thon hast ydo thy cuyre and wolt awake him: take vinegar an salt and waschewel his temples...and he schal awake anon ryst"[8]. Again this author (probably his name was Eawardus) used plants, that were available in England, and we find the same combination of analgetic and psychotropic drugs, and also description of how to wake He patient up after the surgical treatment. Husemann proved 1900 the proof, that the English 'dwale drunk' was the same as the "doll drunk" of Hieronymos of Brunschwigk with one exception: the German preferred flavored aromatic admixtures, the English author the gall of a swine according old Latin recommendations by Galen.

A number of medical historians are convinced that these recipes are just copied from antique sources without authentic or own experience being included[14,17]. The abovementioned variations of their components, for example the substitution of plants available only in the Mediterranean by native solanaceae (e.g. thorn-apple) prove that intraoperative analgesia was actually induced with these substances[7,8,13]. When compared to ancient scripts, specific modifications required for their application as a sleeping sponge favour the idea that intraoperative analgesia was actually carried out in this manner. The sleeping sponge was an invention of the famous surgical school of Salerno , the oldest description was made about 1300[7]. It is very unlikely that non-scholars and physicians - like Hans von Gersdorf or Heinrich von Fulspoint - would have taken the trouble to find a recipe including detailed instructions for the induction of anaesthesia as well as a method for its reversal if it was not of any relevance to them.

Another hint pointing to experience with anaesthesia and analgesia in mediaeval times are detailed comments regarding possible complications as well as strategies to overcome these, Henri de Mondeville (ca. 1250-1320). He writes: ".. if you weake opium and mandrake.. by other agents and give those systemically, they will numb and make (the patient) unconsciousness, but if you give a great amount and without other agents, they will kill.. and relief pain, because the dead feel no pain... Beware of strong narcotics and give them only in small amount and only in danger of life"[11]

Those specific warnings seem to be based on personal experience. The authors noted the risks of different opium and solanaceae dosages down in detailed lists. Therefore, mediaeval physicians did not apply these drugs against general recommendations, Guy de Chauliac was aware of the rsiks, however because of a lack of personal experience, he was not able to suggest, how to overcome them. One hundred years before, his predecessor Henry de Mondeville, recommended the combination of two substances "in small amounts only, and in a weaker concentration". In this context he mentions a combination of hypnotics with other preparations that have an analeptic effect. The recommendation keep the dose of all drugs required for narcosis as low as possible with the help of suitable combinations, is still valid today. This is the basis of balanced anaesthesia. One analeptic substance recommended by mediaeval authors is - among others - camphor in its injectible form. This preparation was applied up to the 20th century.

Last not least, we find evidence for intraoperative anaesthesia and analgesia in the fine arts of the Middle Ages. A very famous example[11] is the grave of Henry II, which has been created by the well-known mediaeval woodcarver Tilman Riemenschneider. It depicts an episode of the year 1000 when the duke, physically weakened by a chronic cystic bladder stone and consecutive renal failure, arrived at the famous monastery Montecassino to undergo surgery. When he was informed that the corpse of St. Benedikt had already been transfered, he was disappointed and went to rest for the night. The legend says that he awoke without any symptoms the next morning, holding the bladder stone in his hand. There are two possible explanations: One was a miracle; the fact that the duke never had any children - a classical complication of lithotomies those days - does not favor this version. The monks at this monastery were famous for their art of handling sleeping sponges and potion. As we all know, solanaceae can induce amnesia. It is conceivable that, a morphine-scopolamine-narcosis had been administered and the patient was operated free of pain and without memory of the procedure. Obviously, Tilman Riemenschneider was aware of this second version, as the cup placed in the niche suggests. We find the same cup in a picture chronic of 1513: the painting illustrates a monk handing a draught to his fellow-brother before the wound stigmata of Christ are inflicted onto him[15].

There are also literary illustrations of intraoperative analgesia. One well-known example can be found in the tenth novella on the 4th day of Decamerone of Bocaccio telling the story of the love affair between a physician's wife and a young man. She was married to an excellent surgeon - probably Roger of Salerno - who neglected his young wife. The surgeon had treated a sick man who was probably suffering from a gangrene. Prior to that he had convinced himself that an operation (meaning an amputation) was not indicated as the patient would not be able to bare the pain. Therefore, in the morning he prepared a liquid containing special ingredients which would be able to "keep the suffering man sleeping as soon as he had drunk it, and for a period long enough for the surgeon to do the cutting". When this liquid was prepared the surgeon had to leave his home for an emergency case, with the potion still standing around. The surgeon's wife sent for her lover and asked him to wait in her bedroom. The young man became thirsty, drank the liquid, the woman found him sleeping deeply and panicked. You should read the book in order to find out how the stroy ends. In this context it is of significance that, Bocaccio knew details about medical procedures in those days.

But why did this knowledge vanish and lead to of medical helplessness was depicted in the beginning ? We find very early evidence that in mediaeval times the application of substances suitable for anaesthesia - particularly alkaloids and solanaceae - was punished by government and clerical institutions. In the constitution of Melphi from 1231 the following reference is given: "anyone administering evil and harmful substances which confuse your senses or poisons shall be sentenced to death"[11]. The disappearance of knowledge about intraoperative analgesia coincides with the birth of inquisition and, witch hunt. Witchcraft was proved by confessions obtained through torture, the victims experiencing hallucinations induced by high-dosed solanaceae ointments. Unprejudiced scientists and physicians mention explicitly that the witch ointments contained the following substances (according to the report of Andreas de Laguna (1499-1560, Physicain of Karl Vth and of the Popes Paul III and Julius III: Solanum (Belladonna), Cicuta (Hemlock), Hyoscyamus (Henbane), Mandragora (Mandrake), that were well-known for their narcotic effect in medical practise[4,7,8,11]. Despite of objections most physicians became entangled in this scenery and atmosphere of prosecution. Only a few - like the physician in ordinary to the Duke of Jülich, Johannes Wier, in the beginning of the 16th century - were willing to state in public that witches were sick people, victims of old age depression and melancholy whose alleged experience was based on imaginations clearly induced by ointments known and used medically as "sleep-making ointments" (cited from[11]).

Hence, it appears plausible that fear of denunciation by the inquisition and by witch hunters prevented physicians from administering such medications in patients. For whatever reasons, Ambros Paré knew about the application of narcotics only by hearsay and described them as the practise of former physicians, listing possible adverse effects of these medications in a far less differentiated manner than Henry de Mondeville in earlier times. Among the analgesics of early modern times - described, by Paracelsus and Thomas Sydenham - we only find flavoured opiates. These medications were not used for intraoperative analgesia, but as sleeping pills.

Another reason for analgesia vanishing is the decline of scientific surgery in Europe towards the end of the Middle Ages[14]. It all began with the resolution of the Fourth Lateran Council under Innozenz III in 1217, deciding that the Church shrinks back from blood, a consensus resulting in the prohibition of monks to cut and burn. This was a considerable setback for the development of surgery, because only monks were in possession of important scientific sources from ancient and mediaeval times. Influenced by scholasticism the Italian medical schools lost significance, later even the French schools were ruined.

For whatever reason we do not find traces of the knowledge regarding intraoperative pain alleviation. In summary, we can consider that 1846 to be the year of birth of modern anaesthesia. Before these days there was not only agony, but within a close compass and involving concrete risks there were measures available for intraoperative analgesia, based on the inhalational administration of opium and extracts from solanaceae. In fact, we should rather talk of rebirth rather instead of birth.

References:

[1] Baader G, Keil G: Einleitung. In: Baader G, Keil G (Eds.): Medizin im mittelalterlichen Abendland. Wissenschaftliche Buchgesellschaft, Darmstadt, 1982, p. 1-44

[2] Brandt L: Geschichte der Anaesthesie. Repetitorium Anaesthesiologicum. Mayrhofen 1995

[3] Darmstaedter E: Anfänge und Entwicklungslinien der modernen Schlafmittel. Schmerz, Narkose, Anästhesie 1934/35; 7: 101-111

[4] Darmstaedter E: Hexen, Hexenmedizin und Narkose. Med Welt 1930; 4: 1851-54.

[5] Dragendorf G: Die Heilpflanzen der verschiedenen Völker und Zeiten. Fritsch Verlag, München 1967

[6] Fuehner W: Solanazeen als Berauschungsmittel. Arch exp Pathol Pharmakol 1925; 111: 281-294

[7] Husemann T: Die Schlafschwämme und andere Methoden der allgemeinen und örtlichen Anaesthesie im Mittelalter. Ein Beitrag zur Geschichte der Chirurgie. Dtsch Zschr f Chir 1896; 42: 517-596

[8] Husemann T: Weitere Beiträge zur chirurgischen Anästhesie im Mittelalter. Dtsch Zschr f Chir 1900; 54: 503-550

[9] Gersdorf, H v: Feldbuch der Wundarznei. Reprint der Orginalausgabe Darmstadt 1967

[10] Klein G: Historisches zum Gebrauche des Bilsenkrautextraktes als Narkotikum. Muench Med Wschrift 1907; 54: 1088 ff.

[11] Kuhlen, F J: Zur Geschichte der Schmerz-, Schlaf- und Betäubungsmittel im Mittelalter und frueher Neuzeit. Deutscher Apotheker Verlag, Stuttgart 1983

[12] Paracelsus: Herausgegeben von K. Sudhoff. Bd. 14, S. 12 (1933)

[13] Randolph, C B: The mandrake of the ancients in folklore and medicine. Proceedings of the American Academy of Arts and Sciences 1904; 40: 487-537

[14] Rüster D: Alte Chirurgie. Legenden und Wirklichkeit. Verlag Gesundheit, Berlin 1991

[15] Schadewaldt H: Hellmut Weese-Gedächtnisvorlesung. Von Galens "Nárkosis" zur modernen "Balanced anesthesia". Anästh Intensivmed 1978; 27:589-601

[16] Schipperges H: Der Garten der Gesundheit. Medizin im Mittelalter. Dtv München 1990

[17] Steudel H: Vorwort zum Neudruck des Feldbuchs der Wundarznei des Hans von Gersdorf. Reprint der Orginalausgabe Darmstadt 1967, p. VI-VII

[18] Wenzel M: Ueber die chemische Bestandteile der Mangragorawurzel. Inauguraldissertation, Berlin 1900

I have to thank Mrs. Judith Schönhoff, M.A. (Institut for German Philology, Department of Mediaeval Literature, Westfälische Wilhems-Universität Münster, Germany) for her assistance, translating the mediaeval sources into German, and Mrs. Suliko Berndt MD (Department of Surgery, University of Lübeck, Germany) for translating this manuscript.

On the History of Resuscitation

P. Safar
From the Safar Center for Resuscitation Research, Department of Anesthesiology and Critical Care Medicine, University of Pittsburgh, USA

Abstract

The development of modern cardiopulmonary-cerebral resuscitation (CPCR), consisting of 3 steps each for basic, advanced, and prolonged life support, began in the 1950s. Modern CPR has given every person the ability to challenge death anywhere. The majority of nine steps of CPCR and their assembly and implementation have been pioneered by anesthesiologists. Cerebral resuscitation *after* cardiac arrest, researched since around 1970, extended CPR to CPCR. Neither CPR nor CPCR was "discovered" by one person. Despite sparks of knowledge and occasional applications of possibly effective lifesaving efforts since antiquity, the possibility to reverse acute terminal states (such as asphyxiation or exsanguination) and clinical death (apnea and pulselessness) by modern, physiologically sound, and effective measures did not become possible until around 1900 inside hospitals, and around 1960 outside hospitals. Around 1900, the opportunity to assemble existing bits of knowledge into an effective resuscitation system existed, but was missed. This should be a warning for those who will lead CPCR into the 21st century. History has shown the need for continuing communication and collaboration among investigators of different countries, and between laboratory researchers, clinicians of various disciplines, and prehospital rescuers. Challenges for the near future include: research and development of "ultra-advanced life support" for external CPR-resistant cases, suitable for initiation outside the hospital; implementation of cerebral resuscitation to achieve complete recovery after 10 to 15 minutes of normothermic cardiac arrest without blood flow; and novel traumatologic resuscitation potentials.

Introduction

Modern anesthesia began during and after World War II, 100 years after the widely researched discovery of ether *analgesia* in the mid 19th century. Making people analgesic was easy and safe, but providing full unconsciousness and immobilization with deep general *anesthesia* required physiologic life support which did not come about until anesthesiologists became reanimatologists and intensivists, skilled in emergency resuscitation and long-term life support.

This paper based on previous publications[134, 135] summarizes some important points in the history of *modern* resuscitation and life support. I apologize for focusing on vignettes from my and my associates' experiences.

For millennia, death was accepted as an act of God. Since the enlightenment, some people were *willing* to challenge death[134, 135]. They tried to turn around dying processes, with few successes. Since around 1900, the knowledge existed to reverse airway obstruction, apnea and pulselessness, at first only inside surgical operating rooms. Only since the 1950s have physicians and non-physicians been able to reverse clinical death inside and outside the hospital in a systematic manner[3, 159].

Every innovator stands on the shoulders of predecessors. History of the same event, written by different observers or participants, will differ in details, priorities, and credits given. Relying merely on historic literature misses unpublished "firsts." Such first, seemingly novel ideas on lifesaving, with or without experimental or clinical trials, have been many in the past. Most were not pursued. Therefore, credit should be given to those who not only expressed novel ideas, but who also recognized their scientific or clinical importance, documented them, and convinced the world. We should seek out lessons from history. Those who cannot remember the past are condemned to repeat it *(Santayana).*

More detailed histories of emergency resuscitation since antiquity have been published [134, 185]. I apologize for not recognizing in this summarizing talk many important contributors to the history of CPCR, because of space constraints or lack of knowledge about their contributions. Input on this subject from readers of this paper is hereby invited. Resuscitation from cerebral ischemia, trauma or hemorrhagic shock, emergency medical services, and intensive care medicine, each has its own history, merely mentioned here.

Some Definitions. "Resuscitare" means restoring life. "Reanimatology," a term introduced by Negovsky of Moscow[108, 109, 110], focuses on "anima," the mind or spirit, which is located in the brain, the target organ of resuscitation. Reanimatology is the study of the pathophysiology and reversibility of acute terminal states (such as asphyxia or shock) and clinical death (i.e., potentially reversible cardiac arrest). This talk will focus on the history of emergency resuscitation methods outside the hospital – from basic life support (BLS) consisting of airway control (step A), breathing control (step B), and circulation support (step C); via advanced life support (ALS) consisting of steps D, E and F (drugs, electrocardiography, fibrillation treatment [defibrillation]) for rapid restoration of spontaneous circulation (ROSC); to prolonged life support (PLS), i.e., intensive care. That we have labelled G (gauged), H (humanized, i.e., brain-oriented, e.g., by hypothermia), and I (intensive care)[147]. [Fig. 1]

Standard external CPR was initiated around 1960 in Baltimore. In 1961, in Pittsburgh, we extended CPR to cardiopulmonary-*cerebral*-resuscitation (CPCR)[159] to make long-term survival with human mentation the goal. Cerebral resuscitation after cardiac arrest has been researched since around 1970[162].

We must differentiate between *protection,* which is treatment initiated before the insult (which continues into *preservation* during the insult), and *resuscitation,* which is to reverse the insult and support recovery.

Early Respiratory Resuscitation

The biblical story about *Elisha* having put his mouth on the mouth of a suddenly dead child is frequently quoted as the first description of mouth-to-mouth ventilation. There was no mention of blowing. However, the Hebrew midwife Puah, was reported to have "breathed into the baby's mouth to cause the baby to cry" (Exodus 1:15-17). *Egyptians* were preoccupied with life *after* death. Did they try to reverse dying? Ancient Chinese physicians felt the pulse, cauterized wounds, and used herbal drugs. *American Indians'* medicine seemed dominated by religion and use of plants; in spite of human sacrifice, they seemed to lack knowledge of anatomy.

Hippocrates, about 400 BC, published a book in Alexandria which includes suggestions of titrated care in contrast to speculation. At about the same time *Aesculapius* became the god of healing. *Galen,* the Greek physician in Rome around 200 A.D., dominated medical rituals. He did, however, observe the importance of the medulla for breathing and that arteries contained blood rather than air. Europeans established Christian hospitals for nursing care of those wounded in the crusades. The Arabs ligated bleeding vessels. *Leonard da Vinci* brought enlightenment through knowledge of anatomy.

The first known breakthrough about effective respiratory resuscitation came from *Andreas Vesalius*[190]. In the mid-1500s he wrote "...that life may be restored to the animal, an opening must be attempted in the trachea, into which a tube of reed or cane should be put. You will then blow into this, so that the lungs may rise again and the animal can take in air. The lungs will swell ... the heart becomes strong ... When the lung has collapsed, the beat of the heart and arteries appears wavy. But when the lung is inflated, the heart becomes strong ... When the lung is inflated at intervals, the motion of the heart and arteries does not stop... I have seen none in all of anatomy that has afforded me greater joy"[190]. He obviously appreciated the importance of his discovery. Conservative colleagues declared him mad. He did an autopsy on a Spanish nobleman and found his heart still beating, or made it beat by his ventilation efforts. To avoid execution by the Inquisition, he made a pilgrimage and died in a shipwreck. His discoveries did not catch on.

Despite the breakthrough discovery of the circulation by William *Harvey* of Britain, around 1600, physicians and the public seemed not to appreciate the dynamics of acute dying for another 200 years. Particularly, the rapidity with which non-viability occurred, and other important pathophysiologic facts, were not appreciated. This gap in knowledge continued in spite of the discovery of oxygen, and of auscultation and percussion. The Napoleonic wars stressed rapid amputation, but hypovolemic shock and airway control in coma apparently were not appreciated.

While airway control and circulation support were poorly understood and ignored, artificial breathing was actively pursued since the 1500s[190]. *Paracelsus,* a Swiss-Austrian alchemist, pharmacologist, and chemotherapist, was probably the first to write, in the mid 1500s, about the use of bellows for resuscitating people[159]. Intermittent positive pressure ventilation (IPPV), however, was forgotten until the 1700s, when the *Humane Societies* came close to implementing it. They prescribed resuscitation attempts, mostly for drowning victims, which seemed rational. These attempts ranged from mouth-to-mouth inflations in children and mouth-to-nasal tube inflations in adults, to the use of bellows – unfortunately without effective valving. These rational acts were often supplemented by irrational acts, such as smoke insufflation into the rectum, venous hemorrhage, warming, and various forms of external stimulation.

On the positive side, *Herhold* and *Rafn* in Copenhagen and *Kite* in England apparently insufflated through laryngeal cannulae; and *Hunter* and *Newby* instructed midwives in mouth-to-mouth ventilation[134]. *Tossach,* a British surgeon, having successfully resuscitated a coal miner with mouth-to-mouth breathing in 1732 seems to have given the first account of mouth-to-mouth ventilation on an adult[187]. In the mid-1800s, the French introduced airway control by tracheotomy for diphtheria-induced obstruction. Until the mid-1800s, there was no experimental documentation of the many different recommended and erratically practiced resuscitation methods. That might explain the coexistence of logical exhaled air ventilation with illogical rituals.

On the negative side, artificial ventilation experienced in the mid 19th century a setback for 100 years. The London physician *Hall,* who died in 1857, contributed to society as the founder of the journal *Lancet* and as an opponent to slavery. He erred, however, on artificial ventilation. Because of exaggerated reports about barotrauma to the lungs from positive pressure insufflation via mouth-to-mouth or bellows-to-trachea, he initiated a century of chest pressure enthusiasm. He and his followers also believed that the prone position relieves airway obstruction by vomitus. Some suspected obstruction by the tongue. *Howard's* chest pressure methods included a suggestion for a second operator to pull the tongue forward. *Silvester,* another physician of London, who immediately followed Hall, recommended chest-pressure arm-lift (supine)[177]. The Viennese physician Brosch[26,139] added elevation of the supine victim's shoulders during performance of chest-pressure arm-lift (supine), so that the head remains tilted backward. Around 1900, *Schafer* turned the patient prone again and only pushed on the chest, without arm-lift[170]. His method was taught by the American Red Cross from 1910 to 1952. Denmark's Colonel *Holger Nielsen* added arm-lift to Schafer's method, because in *conscious* spontaneously breath-holding humans that increased the tidal volume. *Holger Nielson's* back-pressure arm-lift (prone) method was taught by many Red Cross societies around the world in the 1950s, based on *Archer Gordon's* results with unconscious, relaxed, *intubated* humans[61]. *Holger Nielsen* died in 1955, two years before *Safar* documented the failure of these methods in *unconscious,* relaxed, *not* intubated humans[139].

Early Cardiopulmonary Resuscitation

After the discovery of *general analgesia* in the 1840s, there was little incentive at first to search for effective steps A, B, and C. In the 1860s, however, antisepsis followed by asepsis allowed intra-abdominal operations. This required deep *general anesthesia* with ether or chloroform, which provoked surgeons for the first time into searching for airway control, artificial respiration, and artificial circulation. Chloroform anesthesia-induced deaths were first reported by *Snow.* Empirical use of jaw thrust for airway control under general anesthesia was included in the surgical textbooks by *Esmarch* and *Heiberg* of the 1870s.

The late 1800s were full of contrasts. Positive examples include: Some prehospital care by ambulance personnel in Vienna under *Billroth* and *Mundy;* intensive nursing care by Florence *Nightingale;* and initiation of the specialties of pathology, medicine, surgery, and roentgenology. Negative examples include the practice to declare the patient dead when he or she became apneic or pulseless, even when it occurred in the operating room.

The first reports on successful *open-chest* CPR were: in animals with chloroform arrest in 1874, by *Schiff* of Switzerland[171]; and in surgical patients in 1901 by surgeon *Igelsrud* of Norway[134] and others[66]. In the 1950s, *Stephenson* of Missouri reported on remarkable intra-operating room successes with open-chest CPR during the first half of the 20th century[182].

The first reports on successful *closed-chest* CPR were: in cats with potassium arrest in 1874, by *Boehm* of Dorpat[20]. He aimed for artificial ventilation and happened to also produce artificial circulation. Credit for the first successful closed-chest cardiac massage plus artificial respiration attempt in humans goes to *Koenig* and his associate *Maass* of Goettingen[98]. In his historically important paper of 1892[98], *Maass* describes the case of a 9-year-old boy who, during an operation on the palate, developed cardiac arrest under chloroform. Maass pulled the tongue forward and applied chest compressions in the supine position. The pupils constricted and gasping returned. He continued this for 1 hour, until he felt a fluttering movement of the carotid and a return of the radial pulse. The boy slept until the next morning and recovered completely. This was a single episode, as nobody followed it up. Did Maass recognize the importance of this case? He later emigrated to America and died as a disappointed man. In 1997, *Goerig* (anesthesiologist in Hamburg) and *Safar* visited a great-grand uncle of *Maass* in Bremen, to learn more about him.

On sudden cardiac death, ventricular fibrillation (VF) was not understood. *Ludwig* and *Hoffa* described VF already around 1850, but there was no way to reverse it. *Kite* played with electric shock experiments, but the currents were too low to defibrillate[47, 58].

Much of the *knowledge* on which modern external CPR is based had been acquired already by *1900*[134]. Why did no-one put together then the experiences by *Vesalius*[190] and *Maass*[98]; by *Crile*[34] who was the first to use adrenaline[114] for "cardiac stimulation"; by *Einthoven* who invented the electrocardiogram (ECG)[45]; by *Kuhn* who introduced tracheal intubation[89]; and by *Prevost* and *Batelli*[125] of Geneva who observed in animals that electrically induced VF can be defibrillated with higher currents? By 1900, *Ringer, Starling,* and *Kuemmel* had initiated fluid resuscitation and Landsteiner of Vienna had discovered the blood groups. The latter should have led to blood banking and transfusions 50 years before it actually happened. Why did all this lay dormant for 50 years? I explain this hiatus by the lack of scientific proof; a lack of communication among laboratory researchers, clinicians, and prehospital rescuers; authoritative thought-control by conservative medical leaders; and the defeatist attitude of the public that nothing can be done when someone suddenly dies.

Guthrie, Professor of physiology and pharmacology at the University of Pittsburgh between the two world wars, did chest compressions for ventilation and circulation on laboratory animals that accidentally died during experiments[12, 183]. So did other physiologists. Guthrie recognized the importance of bringing the brain to recovery[72, 120]. He also co-initiated vessel anastomoses, transplanted organs, and transplanted even the head of one dog to another. For all this he should have shared the Nobel Prize with Carrel[183].

In 1937, *Negovsky* of Moscow started the world's first resuscitation research laboratory and animal models[109]. During the siege of Moscow by the German Army in winter 1941/42, Negovsky's team resuscitated some clinically dead exsanguinated soldiers by pumping oxygenated blood with epinephrine into their arteries. He considered the brain the target organ of resuscitation, introduced terms and concepts in reanimatology, and defined the postresuscitation disease[110]. This was later also called "secondary post-insult derangements"; and part of it "reoxygenation injury." In 1962, at the First European Congress of Anesthesiologists (in Vienna), under the aegis of *Mayrhofer,* (pioneer of Central European anesthesiology), Safar organized and chaired a panel on "controversial aspects of resuscitation"[146]. This became the first penetration of the iron curtain by reanimatologists, because of the participation of Negovsky and of *Keszler* and *Pokorny* from Czechoslovakia. Lifelong friendships between Safar and these colleagues from Eastern Europe and their associates developed. They practiced glasnost throughout the cold war.

In the 1940s, *Beck* of Cleveland, a thoracic surgeon, was the first to point out that sudden cardiac death is usually the result of VF in "hearts too good to die"[8, 9]. In 1947, based on animal studies by *Wiggers*[198], Beck performed the first successful electric defibrillation of a human heart, via thoracotomy, in the operating room[7]. He also successfully used open chest CPR to resuscitate a colleague who collapsed at the hospital entrance.

Why did it take until the 1940s to defibrillate a human heart? *Pechlin* had observed VF in a man dying with an open-chest wound 200 years earlier, the German physiologists *Hoffa* and *Ludwig* and Britain's *MacWilliam* and *Hoffmann* observed VF, and *Hooker* and *Kouwenhoven* studied in animals electrically induced VF and immediate countershock since the 1920s[47, 58, 134]. Maybe the setback was because of what *Eisenberg calls electroquackery*[47]. There also was no communication among electricity specialists, clinicians, and physiologists. There were no controlled cardiac arrest animal models. Focal myocardial ischemia-induced VF as the cause of sudden cardiac death was not appreciated until observations by *Beck*[8, 9] in the 1940s.

In 1950-52, when I was resident with *Dripps* at the University of Pennsylvania in Philadelphia, we responded hospital-wide with bellows, intubation equipment, emergency drugs, and sterile scalpel, to perform open-chest CPR even outside the operating room[41]. We did not appreciate then that VF is often the cause of sudden death in the absence of frank myocardial infarction.

Progress requires more than a new idea, observation, or discovery. It also requires recognition of an idea's clinical importance. What counts most are *results*. Players to fill the multiple roles required to assemble an effective resuscitation system merged in the 1950s – a few anesthesiologists, cardiac surgeons, and electrical engineers. Cardiologists joined much later.

Modern External Cardiopulmonary Resuscitation

Elam was the first to explore exhaled air ventilation scientifically, first when he was anesthesiologist in St. Louis, and later in Buffalo. *Elam* had shown in the early 1950s[48] that blowing *exhaled air* into the normal lungs of anesthetized patients via tracheal tube or mask and pharyngeal airway can maintain normal blood oxygen and CO_2 values in himself and the patient, provided he used twice normal tidal volumes. In October 1956, at the end of the American Society of Anesthesiologists meeting in Kansas City, *Elam* hitched a ride with *Safar* on return to their homes in Baltimore. *Safar* was then chief anesthesiologist at the Baltimore City Hospital. *Elam* was then with the U.S. Army's chemical warfare center near Baltimore. They talked about first aid and resuscitation for 2 days.

Elam's data[48] "sparked me" from resuscitation teaching and practice into lifelong resuscitation research. *Elam* also aroused my interest in out-of-hospital resuscitation[51, 155]. We anesthesiologists instinctively had practiced mouth-to-tracheal tube ventilation occasionally when the anesthesia machine was not immediately available. I was surprised that Elam had not taken his data on mouth-to-mask ventilation to implementation by first aid organizations[48]. The artificial ventilation methods taught at that time were still the back (or chest)- pressure arm-lift method[61]. I told Elam that they cannot be effective without controlling the airway by backward tilt of the head or jaw thrust or both. To make mouth-to-mouth acceptable, I suggested to compare mouth-to-mouth (without tubes or masks) with the manual methods, in comatose apneic adults, with mouth-to-mouth performed by lay persons and the manual methods performed by trained rescuers. I told him that I can perform these studies and asked him to join; he continued independently.

First came *step A*, airway control without devices. Starting in November 1956 at Baltimore City Hospital, I studied airway control by roentgenograms and spirograms in patients and human volunteers[105, 138, 140]. We documented how the tongue and epiglottis obstruct the air passage during coma, unless the head is tilted backward, which opens the airway. Some subjects needed, in addition, jaw thrust[52, 74] and mouth opened, the "triple airway maneuver"[105, 138]. Also important was the finding that the prone position did not improve this airway obstruction pattern; the tongue does not simply fall forward[140]. My observations[140] were subsequently confirmed by Elam[49, 50] and Ruben[133].

At the same time, I pursued *step B*, breathing control. Elam participated in some of the early experiments. I personally controlled life support and measurements of all "victims" in ultimately 49 experiments[136-141]. *Human volunteers* (physicians and medical students) were sedated and curarized for many hours, and studied on the floor, *without* tracheal tube. This was the only way meaningful data could be obtained, because animals have straight airways and more elastic thoraxes, and conscious humans do not obstruct and breathe with maneuvers[141]. Felix *Steichen,* a resident in surgery, and Richard *Fredrick,* a resident in pathology, volunteered several times. The manual methods failed to produce adequate tidal volumes because they do not control the unintubated airway and do not produce an adequate force for lung inflation[137, 138]. These and our subsequent CPR studies of 1956-69[155] were supported by the U.S. Army.

During performance of the *manual* methods, spirograms were obtained via taped-on masks; there were various airway obstruction patterns, resulting in no or minimal ventilation in the majority of the subjects[137, 138, 139]. During performance of direct *mouth-to-mouth* ventilation or mouth-to-S tube ventilation[136], pneumograph tracings showed large tidal volumes. Ear oximetry values, reduced during apnea of 1 to 2 minutes (SaO_2 values decreased from 98 to 83%), showed complete reoxygenation with 5-7 direct exhaled air inflations[138, 141].

In 1957/58, after our first human data were presented at the National Research Council, *Gordon* confirmed the efficacy of mouth-to-mouth ventilation without tracheal tube in children[62]. A documentary film of our human experiments[141] and training films by Gordon[63] helped sell the change of First Aid guidelines from manual to mouth-to-mouth ventilation in one year worldwide. Gordon later tried to clarify the foreign body clearing maneuvers of back blows and thrusts[64]. The Heimlich maneuver[75] is still controversial.

Our data on steps A and B of what soon became external CPR, were presented first in the U.S.A. at the American Society of Anesthesiologists meeting in Los Angeles in 1957 (during the week when the Soviets launched Sputnik), and first in Europe at the Scandinavian Society of Anesthesiologists meeting in Gausdal, Norway, in 1958.

The histories of respiratory resuscitation and monitoring *devices* are major topics in themselves. In the late 1950s, Henning *Ruben* of Denmark introduced the self-refilling bag-valve-mask unit[132] which replaced the bellows-valve-mask unit of World War II[88]. For general anesthesia and resuscitation with minimal equipment, the bellows-vaporizer unit[100] we modified with the Ruben bag[117].

The histories of *tracheal intubation*[79, 89, 99, 191, 101], and *tracheotomy*[134, 145, 159], are also separate topics. In the U.S.A., tracheal intubation had been taken into the prehospital arena by anesthesiologist *Flagg* in the 1940s[54]. This was not taken up again until the 1970s. *Apgar* pioneered newborn evaluation and resuscitation by mouth-to-tracheal tube puffing in the 1950s, which were accepted immediately[5]. The history of high frequency jet ventilation began before the 1970s[84].

Since the 1930s, Kouwenhoven, Professor of electrical engineering at the Johns Hopkins

University, had conducted electric fibrillation and immediate defibrillation experiments on dogs[87]. In 1957 he visited me at Baltimore City Hospital to observe one of our human volunteer experiments on steps A and B. We discussed, but could not decide, how one might produce *artificial circulation* without opening the chest. I asked my associate Redding to try it in dogs with high pressure IPPV, as suggested earlier by Waters. As that moved only trickle flow, we gave it up.

In 1958, *external cardiac* massage was re-discovered by chance[81, 85, 86, 134] – re-discovered because no-one then knew about Maass[98] having done it 65 years earlier in humans, and Gurvich in animals in the 1940s[71]. The same observations by physiologists[72] had been forgotten. During ventricular fibrillation and immediate defibrillation experiments in dogs, Kouwenhoven's fellow *Knickerbocker,* also an electrical engineer, made the crucial observation: when he pressed the defibrillator paddles on the dog's chest, he observed an arterial pulse wave[86]. Kouwenhoven and Knickerbocker documented in dogs that sternal compressions can produce fair arterial pressures and some (although low) blood flow[86]. After these dog experiments, surgery resident *Jude,* at the Johns Hopkins Hospital, conducted the first clinical trials[80]. The introduction of halothane without precision vaporizers at that time, conveniently provided transiently pulseless patients[80], as did chloroform for Maass[98]. The landmark article on Step C[86] took steps A and B for granted, because anesthesiologist *Benson's* team provided tracheal intubation and ventilation.

In 1960, our group at Baltimore City Hospital documented that with or without cardiac arrest, sternal compressions alone can ventilate animals with or without tracheal tubes (animals have straight upper airways), but not patients without tracheal tubes (humans have kinked airways), and not even patients in cardiac arrest with tracheal tubes[143]. The latter probably was due to the fact that cardiac arrest patients often have stiff lungs, sternal compressions cause closure of bronchioles, and inflation by mere elastic recoil of the chest to resting lung volume is weak. We, therefore, combined step C with the previously established steps A and B, into phase I, BLS by external CPR[143, 147, 156]. The 1:5 and 2:15 ratios of ventilation:sternal compressions, we documented in dogs in studies by Harris[73]. These rates and ratios are merely a compromise. The first external CPR publication in German followed soon[55].

Kouwenhoven[86], *Redding*[126], *Harris*[73], and others, documented in dogs, and *DelGercio* in patients[39] that blood flows produced by external chest compressions are unpredictably low – between 0 and 30% of normal cardiac output. We tried to improve flow through pneumatic modifications and gave up. In the 1980s, sophisticated experimental re-evaluations of such modifications by the Johns Hopkins cardiologists group[195], and by others, documented that sternal compressions produce variable blood flow not only by heart compression, but also by overall intrathoracic pressure fluctuations. Pneumatic modifications such as simultaneous ventilation/compression CPR (SVC-CPR), active compression/decompression CPR (ACD-CPR), or vest CPR are clinically unrealistic because of the need for complex or bulky devices. Only intermittent abdominal compression CPR (IAC-CPR) is BLS without devices. In comparative studies, open-chest CPR proved physiologically more effective than standard external CPR in dogs[17, 18] and humans[39].

Obviously, to achieve ROSC as rapidly as possible is of paramount importance. In 1959 *Safar* and *Jude* transferred *advanced life support* (ALS) (steps D, E and F) from open-chest to closed-chest CPR. In 1956, *Zoll* of

Boston had performed the first successful closed-chest AC defibrillation in humans[200]. He also pioneered external and internal pacing[201, 202]. By 1960, *Gurvitch* of Moscow[71] and Peleska of Prague[118] had produced the first portable DC defibrillators for prehospital use. Gurvitch of Negovsky's laboratory had developed external DC defibrillation in animals already in the 1940s[71]. The cold war delayed communication. In the early 1960s, Lown took the initiative to introduce external DC defibrillation in the U.S.A.[95].

On epinephrine, my associate, *Redding*, whom I stimulated into resuscitation laboratory research in 1958 at Baltimore City Hospital, showed that epinephrine helps restart the heart beat through systemic vasoconstriction, not heart stimulation[128]. He, our group in Pittsburgh, and others examined buffer therapy for CPR, which remains a controversial topic. Modern external CPR[86, 143] we used already in 1959 at Baltimore City Hospital for resuscitation of dogs from lethal drowning[127].

After BLS, and ROSC by ALS, the still comatose patient needs *prolonged life support* (PLS), i.e., intensive care, as do many more patients who did not have a cardiac arrest. Some small specialized 24 hour recovery rooms existed since the 1930s[37]. Then came cardiothoracic surgery units[33]. Respiratory ICUs were initiated in Scandinavia in the early 1950s by *Nielssen*[43, 112] for barbiturate overdose cases; and by *Ibsen*[78] for poliomyelitis cases. The Scandinavians switched from use of the iron lung to manual IPPV while they created the first ICU ventilators. General medical/surgical ICUs were initiated in America in 1958, when *Safar* at *Baltimore City Hospital* initiated a physician-staffed ICU for cases of respiratory *and* multiple organ failure[144]. In 1960 the last poliomyelitis epidemic in the U.S.A. hit Baltimore. Many unvaccinated adults overwhelmed our ICU at Baltimore City Hospital[142, 145]. This challenge led in the U.S.A. to the first total switch from use of Drinker's tank ventilators to the more effective mechanical IPPV. We used mainly Moerch piston ventilators and tracheostomy tubes with large, soft, atraumatic cuffs[145, 148]. Moerch[104] pioneered controlled ventilation for crushed chest. Coronary care units (CCU), primarily for EKG monitoring and prevention of cardiac arrest in infarction patients, began in the early 1960s[38].

Pediatric medical/surgical ICUs in the USA began in Philadelphia[6] and Pittsburgh[82]. *Neonatal* intensive care experienced a breakthrough with spontaneous continuous positive pressure breathing[68], which was transferred also to use in adults[67]. In the early 1960s, the initiation of ICUs mushroomed in many industrialized countries[12, 53, 76, 90, 122, 113, 181]. The establishment of modern respiratory therapy and respiratory therapy training programs, with emphasis on resuscitation and critical care, was aided by the first text books, and one focused on techniques[148], the other on physiology[12].

Severinghaus contributed to the history of resuscitation more than the tri-electrode blood gas measurement unit[174]. His science and teaching enabled resuscitation from pulmonary and cardiovascular failure to be monitored. He also studied the insulted brain. He made broad technologic, scientific, and conceptual contributions without which intensive care may still be more empirical and less effective.

In *Pittsburgh,* starting in 1962, the first physician fellowship in *critical care medicine* (CCM) was initiated and directed in the 1960s by Safar[149] and led since 1970 by *Grenvik*[153]. By 1998, this first CCM program will have trained 500 physicians of various base specialties. Safar coined the term "intensivist" around 1960[144]. The idea that every "complete" anesthesiologist should also be a reanimatologist and intensivist[149], has been implemented in Europe, but only in very few places in the U.S.A.

Pittsburgh's CCM program also became the hub for the implementation of brain death determination and certification[192] simultaneously with the Harvard Group's brain death criteria[10], "letting die" in persistent vegetative state, i.e., critical care triage[44, 69, 106], as well as organ donation for transplant surgery[70].

CCM was initiated as a multidisciplinary subspecialty (or superspecialty) in 1968, jointly by anesthesiologist *Safar,* internist *Weil,* and surgeon *Shoemaker.* Their joint conclusion that a multidisciplinary society of CCM is needed, led to the Society of Critical Care Medicine (SCCM) in 1971. Guidelines for ICU organization[179] and physician education[180] were drafted by Safar and Grenvik in 1970.

Implementation

In 1963, *Elam, Jude, Gordon,* and *Safar* had initiated the first American Heart Association CPR Committee, to develop *national CPR guidelines*[3]. Pittsburgh developed the first *international CPCR guidelines,* endorsed by the World Federation of Societies of Anaesthesiologists (WFSA)[159]. These WFSA guidelines go beyond the American Heart Association guidelines by including trauma and cerebral resuscitation.

The weakest link of the life support chain[4] still is the initiation of resuscitation by lay *bystanders*. Resuscitation *training* was made possible, since the late 1950s, through dollmaker Asmund *Laerdal* of Stavanger, Norway. The other pioneering company was Ambu of Copenhagen, Denmark. *Life supporting first aid* (LSFA), conceptually initiated by A. *Laerdal* and *Safar,* should include CPR steps A-B-C plus control of external hemorrhage and positioning for coma or shock[159]. *Lind*[93] and the Pittsburgh group[15, 164, 199] conducted the first education research on resuscitation in the 1960s and 1970s. Use of self-training systems proved more effective than instructor courses, which agencies like because they can charge for courses, and instructors get ego trips. Self-training is essential to reach millions, namely the whole world population starting at age 10-12.

Life support during transportation did not exist until the 1950s. In the late 1950s, in Baltimore, *Safar* and fire department ambulance chief *McMahon* designed a *mobile ICU ambulance* vehicle; that design was further developed in Pittsburgh in the early 1960s[150, 151]. The new vehicles had a seat at the vertex, strong suction and various devices for resuscitation by fire fighters or doctors. Between 1967 and 1975, the training guidelines for BLS by emergency medical technicians (EMTs) and BLS plus ALS by paramedics, were pioneered by Pittsburgh's *Benson* and *Caroline*. They gave medical direction to Pittsburgh's historic Freedom House Ambulance program[14, 29]. This trained "unemployable" blacks to paramedics level and tested the national guidelines developed by the National Research Council in Washington. These efforts in the U.S.A. were preceded by *Prague* and *Moscow,* which had around 1960 the first physician-staffed mobile ICU ambulances. These delivered intubation, infusion, medication, and countershocks on any dying or dead victim. This pattern was followed by *Frey, Ahnefeld* and *Dick* in Mainz and Ulm, starting in 1963. In 1970, *Nagel* of Miami introduced physician guided paramedics with telemetry and voice guidance[107]. In the early 1970s, *Cobb* became the first to prepare a major community, Seattle, for CPR A-B-C to be initiated by bystanders[31]. *Eisenberg* pioneered the epidemiology of CPR for sudden cardiac death[46]. Both were the first to teach CPR-ALS to paramedics.

The experiences in Belfast in the mid 1960s[116], followed by New York[65], were mostly for cardiology fellows going to the scene to prevent cardiac arrest in myocardial infarction patients. Physician-staffed mobile ICUs in Europe have had, so far, longer response times than paramedic staffed ambulances in the U.S.A. The former seemed to get better results in cases of trauma, while paramedics under radio guidance have had better results with cardiac arrests. *Cummins* recently pioneered the implementation of automatic external defibrillation[35], a technology by Diack, et al[40], based on Mirowsky's earlier automatic internal defibrillation[103].

Manuals and books on modern resuscitation began in Baltimore in the 1950s[156]; and internationally through the World Federation of the Society of Anaesthesiologists (WFSA) since the 1960s[159]. The WFSA publications were translated into 12 languages under support by Laerdal. In the mid-1970s, the first textbooks on emergency medicine[172] and CCM[175] were published.

EMS organization guidelines for communities were first drafted in the early 1960s for Pittsburgh[152], and published by Safar in *JAMA* in 1968 under the auspices of the American Society of Anesthesiologists (ASA)[4]. Community-wide EMS guidelines include life support from the scene via transportation to the most appropriate hospital's emergency department, operating room and ICU. The "chain of survival" is the sequence of CPCR BLS-ALS steps (Fig. 1) to be delivered by the EMS system[4]. Also in the 1960s, *Ahnefeld* implemented EMS organization in Europe as the EMS Rettungskette (life support chain). Traumatology-oriented EMS with helicopters began in the 1970s[32]. Basic traumatologic resuscitation guidelines were "pushed" by anesthesiologists[4, 159] but for advanced trauma life support (ATLS) training of physicians, the American College of Surgeons developed an extensive system[2, 173]. The first international conference on EMS was held in 1973 in Mainz, Germany[56]; at that time, Frey discussed his idea of the "Club of Mainz" with Safar[57].

On resuscitation in *disasters,* there was nothing published until the 1970s. Disaster medicine before the 1970s had been the concern of public health specialists, engineers, organizers, sociologists, and other non-physicians. In 1972, *Frey* of Mainz introduced the idea to create the "Club of Mainz for Emergency and Disaster Medicine"[57]. The multidisciplinary Club of Mainz, founded in 1976, was renamed World Association for Disaster and Emergency Medicine (WADEM) in 1983. It created the world's first journal on disaster medicine, and "disaster reanimatology" as a new field of research[163, 165]. Anecdotal reports were thus followed by semi-quantitative retrospective interview studies starting in the 1980s[124].

Cerebral Resuscitation Research

Cerebral resuscitation after cardiac arrest, considered and promoted for research already before 1970 by Negovsky[108-110], Guthrie[183, 120] and others, has been systematically researched only about 1970[158, 162]. Earlier research on cerebral protection *during* ischemia or the trauma of brain or heart operations, gave some clues, particularly as it concerned protection-preservation by hypothermia. Barbiturate therapy was also considered early for focal brain ischemia (stroke). Life saving after severe brain trauma was pioneered by intracranial pressure (ICP) monitoring and control[97]. For "brains too good to die" (Safar) after cardiac arrest, cutting edge research started around 1970[77, 94, 111, 158, 178] and has come to fruition only in the 1990s[162, 188]. By 1971, Hossman had shown in cats that most but not all cerebral neurons can resume electric activity after up to one hour of complete normothermic global brain ischemia[77]. The

Pittsburgh group documented in dogs for the first time, after cardiac arrest, the delayed and prolonged cerebral hypoperfusion[94, 178]. Using new, clinically realistic outcome models with intensive care in large animals[111, 161, 167], the Pittsburgh group has sought since 1970 to achieve functional and histologically normal brains after 10 minutes of normothermic no-flow[160]. This could be a breakthrough, because response times of advanced life support ambulances cannot be reduced below about eight minutes. The heart-lung machine[59] was adapted for emergency use and as an experimental tool[167].

The first multicenter international randomized clinical CPCR study, the Brain Resuscitation Clinical Trial (BRCT), found thiopental loading[21, 25, 44], calcium entry blocker therapy[22, 23], and titrated high dose epinephrine[24] to be only marginally (in subgroups) effective. More important are clues from examining its vast database from 20 research groups in 7 countries for numerous other unanswered questions on sudden death and CPCR, and the realization that randomized clinical trials for clinical death research have limitations because of the numerous unrecognized and uncontrollable factors involved. An important spinoff of these BRCT studies has been international collegiality of reanimatologists, the Belgian country-wide registry of CPCR cases[106], and the Utstein criteria for EMS resuscitation evaluations in communities[36].

Cerebral resuscitation research has been catalyzed by researchers' symposia in the 1970s[160], 1980s[166], and 1990s[168], as has CPR research been catalyzed first by international researchers' conferences in the 1960s[96, 123], and then by the so called "Wolf Creek Conferences" in 1975[154], which included historic vignettes[51, 81, 85, 91, 155]; in 1980[129]; in 1985[115]; and in 1996[194].

Trials of numerous *pharmacologic* cerebral resuscitation potentials by us and others, over so far 25 years, have resulted in very few statistically significant improvements in outcome[189], without clinically significant breakthrough effects[162]. In contrast, two *physical* cerebral resuscitation potentials have shown breakthrough effects on survival and cerebral outcome in dogs: a) post-arrest blood flow promotion by emergency (portable) cardiopulmonary bypass (CPB)[167] or hypertension with hemodilution[158, 184]; and b) mild resuscitative hypothermia (34°C) which is safe and easy to induce[92] – best a combination of both[169]. The realization that the post-ischemic encephalopathy has a multifactorial pathogenesis[162, 176] which needs multifaceted therapeutic approaches[60] began in the 1970s.

Therapeutic hypothermia for protection-preservation has been established since the 1950s[16, 42, 130, 131, 197]. Modern resuscitative (post-insult) hypothermia began in the 1950s with short-term dog experiments[130] and uncontrolled case reports[13]. Management problems and side effects, however, made moderate resuscitative hypothermia (30°C) become dormant. In 1987, we discovered in dogs with cardiac arrest that mild protective-preservative hypothermia (34°C) is sufficient to achieve benefit[166, 167]. This led to resuscitative mild hypothermia documentation *after* normothermic cardiac arrest in dogs[92, 169]. Simultaneously and independently, two other groups documented benefit from mild protective and resuscitative hypothermia in rat models of incomplete forebrain ischemia, which served valuable mechanism studies. Clinical trials of mild hypothermia after cardiac arrest have begun.

Resuscitative moderate hypothermia *after* traumatic brain injury (TBI) or focal brain ischemia was researched first in the 1950s in dogs by Rosomoff[130]. Patient experiences of the 1960s remained anecdotal[131]. The outcome benefit of resuscitative moderate hypothermia (32°C) after TBI has most recently been scientifically documented in dogs[121], rats[30], and patients[102]. Resuscitative hypothermia after spinal cord injury was found effective in animal models by Albin and White[1, 196], but has not become established in patients – for unknown reasons.

Future and Conclusions

The future of resuscitation medicine will be based on current cutting edge research and development. Developments of modern resuscitation medicine focused in the 1950s on respiratory resuscitation, in the 1960s on CPR, since the 1970s on cerebral resuscitation, and in the 1980s and 1990s on epidemiologic studies, guidelines and community programs for sudden death and traumatology. Around 2,000 A.D., I expect that breakthroughs in knowledge about how vital organ systems' cells die after anoxic or traumatic insults can lead to new breakthroughs in the reversibility of increasingly long periods of terminal states or clinical death.

We must learn from history. Some clinical breakthroughs might be discovered and implemented, as in the past, without the knowledge of their specific mechanisms of action. Examples include anesthesia, insulin, antibiotics, and corticosteroids.

Traumatologic resuscitation developments are a wide-open field for new breakthroughs. Numerous investigators have studied so-called irreversible post-traumatic shock with or without sepsis[19, 193]. Future breakthroughs in traumatologic resuscitation medicine should include an extension of the golden hour of hemorrhagic shock tolerance by treatments in the field which protect the viscera against ischemia[27, 83].

A novel approach is needed for temporarily unresuscitable but ultimately potentially repairable sudden death situations. Examples involve combat casualties with penetrating thoracic or abdominal injuries who have died from internal exsanguination within 5 to 10 minutes of being hit, some civilian trauma cases which are unmanageable in the field (e.g., Martin Luther King, President Rabin, Princess Diana), and sudden cardiac death patients in whom a brief vigorous attempt at ROSC with standard CPR ALS has failed. For such conditions we are researching "suspended animation for transport and repair in clinical death, with resuscitation two or more hours later"[11, 28, 186]. These and other challenges will have to be pursued by goal-oriented multicenter laboratory programs, with well coordinated mechanistic and outcome studies. Serendipitous treatment trials may come from clues of results at the molecular and cellular levels, as well as from clinical observations.

Since the 1980s, an increasing number of focused researchers have become involved in resuscitation oriented studies on one or the other organ system, insult, method, device, or specialty. Only two research programs have pursued dying and resuscitation with a multidisciplinary, international, global, whole organism-oriented approach, namely, the center in Moscow led by Negovsky[109], and that in Pittsburgh led by Safar (1956-1994)[157] and Kochanek (1994-). The Pittsburgh center has pursued questions "from cell to community" and recently even from "DNA to disasters." A few of such globally oriented research centers are needed in addition to a larger number of focused research programs. All should be in constant communication.

Modern resuscitation medicine has created *ethical dilemmas*, which require ongoing dialogue. Law must follow ethics. Dialogues on the ethical dilemmas of resuscitation medicine were started by European anesthesiologists in the 1950s, when they discussed brain death and persistent vegetative state issues with the Pope. Most recently, debates on ethical dilemmas have included research topics such as how to conduct clinical feasibility, side effect, and outcome trials without being able to obtain prospective informed consent; and which treatments can be randomly withheld in control groups of randomized clinical outcome studies, if large animal outcome studies' results show a breakthrough effect. What is the best time to recommend a novel treatment for general clinical use? Clinical feasibility and side effect studies will always be needed.

Resuscitation defends the human brain, seat of the human mind, which is the tip of the arrow of evolution according to the philosopher Teilhard de Chardin. Resuscitation imposes the value of a single human life on the random chances of the universe. Resuscitation has as its ultimate goal "mens sana in corpore sano" – the reversal of unexpected acute dying to survival with a healthy mind in a reasonable healthy body.

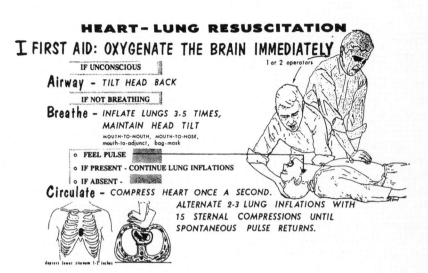

The first assembly of the cardiopulmonary cerebral resuscitation (CPCR) system in 1960[147], with 3 phases of 3 steps each. Note "H" for hypothermia later changed to "humanized (i.e., brain-oriented) intensive care"[159].

References:

1. Albin MS: Resuscitation of the spinal cord. Crit Care Med 1978; 5: 270
2. American College of Surgeons Committee on Trauma (Collicott PE, et al): Advanced Trauma Life Support Course for Physicians. American College of Surgeons, Chicago, IL, 1984
3. American Heart Association and National Academy of Sciences-National Research Council: Standards for cardiopulmonary resuscitation and emergency cardiac are. JAMA 1966; 198: 373, 1974; 227 (suppl): 833, 1980; 244 (suppl): 453, 1986; 255 (suppl): 2843, 1992; 268: 2171. Planned 2000
4. American Society of Anesthesiologists, Committee on Acute Medicine: Community-wide emergency medical services. JAMA 1968; 204: 595
5. Apgar V: A proposal for a new method of evaluation of the newborn infant. Anesth Analg 1953; 32: 260
6. Bachman L, Downes JJ, Richards CC, et al: Organization and function of an intensive care unit in a children's hospital. Anesth Analg 46:570, 1967
7. Beck, CS, Pritchard WH, Feil HS: Ventricular fibrillation of long duration abolished by electric shock. JAMA 1947; 135: 985
8. Beck CS, Weckesser EC, Barry FM: Fatal heart attack and successful defibrillation. New concepts in coronary artery disease. JAMA 1956; 161: 434
9. Beck CS, Leighninger DS: Death after a clean bill of health. JAMA 1960; 174: 133
10. Beecher H (Chairman, Harvard Medical School Ad Hoc Committee to examine the definition of brain death): A definition of irreversible coma. JAMA 1968; 205: 337
11. Bellamy R, Safar P, Tisherman SA, et al: Suspended animation for delayed resuscitation. Crit Care Med 24/S:S24, 1996
12. Bendixen HH, Egbert LD, Hedley-Whyte J, et al: Respiratory Care. CV Mosby, St. Louis, 1965
13. Benson DW, Williams GR, Spencer FC, et al: The use of hypothermia after cardiac arrest. Anesth Analg 1959; 38: 423
14. Benson DM, Esposito G, Dorsch J, et al: Mobile intensive care by "unemployable" blacks trained as emergency medical technicians (EMTs) in 1967-69. J Trauma 1972; 12: 408
15. Berkebile P, Benson D, Ersoz C, et al: Public Education in Heart-Lung Resuscitation. Evaluation of three self-training methods in teenagers. (a) Crit Care Med 1973; 1: 115. (b) Proc National Conf on CPR 1973, Dallas, Amer Heart Assoc, 1975. (c) Crit Care Med 1976; 4: 134 (abstract)
16. Bigelow WG, Lindsay WK, Greenwood WF: Hypothermia: Its possible role in cardiac surgery. Ann Surg 1950; 132: 849
17. Bircher N, Safar P: Open-chest CPR: an old method whose time has returned. Am J Emerg Med 1984; 2: 568
18. Bircher N, Safar P: Cerebral preservation during cardiopulmonary resuscitation. Crit Care Med 1985; 13: 185
19. Blalock A: Principles of Surgical Care, Shock and Other Problems. St. Louis, Mosby, 1940
20. Boehm R: Ueber Wiederbelebung nach Vergiftungen und Asphyxie. Arch Exp Pathol Pharmakol 1878; 8: 68
21. Brain resuscitation clinical trial (BRCT) I study group: Randomized clinical study of thiopental loading in comatose survivors of cardiac arrest. N Engl J Med 1986; 314: 397
22. Brain Resuscitation Clinical Trial (BRCT) II Study Group: A randomized clinical study of a calcium-entry blocker (lidoflazine) in the treatment of comatose survivors of cardiac arrest. N Engl J Med 1991; 324: 1225
23. Brain Resuscitation Clinical Trial (BRCT) II Study Group: Simpson's paradox and clinical trials: What you find is not necessarily what you prove. Ann Emerg Med 1992; 21: 1480

24. Brain Resuscitation Clinical Trial (BRCT) III Study Group: A randomized clinical trial of escalating doses of high dose epinephrine during cardiac resuscitation. Crit Care Med 1995; 23: A178

25. Breivik H, Safar P, Sands P, et al: Clinical feasibility trials of barbiturate therapy after cardiac arrest. Crit Care Med 1978; 6: 227

26. Brosch A: Die wirksamste Methode der kuenstlichen Athmung. Wien Klin Wschr 1896; 9: 1177

27. Capone AC, Safar P, Stezoski W, et al: Improved outcome with fluid restriction in treatment of uncontrolled hemorrhagic shock. J Am Coll Surg 1995; 180: 49

28. Capone A, Safar P, Radovsky A, et al: Complete recovery after normothermic hemorrhagic shock and profound hypothermic circulatory arrest of 60 minutes in dogs. J Trauma 1996; 40: 388

29. Caroline NL: Medical Care in the streets. JAMA 1977; 237: 43

30. Clifton GL, Jiang JY, Lyeth BG, et al: Marked protection by moderate hypothermia after experimental traumatic brain injury. J Cereb Blood Flow Metab 1991; 11: 114

31. Cobb LA, Werner JA, Trobaugh GB: Sudden cardiac death. I. A decade's experience with out-of-hospital resuscitation; II. Outcome of resuscitation management and future directions. Modern Concepts of Cardiovasc Dis (Am Heart Assoc) 1980; 49: 31

32. Cowley RA: The total emergency medical system for the state of Maryland. Maryland State Med J, July 1975.

33. Crafoord C: Pulmonary ventilation and anaesthesia in major chest surgery. J Thorac Surg 1940; 9: 237

34. Crile GW, Dolley DH: An experimental research into the resuscitation of dogs killed by anesthetics and asphyxia. J Exp Med 1906; 8: 713

35. Cummins RO, Eisenberg MS, Graves JR, et al: Automatic external defibrillators used by emergency medical technicians: A controlled clinical trial. Crit Care Med 1985; 13: 945

36. Cummins RO, Chamberlain DA, Abramson NS, et al: Recommended guidelines for uniform reporting of data from out of hospital cardiac arrest: the Utstein style. Circulation 1991; 84: 960

37. Dandy WE: Surgery of the brain. Hagerstown, MD, W.F. Prior Company, 1945.

38. Day HW: History of coronary care units. Am J Cardiol 1972; 30: 405

39. Del Guercio LRM, Feins NR, Cohn JD, et al: A comparison of blood flow during external and internal cardiac massage in man. Circulation 1964; 30: 63

40. Diack AW, Welborn WS, Rullman RG, et al: An automatic cardiac resuscitator for emergency treatment of cardiac arrest. Med Instrum 1979; 13: 78

41. Dripps RD, Kirby CK, Johnson J, et al: Cardiac resuscitation. Ann Surg 1948; 127: 592

42. Dripps RD (ed): The physiology of induced hypothermia. Washington DC National Academy of Sciences 1956.

43. Eckenhoff JE: The care of the unconscious patient. JAMA 1963; 186: 95

44. Edgren E, Hedstrand U, Kelsey S, et al: Assessment of neurological prognosis in comatose survivors of cardiac arrest. Lancet 1994; 343: 1055

45. Einthoven W, Fahr G, DeWaart A: On the direction and manifest size of the variations of potential in the human heart and on the influence of the position of the heart on the form of the electrocardiogram. Pfluegers Arch Physiol 1913; 150: 275. Also, English: Am Heart J 1950; 40: 163

46. Eisenberg MS, Horwood BT, Cummins RO, et al: Cardiac arrest and resuscitation: A tale of 29 cities. Ann Emerg Med 1990; 19: 179

47. Eisenberg MS: Life in the balance. Emergency medicine and the quest to reverse sudden death. Oxford Univ Press, New York, 1997

48. Elam JO, Brown ES, Elder JD, Jr: Artificial respiration by mouth-to-mask method: a study of the respiratory gas exchange of paralyzed patients ventilated by operator's expired air. New Engl J Med 1954; 250: 749

49. Elam JO, Greene DG, Brown ES, et al: Oxygen and carbon dioxide exchange and energy cost of expired air resuscitation. JAMA 1958; 167: 328

50. Elam JO, Greene DG, Schneider MA, et al: Head-tilt method of oral resuscitation. JAMA 1960; 172: 812

51. Elam JO: Rediscovery of expired air methods for emergency ventilation. In Safar P, Elam J (Eds): Advances in Cardiopulmonary Resuscitation. New York, Springer-Verlag, 1977, page 263-265, chapter 39

52. Esmarch JF: The Surgeon's Handbook on the Treatment of Wounded in War. Schmidt, New York, 1878

53. Fairley HB: The Toronto General Hospital respiratory unit. Anaesthesia 1961; 16: 267

54. Flagg PJ: The Art of Resuscitation. New York, Reinhold, 1944

55. Frey R, Jude J, Safar P: External cardiac resuscitation. Indication, technique and results. Deutsche Med Wchschr 1962; 17: 857

56. Frey R, Nagel E, Safar P (Eds): Mobile Intensive Care Units. Advanced Emergency Care Delivery Systems. International Symposium, Mainz 1973. Anesthesiology and Resuscitation Series. Vol. 95. Berlin, Springer-Verlag, 1976

57. Frey R: The Club of Mainz for improved worldwide emergency and critical care medicine systems and disaster preparedness. Crit Care Med 1978; 6: 389

58. Frye WB: Ventricular fibrillation and defibrillation: historical perspectives with emphasis on the contributions of John MacWilliam, Carl Wiggers, and William Kouwenhoven. Circulation 1985; 71: 858

59. Gibbon JR Jr: Application of mechanical heart and lung to cardiac surgery. Minn Med 1954; 37: 171

60. Gisvold SE, Safar P, Saito R, et al: Multifaceted therapy after global brain ischemia in monkeys. Stroke 1984; 15: 803

61. Gordon AS, Sadove MS, Raymon F, et al: Critical survey of manual artificial respiration. JAMA 1951; 147: 1444

62. Gordon AS, Frye CW, Gittelson L, et al: Mouth-to-mouth versus manual artificial respiration for children and adults. JAMA 1958; 167: 320

63. Gordon AS: CPR training films. (a) Breath of Life (Steps A and B); (b) Pulse of Life (Steps A, B and C); (c) Prescription for Life (Steps A-D); and (d) Life in the Balance (Cardiac Care Unit). Am Heart Assoc, Dallas, TX, 1960s; 1980s. Also from Pyramid Films, Santa Monica, CA, 1986

64. Gordon AS, Belton MK, Ridolpho PF: Emergency management of foreign body airway obstruction. In Safar P, Elam J (eds): Advances in Cardiopulmonary Resuscitation. New York, Springer-Verlag, 1977, page 39-50, chapter 7

65. Grace WJ, Chadbourn JA: The first hour in acute myocardial infarction. Heart Lung 1974; 3: 736

66. Green TA: Heart massage as means of restoration in cases of apparent sudden death, with a synopsis of 40 cases. Lancet 1706, 1906

67. Greenbaum DM, Millen JE, Eross B, et al: Continuous positive airway pressure without tracheal intubation in spontaneously breathing patients. Chest 1976; 69: 615

68. Gregory GA, Kitterman JA, Phibbs RH, et al: Treatment of idiopathic respiratory distress syndrome with continuous positive airway pressure. N Engl J Med 1971; 184: 1333

69. Grenvik A, Powner DJ, Snyder JV, et al: Cessation of therapy in terminal illness and brain death. Crit Care Med 1978; 6: 284

70. Grenvik A: Ethical dilemmas in organ donation and transplantation. Crit Care Med 1988; 16: 1012

71. Gurvich NL, Yuniev SG: Restoration of a regular rhythm in the mammalian fibrillating heart. Am Rev Soviet Med 3:236, 1946.

72. Guthrie CC: Experimental shock. JAMA 1917; 17: 1394

73. Harris LC, Kirimli B, Safar P: Ventilation-cardiac compression rates and ratios in cardiopulmonary resuscitation. Anesthesiology 1967; 28: 806

74. Heiberg J: A new expedient in administering chloroform. Med Times Gazette, January 10, 1874
75. Heimlich HG: A life-saving maneuver to prevent food chocking. JAMA 234:398, 1975.
76. Holmdahl MH: Respiratory care unit. Anesthesiology 1962; 23: 559
77. Hossmann KA, Kleihues P: Reversibility of ischemic brain damage. Arch Neurol 1973; 29: 375
78. Ibsen B: The anaesthetist's viewpoint on the treatment of respiratory complications in poliomyelitis during the epidemic in Copenhagen, 1952. Proc R Soc Med 1954; 47: 72
79. Jackson C: The technique of insertion of intra-tracheal insufflation tubes. Surg Gynecol Obstet 1913; 17: 507
80. Jude JR, Kouwenhoven WB, Knickerbocker GG: Cardiac arrest: report of application of external cardiac massage on 118 patients. JAMA 1961; 178: 1063
81. Jude JR: Rediscovery of external heart compression in Dr. William Kouwenhoven's laboratory. In Safar P, Elam J (Eds): Advances in Cardiopulmonary Resuscitation. New York, Springer-Verlag, 1977, page 286-291, chapter 43
82. Kampschulte S, Safar P: Development of multidisciplinary pediatric intensive care unit. Crit Care Med 1973; 1: 308
83. Kim SH, Stezoski SW, Safar P, et al: Hypothermia and minimal fluid resuscitation increase survival after uncontrolled hemorrhagic shock in rats. J Trauma 1997; 42: 213
84. Klain M, Smith BR: High frequency percutaneous transtracheal jet ventilation. Crit Care Med 1977; 5: 280
85. Knickerbocker G: Contributions of William B. Kouwenhoven - reminiscences. In Safar P, Elam J (Eds): Advances in Cardiopulmonary Resuscitation. New York, Springer-Verlag, 1977, page 255-258, chapter 31
86. Kouwenhoven WB, Jude JR, Knickerbocker GG: Closed-chest cardiac massage. JAMA 1960; 173: 1064
87. Kouwenhoven WB, Langworthy OR: Cardiopulmonary resuscitation. An account of forty-five years of research. JAMA 1973; 226: 877
88. Kreiselman J: A new resuscitation apparatus. Anesthesiology 1943; 4 :608
89. Kuhn F: Die Perorale Intubation. S. Karger, Berlin, 1911
90. Lawin P: Praxis der Intensivbehandlung. Stuttgart, Thieme, 1975, 1981
91. Leighninger DS: Contributions of Claude Beck. In Safar P, Elam J (Eds): Advances in Cardiopulmonary Resuscitation. New York, Springer-Verlag, 1977, 259-262, chapter 38
92. Leonov Y, Sterz F, Safar P, et al: Mild cerebral hypothermia during and after cardiac arrest improves neurologic outcome in dogs. J Cereb Blood Flow Metab 1990; 10: 57
93. Lind B: Teaching mouth-to-mouth resuscitation in primary schools. Acta Anesth Scand 1961; 9: (suppl.) 63
94. Lind B, Snyder J, Safar P: Total brain ischemia in dogs: Cerebral physiological and metabolic changes after 15 minutes of circulatory arrest. Resuscitation 1975; 4: 97
95. Lown B, Neuman J, Amarasingham R, et al: Comparison of alternating current with direct current electroshock across the closed chest. Am J Cardiol 1962; 10: 233
96. Lund I, Lind B (Eds): International Symposium on Emergency Resuscitation. Oslo, Norway, 1967. Acta Anaesth Scand (Suppl) 29, 1968
97. Lundberg N: Continuous recording and control of ventricular fluid pressure in neurosurgical practice. Acta Psychiatr Neurol Scand 1960; 36: (suppl 149)
98. Maass F: Die Methode der Wiederbelebung bei Herztod nach Chloroformeinathmung. Berlin Klin Wochenschr 1892; 12: 265
99. Macewen W: Clinical observations on the introduction of tracheal tubes by the mouth instead of performing tracheotomy or laryngotomy. Br Med J 1880; 2: 122
100. Macintosh RR: Oxford inflating bellows. Br Med J 1953; 2: 202

[101] Magill IW: Endotracheal anaesthesia. Proc R Soc Med 1928; 22: 1

[102] Marion DW, Penrod LE, Kelsey SF, et al: Treatment of traumatic brain injury with moderate hypothermia. New Engl J Med 1997; 336: 540

[103] Mirowski M, Reid PR, Mower MM, et al: Termination of malignant ventricular arrhythmias with an implanted automatic defibrillator in human beings. N Engl Med 1980; 303: 322

[104] Moerch ET, Avery EE, Benson DW: Hyperventilation in the treatment of crushing injuries of the chest. Surg Forum 1956; 6: 270

[105] Morikawa S, Safar P, DeCarlo J: Influence of head position upon upper airway patency. Anesthesiology 1961; 22: 265

[106] Mullie A, Verstringe P, Buylaert W, et al: Predictive value of Glasgow coma score for awakening after out-of-hospital cardiac arrest. Lancet i:137, 1988

[107] Nagel EL, Hirschman JC, Nussenfeld SR, et al: Telemetry-medical command in coronary and other mobile emergency care systems. JAMA 1970; 214: 332

[108] Negovsky VA: Resuscitation and Artificial Hypothermia (USSR). New York, Consultants Bureau, 1962

[109] Negovsky VA: Fifty years of the Institute of General Reanimatology of the USSR Academy of Medical Sciences. Crit Care Med 1988; 16: 287

[110] Negovsky VA, Gurvitch AM, Zolotokrylina ES: Postresuscitation Disease. Elsevier, Amsterdam, 1983

[111] Nemoto EM, Bleyaert AL, Stezoski SW, et al: Global brain ischemia: a reproducible monkey model. Stroke 1977; 8: 558

[112] Nilsson E: On treatment of barbiturate poisoning. A modified clinical aspect. Acta Med Scand 1951; 253: (suppl)1

[113] Norlander OP: The use of respirators in anesthesia and surgery. Acta Anaesth Scand:(suppl) 30, 1968

[114] Oliver G, Schafer EA: The physiologic effects of extracts from the suprarenal capsules. J Physiol (Lond) 1895; 18: 232

[115] Otto CW, Eisenberg MS, Bircher NG (Eds): Wolf Creek Conference on CPR Research #3 in 1985. Crit Care Med 1985; 13: 881

[116] Pantridge JF, Geddes JS: A mobile intensive care unit in the management of myocardial infarction. Lancet 1967; II: 271

[117] Pearson J, Safar P: General anesthesia with minimal equipment. Anesth Analg 1961; 40: 644

[118] Peleska B: Transthoracic and direct defibrillation. Rozhl Chir (CSSR) 1957; 36: 731

[119] Petty TL, Ashbaugh DG: The adult respiratory distress syndrome. Chest 1971; 60: 233

[120] Pike FJ, Guthrie CC, Stewart GN: The return of function in the central nervous system after temporary cerebral anaemia. Am J Physiol 1908; 22: 490

[121] Pomeranz S, Safar P, Radovsky A, et al: The effect of resuscitative moderate hypothermia following epidural brain compression on cerebral damage in a canine outcome model. J Neurosurg 1993; 79: 241

[122] Pontoppidan H, Geffin B, Lowenstein E: Acute respiratory failure in the adult. New Engl J Med 1972; 287: 690

[123] Poulsen H (Ed): International Symposium on Emergency Resuscitation. Stavanger, Norway, 1960. Acta Anaesth Scand (Suppl) 9, 1961

[124] Pretto EA, Ricci E, Klain M, et al: Disaster reanimatology potentials: A structured interview study in Armenia. III. Results, conclusions, and recommendations. Prehosp Disaster Med 1992; 7: 327

[125] Prevost JL, Batelli F: On some effects of electrical discharges on the hearts of mammals. Compt Rend Acad Sci (Paris) 1989; 129: 1267

[126] Redding J, Cozine R: A comparison of open-chest and closed-chest cardiac massage in dogs. Anesthesiology 1961; 22: 280

[127] Redding JS, Cozine RA, Voigt GC, et al: Resuscitation from drowning. J Am Med Assoc 1961; 178: 1136

[128] Redding JS, Pearson JW: Evaluation of drugs for cardiac resuscitation. Anesthesiology 1963; 24: 203

129. Redding JS (Ed): Wolf Creek Conference on CPR Research No. 2 in 1980. Crit Care Med, 1981; 9: 357

130. Rosomoff HL, Shulman K, Raynor R, et al: Experimental brain injury and delayed hypothermia. Surg Gynecol Obstet 1960; 110: 27

131. Rosomoff HL, Kochanek PM, Clark R, et al: Resuscitation from severe brain trauma. Crit Care Med 1996; 24/S: S48

132. Ruben H: Combination resuscitator and aspirator. Anesthesiology 1958; 19: 408

133. Ruben H, Elam JO, Ruben AM, et al: Investigation of upper airway problems in resuscitation. Anesthesiology 1961; 22: 271

134. Safar P: History of cardiopulmonary-cerebral resuscitation. In: Kaye W, Bircher N (Eds): Cardiopulmonary Resuscitation. New York, Churchill Livingstone, 1989. Chapter 1, pages 1-53

135. Safar P: On the history of modern resuscitation. Crit Care Med 1996; 24/S: S3

136. Safar P: Mouth-to-mouth airway. Anesthesiology 1957; 18: 904

137. Safar P, Escarraga LA, Elam JO: A comparison of the mouth-to-mouth and mouth-to-airway methods of artificial respiration with the chest-pressure arm-lift methods. N Engl J Med 1958; 258: 671

138. Safar P: Ventilatory efficacy of mouth-to-mouth artificial respiration. Airway obstruction during manual and mouth-to-mouth artificial respiration. JAMA 1958; 167: 335

139. Safar P: Failure of manual artificial respiration. J Appl Physiol 1959; 14: 84

140. Safar P, Escarraga LA, Chang F: Upper airway obstruction in the unconscious patient. J Appl Physiol 1959; 14: 760

141. Safar P: Introduction to Respiratory and Cardiac Resuscitation. A Documentary Film of Human Volunteer Research. Produced by US Walter Reed Army Institute of Research, Washington, DC, USA. Army film PMF5349, 1960

142. Safar P: Introduction to Prolonged Artificial Ventilation. A Documentary Film of Patient Research. Produced by Walter Reed Army Institute of Research, Washington, DC. Army Film PMF5348, 1960

143. Safar P, Brown TC, Holtey WJ: Ventilation and circulation with closed-chest cardiac massage in man. JAMA 1961; 176: 574

144. Safar P, DeKornfeld TJ, Pearson JW, et al: The intensive care unit. Anaesthesia 1961; 16: 275

145. Safar P, Berman B, Diamond E, et al: Cuffed tracheotomy tube vs. tank respirator for prolonged artificial ventilation. Arch Phys Med Rehabil 1962; 43: 487

146. Safar P (Ed): Resuscitation: controversial aspects. International Symposium, Vienna 1962. Anesthesiology and Resuscitation Series. Vol. 1. Berlin, Springer-Verlag, 1963

147. Safar P: Community-wide cardiopulmonary resuscitation. J Iowa Med Soc Nov:629, 1964.

148. Safar P (ed): Respiratory Therapy. FA Davis, Philadelphia, 1965

149. Safar P: The anesthesiologist as "intensivist." In, Eckenhoff JE (ed): Science and Practice in Anesthesia. Philadelphia, JB Lippincott, 1965

150. Safar P, Brose RA: Ambulance design and equipment for resuscitation. Arch Surg 1965; 90: 343

151. Safar P, Esposito G, Benson DM: Ambulance design and equipment for mobile intensive care. Arch Surg 1971; 102: 163

152. Safar P, Benson DM, Esposito G, et al: Emergency and critical care medicine: local implementation of national recommendations. In Safar P (Ed): Public Health Aspects of Critical Care Medicine and Anesthesiology. Philadelphia, F.A. Davis, 1974, pages 65-126

153. Safar P, Grenvik A: Organization and physician education in critical care medicine. Anesthesiology 1977; 47: 82

154. Safar P, Elam J (Eds): Advances in Cardiopulmonary Resuscitation. Wolf Creek Conference on CPR Research No. 1 in 1975. New York, Springer-Verlag, 1977

155. Safar P: From back-pressure arm-lift to mouth-to-mouth, control of airway, and beyond. In Safar P, Elam J (Eds): Advances in Cardiopulmonary Resuscitation. New York, Springer-Verlag, 1977, pages 266-275; chapter 40

156. Safar P, McMahon M: Resuscitation of the unconscious victim. A manual. Baltimore, MD, Fire Department, 1957. Springfield, IL, Charles C. Thomas, 1959, 1961

157. Safar P: Resuscitation Research Center, University of Pittsburgh. Resuscitation 1979; 7: 69

158. Safar P, Stezoski SW, Nemoto EM: Amelioration of brain damage after 12 minutes cardiac arrest in dogs. Arch Neurol 1976; 33: 91

159. Safar P, Bircher NG: Cardiopulmonary Cerebral Resuscitation. World Federation of Societies of Anaesthesiologists. Stavanger, A. Laerdal, and London, WB Saunders, 1968 (1st edition); 1981 (2nd edition); 1988 (3rd edition)

160. Safar P (Ed): Brain resuscitation. Special symposium issue. Crit Care Med 1978; 6: 199

161. Safar P, Gisvold SE, Vaagenes P, et al: Long-term animal models for the study of global brain ischemia. In: Wauquier A, et al, eds: Protection of Tissues Against Hypoxia. Amsterdam, Elsevier, 1982, pages 147-170

162. Safar P: Resuscitation of the ischmic brain. In, Albin MS (ed), Textbook of Neuroanesthesia with Neurosurgical and Neuroscience Perspectives. New York, McGraw-Hill, 1997, pages 557-593

163. Safar P (Ed): Disaster Resuscitology. Prehosp Disaster Med 1:(suppl I), 1985

164. Safar P, Berkebile P, Scott MA, et a: Education research on life-supporting first aid (LSFA) and CPR self-training systems (STS). Crit Care Med 1981; 9: 403

165. Safar P: Resuscitation potentials in mass disasters. Prehosp Disaster Med 1986; 2: 34

166. Safar P, Grenvik A, Abramson NS, et al (Eds): International resuscitation research symposium on the reversibility of clinical death, May 1987. Crit Care Med 1988; 16: 919

167. Safar P, Abramson NS, Angelos M, et al: Emergency cardiopulmonary bypass for resuscitation from prolonged cardiac arrest. Am J Emerg Med 1990; 8: 55

168. Safar P, Ebmeyer U, Katz L, Tisherman S (Eds): Future directions for resuscitation research. [Resuscitation Researchers' Conference, Pittsburgh, May 1994.] Crit Care Med 1996; 24/2: S1-S99, Supplement

169. Safar P, Xiao F, Radovsky A, et al: Improved cerebral resuscitation from cardiac arrest in dogs with mild hypothermia plus blood flow promotion. Stroke 1996; 27: 105

170. Schafer EA: Description of a simple and efficient method of performing artificial respiration in the human subject. Med Chir Trans 1904; 87: 609

171. Schiff M: Ueber direkte Reizung der Herzoberflaeche. Arch Ges Physiol 1882; 28: 200

172. Schwartz G, Safar P, Stone J, et al (Eds): Principles and Practice of Emergency Medicine. Philadelphia, WB Saunders, First edition, 1978

173. Seeley S: Accidental Death and Disability: The Neglected Disease of Modern Society. Committee on Trauma and Committee on Shock, Division of Medical Sciences. National Academy of Sciences, National Research Council, Washington, D.C., 1966

174. Severinghaus JW, Bradley AF: Electrode for blood PO2 and PCO2 determination. J Appl Physiol 1958; 13: 515

175. Shoemaker WC, Thompson WL, Holbrook PR, (Eds): The Society of Critical Care Medicine: Textbook of Critical Care. Philadelphia, WB Saunders, First edition, 1984.

176. Siesjo BK: Mechanisms of ischemic brain damage. Crit Care Med 16:954, 1988.

177. Silvester HR: A new method of resuscitating still-born children and of restoring persons apparently dead or drowned. Br J Med 2:576, 1858.

178. Snyder JV, Nemoto EM, Carroll RG, et al: Global ischemia in dogs: intracranial pressures, brain blood flow, and metabolism. Stroke 6:21, 1975.

[179] Society of Critical Care Medicine: Guidelines for organization of critical care units. JAMA 1972; 222: 1532

[180] Society of Critical Care Medicine: Guidelines for training of physicians in critical care medicine. Crit Care Med 1973; 1: 39

[181] Spence M: An organization for intensive care. Med J Australia 1967; 1: 795

[182] Stephenson HE Jr, Reid LC, Hinton JW: Some common denominators in 1200 cases of cardiac arrest. Ann Surg 1953; 137: 731

[183] Stephenson HE Jr: Charles Claude Guthrie's contribution to cardiac resuscitation. Crit Care Med 1981; 9: 428

[184] Sterz F, Leonov Y, Safar P, et al: Hypertension with or without hemodilution after cardiac arrest in dogs. Stroke 1990; 21: 1178

[185] Thangan S, Weil MH, Rackow EC: Cardiopulmonary resuscitation: a historical review. Acute Care 1986; 12: 63

[186] Tisherman SA, Safar P, Radovsky A, et al: Profound hypothermia (<10°C) compared with deep hypothermia (15°C) improves neurologic outcome in dogs after two hours' circulatory arrest induced to enable resuscitative surgery. J Trauma 1991; 31: 1051

[187] Tossach WA: A man dead in appearance recovered by distending the lungs with air. Med Essays Observations. 1744; 5: 605

[188] Traystman RJ, Kirsch JR, Koehler RC: Oxygen radical mechanisms of brain injury following ischemia and reperfusion. J Appl Physiol 1991; 71/4: 1185

[189] Vaagenes P, Cantadore R, Safar P, et al: Amelioration of brain damage by lidoflazine after prolonged ventricular fibrillation cardiac arrest in dogs. Crit Care Med 12:846, ,1984.

[190] Vesalius A: De corporis humani fabrica. Libri Septem. 1543, Cap IXX, Basel, 1555

[191] Waters RM, Rovenstein EA, Guedel AE: Endotracheal anesthesia and its historical development. Anesth Analg 1933; 1: 196

[192] Wecht C, Grenvik A, Safar P, et al: Determination of brain death. Bull Allegheny Co Med Soc (Pittsburgh, PA, U.S.A.), Jan 25, 1969

[193] Weil MH, Shubin H (Eds): Diagnosis and Treatment of Shock. Baltimore, Williams & Wilkins, 1967

[194] Weil MH (Ed): Wolf Creek IV Conference on CPR (in 1996). New Horizons 5/2:97, 1997 (Soc. Crit. Care Med.)

[195] Weisfeldt ML, Chandra N, Fisher J, et al: Mechanisms of perfusion in cardiopulmonary resuscitation. In, Shoemaker WC, Thompson WL, Holbrook PR (Eds): Textbook of Critical Care. Philadelphia, WB Saunders, 1984, pages 31-

[196] White RJ, Albin M, et al: Spinal cord injury. Sequential morphology and hypothermia stabilization. Surg Forum 1969; 20: 432

[197] White RJ: Hypothermic preservation and transplantation of brain. Resuscitation 1975; 4: 197

[198] Wiggers CJ: Cardiac massage followed by countershock in revival of mammalian ventricles from fibrillation due to coronary occlusion. Am J Physiol 1936; 116: 161

[199] Winchell SW, Safar P: Teaching and testing lay and paramedical personnel in cardiopulmonary resuscitation. Anesth Analg 1966; 45: 441

[200] Zoll PM, Linenthal AJ, Gibson W. et al: Termination of ventricular fibrillation in man by externally applied electric countershock. N Engl J Med 1956; 254: 727

[201] Zoll PM: Historical development of cardiac pacemakers. Prog Cardiovasc Dis 1972; 14: 421

[202] Zoll PM: The first successful external cardiac stimulation and A-C defibrillation. In Safar P, Elam J (Eds.): Advances in Cardiopulmonary Resuscitation. New York, Springer-Verlag, 1977, page 281-285, chapter 42

Acknowledgements

Thanks go to Prof. Dr. J. Schulte am Esch and Dr. Michael Goerig of Hamburg for their invitation to submit this talk and paper, and for their suberb "history of anesthesia" catalogue at the exhibition on anesthetic equipment in the history of German anesthesia, presented in Hamburg, May 1997. The author also wishes to thank Ms. Valerie Sabo and Ms. Fran Mistrick for their help in preparing the manuscript and finding references; and Ms. Lisa Goetz for her help in editing.

Misleading Developments in Anesthesia Techniques as an Impediment of Progress in Surgical Anesthesia.

E. A. M. Frost,
Department of Anesthesiology, New York Medical College, USA

It is not difficult to realise how little real progress was made in surgery before the discovery and application of anaesthesia in the 19th century. Prior to 200 years ago methods to alleviate pain differed greatly. Around the time of the writing of the Edwin Smith papyrus (~3,000 B.C.) the physician was advised "to palpate ... wound, although he shudders exceedingly..." The rationale was that pain, associated only with an injury could not be intensified by anything the surgeon did and therefore could not be relieved by him. The ancient Greeks suggested that pressure on the carotid arteries (Karoun = to plunge into sleep) caused unconsciousness. Paul of Aegina (625-690 A.D.) advised stuffing the patient's ears with wool. Theodoric, a surgeon from Bologna in the 13th century described a sporific sponge of opium, unripe mulberry, hyoscyamus, hemlock, mandragora, wood ivy, and dock and water hemlock seeds. However, the surgeon himself apparently had little faith in his concoction and advised that the patient be firmly tied down.

Throughout the middle ages little reference is made to anesthesia because pain is mentioned so frequently in religious teachings and is envisioned somewhat akin to a "noble" state. Rather, theologic doctrine held that pain serves God's purpose and should not be alleviated.

And so it was difficult even with the dawning of anesthesia in the 19th century to generally realise the potential for surgical advance. Dr. John Erichsen from University College Hospital in London wrote in his textbook "The Science and Art of Surgery" in 1869 - "The employment of anaesthetics in surgery is undoubtedly one of the greatest bonus even conferred upon mankind ... Anaesthesia is not, however, an unmixed good ... We cannot purchase immunity from suffering without incurring a certain degree of danger ... many of the deaths that have followed the inhalation of anaesthetics have resulted from want of knowledge or of due care on the part of the administrators."

However, over the past 200 years it is interesting and even comical to see how some strange developments, often heralded as major anaesthetic advances, either did not work or caused such major complications that successful surgery was not possible.

Mesmerism

Heralded as the „last of the magicians" Franz Friedrich Anton Mesmer a sometime student of divinity, law and medicine claimed the power of working miracles with his "vital energy". Born in Germany in 1734, Mesmer was educated mainly at the University in Vienna where he lived affluently, counting such court figures as Mozart, Gluck and Hayden among his friends. Through his association with a Jesuit priest, Pater Hell who was professor of astronomy at the University, Mesmer became convinced that the lodestone was useful in the treatment of certain ailments. He believed that the magnet could attract human ills as it attracted iron. After much experimentation, be applied his

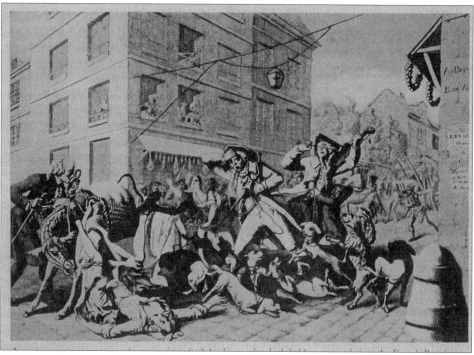

Fig. 1

theories to patients and apparently had some miraculous cures by placing 2 magnets in contact with the body. He was lauded by the Augsburg Academy in 1776 and was made a member of the Academy of Science of Electoral Bavaria. However, the medical profession was less convinced and withheld its recognition. He left Vienna for Paris in 1778 where his animal magnetism continued to cause controversy. He built a wooden tub (boquet) with a double series of charged bottles that converged upon a steel rod from which conductors extended to the painful or afflicted part of the body. He devised other means of mass healing including magnetizing mirrors, wash basins, gardens, parks and even whole forests. When Lafayette went to America at the end of the 18th century he told Washington that, besides munitions of war, he was bringing the United States a most important gift known as mesmerism, "a marvellous weapon against illness and pain." Despite Mesmer's enormous popularity, most physicians in France refused to acknowledge his claims as scientific. King Louis XVI persuaded the Medical Society to hold an enquiry. A committee was appointed that included Guillotin, Benjamin Franklin, Lavoisier (the chemist) and Jussieux (the botanist) to investigate animal magnetism. The commission concluded that Mesmer's activities were inexplicable and not devoid of value but science could not approve what it could not explain. Mesmer retired to Lake Constance where he died in 1815.

One of his disciples, Count Maxime de Puységer of Busancy had a lime tree magnetised in his park by Mesmer. Peasants came to it regularly for cures of whatever ailed them. On one occasion, a 23 year old man had been tied to the tree. The Count in an attempt to increase the magnetic influence of

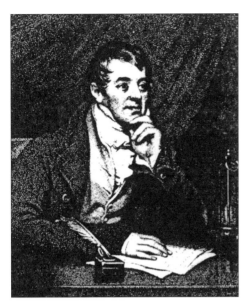

Fig. 2: Sir Humphrey Davy (1778-1829) recognized the analgesic properties of nitrous oxide but failed to understand significance of exhaled carbon dioxide.

the tree, passed his hands over the body. A hypnotic trance was induced in the young man. Puységer repeated the process on many other individuals before he made his disco

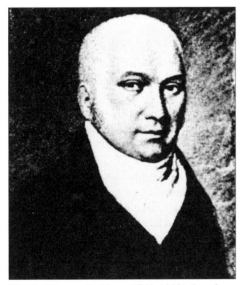

Fig. 3: Thomas Beddoes (1760-1808), founder of the Pneumatic Institute.

very of this state of unawareness known. Baron de Potel, a surgeon and one of his friends, tried the technique for painless operations. His example was followed by Récamier in France and by Jules Cloquet who performed a mastectomy on April 12, 1829. Somnambulism was born and heralded as a new era for surgery.

In the same year, 1829, John Elliotson became interested in mesmerism through the influence of Chenevix who has practised in Paris and later given demonstrations in London. At Elliotson's invitation, the latter attended St. Thomas's Hospital. Some years later, in 1837, Dupotet who had long used mesmerism in Paris also came to London and influenced Elliotson to adopt the technique. Elliotson was a very prominent physician in England - being the first Professor of the Practice of Medicine at the new University of London and senior physician at the College Hospital. He was instrumental in introducing the stethoscope and was known for his progressive attitude. Thus, when he promoted this practice, much attention was paid to his opinions. His demonstrations attended by such notables as Charles Dickins and Thomas Moore were, however, attacked as „humbug". By the end of 1838, a resolution was passed by the Council of University College forbidding the further practice of mesmerism. Elliotson who continued to passionately believe in the practice resigned. In 1843, he started a journal – the Zoist: A Journal of Cerebral Physiology and Mesmerism and their Application to Human Wellfare. The publication lated for 12 years and covered such issues as mesmerism, phrenology and a host of social problems. Many reports of numerous operations performed painlessly during a trance appeared in the Zoist. Elliotson's „anaesthetic" technique was very involved and required that the subject rest in a dark room for about an hour while he made passes over the body and breathed on the vertex of the patient's head.

An ardent follower of Elliotson, James Esdaile, also from Edinburgh, was another strong believer in mesmerism as an anesthetic. While in charge of the Native Hospital at Hooghly, India, Esdaile reported 73 painless surgical operations in January 1846 with the aid of mesmerism. When the Zoist reported on the successful use of ether 10 months later, Esdaile used the agent also in Calcutta. He wrote, "By cautious and graduated doses and with a knowledge of the best antidotes, I think it is extremely probable that this power will soon become a safe means of procuring insensibility for the most formidable surgical operations even. All mesmerists – will rejoice at having been the means of bringing to light one truth more, especially as it will free them from the drudgery required to induce mesmeric insensibility to pain." And so apparently, Esdaile not only realised but was prepared to admit that mesmerism was not always conveniently successful.

Nevertheless, during his 6 year tour in India, Esdaile, according to his reports, performed some 7,000 operations under mesmerism. On his return to Scotland, the local clientele appeared to be less amenable subjects. Attempts to achieve similar pain free surgery by Strohmeyer in Vienna, Auguste Nélaton in France and John Collins Warren in Boston all failed.

One last variation in mesmerism in anaesthesia came about later, during the 1840's. Jame Braid, an Edinburgh surgeon, while interested in mesmerism, did not ascribe to the theory of animal magnetism. In his "Neurpnology or the Rationale of Nervous Sleep" he described how the mesmeric phenomena could be due to suggestion and substituted the term, "hypnotism".

Nevertheless mesmerism was a widespread cult, persued by many important and far thinking individuals. Although a misleading development in that claims were made that were only sporadically realised, the technique did indicate that painless surgery could be achieved - a belief that until the middle of the 19th century was not realised.

Pneumatic Medicine

It is obvious today that anaesthesia may be achieved by the inhalation of gases or vapors. For centuries, men have believed that ailments may be cured and pain relieved by breathing something. The question was „what" ? The pioneer who discovered carbonic acid, oxygen (1771) and nitrous oxide (1772) was Joseph Priestley - a dissenting Unitarian minister who was forced to leave England for America in 1794 because of his sympathies for the French Revolution. He believed that the inhalation of oxygen might be beneficial for diseases of the lungs - a suggestion that led members of the medical profession and others to develop "pneumatic medicine". This treatment fad promoted the inhalation of not only oxygen but also hydrogen and nitrogen as a cure for asthma, tuberculosis, paralysis, scurvy, hysteria and cancer among other diseases. One American physician, Lantham Mitchell, used nitrous oxide in animals. As they all died, he assumed it was a very poisonous gas and believed that it was the contagion for the spread of epidemics. As a prominent figure and doctor, his reports were accepted without disagreement and for years no-one dared to inhale nitrous oxide. However in 1795 Humphrey Davy, then aged 17, and apprenticed to John Bingham Bolase, a surgeon in Penzance tried the gas. By inhalation, after he had dipped his finger in it and had suffered no ill effects, he felt many pleasurable sensations including relaxation, an acuity of hearing and a desire to laugh. Later he used the inhalation of nitrous oxide to relieve the pain he suffered when he cut his wisdom teeth. In his book,

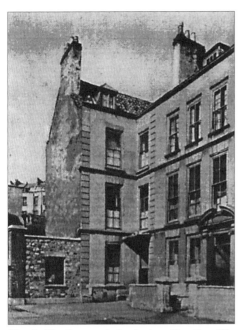

Fig. 4: The Pneumatic Institution. Nos. 6 and 7 Dowry Square in 1948.

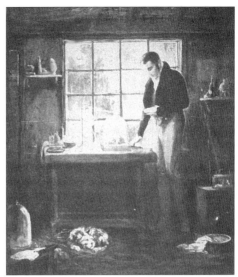

Fig. 5: Henry Hill Hickman experimenting with anesthesia on animals (From an oil painting in the Wellcome Historical Medical Museum)

"Medical Vapors" he wrote later - "As nitrous oxide in its extensive operation appears capable of destroying physical pain, it may be used with advantage during surgical operations in which no great effusion of blood takes place."

Unfortunately Davy made rather too much use of nitrous oxide. He and later his master, Bolase, inhaled it rather frequently and afterwards tended to patients with more merriment than the latter felt to be appropriate. The town of Penzance began to complain of the "devilish gas". A visitor to the town, Dr. Giddy, later to become president of the Royal Society, heard of Davy and recommended him to Beddoes at Bristol. Beddoes invited Davy to become superintendent of his Penumatic Institute at Clifton in 1799. Dr. Beddoes was one of the first to devote himself to making available for medical use the gases discovered by Priestley. The Institute was founded "for the treatment of disease by inhalation". A 10-bed hospital and out patient department were attached. However, it was noted that several patients who inhaled the gases became bradycardic and giddy; many did not get better; some charges of improprieties regarding young ladies were raised.

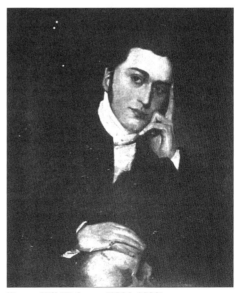

Henry Hill Hickman (1800-1830)

315

The Institute fell into dispute. But not before Davy's 580 page treatise "Researches ... concerning Nitrous Oxide" was written (at that time he was 21) including drawings of his gas machine. Although brilliant and so much before his time in so many areas, Davy made one large error.

"Of respirable gases ... one only has the power of uniformly support life; atmospheric air. Some as nitrogen and hydrogen, effect no positive change in the venous blood. Animals immersed in these gases die of a disease produced by privation of atmospheric air. Oxygen...finally destroys life."

Had he devised a means to supply imprisoned animals with oxygen and remove carbon dioxide his findings would have been more extensive. Instead post mortem findings on all animals showed a pattern which led Davy to the conclusion that the lungs of animals destroyed by nitrous oxide are the same as those destroyed by oxygen. Although he had confirmed the findings of Lavoisier that inspired air contained more oxygen and less carbon dioxide than expired air, he did not adopt this fact to his work and thus was delayed the implementation of a critical part of the anaesthetic puzzle for decades.

Another English physician, Henry Hill Hickman was very concerned about the pain of surgery. Born near Ludlow in 1800, he trained in medicine in Edinburgh before returning to practice in his home town. In 1824, he went to Shifnal, the birthplace of Beddoes where he may have learned of the pneumatic researches of the latter. Hickman conducted many experiments on administration of different gases to animals confined under glass domes. When they become unconscious (presumably from asphyxia) he operated on them in what was apparently a painfree state. Hickman tried repeatedly to get permission to try his experiments on humans but neither Davy nor his assistant Faraday would bring up the matter to a committee of the Royal Society. Hickman later petitioned Charles X of France to bring his proposals to the Royal Academy of Medicine.

At a meeting of the Academy on December 28, 1828, the leaders of French medicine declared that "Operate under laughing gas ... it would be nothing but a crime to expose a human being to such needless perils." Only Baron Dominque Larrey, army surgeon to Napoleon voted against the others noting that he "would be willing for Mr. Hickman to administer laughing gas to me and see what would happen."

Defeated Hickman returned to Shiffnal. He died prematurely on April 5, 1830, age 29. Thus the early 19th century medical authorities of both the United Kingdom and France may be held liable for delaying discovery of surgical anesthesia and advancing surgery for some 20 years.

Rather, other techniques to relieve operative pain were described. In 1846, Dr. J. F. Malgaigne of the Faculté de Médicine in Paris wrote a Manual of Operative Surgery. A chapter on means to dimish pain includes the use of narcotics, mesmerism, cutting the nerve supply to the area or excessive venesection. Malgaigne also relied on James Moore's experiments using a Dupuyten compressor to exert sufficient pressure to damage a nerve and render the incised area anaesthetic.

Inhalation Anesthesia after 1846

The introduction of inhalation anesthesia in 1849 did not automatically make surgery safe and reliable. Indeed the number of surgical deaths rose sharply in the 19th century for several reasons. Procedures were attempted on patients who would have otherwise died; potent agents were given without any ability to control dosages; hypoxic mixtures were the rule; training in anaesthe

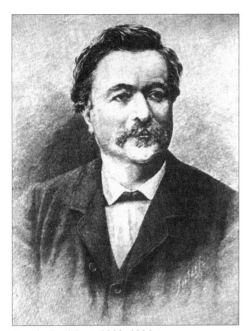

Fig. 6: Paul Bert (1833–1886)

tics was almost non-existent; muscles were often cut hampering recovery and the germ theory was not widely accepted. Over one third of John Snow's text on chloroform published in 1858 is devoted to the complications of its administration.

Nitrous oxide although considered inert was the cause of many deaths. The dentist Colten, had re-established the popularity of the gas for dental extractions in the 1860's. His method consisted of breathing the gas until unconsciousness supervened and then removing the mouth piece and quickly extracting the teeth. When others tried to extend the inhalation and push for longer periods of unconsciousness sudden death was not uncommon - especially in healthy individuals. In 1868, Edmond Andrews, the Chicago surgeon, advised the use of oxygen with nitrous oxide but little attention was paid to his suggestion. By 1924 Gwathmey advised against the use of nitrous oxide altogether and in 1939, Dr. C.B. Courville published an entire book related to the untoward effects of nitrous oxide - mainly those of anoxia.

Paul Bert tried to solve the problem of nitrous oxide anaesthesia (i.e. to allow the gas to induce anaesthesia in something other than a hypoxic mixture). During the 1880's he constructed a special tank, large enough to include the operating table with patient and staff in which he could increase the atmospheric pressure. The idea sounded feasible but did not work. Apart from being cumbersome and very expensive, those inside were subject to the „bends" on decompression.

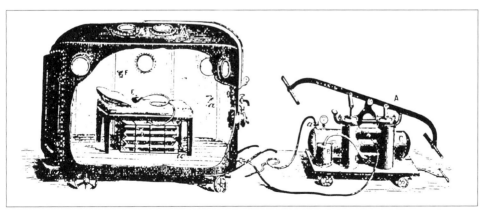

Fig. 7: An ambulatory adaption of Paul Bert's chamber allowed the administration of nitrous oxide at 2 atmospheres.

By the middle of the 20th century, ether and cyclopropane were widely used. However, they were both explosive. The electrocautery had been introduced to coagulate vessels. The danger to patients and practitioners was not inconsiderable.

Woodbridge in the United States gave an explosion rate of 2-4/100,000 anaesthetics. Pinson, in 1930, stated that about 100 cases of burns due to ether fires or explosions occurred annually in Great Britan. However, the incidence was undoubtedly much higher as unless a patient or staff were killed or badly burned, a report was probably not made. (Similar to under reporting). Before the use of conductive rubber materials, static electricity was considered most dangerous especially during cyclopropane anaesthesia. Ether at 4% concentration required a 45 times greater spark energy to ignite then did cyclopropane.

To provide a „non-explosive" ether, especially during neurosurgical procedures when surgeons demanded that spontaneous respiratory patterns be monitored, Van Poznak and Artusio developed methoxyflurane. However this inhalation agent was metabolized up to 50%, caused renal damage and was extremely long acting. These two anesthesiologists then introduced teflurane - a non-explosive cyclopropane (i.e. very rapid action). Teflurane indeed caused an almost instant on and off anaesthetic. However, the incidence of intraoperative ventricular tachycardia and fibrillation was extremely high and further trials with the agent were abandoned.

Acupuncture Anaesthesia

After the establishment of the People's Republic of China in 1949, traditional Chinese medicine, which had fallen into disrepute by the 2nd half of the nineteenth century and which was officially banned during the 1st half of the 20th century received new attention.

Some Chinese physicians considered whether acupuncture, long used to treat pain could prevent pain. A technique of "acupuncture anaesthesia" was developed. The first reported use of acupuncture instead of anaesthesia took place in China in 1958. The operation was a dental extraction. The technique was used sporadically from 1958 to 1968. Then with the Cultural Revolution and succession of Chairman Mao in 1966, reports indicated successful use of acupuncture anaesthesia in over 1/2 million cases. Despite this impressive figure, Dr. John Bonica estimated the total number of cases performed under acupuncture anaesthesia to be less than 1%.

In 1971, New York Times reporters, James Reston and Seymor and Audrey Topping visited China and witnessed surgery performed under acupuncture anaesthesia. Their stories generated a great deal of interest and speculation in the West. Several studies were undertaken as the idea of a drug free anaesthetic state - more reliably induced than by hypnosis - was appealing to many patients and physicians. By the early 1980's after many failed attempts, it was apparent that acupuncture was ineffective for surgical purposes, certainly in Western Countries.

Anaesthesia continues to develop in fits and starts. Alleviation of pain and hence the ability to perform more and increasingly complex surgical procedures has not taken a straight path. However, the safety of our drugs today, the reliability of our delivery and monitoring systems, the level of our training gives credence to the statement ...

"If the patient can withstand the surgical procedure, he can do so more safely under anaesthesia."

Further Reading

1. The Edwin Smith Papyrus: in Breated G.H. (trans ed.): University of Chicago Institute Pub., Chicago, University of Chicago Press, 1930
2. Paul of Aegina. The Seven Books of Paulos Aeginata (3 volumes). Adam F (trans.) London, Sydenham Society, 1844
3. Raper HR: Man against Pain. Prentice Hall, New York 1945
4. Erichsen JE: Science and Art of Surgery. Henry C. Lea, Philadephia 1869
5. Cartwright FF: The English Pioneers of Anaesthesia (Beddoes, Davy, Hickman). John Wright and Sons, Bristol 1952
6. Davy H: Researches, Chemical and Philosophical chiefly concerning Nitrous Oxide or dephagisticated nitrous air and its respiration. London printed for J Johnson by Biggs and Cottle, Bristol, 1800. Printed in Great Britain in Facsimile by Butterworth & Co., 1972
7. Snow J: On Chloroform and other Anaesthetics. John Churchill, London 1858
8. Robinson V: Victory over Pain. Henry Schuman, New York 1946
9. Fülop-Miller R: Triumph over Pain. Bobbs-Merrill Co., Indianapolis 1938
10. Keys TE: The History of Surgical Anesthesia. Henry Schuman, New York 1945
11. Bert P: Ser la possibilité d'obtenir, à l'aide du protoxyde d'azote, une mis-ensibilité de long durée et scev l'innocuité de cet anesthésique. Compt. Rend. Acad. d. sc. 87:728-730, 1878
12. Courville CB: Untoward Effects of Nitrous Oxide Anesthesia. Pacific Press Pub. Assoc. Mountain View, California 1939
13. Keating V. Anaesthetic Accidents. The Year Book Publishers, One. Chicago 1956
14. Robbins BH: Cyclopropane Anesthesia. The Williams & Wilkins Co., Baltimore 1940
15. Acupuncture Anesthesia Monograph, presented by Roerig from the film "Acupuncture Anaesthesia", produced by the Shanghi Film Studio - The People's Republic of China.
16. Frost E, Hsu CY, Sadowsky D. Acupuncture therapy, comparative values in acute and chronic pain. NY State J Med 76:5:695-697, 1976

Albert Niemann and Cocaine Research in Goettingen

U. Braun and Th. Riedl
Department of Anesthesiology, Emergency- and Intensive Care Medicine
Georg August University of Goettingen, Germany

Introduction

The University of Goettingen has been founded in 1737 by Georg August of Hannover, also known as King George II of England. This was the place where Albert Niemann isolated cocaine from the coca leaves in 1860. This presentation is an excerpt from the doctoral thesis of Thomas Riedl carrying the same title (4).

The Life of Albert Niemann

Albert Niemann was born on May 20th, 1834 in Goslar/Harz. This city is located about 50 km north-east of Goettingen at the northern border of the mountain site Harz in central Germany. Goettingen can be found 120 km south of Hannover. The father of Albert Niemann was the local school headmaster. A picture (Fig. 1) shows the grammar school in Goslar at that time, when Albert Niemann was born and where his family lived. There were four brothers and one sister in the family, of which Albert was the youngest son. He attended the grammar school in Goslar and started an apprenticeship at a pharmacy in Goettingen in 1849. The building

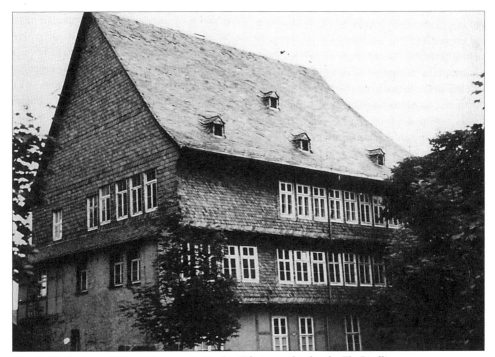

Fig. 1: Birth place of Albert Niemann in Goslar (Photograph taken by Th. Riedl)

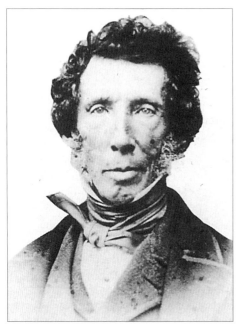

Fig. 2: Photograph of Friedrich W. Woehler

holding this pharmacy still exists (Rathsapotheke, at the town hall square, center of the old town). At the age of eighteen years in the summer of 1852 he matriculated as a student of pharmaceutics, which was a discipline of the philosophical faculty. Among others he heard lectures of Professor Friedrich W. Woehler. He continued his career in pharmacy in Hannover as an assistent pharmacist in 1853 to get prepared for his examination in pharmacy, which he took in 1858. He joined the university again in the same year in Goettingen and built up a close contact with Friedrich Woehler. The young student Albert Niemann was then instructed by his teacher to carry out the following two investigations:
1. The chemical reaction of sulfur chloride (S_2Cl_2) with Ethylene (C_2H_4). This reaction generates mustard gas, a compound not known at the time of the investigation. It was used as a chemical weapon later in World War I.
2. The isolation of the chemical compound of the coca leaves.

Albert Niemann must have become intoxicated by the mustard gas, inhaling the substance during the early experiments. He died on January 24th, 1861 at home in Goslar at the age of 26 years from pneumonia. He successfully conducted the experiments with the coca leaves after having been contaminated. Looking back, he has to be considered an early victim of scientific research and probably as the first fatal case following an intoxication with mustard gas.

Friedrich Wilhelm Woehler

The famous scientist Friedrich W. Woehler was born in 1800 and expired at the age of 82 years (Fig 2.). He was a professor of the philosophical faculty and occupied the chair of chemistry and pharmaceutics from 1836 until his death. His fame was rooted in original scientific work in different areas of chemistry and pharmaceutics. He was able to isolate pure aluminium (1827) and synthesized urea (1828). On top of this he worked on metals and was the first to describe isomerism and radicals. He conducted successful investigations on silicium, organic chemistry and bases of opium. In his laboratory, cocaine was isolated. Justus von Liebig, another famous German chemist, described his friend Woehler in a letter to him: "In your work you look to me like the man from an Indian fairy tale. Bouquets of flowers kept pouring from his mouth when he laughed". The reason that made Woehler instruct Niemann to work on the isolation of the chemical compound of the coca leaves was, that his investigations on the chemical reaction of sulfur chloride and ethylene had been very successful.

Isolation of Alkaloids

Friedrich Wilhelm Sertuerner, a pharmacist from Paderborn, was the first to isolate morphine from opium in 1804. He published his results in 1806, mentioning the induction of sleep after the administration of morphine and describing the alkaline character of the substance, though this early work remained unnoticed. A more detailed paper was published in 1817. At the same time Pelletier and Magendie were able to isolated emetine. Pelletier and Caventou separated strychnine in 1818. Runge isolated caffeine (1819), Posselt and Reimann nicotine (1828) and Lorenz atropine (1831). Many more alkaloids were discovered in the following years. Alkaloid chemistry was based on sound chemical methods in 1860, but still every new discovery lead to excitement.

Cocaine

In September 1859 Dr. Karl Scherzer, who had been on an expedition to Lima, supplied Woehler with a great number of coca leaves. This expedition had been organized by W. Haidinger, a mineralogist and zoologist from Vienna. Since Woehler himself could not do the work due to loads of duties, he asked Niemann to perform the investigations.

Albert Niemann sat the coca leaves in 85% alcohol, containing 1/50 of sulphuric acid. The percolate was treated with milk of lime and neutralized by sulfuric acid. The alcohol was then removed by distillation, leaving a syrupy mass, from which resin was separated by water. The liquid, which was then treated with carbonate of soda to precipitate alkaloid, smelled like nicotine. A substance was deposited, which was extracted by repeated shaking with ether, in which it was dissolved and from which it was regained by distillation. The net gain was 0,25% of alkaloid. The yellowish brown mass with the unbearable smell was then mixed with the substance. It could be removed by repeated washings in alcohol. The colourless crystals were made of the alkloid in form of it's sulfuric salt.

Albert Niemann named the substance "Coca-in", the substance within the plant (english: "cocaine". The structural formula, that he found ($C_{16}H_{20}NO_4$), was not correct as could be proven in the same laboratory by Lossen (1). Cocaine was then supposed to be composed as $C_{17}H_{21}NO_4$. Niemann observed, that there was a peculiar numbness of the tongue when it was brought into contact with cocaine. He mentioned this observation in his thesis.

History of Cocaine

Lossen, who had corrected the structural formula of cocaine also improved the procedure for isolating the substance from it's leaves. With his improved method the hydrochloric salt of the alkaloid was separated from the leaves in 1862. The Merck-company in Darmstadt manufactured some cocaine the same year although it was not known at the time, if the substance carried any therapeutic value. Schroff from Vienna observed, that the skin was insensitive to painful stimuli under the influence of cocaine (1862). Von Anrep in Wuerzburg performed a subcutaneous injection with a cocaine solution into the skin of his forearm. He experienced a feeling of local warmth and an insensitivity to pin prick stimuli (1879). In 1884 the young Sigmund Freud from Vienna wrote a famous article about coca, including all of the available information (5). He took some cocaine himself without becoming addicted and applied the alkaloid in some of his patients for different reasons like general stimulation and morphine withdrawal. He contacted his colleague Koenigstein at the department of ophthalmology in order to administer cocaine to patients suffering from an infection of the eye to achieve relief of pain. Everybody was pleased when they learned that this procedure worked. At the same time and in the same clinical institution, Carl Koller observed a well defined local anaesthetic effect of the cornea and conjunctiva in animals and patients. He presented his data in Heidelberg on September 15th, 1884, which was the birth of local anaesthesia.

The Picture of Albert Niemann

Albert Niemann is almost unknown in the medical literature. He and his discovery are mentioned in the famous book of W. G. Mortimer (2) about the "History of Coca". There is also a picture of A. Niemann (Fig. 3). It shows a man at the age of approximately 50 years. It is very unlikely that this photograph shows Niemann, since he died at the age of 26 years. W.G. Mortimer must have visited the copperplate section of the Bibliothèque Nationale in Paris, France. There are two signatures "Albert Niemann" one with the index "chanteur allemand" (German singer), the other without any additional remark. Having evolved from a mistake of the bibliothèque nationale, both signatures apply to the same person, the court opera singer A. Niemann. So Mortimer mistook the singer to be the same person who discovered cocaine. A picture of Albert Niemann the scientist does not exist.

Conclusions

The alkaloid cocaine was isolated by Albert Niemann in the laboratory of Friedrich W. Woehler at the University of Goettingen in 1860. At this time chemical science was flourishing in Germany and some alkaloids had already been separated from plants, leading to a growth in the knowledge about chemical substances and reactions. Albert Niemann died at the age of 26 years after he

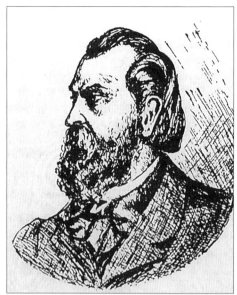

Fig. 3: Reproduction of Albert Niemann showing the court opera singer instead of the scientist (from WG Mortimer, 2)

had been intoxicated with mustard gas, which he had generated during an earlier investigation. The toxic effect of the substance was unknown and there were no safety precautions. Albert Niemann was a victim of scientific work and his death may be considered to be the first person poisoned with mustard gas, which was later used as a chemical weapon. The therapeutic value of cocaine became obvious only after it had been manufactured, after some clinical observations with the new drug had been made, and because of the intervention of the young Sigmund Freud in 1884, when Carl Koller discovered the local anesthetic effect. The isolation of cocaine was not only a mile stone in the evlution of local anesthesia, but also a major step towards widespread misuse of the drug.

References:

[1] Lossen W : Ueber das Cocain. Phil. Diss. Goettingen 1862

[2] Mortimer WG: History of Coca, the Devine Plant of the Incas. J.H. Vail-Press New York 1901, reprint AMS Press, New York 1978

[3] Niemann A: Ueber eine neue organische Base in den Cocablaettern. Phil. Diss. Goettingen 1860a

[4] Riedl Th: Albert Niemann und die Kokainforschung in Goettingen. Diss. FB Medizin, Goettingen 1989

[5] Freud S: Ueber Coca. Centralblatt fuer die gesamte Therapie (Wien), August 1884, p 289-314

Spinal Block for Surgery above the Diaphragm

R. Atkinson, Southend General, U.K.

In 1998 it will be 100 years since the first clinical use of spinal anaesthesia. For many years after that general anaesthesia was relatively primitive. Deep anaesthesia was considered harmful for sick patients and the alternative of spinal block using a local agent which did not itself affect consciousness appealed to surgeons who had to work on patients with systematic disease and often without specialised anaesthetist help.

Theoretically spinal block could extend as high as the first cervical segment, which would cover much of the scalp. In practice, however, there was the danger of causing paralysis of the phrenic nerves. The intercostal nerves would be already paralysed and spontaneous respiration would crease.

It was in the field of thoracic surgery that spinal techniques had an appeal. Before the introduction of controlled respiration with cyclopropane and muscle relaxant drugs the pressure chambers advocated by men like Sauerbruch seemed a possible way of preventing lung collapse. Spinal methods did not prevent lung collapse, but they did obviate the need for deep general anaesthesia and allowed the conscious patient, often with copious sputum to maintain his cough reflexes. Tuberculosis, before the days of chemotherapy, was a major problem and surgery in the nature of thoracoplasty and lung resection and some success was obtained with the help of spinal methods.

High spinal block for thoracic surgery was carried out in North America by Shields of Toronto. Morphine gr 1/4 and nembutal gr 3 were given preoperatively. The patient lay on the affected side and about 200 mg of procaine dissolved in 10 ml spinal fluid was injected in the lumbar region for thoracoplasty and up to 300 mg for intrathoracic surgery. Operating time was short, of the order of 45 to 60 minutes for thoracoplasty with the smaller doses, and up to twice this when bigger doses were used. An intravenous saline infusion was set up in the long saphenous vein. If analgesia was inadequate, intercostal block was carried out. The observations made showed that analgesia of the entire body surface did not occur and was inadequate in 20% in a series of 39 cases. Severe dyspnoea or air hunger was not prominent factor and there was no real evidence of phrenic involvement. Circulatory depression was no greater than that encountered in upper abdominal surgery and there was an almost complete absence of vomiting on the table. A disadvantage was that the patient had to be turned before surgery could begin.

"Light" spinal analgesia with percaine was also used. A dose not exceeding 15 ml 1 in 1,500 percaine was injected with the patient in the ventral position with the upper dorsal vertebrae at the highest point. After 6 minutes to secure bilateral sensory block the patient was positioned for surgery. The Etherington-Wilson technique was also used with the patient sitting for 55 to 60 seconds after the spinal injection of 15-17 ml.

In England, Hewer employed unilateral spinal block with the patient lying on his sound side with the highest point at the level of D5. About 10 ml in 1,500 percaine was injected. Hewer found that motor and sensory block was more or less confined to the affect side. The patient did not have to be moved before surgery, fall in blood pressure was not so marked, while coughing was more effective as there was less motor paralysis. Analgesia lasted from 1 and a half to 3 hours. However, he emphasised that safety margins were low. The patient's position must be correct. Oxygen or helium-oxygen were to be given if any respiratory embarrassment occurred. Ephedrine should be available to treat excessive blood pressure falls.

On a personal note, I would add that I have been present, as a junior doctor, when the surgeon demanded high spinal block before thyroidectomy. In the early days there was little preoperative treatment for thyrotoxicosis other than Lugol's iodine. High spinal block allowed light supplementary general anaesthesia while providing sympathetic block with a slowing of the pulse rate.

Another experience of my junior days was the use of large volumes of dilute lignocaine for paravertabral block combined with modified cervical plexus block for thoracoplasty. Some of the lignocaine solution must have occupied the extradural space. One day I saw a senior colleague insert the needle in the cervical region. Cerebrospinal fluid dripped out from the needle end. The result was that in minutes the patient lost consciousness and stopped breathing. Immediate ventilation of the lungs with oxygen quickly restored the situation and the patient recovered consciousness and spontaneous respiration within about 20 minutes. Once calm had been restored the operation was commenced, the surgeon remarking on the excellent surgical field!

References:

[1] Shields H J: Spinal Anaesthesia in Thoracic Surgery. Anesthesia and Analgesia 1935; 14: 193-198

[2] Hewer C L: Recent Advances in Anaesthesia and Analgesia. 3rd edition Churchill, London, 1939

Ryszard Rodziński – a Pioneer of Combined Spinal-Epidural Analgesia (CSE)

K. Duda, A. Kubisz,* M. Ziętkiewicz
Surgical Intensive Care Unit, Institute of Oncology, Cracow.
* Department of Anesthesiology and Intensive Care.,
  Collegium Medicum, Jagiellonian University, Cracow, Poland.

Substitution of toxic cocaine with less toxic novocaine at the beginning of the 20th century was an important cause of the development of local anesthesia (Fig. 1). Another theoretical support for this method of anesthesia was the term "a-noci-association" introduced by Crile in 1911[1,2]. It means, that the central nervous system is protected against surgical trauma not only by general anesthesia, but primarily by blocking the conductivity from injured tissues by local analgetic agents[1,2,3,4].

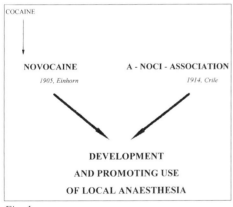

Fig. 1

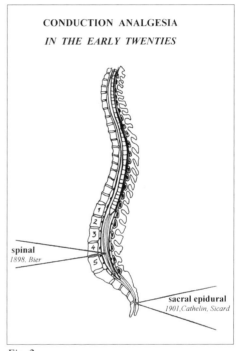

Fig. 2

In the early twenties conduction analgesia used for operations on body regions below the umbilical line was either spinal analgesia (introduced into clinical practice by Bier in 1898), or epidural sacral analgesia (Cathelin and Sicard, 1901). Epidural analgesia from lumbar access was unknown (Fig. 2).

Both methods of analgesia involved many dangers and side effects. Statistics concerning patients anesthetized spinally showed a higher mortality rate as compared to general anesthesia, an average ratio was 1:2500 in comparison with 1:6000[6]. Persistent headaches associated with the loss of the cerebrospinal fluid was the reason to search for new procedures, like epidural anesthesia. The effectiveness of sacral epidural analgesia was insufficient in operations on lower abdomen. This insufficiency was due to:

1) usual doses 30-40 ml of 1% Novocain practically caused a saddle block

329

2) administering of 60-80 ml and even up to 100 ml of 1% Novocain often caused toxic effects (Fig. 3).

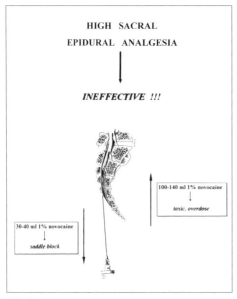

Fig. 3

Arthur Läwen, a disciple of H. Braun and F. Trendelenburg warned against administration of so called "high" sacral analgesia and exceeding the dose of 30-40 ml of 1% novocaine[6]. A Polish surgeon from Lvov - R. Rodziński in his paper entitled: "On local anesthesia" presented at 18th Meeting of Polish Surgeons in Warsaw (3-5 October, 1921) considered the problem why sacral epidural analgesia was ineffective in abdominal operations[7]. He tried to explain the difficulties of analgesia above the navel line mechanically:
1) by compression of dura mater sac and such dislocation of cerebrospinal fluid "... which does not allow sufficient spread upwords of the injected fluid ..." and
2) "... in the upper regions of supraspinal cavity (= epidural) a nerve radicle segment, which should be affected by the novocaine, is too short and covered by a so thick dura mater sleeve, that novocaine is unable to impregnate it ...".

While trying to widen the range of sacral analgesia according to his own theory of the pressure changes in the vertebral canal, Rodziński let off 15 ml of cerebrospinal fluid. This procedure was only partly successful. He tried four times to administer lumbar epidural bloc, as "having practised on cadavers the way of access to supraspinal cavity on any level, I was able to introduce the fluid on the level of 7th vertebra ...". Unfortunately, the trials proved a failure[7].

At the 19th Meeting of Polish Surgeons (29-30 June and 1 July, 1922) in Warsaw, Rodziński presented his paper entitled: "On combined lumbosacral analgesia"[8] in which he described a combination of two types of conduction analgesia, used by the Lvov clinic since October 1921 during operations on lower extremities and hypogastrium (Fig. 4).

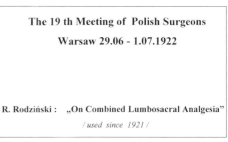

Fig. 4

The formula included:
- 3-4 ml of 1% novocaine administered spinally and
- 30-40 ml of 1% novocaine administered epidurally (via sacral route) (Fig. 5)

He valued this combination as much more effective in comparison to "high" epidural analgesia from the sacral access. Rodziński emphasized, that there is no need to use higher doses or concentrated solutions of novocaine, and that the cerebrospinal fluid must be

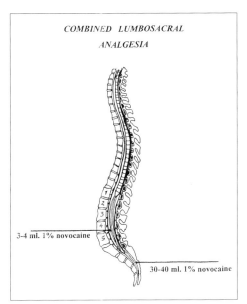

Fig. 5

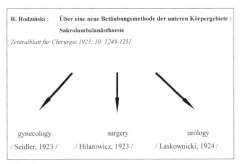

Fig. 6

prevented from leaking out, as it may cause headaches. In premedication, besides morphine he postulated the use of Veronal which acts protectively and enhances novocaine tolerance.

At the same time Rodziński and Tychowski conducted experiments (on cadavers, dogs and finally in 7 clinical cases) on the influence of supradural administration of 40-70 ml of fluid from the sacro-coccygeal access on cerebrospinal fluid pressure measured on L3-L4 level. A visible, increased CSF pressure lasting 4 to 8 minutes was observed[9].

After the publication of the modern technique "analgesia of lower body areas" in both Polish[7,8,10] and German[11] literature, Rodziński suggested testing it, also in the obstetric-gynecological clinic and later in general surgery and urology clinics in Lvov (Fig. 6).

In 1924 Laskownicki mentioned Rodziński technique among local anesthesia methods used in urologic operations on ureters and the bladder[12]. At the same time, while visiting Prof. Marion's clinic in Paris, he was surprised that in the country of origin sacral analgesia, the method was so rarely applied. In his article published in French[13] he presented his experiences concerning various types of analgesia used in urology. He writes, that to obtain sufficient anesthesia" ... we applied analgesia called sacrolumbar, as described in 1923 by Rodziński, an assistant at our clinic. It consists of subdural administration of a small dose of novocaine 1% (4 ml) and supradural administration of 40 ml of 1% novocaine, the method is devoid of all danger ...". Further he writes: "we always begin with spinal analgesia, because supradural administration (as shown by Rodziński on cadavers and animals) pushes proper dura mater from the vertebral arch and then it is difficult to find dura mater sac ...". The sequence of administration of local analgesic agents was interpreted differently and did not play so important role in the development and extent of the blockade as Rodziński had supposed[10]. He was afraid that the introduction of 40 ml of the fluid extraduraly would push out spinally administered analgesic into the upper regions of the spinal canal. However, one should appreciate the attempts at diminishing the risk of analgesia through a decrease in novocaine doses concentrations, and accurate descriptions of the method and detailed observation of the patients[7,8,9,10]. With the lack of information about spinal block pathophysiology, the influence of vascular diseases (atherosclerosis, diabetes mellitus) and with a standard doses of applied local analgesia, the statistics of complications naturally evoked particular caution.

R. Rodziński played a great role not only in investigating the methodology of the new local analgesia techniques and their combinations, but also perfecting them with respect to efficacy and safety.

A renaissance of the combination of both described analgesia methods was observed in 1981 with development of obstetrician anesthesia techniques, particularly for cesarean section (Fig. 7).

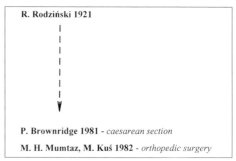

P. Brownridge 1981 - *caesarean section*
M. H. Mumtaz, M. Kuś 1982 - *orthopedic surgery*

Fig. 7

At present the most popular combination consists of spinal analgesia with continuous epidural analgesia with a simultaneous use of a catheter for postoperative analgesia.

References:

[1] Crile GW: Nitrous oxide anesthesia and a note on anociassociation, a new principle in operative surgery. Surg Gynec and Obstet 1911; 13: 170-173

[2] Crile GW: The kinetic theory of shock and its prevention through anoci-association (shockless operation), Lancet 1913; 11: 7-16

[3] Crile GW, Lower W.E.: Anociassociation Sannders, Philadelphia, 1914

[4] Labat GL: Regional short review of the general principles. Annals of Surgery 1921; 73: 165-169

[5] Katz J.: George Washington Crile, anoci-association and preemptive analgesia. Pain 1993; 54: 243-245

[6] Braun H, Läwen A: Die örtliche Betäubung, 9 Aufl. Johann Ambrosius Barth Verlag, Leipzig 1951

[7] Rodziński R: O znieczuleniu miejscowem. Polski Przegląd Chirurgiczny 1922, 1: 107-118

[8] Rodziński R: O kombinowanem znieczuleniu ledzwiowo-krzyzowem. Polski Przeglad Chirurgiczny 1923; 2: 39-47

[9] Rodziński R, Tychowski W: Badania doświadczalne nad znieczuleniem krzyzowem. Polska Gazeta Lekarska 1923, 2: 51-55

[10] Rodziński R: O nowym sposobie znieczulenia dolnych obszarow ciala. Polska Gazeta Lekarska 1923; 2: 296-299

[11] Rodziński R: Über eine neue Betäubungsmethode der unteren Körpergebiete: Sakrolumbalanästhesie. Zbl f Chir., 1923, 50: 1249-1251

[12] Laskownicki S: Znieczulenie miejscowe w urologii. Polska Gazeta Lekarska 1924; 3: 736-739

[13] Laskownicki S: Anesthésie épidurale et anesthésie sacrolumbaire en urologie. Journal d'Urolgie, 1926, 390-394

[14] Brownridge P: Epidural and subarachnoid analgesia for elective caesarean section. Anaesthesia 1981; 36: 70

[15] Duda K, Mizianty M: Łączona analgesia podpajęczynowkova z ciągłą zewnątrzoponową do dlugotrwalych operacji onkologicznych. Anestezja Intensywna Terapia, 1992, 24: 167-170

Martin Kirschner's "Spinal Zone Anaesthesia placed at Will and Dosage Individually Graded" Technique – Recent Importance

Ch. Weißer
Chirurgische Universitätsklinik Würzburg/Institut für Geschichte der Medizin, Würzburg, Germany

Martin Kirschner (1879-1942) (Fig. 1) was one of the outstanding German surgeons of the early 20th century. He had a great influence on all fields of surgery, as well as on anaesthesiological problems. Orthopedic surgeons for example are familiar with the "Kirschner wire" even today.

The most important mile stones in Martin Kirschner's life were the three surgical chairs he held at Koenigsberg, Tuebingen, and Heidelberg. Born on October 28th, 1879 in Breslau, he grew up in Berlin being the son of the mayor of the capital of Germany. From 1899 till 1904 he studied medicine at Freiburg, Zurich, Munich and Strasbourg, where he graduated with the degree of a medical doctor in 1904. After his fellowship in internal medicine and surgery in Berlin, Greifswald and Königsberg he became "Privatdozent" in 1911. In the time between 1916 and 1921 he worked as a professor in Koenigsberg, from 1928 until 1934 in Tuebingen, and in the period of 1934 to 1942 in Heidelberg. He died on August 30th,1942 in Heidelberg having suffered from gastric cancer.

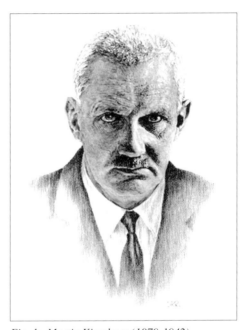

Fig. 1: Martin Kirschner (1879-1942)

Theoretical Aspects of Spinal Anaesthesia

Some important peculiarities of lumbar anaesthesia were criticized by Martin Kirschner. His objections towards the contemporary technique were based on the following reasons: 1. in order to obtain a sufficient degree of anaesthesia a great quantity of anaesthetic has to be injected; 2. a big part of the whole body is anaesthesized unnecessarily leading to a disturbance of the blood circulation; 3. in spite of a completely identical injection technique different effects could be observed on the examination of different individuals; 4. in some individuals the ascend of the anaesthetic came out of control.

As a means to improve the technique of spinal anaesthesia, he set the following stipulations: 1. the diffusion of the anaesthetic within the dural sack had to be limited; 2. a

333

DER CHIRURG

3. JAHRGANG 15. JULI 1931 HEFT 14

Eine gürtelförmige, einstellbare und individuell dosierbare Spinalbetäubung.

Von Prof. Dr. **Kirschner.**

Aus der Chirurgischen Universitätsklinik zu Tübingen. — (Direktor: Prof. Dr. *Kirschner.*)

A. Kritik der bisherigen Spinalanästhesie.

Die Unsicherheit und die üblen Zufälle der bisherigen Lumbalanästhesie finden in *grundsätzlichen Unvollkommenheiten* dieses Verfahrens ihre ausreichende Erklärung. Das Unzweckmäßige des üblichen Vorgehens liegt in folgendem:

1. Um den Liquor spinalis an einer *begrenzten* Stelle des Arachnoidalsackes in eine ausgekierten Weg, ohne das Steuer sicher in der Hand zu haben: die Schiffbrüche rechts und links bleiben daher nicht aus.

2. Aber auch wenn die soeben gekennzeichneten ungünstigen Ereignisse nicht eintreten, sind die Gefahren der heutigen Spinalanästhesie nicht erschöpft: Statt *allein das Operationsgebiet* zu betäuben, müssen wir *große Abschnitte des Körpers*, wo wir die

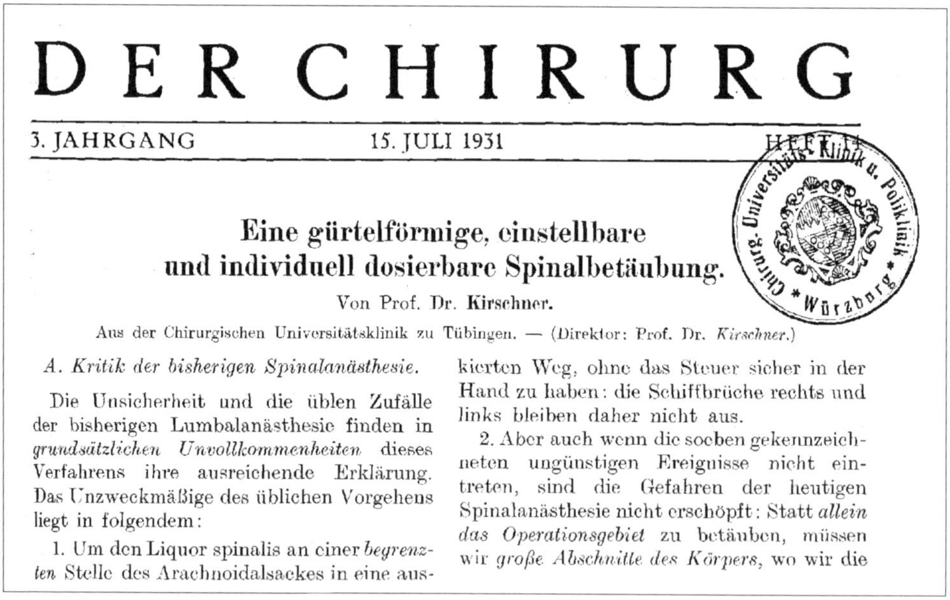

Fig. 2: Title-page of Kirschner`s paper of 1931

spread of the anaesthetic cranially had to be prevented; 3. the anesthesized segment ought to be at the desired level; 4. the dosage of anaesthetic ought to be adjusted as required.

Experimental Basis

Kirschner started his attempts to improve the technique of lumbar anaesthesia with theoretical considerations based on extensive experimental studies. The first task was to find an anaesthetic that would not blend with cerebrospinal fluid. In case of using an hypobaric anaesthetic, the drug would move to the highest position inside the dural sack thus getting out of control. Considering this, he had the idea to elevate the caudal part of the dural sack and to replace a big amount of CSF by air, in order for the anaesthetic to float on top of the CSF as a "plug".

He discovered that a mixture of Percain 0.125 g, Dextrin 0.90 g, alcohol (100 %) 11.60 g, aq. dest. ad 100.00 ml provided the most suitable properties for this "plug". This mixture had a specific gravity of 986,65, did not blend with cerebrospinal fluid, and remained in situ, if it was injected into a bubble of air placed above the surface of the CSF.

The closed end of the glass tube model (Fig. 3) represents the spinal canal, and the open cone for pressure compensation serves as the cerebral liquor space. A lateral rubber

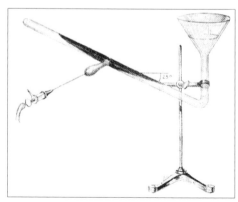

Fig. 3: Glass tube model of the spinal and cerebral liquor space: spread of hypobaric anaesthetic without insufflating air [3]

cap allowes the "puncture" of the glass tube filled with cerebrospinal fluid. For the investigation of the distribution of the anaesthetic, Kirschner created a simple, but very efficient model of the spinal and cerebral fluid space.

Kirschner tested his experimental results in vivo by medullographic studies: insufflating air (10/20/30 ml) made a swimming contrast medium "plug" move upwards. This could be observed using X-rays. The airbubble inside the dural sack is essential for moving the "plug".

Technical Reflections

In order to be able to employ this mode of anaesthesia, Kirschner developed specific instruments. The puncture and injection cannula (Fig. 4) designed for lumbar puncture is oblique closed at its tip and opened to one side. The idea of this shape based on the consideration, not to punch out a cylinder of tissue and to be able to inject the anaesthetic towards the desired direction.

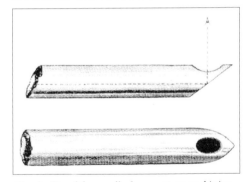

Fig. 4: Tip of the needle for puncture and injection [2]

The device of the syringe that allowed draining the CSF, injecting air and the anaesthetic mixture consisted of two tightly connected cylinders: the smaller one (10 ml) contained the anaesthetic, the other one (50 ml) holding the air. The pistons were to be moved by screws permitting exact dosage,

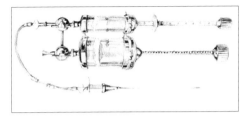

Fig. 5: Double cylinder syringe device [3]

while a rubber tube between the syringe and the needle allowed little movement of the syringe. Each cylinder could be connected to the tube and the needle by two taps.

Technical Performance of Kirschner's Spinal Anaesthesia

The *first step* Kirschner took to perform a lumbar puncture was to insert the needle with the patient being in a lateral position the pelvis being elevated 25 degrees. The puncture site was chosen according to the desired level of analgesia: i.e. L1/2 for "high" (abdominal and thoracic surgery) or L3/4-L4/5 for "low" anaesthesia (lower extremities). However, this did not influence the extent of analgesia.

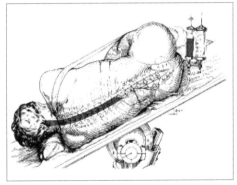

Fig. 6: Technique of Kirschner's spinal anaesthesia [3]

The *second step* was to introduce the bubble of air. The double syringe set was tightly connected to the puncture cannula. Then 15-20 ml of CSF were drained into the

50 ml-cylinder; the cylinder was emptied and filled with air. About 15 ml of air were insufflated into the spinal fluid space: In order to adjust the level of CSF in an exact position according to the desired extent of analgesia, an additional volume of air had to be inserted. Kirschner suggested 10-15 ml of air to achieve analgesia below the umbilicus and 20-25 ml of air for analgesia below the mamillaries. This was how a bubble of air in the sacral part of the dural sack was produced. The tight connection of the two cylinders of the syringe then allowed the injection of local anaesthetic without being forced to disconnect the syringe from the cannula. In case of disconnection, leakage of air would result.

The *third step* he took was to inject the anaesthetic and to position the "plug". Because of the lateral opening of the needle, the direction of the injection of the local anaesthetic could be chosen: e.g. aiming for abdominal anaesthesia the outlet headed cranial ("head shot"), as opposed to analgesia for the legs the opening had to be turned downwards ("pelvis shot"). The first dose of the anaesthetic injected was just as high as required, the hypobaric local anaesthetic now forming the so called "plug" positioned on the top of the CSF just below the sacral bubble of air.

The extent of anaesthesia could be adjusted by adding or omitting air. After a few minutes the area anaesthesized had to be tested. If analgesia was not sufficient or not placed at the desired spinal segments, the dose of the injected anaesthetic was increased or the position of the anaesthetic "plug" was corrected by de- or inflating air. As soon as a sufficient degree of anaesthesia had been obtained, the needle was removed and the patient was put in a supine position. During and after surgery, the patient had to stay in a head-down-position, until analgesia had completely worn off.

Figure 7 sketches the relationship between the extent of anaesthesia and the position of the anaesthetic "plug".

Results

The results Kirschner and his team obtained applying this technique were outstanding, he acquired great experience with this method: about 1000 case reports are available showing excellent results. Each procedure was exactly noted and documented for evaluation; the mortality rate was 1 in 1000 patients; no significant fluctuations in blood pressure occured.

Another important innovation was the so-called "psychic narcotist" who always had to be present in case a patient received spinal anaesthesia.

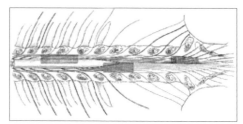

Fig. 8: Spread of analgesia dependent on the localization of the "plug" [3]

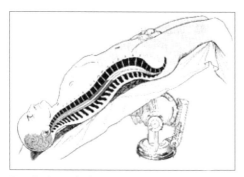

Fig. 7: Spread of anaesthesia [1]

In a diagram of 1932 (Fig. 8) Kirschner exactly illustrates his observations on the extent of analgesia depending on the localization of the anaesthetic "plug": all segments within the bubble of air were spared from anaesthesia. This lead to the conclusion that spinal anaesthesia did not act on the spinal cord itself but on the spinal roots.

Kirschner`s clinical observations remain valuable for the present day discussion of the site of action of local anaesthetics in spinal anaesthesia.

References:

[1] Kirschner M: Versuche zur Herstellung einer gürtelförmigen Spinalanästhesie. Langenbecks Arch klin Chir 1931; 167: 755-760

[2] Kirschner M: Eine gürtelförmige, einstellbare und individuell dosierbare Spinalbetäubung. Chirurg 1931; 3: 633-644

[3] Kirschner M, Stauss: Beiträge zur willkürlichen Begrenzung und zur individuellen Dosierung der Spinalanästhesie. Erfahrungen an über 1000 eigenen Fällen. Langenbecks Arch klin Chir 1932; 173: 322-389

[4] Kirschner M: Spinal zone anaesthesia, placed at will and dosage individually graded. Surg Gynecol Obstet 1932; 55: 317-329

[5] Philippides D: Ein vereinfachtes Verfahren der gürtelförmigen einstellbaren Spinalanästhesie. Langenbecks Arch klin Chir 1937; 189: 445-451

[6] Moritsch P: Die Schmerzverhütung bei chirurgischen Eingriffen. Wien 1949, p. 185-186

[7] Weisser Ch: Martin Kirschners willkürlich begrenzte und individuell dosierbare gürtelförmige Spinalanästhesie. Grundlagen – Technik – aktuelle Bedeutung. Ein Beitrag zur Geschichte der Regionalanästhesie. Würzburger med. hist. Mitt. 1992; 10: 39-52

The Delayed Arrival

A. K. Adams,
Cambridge, UK

In 1800 Humphry Davy wrote "as nitrous oxide appears capable of destroying physical pain, it may probably be used with advantage during surgical operations."[1] It was not until 46 years later that Morton gave ether in public for a surgical operation. A delay of nearly half a century before Davy's observation was followed up seems surprising. The mind of a 20th century doctor cannot comprehend how the search for anaesthesia should not have been under way for hundreds of years. But 200 years ago in Davy's time only very perfunctory attempts were being made solve the problem.

The state of knowledge in the late 18th century.

The Greeks, the Chinese, the Arabs and others all knew of concoctions that produced some degree of stupor and oblivion. Mandrake, opium, alcohol and cannabis were amongst remedies used for their analgesic and soporific actions. Mandrake, containing hyocyamus, was one of the most powerful and hence the most dangerous but it was certainly in use at least until the time of Shakespeare.

Ether was known to Paracelsus, that wayward genius, part superstitious alchemist, part original scientist and almost 20th-century in some of his thinking, a man who quarrelled with everyone and seldom stayed in one place for more than a few months. In 1525 with Valerius Cordus he gave ether in the form of "sweet oil of vitriol" to chickens. He described how they went to sleep, could not be aroused by painful stimuli and woke up none the worse for the experience, a good description of surgical anaesthesia.[2]

The 17th century brought the "age of enlightenment". Science was advancing rapidly with experiments on respiration and combustion. William Harvey described the circulation of the blood and Richard Lower deduced that the lungs absorbed air. Robert Hooke demonstrated that when breathing stopped, life would continue if air was pumped into the lungs, thus confirming the observations of the anatomist Vesalius a century before. The constituents of air were isolated by chemists including Boyle, Priestley, Lavoisier, Scheele and Black. Many of these men pursued science purely as a hobby. Anton Lavoisier, now regarded as the founder of modern chemistry, was a tax collector and social reformer who died on the guillotine for his political beliefs. Joseph Priestley, who had manufactures nitrous oxide in 1772, was a cleric whose radical views forced him ultimately to flee to America, yet it was in his leisure time that he became one of the discoverers of oxygen.

Humphry Davy's contribution.

This was the base of knowledge that Humphry Davy inherited when he came to work with Thomas Beddoes in his Pneumatic Institute in Bristol in 1799. History has been hard on Beddoes, regarding him as important only in that he discovered Davy. But he too was an original thinker, ahead of his time in many ways, including his insistence that controlled trial must precede treatment.³ To support Davy he recruited a strong team, including the engineer James Watt who designed accurate apparatus for Davy's studies of gases on himself and his friends, as well as his patients.

Davy described precisely all the effects of nitrous oxide known today. He inhaled it when he was in pain and observed that his pain was relieved, only to recur as the gas wore off.⁴ In his 500-page treatise it was almost as a throwaway line he speculated that nitrous oxide may probably be used with advantage during surgical operations.

By the year 1800 all the scientific knowledge needed to achieve surgical anaesthesia was in place, yet no-one put ether or nitrous oxide to the service of surgery. More was needed, both the will and the concept. Advances may be conceptual or technical and whilst not belittling technical progress in its contribution to usefulness, conceptual thought and imagination are necessary to appreciate the significance of new knowledge and furthermore, to realise how it can change ways of thinking in addition to allowing practical progress.

Attitudes to human suffering

As the science was there we need to look elsewhere to find why relief of the pain of surgery was not actively being sought. Professor Emmanuel Papper in his scholarly thesis *"Pain, Suffering and the Romantic Period"*[5] gave a clue. Papper claims that traditional inherited Western European attitudes to suffering may have had a major influence and he showed how these changed during the Romantic Period. He noted that the word "pain" is derived from the Greek word for "penalty" and the Latin for "punishment" and that Judeo-Christian beliefs were a curious blend of these two ideas. Pain was seen as a punishment for sin inflicted by a vengeful god, but also, particularly if it was born with fortitude, as a means of atonement and of building up merit for a future life. If little could be done to save life it was more important to die with dignity and hope for a good life eternal, than to treat sickness. These beliefs were strongly held throughout mediaeval life and were slow to be abandoned.

Pain too was deliberately inflicted for various reasons. Anthropologists record how it has long been part of important initiation rites. For example, scarification and circumcision are often ritually inflicted and bearing such pain with stoicism denotes entry into manhood. Also, throughout history brutal punishments such as flogging, branding with hot iron and even death were penalties for trivial offences.

Although doctors might be expected to feel differently, nevertheless they live in their own age, so their attitudes are moulded by the same traditions. Their time was taken up with treating the predominant causes of death and until very recent times these were the various infections. Also, they knew that other diseases in themselves caused suffering worse even than surgery without anaesthesia. Surgical operations were rare, a few such as amputations, cutting for stone and skull trephines were done as a last resort. Many operations were done in the heat of battle when pain may be dulled. Thus whilst small numbers died from surgery, millions perished from infections. Surgeons also convinced themselves that pain served a useful function, acting as a stimulus to survival and preventing shock. So throughout history pain was not necessarily regarded as something which should, even if it could, be avoided. As Greene commented "whilst witches were being burnt in Salem, anaesthesia was not likely to be thought of 20 miles away in Boston".[6]

But because surgeons could not relieve the pain they inflicted it did not follow that they were unaffected by it. Cheselden, skilled surgeon as he was, so dreaded operating that he seldom slept the night before. Abernethy considered that "operations are the reproach of surgery" and Hunter said that "operations are humiliating examples of the imperfections of our science."[7] It is arguable that the surgeons themselves were unlikely to be the discoverers of anaesthesia because their education was against it. Whilst physicians were usually university-educated, surgeons, even after they had emerged from their barber status, were still largely trained by apprenticeship. They had little knowledge of drugs for these were the province of the apothecaries, so surgeons were unlikely to make the conceptual advance.

The Romantic Movement and changing attitudes.

By the 18th century society and its attitudes were changing fundamentally. The rise of the romantic movement coupled with the belief in man's right to freedom, as propounded during the French Revolution, were adopted by young men all over Europe, who focussed attention on the common man whose sufferings had been ignored in the past. The rise of humanitarianism demanded sympathy for the individual. This was shown in other spheres by the emergence of a sense of philanthropy. Important developments took place including the founding of hospitals and schools for the poor, the beginnings of public health and of the campaign to abolish slavery, whilst Parliament passed laws to limit the abuse of workers in the new mines and factories.

Doctors again were caught up in the changing society of their time. Medicine moved away from the Church and came to be dominated by the science of the enlightenment.

Use of ether and nitrous oxide.

Although ether and nitrous oxide were not used in a way which might result in anaesthesia, they were nevertheless used, perhaps surprisingly for social amusement. They were inhaled in "ether frolics" at parties and for theatrical entertainment. Ether also retained a respectable medical use as a soothing anodyne and inhaled for relief of chest diseases as in Beddoes' day.

It is strange that Davy did not follow up his observation, but he too was a man of his times and regarded it more as a scientific curiosity. However he was not an ordinary man and one cannot help wondering why this scientific genius should have failed to see the significance of his findings. He made the scientific but not the conceptual advance. He left Bristol for London for the Royal Institution and was sidetracked into other work and sadly he came to denigrate his earlier studies in Bristol. If it had not been for his change of career anaesthesia might have been introduced 40 years earlier not in Boston, Massachusetts but in Bristol, England by Humphry Davy whilst James Watt, the inventor of the steam engine, might also have been the designer of the first anaesthetic machine.

Hickman, the man who tried.

One man in England did try to provide painless surgery, namely Henry Hill Hickman, a country practitioner born in the year in which Davy published his treatise on nitrous oxide.[8] He tried to produce a state of "suspended animation" during which surgery could be carried out painlessly and he had some success in animals. Unfortunately he seems not to have known of Davy's work and he used not nitrous oxide but carbon dioxide. His attempts to get his observations made known both in Britain and France failed. Whilst he had no influence on the introduction of anaesthesia into clinical practice he must be credited with having thought of it and with making a genuine attempt to abolish the pain of surgery.

341

Success in America.

If all the preliminary work was done in Europe reasons must be sought for success eventually being found in America. Certainly there was no shortage of American physicians coming to study in Europe nor of British doctors going to America. Joseph Priesley himself, when he fled to escape religious persecution, was offered the chair of chemistry in Philadelphia, though he did not accept it. As in Europe the practice of inhaling laughing gas and ether for social and theatrical entertainment was common, so incidentally was mesmerism, though Mesmer himself failed to realise how it might be used for surgery. The men in America who eventually used ether for painless surgery did so having inhaled it themselves for fun and noted its effect in dulling pain.[9] Possibly doctors in a vigorous young country might have been more receptive to new ideas than in the conservative Old World. For whatever reason it was they who made the conceptual advance, they used it for surgery and anaesthesia arrived on the medical scene.

Conclusion.

In retrospect the arrival of anaesthesia seems to have been strangely delayed. Knowledge, attitudes and events coalesced and eventually the time came. History has shown that this is not unique to anaesthesia even though it had such humanitarian appeal. The mere possession of knowledge is not in itself enough. Many factors, sometimes subtle ones, may delay advances for long periods before a new idea comes to fruition.

References:

[1] Davy H: Researches, Chemical and Philosophical; chiefly concerning Nitrous Oxide. London: J Johnson, 1800; 556

[2] Paracelsus: 1605. Quoted by Schullian DM in: Faulconer A and Keys TE Foundations of Anesthesiology, Springfield, Illinois: Charles C Thomas, 1965; 266

[3] Barzun J: Thomas Beddoes on medicine and social conscience. J Amer med Assoc; 220: 50-53

[4] Davy H: Researches, Chemical and Philosophical; chiefly concerning Nitrous Oxide. London: J Johnson, 1800; 456-467

[5] Papper EM: Pain, suffering and anesthesia in the romantic period. Doctoral thesis at the University of Miami, Florida, 1990

[6] Greene NM: A consideration of factors in the discovery of anesthesia and their effects on its development. Aneshesiology 1971; 35: 515-522

[7] Warren JC: The influence of anesthesia on the surgery of the nineteenth century. Trans Amer Surg Assoc 1897; 15: 1-25

[8] Cartwright FF: The English pioneers of anaesthesia. Bristol: Wright, 1952: 265-292

[9] Sims JM: The discovery of anaesthesia. Virginia Med monthly 1877; IV: 19-41

From Ether to Chloroform. The Beginnings of Chloroform Anaesthesia in France

M. Th. Cousin, Paris, France

On november 9th 1847, Doctor Adrien Philippe, first surgeon in Hôtel-Dieu de Reims, corresponding member of Académie de Médecine, made the first trials known in France with chloroform[1]. The serial trials were made in 9 men: five patients and four volunteers. There were five successes. He *hastened* to announce this event to the Académie de Médecine but his letter was only read on november 30th at the moment where all Parisian surgeons had already used chloroform.

Again on december 8th, two major surgical interventions, lithotricy and hip amputation, were solemnly performed by Philippe, in the presence of several witnesses: the president of the hospital, and the administrator, four surgeons and physicians and all the students of the Medical School[2]. His full success was *quickly* and somewhat pompously *(the heroic power of this marvelous agent,* used for *two cases of great surgery)* described in a letter to Académie. Again the letter was only read on december 21th. So was the province's priority obtuned.

How was Philippe informed about chloroform? His first trial occurred the day before Simpson's first communication to the Edinburgh medico-surgical Society. It was not a simultaneous discovery since Philippe paid homage to Simpson and celebrated *"the triumph of Simpson's liquor"*[2]. Up till now no clue has been found about a direct correspondance between Simpson and Philippe or between Scotland and Champagne or about a witness's story of Simpson's experiments.

Chloroform had been known since 16 years ago. Its discovery made nearly simultaneously by Eugène Soubeiran, Samuel Guthrie and Justus von Liebig in 1831 and 1832. The chemist Jean-Baptiste Dumas established its formula in 1835. And in March 1847, the physiologist Marie-Jean-Pierre Flourens observed that chloroform had the same but more powerful anaesthetic properties than ether[3]. However the surgeons did not pay attention to this fact and Velpeau could regret six monthes later: *"So was lost for France the honour of a part of this discovery"*[4]

Dumas, during a trip in Scotland with other French colleagues, witnessed Simpson's chloroformisations for major surgery, on november 15th. When he returned to France, and when at the same time English and French medical journals reported Simpson's experiments, the first Parisian trials took place. In less than a month, all people in the province and in Paris, got to know about chloroform: surgery, obstetrics, veterinary, animal experiences, self administration and volunteers's administration, new apparatus, new chapters in anaesthetic books, all the domains are concerned.

Easy to give, powerful, quick and seemingly without undesirable effects, chloroform becomes the favourite. In some weeks ether seems to be forgotten.

However some voices warn against potential hazards. At first, Flourens, recalling his experiments and announcing new works, declares (4bis): *"I said ether was a marvelous and terrible agent. I'll say chloroform is even more marvelous and more terrible ("il est plus merveilleux et plus terrible encore")"*. This unintentional alexandrine will be remembered when first hazards occur.

It is also Charles E. Sédillot from Strasburg who records on january an 8th, worrying observations[5]: *"Pallor, weak pulse, faint inspirations, cooling are increasing in an alarming way when the administration is stopped. Twice I was seriously frightened by this imminent annihilation of life"*. It is yet Etienne F. Bouisson from Montpellier who alerts people on february 7th to the drastic effects of chloroform[6].

Hannah Greener's death announcement in the Gazette des Hôpitaux civils et militaires[7] did not arouse any concern in French readers. This case is ignored until the publication of the first hazard in France. Gorré the surgeon, reporting his accident, starts with the complete story of Hannah Greener which he had not known until his own occurs on March 26 1848. Gorré's report is read at Académie de Médecine on July 10th[8]: *"Miss Stock, a young woman about thirty years old, (...) was usually in good health"*. (...) He had to open a thigh abcess: *"I put on the nostrils a handkerchief on which were poured at the most 15 to 20 chloroform drops. Scarcely after some inspirations, she puts her hand to the handkerchief to take it away, and cries out in a plaintive voice: "I suffocate". Then immediately, the face is going pale, the features are changing, respiration is difficult, foam is coming to the lips. At the same moment (and certainly less than a minute after inhalation has started) the handkerchief is taken away"*. The surgeon opens the abcess and removes a piece of wood fom the thigh, while (during the infinitely short time used for this little operation) his colleague starts to resuscitate his patient. *"All what is possible to do in such a case was done by my collaegue and myself for more than two hours. (...) Vain efforts"!*

Air was post-mortem found in the venous system and was attributed to putrefaction.

Administrative authorities are worried by this death. A double inquiry is required by the Justice Minister and by the Public Instruction Minister 1) to determine responsibilities in miss Stock 's death and 2) to know if chloroform is totally innocuous[9]. A thirteen academicians committee is formed. The reporter, the surgeon Joseph-François Malgaigne (known as the first to use ether in Paris) gives his report on october 30, definitive conclusions of it are given on february 6th 1849[10,11].

At first, Malgaigne answers the question of penal responsibility in the Gorré`s case [10]. He notes there are many sudden death examples in medicine, with or without surgery, with or without anaesthesia. In this case gaseous emboly is nearly certain, and finally Miss Stock's death may not in any way be attributed to chloroform.

Second, Malgaigne gives an answer to the question of the Public Instruction Minister. He records seven cases of sudden death: Hannah Greener and four other English and American cases, and two French cases. These two cases occurred in two "June Wounded" (it is to say two men wounded by firearms during the 1848 revolutionary days). They died in the same manner at the beginning of a second complementary chloroform administration, one of them being cared for by Doctor Robert, the other by Malgaigne himself. For the first five cases he puts forward asphyxia, due to technical administration errors. In the June-wounded, hemorrhage and infection are advanced. He concludes: *"One can be out of all the dangers by observing administration rules ..."*. Among the rules he gives, we can mention: to supply enough air, to stop inhalation as soon as insensibility sets in.

Many critiques are expressed against the report, some coming even from Committee members! So the surgeon Alfred Velpeau (one of the thirteen members) asks for an amendment to the first part of the report: *"It seems to be not demonstrated that chloroform was or was not the cause of the death"*. He admits he had terrors when he saw „*patients staying in a state as cadaverous, face pallor, cornea withering, all the appearances of death"*[12].

His argumentation reflects the point of view of many surgeons: *"If chloroform has killed, the use of a so dangerous means must be given up, in spite of the hopes it aroused, and the immense service it has given. (...) As for me, I consider it as innocent of all these hazard"*.

The most violent attack against Malgaigne comes from his old enemy Jules Guérin who calls into question the scientific characteristic of the report in which Académie is pledged[13]. *"The report is failing on three points: observation, experimentation and reasoning"*[14]. His more than two hours argumentation can be summed up so: Observation: incomplete, experimentation : nothing, reasoning : weak, conclusions : dangerous, Academy liability : involved. The violent exchanges between the two protagonists were exacerbated as far as to go into a duel of provocations! (what Malgaigne declines ...) Malgaigne's conclusions are voted for by the Académie with a large majority and almost without changes[11].

Just one week after the report definitive conclusions publication, a new sudden death is announced in *Union Médicale*[15], which occurred in Lyon on january 31st 1849, while Academicians in Paris were still disputing about safety of chloroform. For the surgeon Dr. Barrier, until this date fervent supporter of this agent, there is no doubt death is due to chloroform. This event led the Lyonnais to return to ether. Another sudden death occurs in the same year in Langres[16], then two in Strasburg in 1850 and 1852, one in Orléans in 1852, one in Chatellerault in 1853[17], and several near-deaths are not counted.

New committees are formed by Académie des Sciences and by Societé de Chirurgie respectively[18]. The Société de Chirurgie reporter, Docteur Robert, the surgeon of one of the June Wounded, is working during one year: he makes an inventory of all the chloroform associated deaths (78 in 1853) detailing six sudden death cases. He experiments on animals by himself, he makes trials with other drugs and ether-chloroform mixture, he proposes indications and counterindications, methods of administration, accidents management and concludes: *"Chloroform may cause death nearly instantaneously. There is no means to prevent it. Surgeons's cautions may prevent against legal proceedings but not against fatality and patient's death"*.

One must be waiting for fifty years to understand the actual cause of sudden death until Goodman A. Levy demonstrated, in 1911, the adrenalino-chloroformic syncope mechanism[19].

References:

1. Philippe A: Lettre à l'Académie de Médecine sur l'inhalation du chloroforme. Bulletin de l'Académie Royale de Médecine 1847; 13: 427

2. Philippe A: Communication sur les effets du chloroforme. Bulletin de l'Académie Royale de Médecine 1847; 13: 470-473

3. Flourens MJP. Note touchant l'action de l'éther sur les centres nerveux. Compte-Rendus des Séances de l'Académie des Sciences 1847; 24: 340-344

4. Velpeau A: Communications relatives au chloroforme. Séance de l'Académie des Sciences du 13 décembre 1847. Union Médicale 1847; 1: 631

4. Flourens MJP: ibidem. Annonces du 19. novembre 1847 London Medical Gazette 1847; 5: 906

5. Sédillot CE: Nouvelles remarques sur les effets anesthésiques du chloroforme. Séance du 8 janvier 1848. Compte-Rendus des Séances de l'Académie des Sciences 1848; 25: 37

6. Bouisson EF: Emploi du chloroforme et de l'éther sulfurique; de leurs indications respectives; quelques réflexions concernant les cas où il convient de mettre en usage l'éther ou le chloroforme. Séance du 7 février 1848. Compte-rendus des Séances de l'Académie des Sciences. Gazette Médicale de Paris 1848; 3: 128-129

7. Anonymous: Dangers du chloroforme. Gazette des Hôpitaux Civils et Militaires 1848; 10

8. Gorré: Observation sur un cas de mort causée par l'inhalation de chloroforme. Bulletin de l'Académie Nationale de Médecine 1848;13: 1144-60

9. Correspondance officielle: Séance du 25 juillet 1848. Bulletin de l'Académie Nationale de Médecine 1848;13:1209

10. Malgaigne JF. Rapport sur les accidents observés au cours de l'éthérisation par le chloroforme. Séance du 30 octobre 1848. Bulletin de l'Académie Nationale de Médecine 1848; 14:203-248

11. Malgaigne JF: Conclusions du rapport sur le chloroforme. Séance du 6 février 1849. Gazette Médicale 1849; 4: 109

12. Velpeau A: Discussion sur le chloroforme Séance du 14 décembre 1848 à l'Académie de Médecine. Union médicale 1848; 2: 590

13. Guérin J: Discussion sur le chloroforme. Séance du 13 novembre 1848. Bulletin de l'Académie Nationale de Médecine 1848; 14: 289-305

14. Guérin J:Discussion sur le rapport de Malgaigne au sujet du chloroforme. Union Médicale 1849; 3: 24

15. Barrier F. Lettre. Union Médicale 1849; 3: 69-70

16. De Confrevon:Cas de mort par le chloroforme, nouveau moyen anesthésique. Abeille Médicale 1849; 6: 291-293

17. Robert A:Rapport sur un cas de mort par le chloroforme. Bulletin de la Société de Chirurgie 1853; 3: 582-606

18. Discussion sur le Chloroforme. Bulletin de la Société de Chirurgie 1853-1854: 3-4: 209-465

19. Levy AG, Lewis T: Heart irregularities resulting from the inhalation of low percentages of chloroform vapour and their relationship to ventricular fibrillation. Heart, iii, 1911; 99

From Simpson to Livingstonia

A. G. McKenzie, Edinburgh, UK

James Young Simpson (1811-1870) and David Livingstone (1813-1873) were contemporary Scotsmen both of strong resolve, yet very different characters. J. Y. Simpson hailed from the east of Scotland and D. Livingstone from the west. Simpson was of jovial disposition and a natural leader[1]; Livingstone was serious by nature and awkward in social skills[2].

In 1840 Simpson was elected to the Chair of Midwifery at Edinburgh[1]; he became a great teacher of good medical practice[3]. In the same year Livingstone gained the licence of the Faculty of Physicians and Surgeons, Glasgow, was ordained a minister and set sail for South Africa. He went to join Robert Moffat at the London Missionary Society (LMS) mission station at Kuruman, in the far north of Cape Province[4].

On 2 January 1845, Livingstone married Robert Moffat's daughter, Mary, at Kuruman. He took her about 200 miles northeast to Mabotsa, and later a further 80 miles north to Kolobeng (which is in Botswana)[4].

The first use of chloroform in obstetrics by Prof James Young Simpson was reported in the Lancet in 1847[5]. Livingstone had issues of the Lancet sent to him and thus learnt about

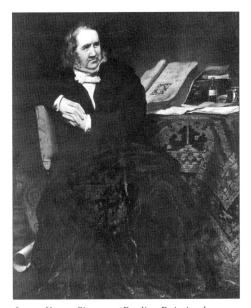

James Young Simpson (Replica Painting by Norman Macbeth, 1879).
Acknowledgement: Edinburgh University Archives

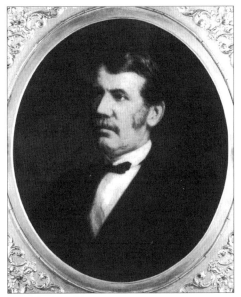

David Livingstone, in his forties.
Acknowledgement: The Council for World Mission, London

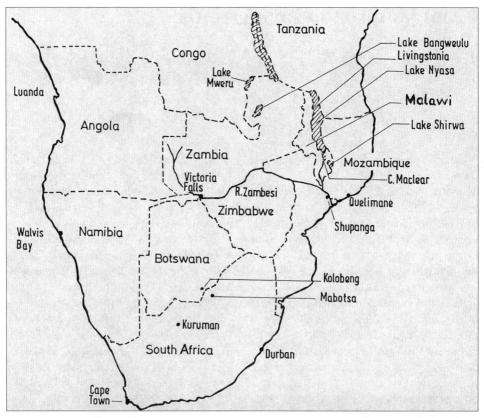

Map of Central & South Africa showing places referred to in text and current political boundaries.

ether and chloroform. It is evident from his letter to Robert Moffat from Kolobeng on 31 January 1849 that Livingstone was enthusiastic about administering chloroform for labour[6].

"Wish much I had some chloroform. From the accounts I see of its operation I expect the old ladies will be wishing they could begin again. It is uniformly safe for both mother and child and the recovery is much accelerated. It is much more speedy in its operation than ether, and has not any of the disagreeable effects of that drug. Half a teaspoonful sprinkled on a handkerchief held to the nose is all that is required. There is no lividity, coughing, but a calm and gentle sleep and the mothers will scarcely believe when they waken that they have a child. Should have attempted to make some by a makeshift retort but fear the heat is too great here and it is very volatile. Could we not procure some chloral from England and a retort? Professor Simpson of Edinburgh has used it in 50 cases with entire success."

At this time Mary Livingstone was pregnant and 5 weeks later her 3rd child was born. It is unknown whether Livingstone obtained chloroform for this labour, but it seems unlikely, for in the preserved fragments of his Kolobeng journal (1849) only the following reference to the birth appears[7]:

"MARCH 7: Mrs L delivered of a son, Thomas Steele - quick recovery. May God accept and save him."

One would like to know Moffat's response to Livingstone's request of 31 January 1849. Unfortunately Moffat's letters to Livingstone during this period have not been preserved - they were probably destroyed in the sack of Livingstone's house at Kolobeng which occurred in 1852[8].

In another letter to the Rev. Moffat from Kolobeng dated 23 March 1849, Livingstone wrote about the birth, but made no mention of chloroform (or ether)[6].

During the next two and a half years Mary Livingstone delivered two more children in Botswana: a daughter at Kolobeng in August 1850, and a son at the river Zouga (now named Botletle) in September 1851. Again Livingstone wrote about these births in letters and in his private journal, but made no reference to administration of chloroform (or ether)[6,7]. In 1852 Livingstone sent his wife and four children back to Britain.

It has been stated in a popular biography that Livingstone helped his wife through several pregnancies with chloroform[2]. The lack of any written evidence for this makes the belief conjectural at best.

Livingstone returned to England on 9 December 1856 - famous! In September 1857 he was granted the Freedom of the City of Glasgow and then of the City of Edinburgh[9]. On September 23 he was entertained to a breakfast in Edinburgh, hosted by the members and friends of the Medical Missionary Society of Edinburgh (EMMS). It was attended by numerous dignitaries including Professor James Young Simpson (whose numerous interests at this time included African customs[3]). Simpson had also been a Director of the EMMS from 1848 to 1854, and was destined to become Vice President in 1866[10]. After the breakfast Livingstone gave a brief address. Prof. Simpson responded by proposing that the British Prime Minister should award Livingstone a substantial pension, and this was reported in The Daily Scotsman as follows[11].

"Professor Simpson rose to make one proposition. Perhaps many ladies and gentlemen know that when Dr. Livingstone came home in the character of a traveller, there were some who expressed doubts as to whether he was taking up the proper duties of a missionary. There were some of them there who thought him the greatest missionary they ever had. (Cheers). He was going out again, and it was the special duty of the friends of the Medical Missionary Society to see that his family should be suitably provided for. He thought that Lord Palmerston should be asked to bestow upon their guest a pension of 300 or 400 pounds a-year, which would make him independent for life - a reward which he so richly deserved. (Cheers)."

Asked to comment on his surgical experience in Africa, David Livingstone gave a resume', including his services in midwifery - which doubtless was of interest to Professor Simpson.

The influence of Simpson may well have played a part in the decision of the British Government 2 months later to sponsor Livingstone's Zambezi Expedition.

In November 1857, Livingstone's book Missionary Travels and Researches in South Africa was published. In Chapter I of this 711 page volume[12] Livingstone described his experience of being attacked by a lion. His reference to chloroform is most notable.

"Growling horribly close to my ear, he shook me as a terrier dog does a rat. The shock produced a stupor similar to that which seems to be felt by a mouse after the first shake of the cat. It caused a short of dreaminess, in which there was no sense of pain nor feeling of terror, though quite conscious of all that was happening. It was like what patients partially under the influence of chloroform describe, who see all the operation, but feel not the knife. This singular condition was not the result of any mental process. The shake annihilated fear, and allowed no sense of horror in looking round at the beast. This peculiar state is probably produced in all animals killed by the carnivora; and if so, is a merciful provision by our benevolent Creator for lessening the pain of death."

Livingstone's left humerus was shattered in this attack and the event is an example of central inhibition of pain by descending nerve tracts. Incidentally the humerus underwent malunion, which served to authenticate his body after it was brought back to Britain in 1874[13].

The Zambezi Expedition arrived at the mouth of that river on 14 May 1858. A young member was Dr. John Kirk, who was appointed as Economic Botanist and Medical Officer. Kirk had graduated MD and LRCS at the University of Edinburgh in 1854 and proceeded to a resident physicianship at the Edinburgh Royal Infirmary in 1854-55. He trained under Professors James Syme and J. Y. Simpson. In 1855 he did voluntary medical service in the Crimean War[14]. On 3 May 1858 (during the sail from Cape Town to the east coast of Africa) Dr. Kirk checked the medical supplies and listed them in his Journal - the list included chloroform[15].

In August 1858 Kirk disembarked from the steam launch at Shupanga (near the Zambesi delta) and befriended the Portuguese camp. He was soon obliged to provide medical services for the Portuguese army, which was campaigning against 'rebels'. A terse statement in his diary dated 2 September reads [16]:

"Have a large hospital of sick and wounded from the front". On the same day his younger colleague, Richard Thornton (who was the appointed Mining Geologist for the Expedition) recorded in his own journal that Kirk attended a soldier who had been shot - a ball had passed through the groin. According to Thornton's journal on that same day Kirk dissolved some gutta percha in chloroform to purify it[17]! Was it just coincidence that Kirk had the chloroform out that very day - or was it at hand because of surgical requirement? Having trained in Edinburgh Kirk would have administered the chloroform by Simpson's method: dripping it onto "a pocket handkerchief, rolled into a funnel shape, and with the broad or open end of the funnel placed over the mouth and nostrils"[5].

In 1861 a Universities Mission joined the Zambezi Expedition. It included James Stewart, a young representative of the Free Church of Scotland, whose remit was to plan a mission for the Shire Highlands[2]. Stewart was to play a decisive role in years to come.

A leather medicine chest apparently used by Livingstone from 1861 was recovered after his death in 1873 and is now preserved in the Science Museum, London. The contents were catalogued and included sulphuric ether[18].

James Young Simpson died in May 1870 and David Livingstone died 3 years later. Both men were commemorated by a memorial in Westminster Abbey, the highest honour which the British nation confers on its heroes. In Edinburgh, both men were commemorated by statues in Princes Street: the statue of Simpson is at the west end and that of Livingstone at the east end!

Touched by Livingstone's funeral at Westminster Abbey in 1874, James Stewart (who had been with him on the Zambesi 12 years before) resolved to start a Free Church of Scotland Mission on the shores of Lake Nyasa[19]. This came to pass in December 1875 when the original Mission named Livingstonia was establisned at Cape Maclear on the southern tip of the Lake[19]. Later Livingstonia was moved to Northern Nyasaland (now Malawi).

The first missionaries at "Old Livingstonia" included Dr Robert Laws, who had studied arts, theology and medicine

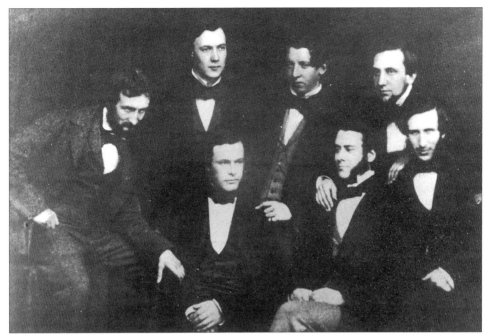

The resident physicians of the Royal Infirmary of Edinburgh, winter 1854-55.
L-R Back Row: J. Beddoe; John Kirk; G. H. Pringle; P. H. Watson.
Front Raw: Joseph Lister; D. Christison; D. Struthers.
Acknowledgement: Edinburgh University Archives

concurrently at the University of Edinburgh. He had completed his medical studies in Aberdeen in April 1875 and then travelled out to Lake Nyasa. At Old Livingstonia on 2 March 1876, Dr. Robert Laws, assisted by George Johnston, administered chloroform to a patient named Koomfonjera, and then proceeded to remove a cystic tumour above Koomfonjera's left eye. The operation was entirely successful and the chloroform anaesthetic was claimed to be the first in Central Africa[20]. However it is more probable that a general anaesthetic was administered in Central Africa much earlier - by David Livingstone or John Kirk. They certainly brought chloroform and ether to that part of the world no later than 1858, and over all the years they spent there, the occasional need for anaesthesia surely arose. These doctors were busy men, deeply involved in exploration, land survey and collecting botanical specimens - to say nothing of daily chlores. Inspection of their journals reveals (usually) concise notes - they would not have felt compelled to record the administration of ether or chloroform for a minor procedure.

The establishment of medical services at Livingstonia was not the last of Simpson's legacy to Central Africa. Simpson's House in Edinburgh (no. 52 Queen Street) was endowed to the Church of Scotland in 1916. Hence it was used by missionaries coming on leave to Edinburgh from overseas[21].

References:

[1] Simpson M: Simpson the Obstetrician. Victor Gollancz, London 1972

[2] Jeal T: Livingstone. Heinemann, London 1973

[3] Duns J: Memoir of Sir James Y. Simpson, Bart. Edmonston & Douglas, Edinburgh 1873

[4] Campbell RJ: Livingstone. Ernest Benn, London 1929

[5] Simpson JY: On a new anaesthetic agent, more efficient than sulphuric ether. Lancet 1847; 2: 549-550

[6] Schapera I: David Livingstone Family Letters Vol. 2 (1849-1856). Chatto & Windus, London 1959

[7] Schapera I: Livingstone's Private Journals (1851-53). Chatto & Windus, London 1960

[8] Northcott C: Robert Moffat: Pioneer in Africa. Lutterworth, London 1961

[9] The Daily Scotsman 18 September 1857 (National Library of Scotland - microfilm)

[10] Edinburgh Medical Missionary Society (personal communication)

[11] The Daily Scotsman 26 September 1857 (National Library of Scotland - microfilm)

[12] Livingstone D: Missionary Travels and Researches in South Africa. John Murray, London 1857

[13] Fergusson W: British Medical Journal 1874; I: 523

[14] Coupland R: Kirk on the Zambesi. University Press, Oxford 1928

[15] Foskett R: The Zambesi Journal & Letters of Dr John Kirk 1858-1863 (Vol. 2). Oliver & Boyd Ltd., London 1965

[16] Foskett R: The Zambesi Journal & Letters of Dr John Kirk 1858-1863 (Vol. 1). Oliver & Boyd Ltd., London 1965

[17] Tabler EC (ed): The Zambesi Papers of Richard Thornton (vol. 1). Chatto & Windus, London 1963

[18] Science Museum, London: personal communication

[19] Wells J: Stewart of Lovedale. Hodder & Stoughton, London 1909

[20] Livingstone WP: Laws of Livingstonia. Hodder & Stoughton, London 1921

[21] Atkinson RS: Simpson House. Anaesthesia 1973; 28: 302-306

Doctor Charles Thomas Jackson's Aphasia

R. Patterson
Department of Anesthesiology, University of California, Los Angeles, USA

On August 28, 1880 Charles Thomas Jackson M.D. died at the McLean Asylum for the Insane, in the Boston suburb of Somerville, where he had been hospitalized for seven years. Subsequent fictionalized accounts of his presumed descent into insanity (his total psychic disintegration and maniacal loss of control necessitating incarceration in chains) have been accepted as biographical facts. The following bizarre accusations are typical of false information repeatedly copied even into present day articles: 1938, "...a raging maniac in front of Morton's Memorial, bound and removed by the police and placed under restraint in the McLean Asylum."; 1962, "... flung himself onto the statue, trying with his fingers to tear it to pieces"; 1995, "Jackson appears to have been obsessed with stealing other people's ideas, and, in the half-mad workings of his mind, we can see some twisted motive for the long vendetta he waged against Morton."; 1996, "...turned hoelessly insane over his frustrations"; 1996, "an uncontrollable psychotic ...serious paranoia, went berserk."

During his lifetime Jackson was not considered insane, even when confronted by spiteful, vindictive disputants: contrariwise no 20th century commentator fails to mention the adverse effect that paranoia had on his contributions in the fields of chemistry, medicine, and geology. Perpetuation of such myths results from neglect of the actual record contained in archival material.

Shortly after ether was introduced into surgical and obstetric practice Dr. Jackson began an association with a division of the Massachusetts General Hospital, the McLean Asylum for the Insane. The superintendent of the asylum, Dr. Luther Vose Bell, a founding member of the Association of Medical Superintendents of American Institutions for the Insane (AMSAII, the forerunner of the American Psychiatric Association), had been treating patients at the asylum with "Haschisch", Cannaby Indica, with disappointing results. He sought the help of Jackson for trials of the inhalaton of ether and chloroform to treat violent insane patients. Jointly Bell and Jackson published their findings.

Jackson was extremely busy the next 25 years; lessening his medical activities while concurrently expanding his teaching of analytical chemistry, chemical consultations for industries, and extensive geological surveys throughout the country.

Throughout his lifetime his personality and temperament remained unchanged. In the intimate circle of family and friends it was considered that he had never fully grown up; throwing himself wholeheartedly into romping with the children, putting on private theatricals, organizing family festivities, and actively participating in town celebrations. He was well-known as an enthusiastic conversationalist, even eloquent in his speech, and fond of story telling. "He was so full of knowledge, wit and charm that the ladies manoeuvered to sit next to him."

On the 5th of March 1873 Jackson was present, as usual, at the regular meeting of the

Boston Society of Natural History, and entered into the discussion of the classification of the rocks of New Hampshire, a subject in which he was quite knowledgeable, having pioneered that state's geological survey 40 years previously.[1] For many years he had been Vice-President of the organization and in 1871 he had been proposed for President in recognition of being "one of the earliest, most constant and devoted of the friends of the society, upon his unwearying interest in its welfare, his liberal contributions to its treasures, his constancy as a presiding officer, and his well-known scientific attainments."[2] He declined the position stating that his health "which is often impaired, especially in the winter months, might be inadequate to the very important duties and constant attention required of the first officer of the Society."[3] Family members were aware that in addition to his bronchitis "his heart sometimes skipped a beat and he took alcohol regularly for that."

April 1873 he was busily occupied with his numerous endeavors; among other matters, performing a chemical analysis of wallpapers for his sister, Lidian, as she mentioned in a letter to her daughter, Ellen:

> "Uncle Charles saved me 85 dollars! and the trifling matter of danger to health by analyzing specimens of all our papers. Five dolls. a specimen is the regular price. I offered him pay today. He laughed & said 'we will settle that matter a hundred years hence not sooner'. And it is fortunate indeed that he did one paper has a teaspoonful of arsenic to the square foot."[4]

Ellen remembered the fateful day in June 1873 when the sudden collapse of her uncle occured:

> "Uncle Charles & Aunt Susan, and Lidian came to the wedding and stayed with us. Lidian stayed to the reception on Mid-Summer Day, he and Aunt Susan went home, she meaning to return the next day, but instead she telegraphed to Lidian to follow, Uncle Charles had fallen down in his study & remained unconscious. The next day mother went to see Uncle Charles. He was conscious but could not talk any intelligible language, he made some new words and used old ones out of their meaning..."[5]

Charles' wife, Susan, writing to a friend recounts the incident:

> "Out shopping, returned to find husband surrounded by doctors who say it is paralysis. He cannot speak but they tell us he will tomorrow."[6]

An acute catastrophe but not a rare medical entity: family members recalled the speech difficulties that followed another relative's shock. The medical professon considered apoplexy to be one of the causes of insanity, grouped along with epilepsy, palsy, and other bodily disorders; other disparate etiological groups were associated with poverty, religon, intemperance, vice and sensuality, politics, excessive study.

Jackson was hospitalized at McLean June 28, 1873. The favorable prognosis put forth by his physicians encouraged his relatives; in July, "still improving"[7]; in August, "is better & better"[8]; later, the report was "still hopeful". However it does not appear that his speech was ever again understandable.

In a letter dated Nov. 28, 1873 Thomas B. Hall, Secretary of the Massachusetts General Hospital, informed Mrs. Chas. T. Jackson:

> "that at a meeting of the Trustees of the Massachusetts General Hospital held yesterday, it was unanimously voted That in recognition of the services of Dr. Charles T. Jackson in connection with

the discovery and use of Ether at the Massachusette General Hospital; and furthermore remembering his many kindnesses during the past years to the patients of the McLean Asylum the Trustees desire to express their sympathy with himself and his family for his present illness, and to consider him while he needs their care as a guest of the Institution from the time of his admission as a patient."[9]

According to its Annual Report the McLean Asylum was essentially a private hospital with "accommodations for those willing and able to pay a high price."[10] The wealthy class lived in well appointed apartments detached from the main building.[11]

It seems that this man who had written hundreds of scientific articles and reports never again read or wrote. There is no mention of residual paralysis nor of abnormal behavior, other than inability to communicate: the signs of incapacitation which he did display over the years at McLean were described by his niece, Ellen:

"Mother & Aunt Susan visited him ... he recognized them & was always overjoyed to see them. He called Aunt Susan Alice (Susan's dead sister) and Mother, I think Lucy (elder sister of Lidia and Charles) and talked to them eagerly all the time they were there, but they could understand nothing. ... what was it that he seemed so earnest in telling them?"[12]

A retrospective summary of Jackson's 1873-1880 hospitalization states:

"From our records it would appear that he was suffering from a mental illness caused by arteriosclerosis and that he suffered with what is now known as cerebral accidents, or in the lay term, "shocks". There is nothing in this record that would indicate in any way that Dr. Jackson was intemperate in the use of alcohol or that he was a "raving maniac" [13].

The Superintendent had been joined by another member of the Asylum in this review who added:

"there was no indication whatever of alcoholism in the clinical record or in the autopsy findings. Examination of the record indicated that Charles was a very cooperative patient and one who left an altogether favorable impression on those who had to do with him. Dr. Wood would have liked to write a much more emphatic letter, but the rules laid down by the Trustees limited him to the bare statement."[14]

Dr. Jackson died August 28, 1880. The Commonwealth of Massachusetts Death Certificate states the immediate cause of death was "insanity". By this time, 1880, the lay public was well aware that the term "insanity" was a wastebasket without real meaning for the newspapers were extensively reporting the rancorous dispute between the Superintendents and the Neurologists which reached an impasse when neither party could even define the term.[15]

1880 was the midpoint of the asylum reform movement that pitted in conflict two very different sections of the medical profession, each claiming responsibility for the care of the insane. In a defensive mode to protect their financial and political power bases the long established AAMSII was accused of providing merely custodial service to those sufficiently ill, aged, or difficult to manage as to require hospitalization. A younger group of physicians emerging in the aftermath of the American Civil War, the neurologists, working with theories drawn largely from French and German sources centered on the diagnosis and treatment of organic disorders, were in attack mode seeking to break the asylum monopoly on patients and gain entry to command the material essential to a thorough clinical and pathological demonstration of insanity. In the end neither group could define "insanity", nor reach agreement on the meaning of the term, or its etiology. To the Superintendents it was a purely mental phenomenon in all aspects, an intangible thing: this was anathema to the Neurologists who were dedicated to medical models of mental disorders, with etiologies based on specific brain leions. Insight valuable to constructing a medical model of mental disorder occured during the 1860s & 70s with the gradual realization that only the primary functions (perceptions) can be referred to specific cerebral areas. All processes which exceed these functions such as thought, consciousness, speech, etc. were concieved to depend on fiber bundles connecting different areas of the cortex.

In Vienna, the search for anatomical localization was given fundemental direction by Theodore Meynert who was motivated to change psychiatry from a descriptive to an interpretive study. Among other advance he distinguished between two cortical fiber systems, each with a different function: the projection fibers "which connect the cortical cells with the sensitive surfaces and the contractile masses of the musculature", and the association fibers "which form connections between different areas of the cortex", the basis of rationalization and ethical motivation. Meynert's endeavors "to deliver psychiatry from the patriarchial impasse of closed institutions and to open it up to the rich new ideas from university life" precipitated his dismissal.[16]

In 1865 in Paris debates on the phenomenon of aphasia brought together Paul Broca, who, in 1861, had described the cortical motor area, with Marc Dax and his son, Gustave, supporters of the localization of the center for speech in the median lobe of the left hemisphere. Inspired by the debates and interested in the physiological foundation of language in the brain, Arnoldus van Rhign finished his medical studies at the University of Leiden in1868 with a dissertation on "Aphasia" wherein he hypothesized that not only anatomical lesions to cortical and subcortical languages-related centers could cause aphasia, but aphasia may also occur as a consequence of a disruption of the fibers connecting various centers.

Working in Meynert's laboratory Carl Wernicke was decisively inspired to research aphasia and in 1874 described a sensory speech area, the auditory association cortex, which when disconnected from Broca's area results in a characteristic aphasia. The manifestations of this sensory aphasia ("a copious, fluent, but confused speech output with transposition of sounds, syllables, words, and phrases") as described by Wernicke in 1874 are those that described Jackson in the family letters of 1873.[17] There is little variation in substance in present day listing of the behavorial features:

> "Speech outputs facile in articulation and sentence structure, tending to be filled with ill chosen words and poorly formed sentences. In severe cases speech output consists only of neologistic jargon; a series of speech sounds without meaning. Auditory comprehension is defective even for the comprehension of common object names (it is even more defective for the comprehension of sentences). Word finding is severely restricted so that free conversation is often circumlocutory and empty. Patient's rate of speech is sometimes excessively rapid."[18]

Jackson was autopsied: a second death certificate filed in the City of Somerville lists as cause of death : insanity, bronchitis with emphysema, and meningitis. The latter implies that the skull was opened and the brain examined. It is not known how familiar those in charge were with Wernicke's treatise in German but they should have seen, as he described, an area of softening and scarring involving the entire left posterior portion of the 1st temporal gyrus, the auditory association cortex, extending posteriorly to include the angular gyrus, involved in the reading and writing disorder. Commonly asylums and psychiatric hospitals preserved these gross brain specimens; it may be that his still exists showing the arteriosclerotic occlusion of the lower division of the left middle cerebral artery and the resultant left superior temporal area lesion.

References:

[1] Jackson C: Remarks on the geological survey of New Hampshire. Proc Boston Soc Nat Hist 15: 309, 1873.

[2] Pickering E: Nomination of CT Jackson. Proc Boston Soc Nat Hist 14: 1, 1871.

[3] Jackson CT: Withdrawal of nomination. (op. cit. ref 2): 2

[4] Emerson LJ: Letter to Ellen T Emerson of 28 April 1873. In: Carpenter DB, ed. The Selected Letters of Lidian Jackson Emerson. Columbia: University of Missouri Press, 1987: 309

[5] Emerson ET: The Life of Lidian Jackson Emerson. Carpenter DB, ed. East Lansing: Michigan State University Press, 1992: 164

[6] Miller ED: Letter to Alexander Forbes of 15 December 1938. In: Alexander Forbes Archives. Countway Library of Medicine, Boston

[7] Emerson LJ: Letter to Ellen T Emerson of 29 July 1873. (op. cit. ref 4)

[8] Emerson LJ: Letter to Ellen T Emerson of 6 August 1873. (op.cit. ref 4) : 311

[9] Hall TB: Letter to Mrs. Susan Bridge Jackson of 28 November 1873. Jackson Archive, Boston Medical Society, Countway Library of Medicine, Boston

[10] Asylums Annual Report. J. Insanity 2: 56, 1845

[11] Asylums Annual Report. J. Insanity 11: 180, 1854

[12] Emerson ET: (op. cit. ref 5) :164

[13] Wood WF: Letter to Alexander Forbes of 12 December 1938. In: Alexander Forbes Archives, Countway Library of Medicine, Boston

[14] Forbes A: Letter to Mrs. Robert N. Miller of 11 January 1939. In: Alexander Forbes Archives, Countway Library of Medicine, Boston

[15] Blustein BE: A hollow square of psychological science. In: A Scull ed. Madhouses, Mad-doctors, and Madmen. Philadelphia: University of Pennsylvania Press, 241-270, 1981

[16] Lesky E: The Vienna Medical School of the 19th Century. Johns Hopkins University Press, Baltimore and London, 1976

[17] Eggert GH: Wernicke's Works on Aphasia. Hague, Paris, New York: Monton Publisher, 1977

[18] Goodglass H: Understanding Aphasia. San Diego: Academic Press, 1993

Early Encounters with a Stranger

L. E. Morris,
Bainbridge Island, WA USA

It is my purpose today to tell you about my first encounters with a stranger identified as one of noble character, "chemically inert", and called by a name which means stranger. The stranger is of course the rare gas Xenon, which name is the Greek word for stranger. Xenon is a normal component of our atmosphere but it is present only as an occasional molecule in the air, one part per twenty million so it is quite unobtrusive.

In 1951 Stuart Cullen and Erwin Gross made the first report of surgical anesthesia by inhalation of the rare gas Xenon[1]. Their interest in the rare gases and the possibility that inhalation would have some anesthetic effect had been stimulated by a previous inconclusive report of animal studies published in 1946[2]. In the early 1950's, I was a member of the medical school faculty at the University of Iowa and had the opportunity to be a "volunteer subject" for breathing some of the rare gases. I remember that the breathing of Krypton gas made me feel that my head was acutely expanding and that I would need a hat of much larger size. Xenon, however, quickly led to a feeling of impending anesthesia. Subsequent trials of the odorless Xenon mixed with 50% oxygen breathed from a closed system spirometer resulted in subjective sensations of incipient loss of consciousness. These results seemed to warrant trials of Xenon for clinical anesthesia.

The First Clinical Trials

The written report by Cullen and Gross described the first clinical use of Xenon in two surgical operations. After partial de-nitrogenation by breathing 100% oxygen for about ten minutes, each of these patients was given an inhalation mixture of 80% Xenon with 20% oxygen. In each instance the surgical incision was made about ten minutes after beginning the inhalation of Xenon and conditions were said to be satisfactory for the surgical event. One of these patients was an eighty-one year old man for an orchidectomy and the other was a thirty-eight year old woman for ligation of the fallopian tubes post delivery. Recovery of consciousness appeared to be more rapid than would have been expected with either nitrous oxide or cyclopropane.

Confirmation by a Small Series

Following this first report of clinical use of Xenon as an anesthetic for surgical procedures, there were during the next year an additional twelve patients for whose operations Xenon was used as the sole inhalation anesthetic. In five of these patients, each of whom had been admitted for elective hernioplasty and was otherwise in good physical condition, basic clinico-pathologic studies of blood and urine were done to determine whether there were any identifiable changes associated with Xenon anesthesia[3]. These studies revealed no evidence of disturbance in either biochemic or physiologic processes that could be attributed to Xenon. The clinical course of each anesthetic was satisfactory and uneventful, although in three of the five patients it was deemed appropriate to use a small amount of intravenous meperidine as a supplement to the Xenon. Each of these patients was anesthetized with Xenon for approximately one hour, although under the conditions of the closed carbon dioxide absorption system being, used at that time the concentration of Xenon was probably not appreciably above the MAC value (71%). Despite the undoubted light anesthesia there was no indication of awareness.

Electroencephalographic Changes

In another group of seven patients anesthetized with Xenon, the principal study purpose was to evaluate the electroencephalographic changes during Xenon anesthesia[4]. Changes did occur but these were not similar to the characteristic six or seven levels of electroencephalographic patterns already established for Cyclopropane or Ether anesthesia. During clinical anesthesia with Xenon, the EEG patterns could be divided into no more than three levels, and the slower frequency of the dominant activity associated with clinical anesthesia produced by Xenon is apparently faster than the slow activity described as characteristic with either Cyclopropane or Ether anesthesia. In no case was there any "suppression" or "burst suppression" in the electroencephalographic tracings during anesthesia with Xenon. Characteristic changes in the encephalogram of a patient anesthetized with Xenon are shown in figure 1. One can see an initial depression of alpha activity and a low voltage fast pattern in the initial stage followed by a rhythmic five to seven per second pattern mixed with other frequencies. As the clinical level of anesthesia presumably became deeper with elapsed time, there tended to be some increase in random two to three second activity and a more prominent four to five second activity but the higher frequencies continued to be apparent. In figure 2 there is presented graphically the dominant patterns and the range of frequencies observed together with changes in heart rate, blood pressure and partial pressure of oxygen in the respired atmosphere during the course of the anesthetic. As can be surmised from the anesthetic record, this was a patient for extraperitoneal caesarean section and subsequent ligation of fallopian tubes. The patient had a copious emesis during induction which led to partial obstruction and temporary laryngospasm. It was quickly decided that it would be wise to ensure the airway and also to reduce to a minimum the loss of Xenon by the use of an endotracheal tube which was facilitated by intravenous administration of 18mg of d-tubocurarine following which the endotracheal tube was placed, the closed system re-established and the operation allowed to begin. Satisfactory and otherwise uneventful anesthesia was provided with Xenon for one hour and fifty-five minutes. Fifty-five minutes after the beginning of Xenon and forty-two minutes after the injection of curare a male infant was delivered who cried lustily and spontaneously before complete removal from the uterus. There was no evidence of any depression. The patient was awake within two minutes of removing the mask from her face. On request she could easily raise her head from the pillow and sustain it. Figure 3 depicts another anesthesia record with the addition of a graphic presentation of the electroencephalographic frequency range and also the dominant frequency. This patient was a fifty-six year old female who weighed two hundred and twelve pounds. She had a diagnosis of carcinoma of the uterus and the procedure was a D & C with insertion of radium. A light level of anesthesia was maintained for about forty-five minutes, during which the operative procedure was conducted under very satisfactory conditions. The patient awoke quickly at the end of the procedure. Pre-medication for both of these patients had been only 0.2 mg and 0.3 mg of scopolamine

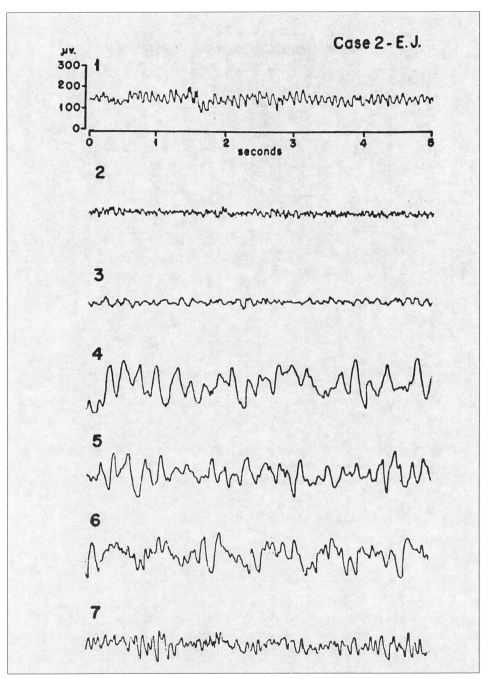

Fig. 1: Selected positions of the EEG tracing: (1) Patient breathing air prior to anesthesia; (2) 4 minutes after start of Xe; (3) 10 1/2 minutes after start of Xe; (4) 18 minutes after start of Xe; (5) 28 minutes after start of Xe; (6) 68 minutes after start of Xe; (7) 7 minutes after discontinuation of Xe anesthesia-patient now responding.

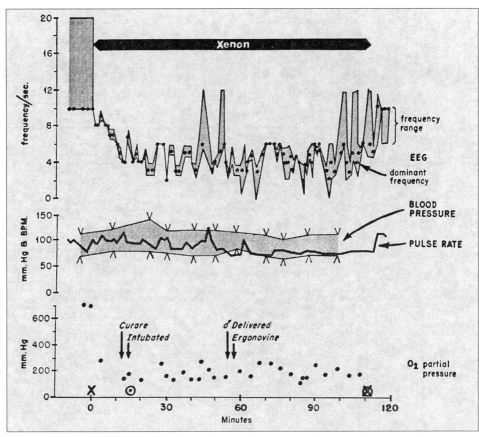

Fig. 2: Changes in EEG frequency range, dominant frequency, blood pressure, heart rate, and partial pressure of oxygen in the respired atmosphere during xenon anesthesia.

respectively by hypodermic injection. In these patients the supplemental use of potent analgesics and barbiturates had been deliberately avoided. Electrocardiographic changes were relatively minimal throughout these anesthetics and none were observed which could be ascribed to the Xenon itself. Determinations of blood oxygen and carbon dioxide during these studies were within normal ranges indicating good oxygenation and adequate ventilation for removal of carbon dioxide.

Satisfactory surgical conditions were provided in these patients by Xenon anesthesia. Although EEG changes were observed during anesthesia with Xenon, the degree and character of the changes appeared to be different from those described for other inhalation agents. It was interesting that the electroencephalographer observing changes in EEG activity was able to predict a change in the level of clinical anesthesia several seconds in advance of demonstrable clinical signs.

Closed System Technique Required

For all fourteen of these clinical anesthetics, Xenon was administered using existing

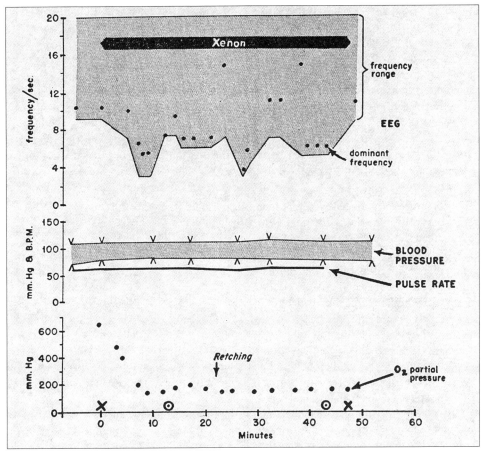

Fig. 3 Changes in EEG frequency range, dominant frequency, blood pressure, heart rate, and partial pressure of oxygen in the respired atmosphere during xenon anesthesia; note the persistence of the high-frequency EEG rhythms throughout the anesthesia.

anesthesia machines in which the compressed gas cylinder of Xenon was hung on an available nitrous oxide yoke. When set at one liter flow, the nitrous oxide rotameter delivered approximately 900 ml of Xenon per minute. In each of these anesthetics a to and fro carbon dioxide absorption closed system technique was used after a period of semi-closed high flow oxygen for up to ten minutes of partial denitrogenation. After this the patient was then given a mixture of 80% Xenon in oxygen which was followed by a minimal metabolic flow of oxygen (±250 ml per minute) and with subsequent intermittent brief additions of Xenon to keep the breathing bag full and to maintain respired oxygen at approximately 20% (range 18-22 percent) as measured by a Beckman-Pauling oxygen meter.

Xenon had been supplied to the Division of Anesthesia at the University of Iowa by the Linde Air Products Company in support of these investigative purposes. It had been collected in a process whereby Xenon gas was retrieved from liquid air by fractional distillation. We were told that this rpocess was quite costly, being estimated at approximately $50 a liter. We calculated that for a one hour anesthetic with Xenon, even in the closed system, about fourteen liters of gas was required for induction and maintenance of anesthesia. Therefore, we had used about $700 worth of Xenon gas in that one hour.

Questions Lead to Further Studies

Following these studies of the electroencephalographic patterns during the light levels of anesthesia produced by Xenon, there was a considerable discussion and some speculation about the differences in the electroencephalographic patterns recorded during Xenon anesthesia as compared with those found to be characteristic during anesthesia with a more potent agent such as Cyclopropane or Ether. Because of the observed differences during the light levels of anesthesia possible with Xenon at atmospheric pressure, it seemed pertinent to find out whether the patterns of electroencephalographic tracings which had been observed by others during anesthesia with more potent anesthetic agents might also result from the inhalation of Xenon at partial pressures sufficiently elevated to produce deeper levels of surgical anesthesia. Deep levels of anesthesia would be attainable at higher total pressure which could be provided by a hyperbaric chamber. Consequently after some considerable planning, studies were undertaken to investigate the electroencephalographic and other pharmacologic effects associated with the deeper anesthesia produced by elevated partial pressures of Xenon which could be achieved in a hyperbaric chamber[5].

Hyperbaric Studies with Monkeys

Because of an apparent lack of objective data related to the clinical effects resulting from the inhalation of anesthetic agents at an increased partial pressure while the partial pressure of oxygen was held at constant level, it was decided to use monkeys as the subjects of this study. There was no hyperbaric chamber at Iowa so it was arranged for three of us at the University of Iowa to go to Rochester, Minnesota, to work with three physicians of the Mayo Clinic staff in their hyperbaric chamber. The pressure chamber was large enough to accommodate the experimental animal and all necessary equipment as well as two anesthesiologists. Electric signals from the interior of the chamber were transmitted to the outside and reciprocal communication was provided between persons within the chamber and those at the outside recording area. Electroencephalographic tracings were simultaneously recorded both graphically on a Grass model IIIC, eight channel pen writing osciligraph and optically as galvinometer deflections on photosensitive paper.

Oxygen and carbon dioxide were determined by the Van Slyke method in an initial sample of arterial blood. The oxygen value was used for calibrating a Waters-Conley oximeter cuvette which was subsequently used for single and double scale cuvette oximetry. Xenon was determined in arterial blood samples by a mass spectrometric method calibrated against recovery from known volumes of Xenon. The partial pressure of oxygen in the respired gases was observed visually on a Pauling oxygen analyzer with continuous sampling and return of the sample through the tail of the breathing bag. Respiration was recorded optically from variations of pressure of the respired atmosphere at the side of a T tube connected to the endotracheal tube. Blood pressure was also continuously recorded optically from a canula placed in one of the femoral arteries of each experimental animal. Electrocardiographic tracings were also recorded.

The experiments were performed on three macacus rhesus monkeys on three successive days. At the beginning of each experiment, all continuous recordings were begun on the alert, restrained monkey breathing pure oxygen at atmospheric pressure. Xenon was then admitted to the rebreathing system until the partial pressure of oxygen had decreased to 200 mm of mercury, the tension which thereafter was kept as constant as possible throughout the experimental hours. After a stabilization of about ten minutes under Xenon anesthesia at atmospheric pressure, the pressure within the chamber was allowed to rise to a peak value and decline at rates comfortable to the human occupants. Intermittent tests of cuvette oximetry were made and blood samples were drawn for subsequent Xenon determinations.

Evaluation of Anesthesia Effect Correlated with Xenon Pressures

The measured volumes of Xenon in the arterial blood samples from these monkeys correlated with the calculated partial pressures of the Xenon gas in the respired atmosphere as a straight line function, which reflects simple solubility. Chamber pressures were elevated to a total of three atmospheres (two additional). Careful observation of physical signs related to depth of anesthesia (changes in muscle tone, reflexes, and respiratory effort) demonstrated that the markedly increased partial pressure of Xenon correlated closely with an increasing depth of anesthesia which became very profound. Corrspondingly, indications of lighter anesthesia returned as partial pressure of Xenon decreased. With respect to respiratory effort, the intercostal activity in each of the three animals disappeared first, the diaphragm activity last. Respiratory effort was deemed inadequate without assistance at a Xenon partial pressure of about 800 mm of mercury. Correspondingly, there was return of feeble respiratory effort at a Xenon partial pressure of about 1000 mm of mercury.

The results of cuvette oximetrey indicated that increasing the depth of anesthesia by increasing the partial pressure of Xenon is not associated with hypoxemia even when the oxygen concentration of the respired gases decreases to less than 9% while maintaining a sustained partial pressure of oxygen at approximately 200 mm of mercury.This supports the early statement of Paul Bert who was first to stress the importance of the partial pressure of oxygen rather that its percent concentration in a respired gas mixture. Hypoxemia does not occur even during the apnoea produced by a profoundly deep anesthesia provided adequate ventilation is maintained.

Observed Electroencephalographic Changes

Fairly consisted electroencephalographic changes were associated with the increasing depth of anesthesia produced by increased pressures of Xenon. These EEG changes can be briefly summarized: there was a decrease in frequency rate of the dominant rhythm; there was a decrease in the overall frequency range; even though a relatively faster frequency might be dominant, a very slow background frequency would often be present; monorhymicity such as has been noted with ether or cyclopropane was generally absent or occurred only occasionally at markedly elevated pressures; burst suppression and total suppression which occur with deep ether anesthesia at ambient pressures (but before cessation of respiration) were not observed at even the highest pressure of two additional atmospheres even though the animals were apnoeic, areflexic and completely flaccid. In the EEG tracings of these three animals there was not a neat categorization of "levels" of electroencephalographic activity which parralled "levels" of anesthesia.

Discussion

These hyperbaric studies in monkeys tend to confirm the observation in human beings that the apparent clinical depth of Xenon anesthesia exceeds an electroencephalographic estimate of depth if that estimate is based on interpretations derived from EEG's obtained during ether or cyclopropane anesthesia. This leads to speculation that possibly Xenon does not act on the same neuro systems nor in the same fashion as do these other anesthetic agents and that this contributes to the lack of comparability.

The original several studies on the anesthetic effect of Xenon by Cullen and the group of investigators at the University of Iowa created a transient surge of interest, perhaps because Xenon seemed to have many of the desired attributes of an "ideal" gas anesthetic. Interest subsided largely because of the excessive cost, which seemed to preclude any serious consideration of popular usage. However, the pharmacologic action of the rare gas Xenon to produce the phenomenon of anesthesia provoked great interest and controversy in theoretical considerations about the mechanisms of general anesthesia[6]. More recently there has been a resurgence of interest in the possible use of Xenon for surgical anesthesia within either a low flow or closed carbon dioxide absorption system[7]. It now also appears that commercial efforts to retrieve and recycle previously used Xenon may become economically feasible and by reducing costs help to make clinical use of Xenon anesthesia a practical reality in future.

References:

[1] Cullen St C and Gross E G: Anesthetic Properties of Xenon in Animals and Human Beings. Science 1951, 113: 580-582

[2] Lawrence J H, Loomis W F et al.: Preliminary Observations on the Narcotic Effect of Xenon with a Review of Values for Solubilities of Gases in Water and Oils. J. Physiol. 1946; 105: p. 197-204

[3] Pittinger C B, Moyers J et al.: Clinico - Pathologic Studies Associated with Xenon Anesthesia. Anesthesiology: 1953, 14: 10-17

[4] Morris L E, Knott J R et al.: Electroencephalographic and Blood Gas Observations in Human Surgical Patients during Xenon Anesthesia. Anesthesiology 1955, 16 (May) p. 312-319

[5] Pittinger Ch B, Faulconer, Jr. A et al.: Electroencephalographic and Other Observations in Monkeys during Xenon Anesthesia. Anesthesiology 1955 16: p. 551-563

[6] Cullen St C and Featherstone R M eds.: Mechanism of Anesthesia. International Anesthesiology Clinic. Vol I, 1963 (August)

[7] Lachmann B, Armbruster S et al.: Safety and Efficacy of Xenon in Routine Use as an Inhalation Anaesthetic. Lancet 1990 (june 16); 335: 1413-1416

The figures, originally published in Anesthesiology, were reproduced here with permission

Helmut Schmidt - an Early Protagonist of Professionalized Anaesthesia in Hamburg

M. Goerig
J. Schulte am Esch
Department of Anaesthesiology, University Hospital Hamburg, Germany

Helmut Schmidt characterized his efforts to establish anaesthesia as a specialty in a still existent curriculum vitae of 1932 like this: "The main goal behind my scientific striving can perhaps best be characterized as the improvement of anaesthesia methods in Germany, further development in inhalational techniques and other methods, the specialized education of students, interns, and nurses at the hospital, the strict organization of anaesthesia and to teach people how to act responsibly and that is why I recommend creating the position of a specialist for anaesthesia at bigger hospitals ...".

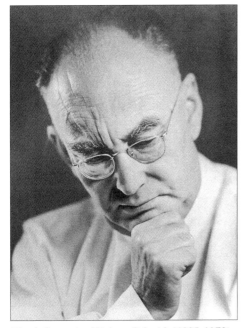

Fig. 1 Portrait of Helmut Schmidt (1895-1979), around 1960[30]

About his biography

Helmut Carl Detlef Schmidt was born in Berlin on 6th of December 1895, where his father - the chemist Dr. Albrecht Schmidt (1886-1959) was working as head of the scientific laboratory of the drug company Schering A.G. (Fig. 1).[30] After graduating in Frankfurt in April 1914 he took up medicine in Marburg but because of the Great War, continued his studies in December 1918. He passed his final examinations in Frankfurt in 1921. After gaining his doctoral degree in Hamburg in 1922 he spent his practical year at the Eppendorf Hospital-Hamburg, which was headed by the internist Rudolph Brauer (1865-1951). After voluntary work at the Department of Pathology for one year Schmidt was employed as surgical resident at the same hospital. The senior surgeons were Hermann Kümmell (1852-1937) and Paul Sudeck (1866-1945). As they were keenly interested in the further development of anaesthesia techniques before and had contributed innovations to the development of our field, it is no surprise that Schmidt became interested in its unsolved problems quite early[10,17]. In 1928 he gained the professor title at the University of Hamburg by publishing an article titled "The efficacy of nitrous oxide anaesthesia during surgery. A comparative study in order to reestablish and promote nitrous oxide anaesthesia in Germany"[35]. This can be perceived as a first hint, that his further scientific efforts were mainly about the improvement of inhalational techniques, especially those involving nitrous oxide. The fact that

Schmidt had become a professor, by publishing on an anaesthesiological topic, was announced nationwide by an editorial published in the first German anaesthesia journal, "Der Schmerz" and was well recognized. An excerpt from the text: "To our knowledge this has been the first time that a German university has issued the privilege to hold lectures exclusively for the important speciality anaesthesia. This fact had found our heartfelt approval"[1].

But Schmidt did not only find out important basics about inhalational techniques. He also did extensive research on spinal anaesthesia during the early thirties. The technique had a bad reputation because of the feared side effects. Schmidt`s still up-to-date concepts have fallen into oblivion, because Martin Kirschner (1879-1942), who was the very influential head of the department of surgery at the University of Tübingen, was interested in this topic as well and had become well-known for his innovative approach[21].

After Schmidt had become chief of the Department of Surgery in a hospital in Remscheid, he got involved in studies concerning anaesthesia only every now and then[30]. But one has to mention that he, in close cooperation with people like the pharmacologist Hellmut Weese (1897-1954), the surgeon Ferdinand Koss (1912-1970) and among others together with the first head of the department of anaesthesiology Martin Zindler (1922-) starting lecturing on clinical anaesthesia from the beginning of winter term 1948/1949 on. He later claimed that these lectures, held at the Medical Academy of Düsseldorf had been "the finest ever"[44]. At his former teacher's hundredth's birthday Schmidt held the lecture "Studium analgeticum nach Sudeck"[44]. There, at the University Hospital of Hamburg, he met Karl Horatz (1913-1996) who had become the first full professor of anaesthesiology in Germany and was in charge of the institutions department of anaesthesiology[45]. In 1979 Helmut Schmidt died, without beeing honored for his lifetime achievements. But he has deserved to be among the first honorary members of our scientific society among others like Hellmut Weese (1897-1954) and Hans Killian (1892-1982) (Fig. 2)[14].

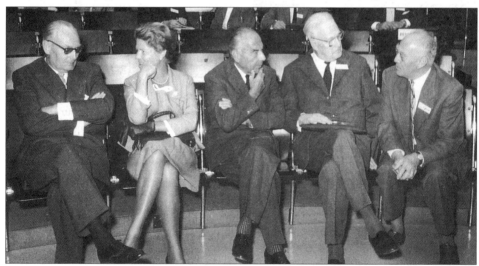

Fig. 2 German "pioneers" of anaesthesia. The photo was taken during Hans Killian`s 80 th birthday ceremony at the University of Mainz. From left to right: the brother of Helmut Schmidt, his wife, the surgeon Kümmerle, Hans Killian and Helmut Schmidt[30]

Helmut Schmidt - a Protagonist of Specialization in Anaesthesia

In 1932 Schmidt described his efforts to establish anaesthesiology as a separate specialist field like this: "The main goal behind my scientific strivings can perhaps best be characterized as the improvement of methods in anaesthesia in Germany" and to "... educate students, interns and nurses ... by strictly organizing anaesthesia". Furthermore he wanted anaesthetists working at bigger hospitals "to have the same rights as the other specialists"[29].

With his idea of establishing anaesthesia in the German speaking nations as a separate and equal field of medicine, he encountered more outright refusal than approval. Well-known German surgeons were against such ideas and published their opions in textbooks: "We do not have specialists for anaesthesia and hopefully won`t get them"[22]. Despite of this widely spread conviction there was a change of mind mostly among younger surgeons, with introduction of modern anaesthesia techniques in the middle of the 1920`s[43]. Particularly the use of the highly explosive narcotic Narcylene required the anaesthetist to have a special qualification, so that nurses could not be entrusted with this task. This was also true for nitrous oxide-oxygen anaesthesia techniques which became more popular as well. Thus "special training" for physicians performing anaesthesia appeared to make sense. The Americans had recognized the need for specialists years before and there were statements regarding this topic like the following: "every hospital, certainly every large hospital should have as a regular member of its staff an attending anaesthetist, whose authority in his special branch should be as complete as that of the attending surgeons in theirs"[23]?

While staying in the U.S. for nearly half a year for scientific reasons in summer 1928, Schmidt personally experienced the advant-

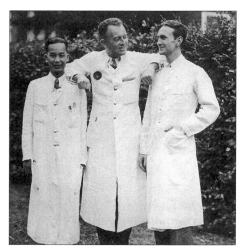

Fig. 3 Helmut Schmidt and two American guests, the surgeons Chen and Roger, around 1930[30]

ages of specialization in anaesthesia. Together with Hans Killian, who at that time was employed at the Department of Surgery at the University in Freiburg/Breisgau, he visited several reputed institutions, learned about the local anaesthesia methods and demonstrated his own abilities, acquired while working in Hamburg. It was due to the contacts he made on this trip that many highly regarded anaesthetists came to visit him there as well (Fig. 3)[3,18,30].

At a congress of anaesthetists in Minneapolis, Schmidt outlined the situation of anaesthesiology in Germany and mentioned his efforts to establish a "school of anaesthesia" at the University Hospital Eppendorf of Hamburg. He stated: "My colleague and I represent the modest beginning of a modern German Society of Anaesthetists. We as surgeons are convinced of the importance of anaesthesia as a speciality. We in Germany hope to make progress ... in the expert methods of anaesthesia. The University of Hamburg is the first in Germany to attempt this and as a lecturer there it will my special desire to develop the eductional aims and progress of this most important branch of medical practice"[37].

In the beginning of his efforts, there were lectures that were part of the general surgery lessons. They were mainly about clinical issues and designed to cause students to become interested in this field of medicine. Most of the attending students were female and this field offered, as he once casually remarked "rewarming and promising perspectives" to them[39].

The first German Congress of Anaesthesia in Hamburg 1928

A few months later, in September of 1928 in Hamburg, there was the 90 th meeting of the "Association of German Natural Scientists and Physicians" in Hamburg (Fig. 4, 5)[24].

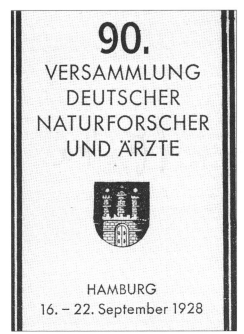

Fig. 4 *Official advertisement for the 90th meeting of the Association of German Natural Scientists and Physicians in Hamburg in 1928; nowadays this meeting is regarded as the first German Congress of Anaesthetists*[14].

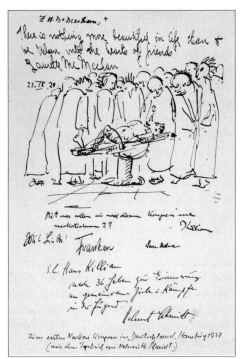

Fig. 5 *"With was we shall anaesthetize after this congress?" This humorons drawing shows doctors attending the first German Congress of Anaesthetists in Hamburg and bears several signatures*[19].

During this congress national and international representatives of the group supporting the specialization in anaesthesia came together, in order to discuss the unanswered question regarding the further fate of anaesthesiology[19]. But Schmidt, who like others, had emphasized the importance, and need for specialists for anaesthesia, if surgery was to be developed further did not succeed. The surgeon Eduard Rehn (1880-1972) from Freiburg, was presiding over the final meeting, vehemently refused the idea of anesthesiology as a separate branch of medicine[28]. Thus another 25 years were to pass before a German Society of Anaesthetists was formed. Right after this had been done Helmut Schmidt, was made an honary member of the German Anaesthesia Society because of his decades of work further developing our speciality field. Other members of honor were Hans Killian and Hellmut Weese[7].

Helmut Schmidt - a Supporter of Inhalational Anaesthesia

Just a few years after Schmidt had started working in Hamburg, the inhalational narcotic Narcylene became available for anaesthetic purpose and he extensively studied its properties. The substance called Narcylen merely was purified acetylene that had been used for welding for decades. The excellent anaesthetic qualities had been discovered by chance when accidents caused by the substance had occured. The gas was found to be totally different from all existent agents used at that time since it had been demonstrated in animal models that is was not toxic and was not metabolized inside the body[12]. Thus, the highly effective and explosive substances rapidly became popular. At the hospital of Eppendorf people were impressed by its properties and within a few months the majority of all anaesthesias were performed using Narcylene. But after several explosions that had obviously been caused by the gas, its further use was prohibited until the end of the investigations[33].

It has to be mentioned that Schmidt had started his own research regarding concentrations of the gas within the theatres in order to find out more about reasons for explosions before the first accidents happened. His studies were supported by the "Chemisch-Technische Reichsanstalt" (National authority for Chemistry and Technical Science) after combustions had taken place. Many safety regulations in operations rooms, like the prescribed grounding of anaesthetic machines, were created then due to his publications and are still in effect, thus further explosions were avoided (Fig. 6, 7)[12].

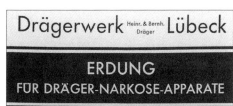

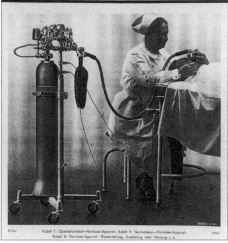

Fig. 6 Advertisement of the Dräger company with some recommendation, how to prevent explosion hazards by earthing[14]

Helmut Schmidt – an Advocate of Nitrous Oxide-Oxygen Anaesthesia

The explosive qualities of Narcylene was the reason why Schmidt studied another inhalational agents, that he had learned about more or less accidentally: nitrous oxide also known as laughing gas[35]. Since his part in reestablishing nitrous oxide oxygen anaesthesia techniques in Germany cannot be overestimated, his achievements are described in separate articles. But in order to provide the reader with a better understanding of the situation it has to be mentioned that the renaissance of nitrous-oxide oxygen anaesthesia techniques use is closely related to his name.

While visiting the Dutch surgeon Jan Hendrik Zaaijer (1876-1932) in Leiden, Netherlands, where he was exspected to teach his Dutch colleagues the new Narcylene

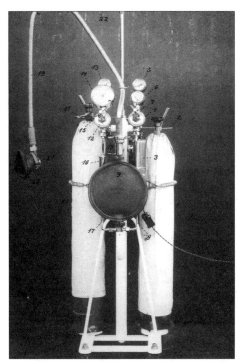

the first serial produced nitrous-oxide-oxygen anaesthetic apparatus ever, called "Modell A", in 1924/1925. The machine was largely responsible for the success of the new technique in Germany (Fig. 8)[15,29,35,46].

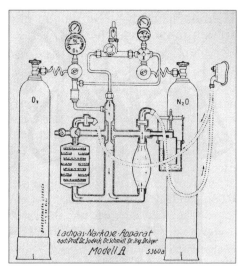

Fig. 7 Dräger´s "Nitrous-Oxygen Anaesthetic Apparatus", the so-called "Modell A". In 1925, this device was constructed in close collaboration with the surgeons Prof. Dr. Paul Sudeck and Dr. Helmut Schmidt from the University Clinics Eppendorf, Hamburg[35].

Fig. 8 Scheme of the first nitrous oxide anaesthesia aparatus made by the firm Dräger, Lübeck. Please note the scheme of the closed circle system, 1925[14]

anaesthetic technique, he found about the local habit of administering a mixture of nitrous oxide and oxygen. The anaesthetic was given using a simple apparatus designed by Zaaijer himself[48]. During his stay in Leiden, the first explosion caused by Narcylene occured in Hamburg, several more followed after his return in the German speaking area[12].

Recognizing the hazards and because of the authorities banning Narcylene from the operation rooms for the time needed to investigate the reasons for the accidents, his chief Paul Sudeck (1866-1945) agreed to experiments with the non toxic and and non explosive nitrous oxide. In close collaboration with the company Dräger of Lübeck, they created

Helmut Schmidt - a Supporter of the Pharyngeal Airway

When describing Schmidts merits, one must not omit his seemingly unspectacular small publication of 1925, which instantaneously made the use of the Mayo-tube popular in Germany. The study was called: "Zur Verwendung der Rachenkanüle während der Narkose" (About the use of a pharyngeal airway during anaesthesia), Schmidt described the device which he had got to know while staying in Leiden as "humane, practical and always working"[60]. After returning from the Netherlands, he convinced the company AD Krauth, a manufactorer of medical instruments from Hamburg, to produce three different sizes of the pharyngeal airway, that was made like the

American model of nickel-plated wire frame[60].

Helmut Schmidt - an Advocate of Spinal Anaesthesia

At the end of the 1920`s Schmidt published many important articles on local anaesthesia and extensively studied lumbar anaesthesia techniques using hypo- and hyperbaric local anaesthetic solutions[40,41]. It is interesting that he got intrigued by this special method after staying in the United States for a few months and encountering personally by the American surgeon George Pitkin (1885-1943)[26].

The Situation of Spinal Anaesthesia in 1925

After a number of case reports on fatal incidents after lumbar spinal anaesthesia had shed a negative light on this technique, many surgeons in Germany refrained from employing the method until the early twenties[8,10,47]. The knowledge about the inferior quality of local anaesthetics added to this. But these common prejudices did not keep surgeons like Martin Kirschner from Tübingen and Helmut Schmidt from developing new techniques of spinal anaesthesia (Fig. 9a). Both men were probably inspired by the publications of Pitkin who managed to achieve a way to gain control over the anaesthesia by adding substances to Procain causing the mixture to be either hypo-or hypobaric[26]. These combinations were sold in Germany as "Spinokain leicht or schwer ("light" or "heavy"), and thanks to them the much feared cases of loss of blood-pressure after the anaesthetics injection could be avoided[40,41]. Moreover Schmidt advocated the combination of the use of the mentioned substances and special positioning of the patient taking into account of the specific weight of the anaesthetic and the desired analgesic effect. Employing a protractor, called "Tiltometer", attached to the

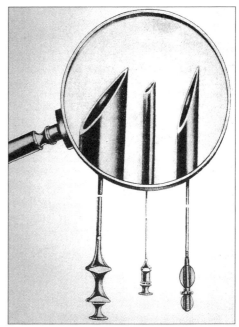

Fig. 9a The "atraumatic" spinal needle, which was used by Schmidt in the late twenties. Please note the different calibers of the needles and the different bevels[40].

operating table, he was able to limit the anaesthetic effect to those spinal nerves that normally innerved the area operated upon. The technique was praised because of the stable hemodynamic situation it provided[26]. In order to further improve his technique, Pitkin regularly subcutaneously injected ephedrine, a vasopressor made of a vegetable extract developed a few months earlier[27].

Schmidt copied Pitkins technique and thus spinal anaesthesia experienced a renaissance after the technique had hardly been used in Hamburg between 1923 and 1927 (Fig. 9b, c)[40,41]. Schmidt also advised him of the possiblity of injecting the ephedrine intravenously, but at the time cautioned him about its use in patients with cardiac problems. It is worth mentioning that the subcutaneous dose of ephedrine was already fixed the day before the operation. Blood pressure on the day and

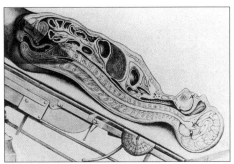

Fig. 9b Spread of spinal anaesthesia in lower extremities anaesthesia and the position of the anaesthetic solution. Please note the "Tiltometer", attached to the operating table[40].

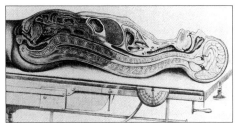

Fig. 9c Spread of spinal anaesthesia in high spinal anaesthesia and the position of the anaesthetic solution[40].

the number of spinal segments to be anaesthetized were taken into account[41]. In 1932, Pantocain was replaced by a the new local anaesthetic: Spinocain[42]. The substance was introduced into clinical practice by Schmidt and was a derivative of Novocaine. Thanks to his father he had a good relationship to the drug company Hoechst and asked to preside over the clinical trails of the new substance. Its anaesthetic effect was 10 fold and its duration of action was three to four times as long. The fact that the new local anaesthetic proved to be more stable than its predecessors, its mode of action was more smoothly and last but not least could be used to anaesthetize mucosa, warranted its popularity in the following years[43].

Helmut Schmidt - a Supporter of Intraoperative Monitoring

Schmidt had realized that, in order to convince his colleagues to be less reserved regarding spinal anaesthesia, he had to prove that his modified spinal anaesthesia technique was "safe" in comparison to the the then used method. Thus he established a regimen of unusual close intra-and postoperative monitoring of surgical patients. He stated " the patient´s heart rate, respiration and colour of skin have to be observed continuously"[41]. To us it may seem the most normal thing on earth but in Germany at that time it was most unusual and revolutionary that the anaesthetist had to "... check the blood-pressure regularly during the operation and write it down on a anaesthesia chart". Schmidt had obviously been convinced of the advantages of this method while staying in the US, where the blood-pressure had been routinely checked and recorded during surgical proce-

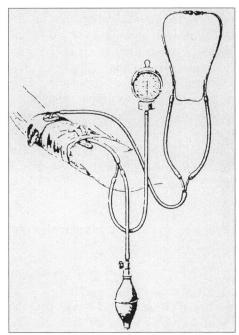

Fig. 10 Blood-pressure device, which was recommended by Helmut Schmidt in an article[36]

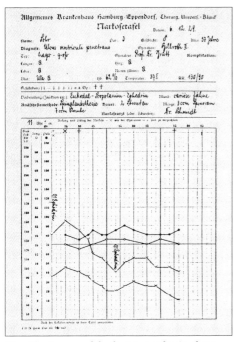

Fig. 11a A copy of the first anaesthesia chart which was used in Germany. Modifications of this type of anaesthesia chart were used for decades at the University Hospital Eppendorf, Hamburg[41]. Front of the anaesthesia chart.

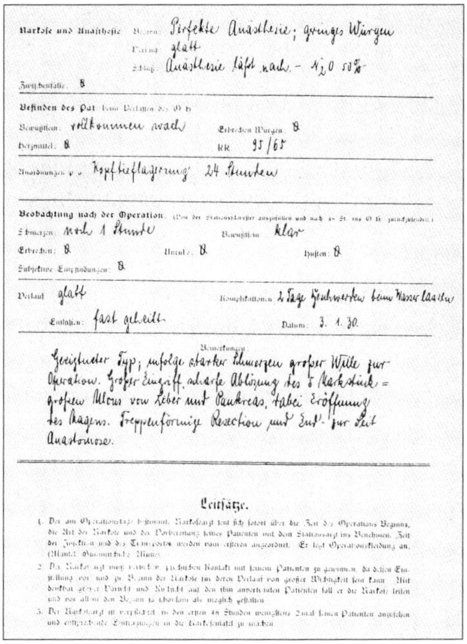

Fig. 11b Back of the anaesthesia chart

dures since the turn of the century[4]. Machines which were able to automatically monitor the patients blood-pressure had been introduced at the congress in Minneapolis in 1928 he had attended and were advertised in anaesthesia journals, but since they were not available in Germany he advocated to check the patient's pressure by auscultating the Korotkoff-sounds. The methods, quote: "involving the palpation of the radial artery or the observation of the oscillation of the pressure gauge" were "significantly less safe"[41].

Thus obviously he copied techniques he had learned about in the United States, and on which the anaesthetist John Henry Evans (1876-1955) from New York had repeatedly reported. He, in fact, had one so at the congress in Minneapolis[9]. He described the advantages of intraoperative blood-pressure monitoring in several publications and added pictures, so that his technique could easily be understood all over the German speaking nations (Fig. 10)[36,38]. He also was the first to create an anaesthesia chart, called "Narkosetafel" (anaesthesia chart) (Fig. 11a, b)[41]. His idea was obviously not taken up by other physicians, because there are no publications on the topic except for those by Schmidt. The textbooks that were sold at that time did not contain hints about recording the patients vital statistics nor show a picture of an anaesthesia protocol. It was not until after World War II, that German anaesthetists, influenced by their American colleagues, started using anaesthesia charts[16].

When looking at Helmut Schmidts scientific achievements, there are several of his concepts still which are still unchanged and up-to-date. In our opinion those are:

- That our field of medicine should be taught at German universities, and that there are regular lectures and practical exercises
- The demand to professionalize anaesthesia by appointing habilitated professors to teach this field at the university
- The use of nitrous-oxide-oxygen mixtures
- His suggestions for safety regulations that were to apply when Narcylen was used, but are still in effect today
- His recommendations to secure the airway, using a Mayo-tube
- His research regarding spinal anaesthesia using hypo-or hyperbaric solutions and blunt non, traumatic cannulas were used
- His advice to closely monitor the patient under anaesthesia, and to record his vital parameters like respiration, heart rate and blood-pressure using an anaesthesia protocol, then called "anaesthesia chart".

References:

1. Anonymous: Zur Tagesgeschichte. Der Schmerz 1928:1

2. Anonymous: Anesthesia and the Hamburg Congress. Anesth & Analg 1929; 16-19

3. Bacon D: Personel communication

4. Barr D: Preliminary note on a new method of recording blood pressure with presentation of a model. Anesth & Analg 1927; 273-277

5. Beecher HK: The first anesthesia records (Codman, Cushing). Surg Gynec Obstet 1940; 689-693

6. Blaschke F, G Hermann: Zur Frage der Hirnnervenschädigung nach Lumbalanästhesie. Med Klin 1925; 45: 1685-1686

7. Bräutigam KH: 40 Jahre "Facharzt für Anästhesie". Anästhesiologie und Intensivmedizin;1993; 9: 259-268

8. Denk W: Die Gefahren und Schäden der Lokal- und Leitungsanästhesie. Wien klin Wochenschr 1920; 29: 630-636

9. Evans J H: Teaching anesthesia in the specialities: ear, nose and throat. Anesth & Analg 1928; 7:264-268

10. Franke M: Über Dauerschädigungen nach Lumbalanästhesie mit Novokain-Suprarenin-Lösung. Dtsch Zschr f Chir 1927; 222: 262-269

11. Goerig M, K Ayisi, J Schulte am Esch: The merits of Ludwig Burkhardt and Hermann Kümmell for the development of intravenous anaesthesia. Anaesthesia History Society, Rotterdam Meeting May, Rotterdam 1991

12. Goerig M, H Böhrer: Narcylennarkose. AINS 1994; 29: 297-299

13. Goerig M, J Schulte am Esch: Hellmut Weese - der Versuch einer Würdigung seiner Bedeutung für die deutschsprachige Anästhesie. AINS 1997; 32: 678-685

14. Goerig M: Collection Goerig

15. Haupt J: Der Dräger-Narkoseapparat - historisch gesehen - Sonderdruck MT 105, Dräger-Werke, Lübeck 1984

16. Henley J: Einführung in die Praxis der modernen Inhalationsnarkose. Walter de Gruyter & Co., Berlin 1950

17. Howat D C: Paul Sudeck - His Contribution to Anaesthesia. Anaesthesia 1989; 44: 847-850

18. Killian H: 40 Jahre Narkoseforschung. Verlag der Deutschen Hochschullehrer-Zeitung, Tübingen 1964

19. Killian H: Reminiscenses of the first German Anaesthesia Congress in Hamburg 1927 and Rolf Frey´s departure to Main. In: Ruprecht J, Lieburg M J van, Lee J A , Erdmann W (Eds) Anaesthesia. Essays on its History. Springer, Berlin-Heidelberg, New-York,Tokyo1985

20. Kirschner M: Häufung über üble Zustände der Lumbalanästhesie. Zbl f Chir 1919; 18: 322-324

21. Kirschner M: Eine gürtelförmige, einstellbare und individuell dosierbare Spinalbetäubung. Chirurg 1931; 14: 633-644

22. Leusden F:Die Bekämpfung des Schmerzes in der Chirurgie. In: Kirschner-Nordmann: Die Chirurgie, Band II, Urban & Schwarzenberg , Berlin-Wien 1926

23. McCormic A S: Some oberservations on anesthesia as a speciality and the anesthetist as a specialist. Am J Surg, Anesth Suppl 1919; 66-71

24. Mc Mechan F H: Anesthesia and the Hamburg Congress. Anesth & Analg 1929; Jan-Febr: 16

25. Plesch J: Über einen neuen selbstregistrierenden Blutdruckapparat. Med Klin 1928; 11: 415-417

26. Pitkin G: Controllable spinal anesthesia. Am J Surg 1928; 5: 537-553

27. Pitkin G : Controllable spinal anesthesia with Spinocain. Anesth & Analg 1929; 3/4:78-90

28 Rehn E: Bericht zur 90. Versammlung Deutscher Naturforscher und Ärzte in Hamburg. Zbl f Chr 1929; 3: 174-178

29 Richter: Mitarbeiter am Staatsarchiv Hamburg, Personalakte von Prof. Dr. med. Helmut Schmidt. (Hochschulwesen, Dozenten- und Personalakten, IV 947) Staatsarchiv Hamburg, Correspondence Oktober 1987

30 Schmidt A: Son of Helmut Schmidt, personel communication concerning Professor Dr. med. Helmut Schmidt 1987-1996

31 Schmidt H: Zur Narzylennarkose. Münch Med Wschr 1925; 21: 841-844

32 Schmidt H: Zur Verwendung von Rachenkanülen während der Narkose. Zbl f Chir 1925; 34: 1884-1885

33 Schmidt H: Der heutige Stand der Gasnarkose in Deutschland. Verhandlungen des Ärztlichen Verein Hamburg. Sonderdruck aus den Mitteilungen fuer die Aerzte und Zahnärzte Groß-Hamburgs 1926. (Hrsg.) Vom Vorstande des Aerztlichen Vereins. Druckerei der Oldenburger Landeszeitung, Oldenburg 1926

34 Schmidt H: Ein Überdruckapparat mit geringen respiratorischen Druckschwankungen. Zbl f Chir 1926; 20: 1269-1271

35 Schmidt H: Die Leistungsfähigkeit der Stickoxydul-Sauerstoffnarkose in der Chirurgie. Eine vergleichende Narkosestudie zur Wiedereinführung der Lachgasnarkose in Deutschland. Abhandlung zur Erlangung der Venia Legendi der Hohen Medizinischen Fakultät der Hamburgischen Universität, Hamburg 1928

36 Schmidt H : Das Ephedrin in der operativen Praxis. Zbl f Chir 1928;51: 3207-3209

37 Schmidt H: Inhalation or injection narcosis ? The development of the speciality of anesthesia in Germany. Anesth & Analg 1929; Jan-Febr: 20-23

38 Schmidt H: Narcosis moderna y narcoticos. Rev Medica Germano Ibero Americano 1929; 2: 371-379

39 Schmidt H:Der Narkosespezialismus in den Vereinigten Staaten. Der Chirurg 1929; 21: 959-964

40 Schmidt H: Pitkins kontrollierbare Spinalanästhesie mit viskotischen, spezifisch leichteren Novocainlösungen. Arch f klin Chir 1929; 157: 206-211

41 Schmidt H:Lumbalanästhesie mit spezifisch leichter viscotischer Novocainlösung (Spinocain) und prophylaktischer Stabilisierung des Blutdrucks durch Ephedrin. Klin Wschr 1930; 16: 748-756

42 Schmidt H: Pantokain zur Lumbalanästhesie. Zbl f Chir 1932; 21: 1321-1331

43 Schmidt H:10 Jahre Forschung und Fortschritt in der chirurgischen Anästhesie, ihre bleibenden und praktischen Ergebnisse. Maschinengeschriebenes Protokoll eines Vortrages vor der medizinischen Gesellschaft in Düsseldorf 19.6.1934

44 Schmidt H : Das Stadium analgeticum der Inhalationsnarkose nach Sudeck. Der Anaesthesist 1967; 16: 270- 274

45 Schmidt H :Gruß an Hans Killian. In: R. Frey et al: Erlebte Geschichte der Anästhesie. Mainz 1972

46 Schulte am Esch J : Karl Horatz-75 Jahre alt. Anaesth Intensivther Notfallmed 1988; 23: 2-3

47 Sudeck P, H Schmidt:Ein neues Modell eines möglichst druckkonstanten Überdruckapparates. Dtsch Zschr f Chir; 197: 1-9

48 Strauss M: Mortalität und üble Zufälle bei der Lumbalanästhesie. Dtsch Zschr f Chir 1922; 172: 296-304

49 Wijhe M van: From Stupefaction to Narcosis. Alkmaar, Slinger 1991

Cardio-Pulmonary Resuscitation in Egypt 5000 Years ago?

A. Ocklitz
Department of Anaesthesiology, St. Gertrauden Krankenhaus Berlin, Germany

Since a large portion of what we know today about ancient Egyptian medicine was handed down in the context of the Cult of the Dead, it is not out of place to examine Cult of the Dead activities regarding their medical content. The U.S. Egyptologist, A. M. Roth, for example, did that and established an astonishing correlation between the death cult and obstetrics. Thus she was able to prove that examination of the mouth of newborn infants for life-threatening deformities was performed 5000 years ago in the Egyptian cult of the dead[1].

In the German medical journal 'Der Anaesthesist' in 1/96 I had the opportunity of showing that the ancient Egyptian's Opening of the Mouth ceremony in particular, as it is depicted in the Hunefer Papyrus, shows considerable similarity to modern emergency procedures up to and including artificial respiration (Fig. 1)[2]. Here you can see these ritual steps being performed on the standing mummy. On the side table, depicted on the bottom right of the Hunefer Papyrus, you can see the tools used. This cult duplicated the resuscitation of the dead Pharaoh for the afterlife. Opening of the mouth with the Chisel of Iron was central to the ritual. But opening of the eyes, in the sense of modern pupillary examination, the extraction of teeth and perhaps also the insertion of a breathing tube were also simulated. It is possible that the so-called Horus fingers, which were very closely connected to the resuscitation of the Pharaoh, were used as breathing tubes. These were golden tubes, and are to be seen on the side table in the Hunefer papyrus above the eye-opening device. This suggests the use of gold tubes as breathing tubes when you take into account that the first tubes used in our times were also made of metal, and that Avicenna reported on an Arabic method of intubation with gold tubes a thousand years ago.

A series of mouth-opening chisels, put in line from left to right, can be seen on the side table in the Hunefer Papyrus. They are laid out in preparation for use, according to mouth size and form, as on a modern anaesthetic table. The German palaeontologist, Pahl, could demonstrate that these devices were used in fact to open the mouths of mummies[3]. Wallis Budge, a legend among Egyptologists, found that the procedures carried out during this ritual were performed on fresh corpse in ancient times. That means that the Egyptians did have experience of resuscitation-like procedures using those obscure instruments.

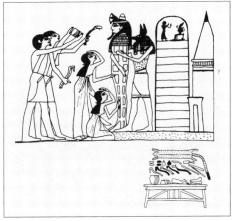

Fig. 1: Papyrus Hunefer. The Opening of the Mouth ceremony.

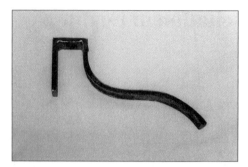

Fig. 2: The Mouth-Opening Device.

Please note the following characteristics of these devices. They all have:
1. two perfect right-angles at the head of the device,
2. a perfectly straight tongue depressor,
3. thickness of almost 10mm,
4. full metal or all-wood form.

The mouth-opening devices are similar to the u-shaped laryngoscope designed by Magill[4]. They are made of nickel iron. This is astonishing since iron probably was first processed in Egypt after 580 BC.

With my reconstruction of this ancient Egyptian mouth-opening device (Fig. 2), I can show that within the framework of their Cult of the Dead, the Egyptians were equipped with a technique that made artificial respiration possible, 5000 years ago. My reconstruction, which I will present in more detail in my video resembles exactly to those shown in the Hunefer Papyrus. I demonstrated its use on a phantom in a video documentation on March 1st at the Vienna Clinical Meeting and at the German Anaesthetics Congress in 1997.[5] A paper on this reconstruction will be published in Der Ansthesist[6]. For the device to function in the sense of emergency medicine, the subject must be in a supine position. There is a painting in the tomb of Nakhtamun in Deir el Medina which may be a depiction of this process (Fig. 3). The mortuary priest, holding the iron device in his hand, assumes a position corresponding to inverse intubation in modern polytrauma management (Fig. 4)[7].

As you can see here (Fig. 5), intubation on a phantom is possible using my reconstructed device without having an extra light source, but a second person is needed for the insertion of the tube. Intubation using modern laryngoscope application methods is unlikely, due to the properties of the material used. Flat rolled steel did not exist then. All figures show a thick, forged instrument, like that depicted in a painting from the 3300 year old tomb of Ankherkah, or rather that from Tutanchamun.

The fact that the ancient Egyptian's experience on emergency medicine was passed on only through Cult of the Dead has probably got to do with the central role played by this cult in the power structure of the early Pharaonic state. The so-called ritual resuscitation of the

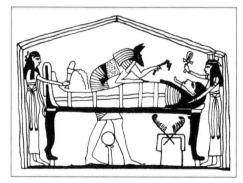

Fig. 3: Tomb of Nekhtamun, 19. Dyn. Deir el-Medineh, Thebes.

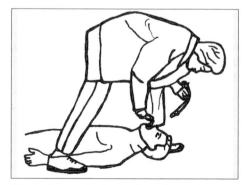

Fig. 4: Inverse intubation in modern polyrauma management.

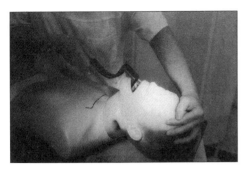

Fig. 5: The mouth-opening with the reconstructed chisel using the ancient method.

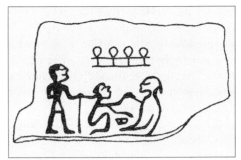

Fig. 6: King Aha's slab.

Pharaoh was originally the responsibility and privilege of the king of the Egyptians only. Thus medical knowledge in connection with resuscitation was monopolised by this elite.

There are, however, sufficient hints to experience with cardio-pulmonary resuscitation beyond the ancient Egyptian Cult of the Dead. Ahnefeld drew attention to the so-called Hebrew method of resuscitation. More than 3000 years ago, midwives in Palestine practised mouth-to-mouth respiration on asphyxiating newborn infants.

Certain depictions from the early Old Kingdom have been linked with the performance of tracheotomy. Here you can see an artist's impression of the so-called King Aha's slab (fig.6)[8]. Vikentiev pointed out that tracheotomy was ritually simulated at the Heb-Sed celebration, a royal anniversary in the Old Kingdom[9].

There is also an astonishing relief in the Abu Simbel Temple, showing the famous battle of Kadesh in 1275 BC (fig.7)[10]. Felkai Peter pointed out that a medical act is depicted in the turmoil of that scene. A badly wounded Hittite prince is being treated by a helper. The rescuer, obviously skilled in medicine, is using an emergency procedure very common today. It is known as the Esmarch-Heiberg grip or head-tilt-chin-lift-method to keep the respiratory tract free. This proves that freeing the airway was common at that time and not limited to the Cult of the Dead.

This finding relates with the achievements of a group of emergency doctors in ancient Egypt. The members of this organisation called themselves exorcists of Serqet after the goddess Serqet, and they adhered to specialist standards. They had been able to treat life-threatening conditions caused by snake bites or scorpion stings for example. The activities of this group are well documented, for example in the sitting statue of the rescuer Djed-Hor in the Egyptian Museum in Cairo.

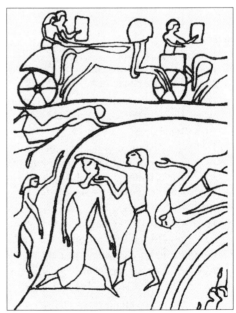

Fig. 7: Relief in the Abu Simbel Tempel, Battel of Kadesh, 1275 BC

Engelmann and Hallof translated the inscription on the statue as follows: 'This is the doctor who prepares the way to revive the dead, who puts air into the closed nose (!) of he who is without breath, to resuscitate him by moving his arms by making use of all the methods of the .... exorcists of Serqet .'[11]

It is not sure whether that all the Serqet exorcists methods form a system of cardiopulmonary resuscitation as we would define it. However, as my reconstruction of the ancient Egyptian mouth-opening device shows, further hints on of this knowledge may be written down in the Cult of the Dead. It is possible that the achievements of the Old Kingdom may have been preserved for all eternity in this way. The Smith and Ebers medical papyri, also found in tombs, are impressive for the seemingly modern systematic manner in the diagnosis and treatment of various diseases. It is possible that these papyri form a fraction of a far more extensive body of scientific knowledge.

All reproductions were made by F. Knolle.

References:

[1] Roth AM: Fingers, stars and the opering of the mouth . J Egypt Archaeol 1993; 79:57-79

[2] Ocklitz A: Künstliche Beatmung mit technischen Hilfsmitteln schon vor 5000 Jahren? Anaesthesist 1996; 1/45: 19-21

[3] Pahl WM: The ritual of opening the mouth: Arguments for an actual body-ritual from the view-point of mummy research. In: Science in Egyptology. Manchester. Manchester Univ Press, 1986, p 211

[4] Pryor WJ, Bush DCT: A Manual of Anaesthetic Techiques. Bristol.Wright & Sons, 1966, p 43

[5] Ocklitz A: Kardio-pulmonale Reanimation in Ägypten schon vor 5000 Jahren? Wiener Klin Wschr. 1997; 109/11: 406-412

[6] Ocklitz A: Rekonstruktion des altägyptischen Mundöffnungsgerätes. Anaesthesist 1997; 7/46: 599-603

[7] Ocklitz A: Deir el-Medina und das Totenritual der Alten Ägypter. Kemet 1996; 5/3:25-27

[8] Pahor AL: Ear, Nose and Throat in ancient Egypt. In: Science in Egyptology, Manchester Univ Press, Manchester, 1986, p 243-249

[9] Vikentiev V: Deux rites du jubilé royal l'époque Protodynastique.

[10] Felkai P. Az jralesztsi kisrletel els nyoma az kori Egyiptomban. Orvosi Hetilap, 1986; 28:1709-1712

[11] Engelmann H, Hallof J: Medizinische Nothilfe und Unfallversorgung auf staatlichen Arbeitspltzen im alten Ägypten. Zeitschr. f. ägypt. Sprache und Altertumskunde 1995; 122/2: 119-120

Pulmonary Resuscitation in Ancient Egypt

W. H. Maleck[1], K. P. Koetter[2]
[1] Department of Anesthesiology, Klinikum, Ludwigshafen, Germany
[2] Neurological Intensive Care Unit, Leopoldina-Hospital, Schweinfurt, Germany

Introduction:

Ocklitz proposed a new interpretation of the Ancient Egyptian funeral ritual of "Opening of the Mouth" as a relic of knowledge of pulmonary resuscitation in the earliest times of Ancient Egypt[1-4].

Methods:

We tried to discover more facts pointing to a knowledge like this, using Medline, newer books on Ancient Egyptian Medicine and its secondary literature.

Results:

Two slabs from protodynastic time (about 3000 BC) show a person pointing a knife to the neck (or upper thorax) of another. One of these was discovered by Petrie in Abydos, the other by Emery and Saad in Saqqara[5-7]. Emery considered this as a captive to be stabbed in the breast in 1938, i.e. ritual sacrifice[6]. In 1949, however, Vikentiev proposed that this could have been a tracheotomy[8]. Ever since there has been a lot of discussion[9-19]. This issue is discussed in detail in another paper by von Hintzenstern and us in this book. It is of interest that one of these slabs dates to the reign of Djer, about whom Manetho (according to Africanus) wrote: "Athotis [or Djer], his [i.e. Menes'] son, [ruled] for fifty-seven years. He built the palace at Memphis, and his anatomical works are extant,for he was a physician"[19].

The surgical Papyrus Smith is known as "Book of Wounds". The preserved copy was written about 1550 BC (early New Kingdom). It is, however, a fragment of a text of which only 48 cases relating to head, neck, arms and thorax have been copied. The original was probably of much older origin. This thesis is based by the egyptologists on the glossary (footnotes) explaining archaic expressions which were unknown to the average reader in the New Kingdom. Westendorf writes "text analysis shows without doubt that the text was written in the Old Kingdom".[20] However, its ancient origin has been recently doubted as Ancient Egyptians sometimes introduced archaic features in their texts to add authority[19].

Anyway, Papyrus Smith is at least 3,500 years old and describes quite modern medicine. Based on medical history taking and physical examination, in each case a diagnosis has been made and one of three possibilities were considered:
- "An ailment which I will treat"
- "An ailment with which I will contend"
- "An ailment not to be treated "[19]

Then (excluding most hopeless cases) a therapy was included:bandage, suture, drugs. In case No. 7, Papyrus Smith describes a head injury with trismus. The physician – in order to feed the patient – "should than cause to be made for him a chisel of wood, padded with linen and placed in his mouth"[19]. Westendorf emphasizes the fact that a chisel was also used for the above mentioned ritual of "Opening of the Mouth"[20].

Two pictures from the Ramesseum (about 1200 BC) show a resuscitation in (near-) drowning. Beside the obsolete inversion method the modern head-tilt-chin-lift-method is shown[21]. Furthermore, Ocklitz mentioned at the symposium the statue of Djed-her-le-Saveur, that possibly refers to mouth to nose breathing. Jelínková-Reymond gave the following French translation of the relevant passage: "celui qui prépare la voie pour faire revivre les morts, pour donner de l'air au nez bouché, pour réanimer l'asphyxie par le geste de ses bras [ainsi que] par tout procédé de 'dompter-le-scorpion'"[22]. However, this statue is of an origin dating back only to the Macedonian period (about 320 BC).

Conclusion

These documents show basic methods for artificial feeding and securing the airway in the New Kingdom (1550-1100 BC) and the Macedonian period. Hints to invasive methods of airway management are only given in the controversial tracheotomy scenes from protodynastic time. We know that in the pyramid age (about 2500 BC) a highly organized medical profession existed.[23] Unfortunately, no medical texts from this era are known. From the medical texts known, Ocklitz' hypothesis can neither be proven nor refuted.

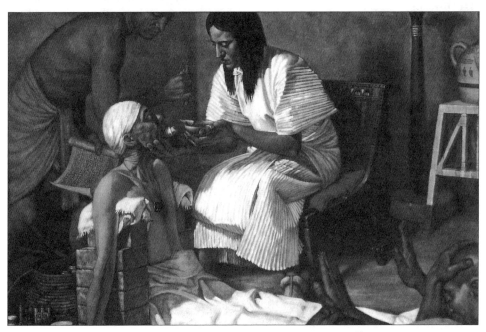

A modern picture of the "Opening of the Mouth" in case 7 of papyrus Smith.[24] With kind permission of Parke-Davis, division of Warner-Lambert company.

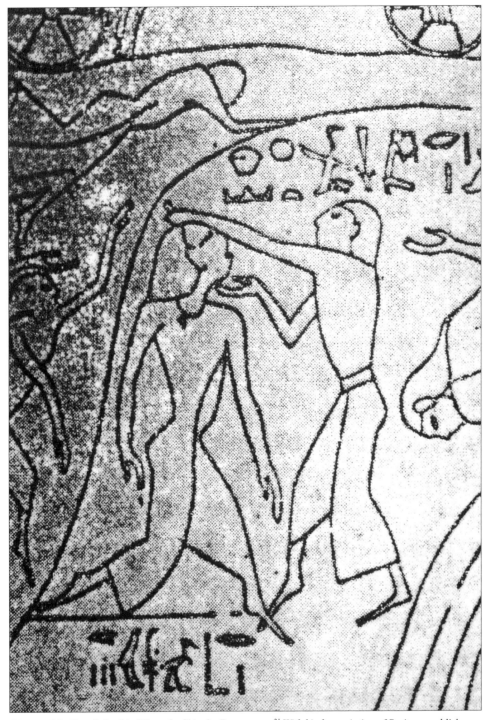

Picture of the "head-tilt-chin-lift-method" in the Ramesseum.[21] With kind permission of Springer publishers.

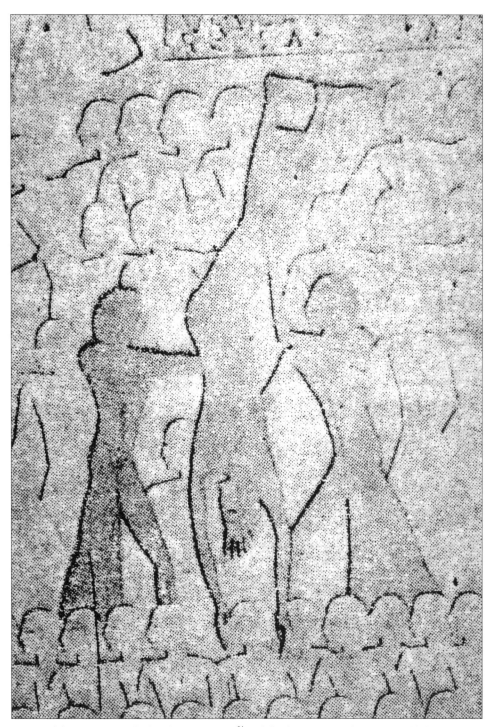

Picture of the inversion method in the Ramesseum.[21] With kind permission of Springer publishers.

References:

1. Ocklitz A: Das Mundöffnungsritual der alten Ägypter. Ancient Skies 1995; 19/1:8-11

2. Ocklitz A: Die Pyramiden: Reanimationskapseln? Ancient Skies 1995; 19/6:7-9

3. Ocklitz A: Das altägyptische Mundöffnungsritual im Licht der modernen Wiederbelebungsmedizin. Kemet 1995; 4/4:31-33

4. Ocklitz A: Künstliche Beatmung mit technischen Hilfsmitteln schon vor 5000 Jahren? Anaesthesist 1996; 45:19-21

5. Petrie WMF: Royal Tombs of the Earliest Dynasties. (= Volume II of Royal Tombs of the first Dynasty) Egypt Exploration Fund, London 1901, Plate III,6

6. Emery WB, Saad ZY: The Tomb of Hemaka. Government press, Cairo 1938, p. 35-36 and Plate 17-18

7. Emery WB: Archaic Egypt. Penguin Books, London 1991, p. 59

8. Vikentiev V: Deux rites du jubilé royal a l'époque protodynastique. Bulletin de l'Institute d'Égypte 1949-50; 32:171-200

9. Hussein MK: Quelques spécimens de pathologie osseuse chez les anciens Égyptiens. Bulletin de l'Institute d'Égypte 1949-50; 32: 11-17

10. Sercer A: 2000 Jahre Tracheotomie. Ciba-Symposium 1962; 10:78-86

11. Weill R: Recherches sur la 1re dynastie. Institut Francais d'Archéologie Orientale, Caire 1961, Vol. 2, Chapter 14

12. Ghalioungui P: Magic and Medical Science in Ancient Egypt. 1st Ed., Hodder&Stoughton, London 1963, p. 93-95

13. Ghalioungui P: The House of Life per Ankh. Magic and Medical Science in Ancient Egypt. 2nd Ed., B.M.Israel, Amsterdam 1973, p. 90-92

14. Shehata MA: History of laryngeal intubation. Middle East J Anaesth 1981; 6:49-55

15. Klippe HJ, Löhr J, Kroeger C: Historische Aspekte zur Entwicklung der endotrachealen Intubation. Praxis der Pneumologie 1981; 35:413-420

16. Biefel K, Pirsig W: Tracheotomien vor 1800. Gesnerus 1988; 45:521-539

17. Pahor AL: Ear, nose and throat in ancient Egypt, Part II. J Laryngol Otol 1992; 106:773-779

18. Stetter C: The Secret Medicine of the Pharaohs. Edition Q, Chicago 1993, p. 36 and 41

19. Nunn JF: Ancient Egyptian Medicine. University of Oklahoma, Norman 1996, p. 25-42, 131, 169, 182

20. Westendorf W: Erwachen der Heilkunst. Die Medizin im Alten Ägypten. Artemis&Winkler, Zürich 1992, p. 129-144

21. Felkai P : Az újraélesztési kisérletek elsö nyoma az ókori Egyiptomban. Orvosi Hetilap 1986; 127: 1709-1712

22. Jelínková-Reymond E: Les inscriptions de la statue guérisseuse de Djed-her-le-saveur. Institut Francais d'Archéologie Orientale, Caire 1956, p. 132-133

23. Ghalioungui P: The Physicians of Pharaonic Egypt. Philipp von Zabern, Mainz 1983, p. 16-23

24. Bender GA, Thom RA: Medicine in ancient Egypt. In: A History of Medicine in Pictures. Parke, Davis & Company, 1957

Pioneers of Cardiac Massage

H. Böhrer and M. Goerig*
Department of Anaesthesia, Universität Heidelberg, Heidelberg, and Department of Anaesthesia, University Hospital Hamburg*, Hamburg, Germany

In the anaesthesia literature, it is generally thought that open-chest cardiac massage to treat patients with chloroform syncope was first attempted by Niehaus in the late 1880s, and that closed-chest cardiac massage, as described by Koenig in 1883 and Maass in 1892, was not used in later years[1]. We would like to clarify several inaccuracies associated with these statements.

Open-chest cardiac massage in humans

When Niehaus is referred to, an article by Zesas is usually quoted[2]. In 1903, Zesas described that in the late 1880s he had witnessed Dr. Niehaus performing a thoracotomy and rhythmic compressions of the heart in a previously healthy 40-year-old patient undergoing thyroid surgery. Anaesthesia was induced in this patient with pure chloroform. Immediately before surgical incision, apnoea occurred, the patient became cyanotic, and no pulse was palpable. After attempting manual ventilation, Niehaus opened the thorax and started direct cardiac massage. However, the patient died despite these efforts. When trying to identify the curriculum vitae of Dr. Niehaus, it became evident that there was a misspelling in Zesas' article. It was found that "Niehaus" should be read "Niehans". Paul Niehans (1848–1912) (Fig. 1) was born in Berne on February 6th, 1848 and attended medical school in his home town. After graduating, he trained in Paris, Vienna, Berlin, London and Edinburgh, before returning to Berne to become a resident and staff member in the surgical department. His main areas of interest were orthopaedic surgery and the effects of massage on muscles and orthopaedic diseases. Paul Niehans died in Berne on November 28th, 1912.

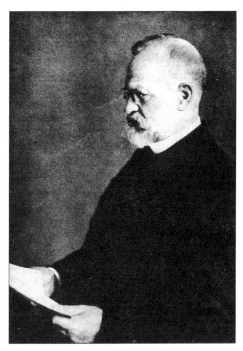

Fig. 1: Paul Niehans (1848–1912)

A second case of open-chest cardiac massage was reported by Carl Langenbuch (1846–1901) at the 16th Congress of the German Surgical Society in Berlin on April 13th, 1887[3]. Langenbuch, who was head of the Lazarus Hospital in Berlin, described a patient who suffered from chloroform syncope immediately after induction of anaesthesia. Artificial manual ventilation had been attempted for at least half an hour when Langenbuch made the decision to perform a lateral thoracotomy. He then grasped the heart of the patient and applied pressure rhythmically. Langenbuch expressed the view that during these compressions the face of the patient regained a healthier colour, and - despite the fatal outcome in his patient - he recommended this technique for the treatment of chloroform syncope.

Closed-chest cardiac massage

Closed-chest cardiac massage for chloroform syncope in cats was first performed by Boehm and co-workers at the University of Dorpat in the 1870s[4]. The first clinical description of external cardiac massage was by Koenig in 1883, who extended the technique of artificial, manual ventilation to compressions over the heart region. Franz Koenig (Fig. 2) was born in Rotenburg on February 16, 1832. He spent most of his medical school years in Marburg. After graduation he became a general practitioner with special interests in surgical problems such as lung injuries. He was then appointed as a full professor of surgery in Rostock. In 1875, he went to Göttingen to become chairman of the surgical department. There he developed his technique of external cardiac massage, which was described in the first edition of his textbook on general surgery published in 1883[5]. He also mentioned that his technique had saved half a dozen patients in whom the pulse had been absent. After 20 years in Göttingen, he was appointed professor of surgery in Berlin. Franz Koenig did not restrict his efforts to surgical problems, but also worked on tuberculosis and cardiovascular disease. He died on December 12, 1910.

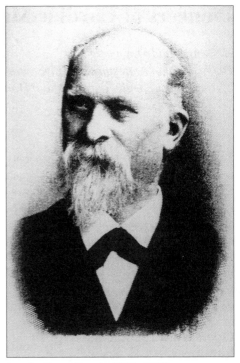

Fig. 2: Franz Koenig (1832–1910)

In 1887, Kraske described the case of a 5 year-old boy suffering from croup who was taken to the hospital in respiratory and cardiac arrest [6]. Following immediate tracheostomy, artificial manual ventilation was initiated, which included rhythmic compressions of the arms on the thorax. Five minutes later, the child´s face and lips gained a healthy colour, so that the bystanders expected the resuscitation to be successful. However, each time the manoeuvres were interrupted for auscultation of the heart, the boy's lips became cyanotic and the pupils dilated again. Resumption of manual resuscitation always resulted in the healthy facial colour being regained. Kraske also noted that the more rapid and vigorous the measures, the earlier the boy´s face recovered. These efforts were finally discontinued after 1 h and 45 min. Kraske concluded from this case that a minimal circulation must have been maintained, and he ascribed this to cardiac compressions resulting from external manual ventilation. He then conducted several experiments in dogs and found that chest compression in his animals maintained minimal circulation. He concluded from his animal experiments that, especially during chloroform syncope, air should not be insufflated via a tracheostomy tube, but that external manual ventilation should be performed to ensure circulatory effects.

Kraske also found that children and animals such as dogs are similar with regard to the circulatory effects of external chest compression. In adults, however, the non-compliant thoracic cage made it necessary for simultaneous abdominal compression to be performed by an assistant in order to maintain minimal circulation. These findings were derived from experiments with adult corpses, in whom he had injected a blue dye solution. In summary, the abdominal compression technique, which has been recommended for cardiopulmonary resuscitation in recent years, was thus already advocated more than 100 years ago.

Koenig's surgical resident Friedrich Maass (Fig. 3) published a report on two cases of successful resuscitation from chloroform syncope in 1892[7]. He used a modification of Koenig's technique (Fig. 4) by increasing the external compression rate to 120 per minute, and verified the efficacy of the massage by palpating the artificial carotid pulse. Friedrich Maass was born on October 14th, 1859. He went to medical school in Halle, Heidelberg and Berlin. After graduation he worked in the anatomy institute before he became a surgical resident in Göttingen. From 1897 until 1914 Friedrich Maass was a surgeon in Detroit and New York. Just before the World War I he returned to Germany and lived in Bremen, where he spent the rest of his life until his death in 1941.

The English-speaking literature conveys the impression that the closed-chest method of cardiac resuscitation was not pursued any further, so that William Kouwenhoven (1886–1975) et al had to re-introduce this technique in 1960[8]. However, according to Keen's report in 1904[9], George Crile used external cardiac massage, which consisted of rhythmic compressions upon the thorax over the heart, in several patients. In addition, Cheever described a 3 year-old girl in whom external heart massage over the third, fourth and fifth left costal cartilages was performed[10].

Following the Maass publication, the technique of external cardiac massage did not fall into oblivion in Germany until several

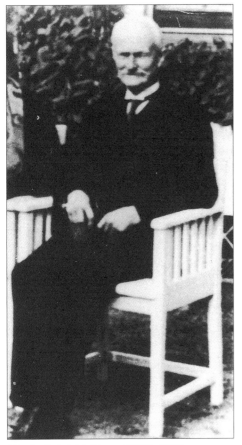

Fig. 3: Friedrich Maass (1859–1941)

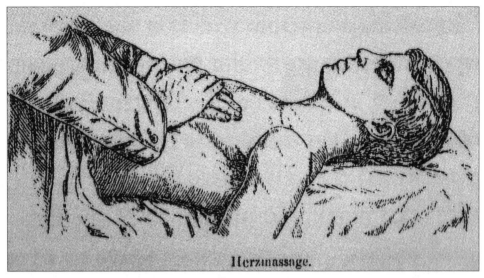

Fig. 4 Extrathoracal cardiac massage, 1896[21]

decades later. The combination of artificial ventilation and external cardiac compression to treat chloroform syncope was mentioned in standard textbooks of general surgery[11]. Both cases of chloroform syncope that occurred in Heidelberg in 1896 were treated with artificial ventilation and closed-chest cardiac massage[12]. In the early years of the 20th century, German surgeons generally performed external cardiac massage for several minutes before changing to the open massage technique [13-15]. In addition, von Cackovic's review article[16] even included the indirect cardiac compressions according to Maass in the list of common resuscitation methods. In his published lecture to medical students on anaesthesia in 1905[17], the surgeon Johannes von Mikulicz (1850–1905) taught the exact technique of handling cardiac arrest due to chloroform syncope; this included artificial ventilation, which had to be combined with external cardiac massage according to Koenig. In Max von Brunn's (1875–1924) textbook on general anaesthesia[18], which was published in 1913, half a page was dedicated to Koenig-Maass' external cardiac massage technique. However, by 1920 this technique had become more unusual in Germany, so that only sporadic use of it can be found in the more recent literature[19, 20].

References:

[1] Jude JR: Origins and evolvement of cardiopulmonary resuscitation, The History of Anaesthesia. Edited by Atkinson RS, Boulton TB. Casterton Hall, Parthenon, 1989, pp 452-464

[2] Zesas DG: Über Massage des freigelegten Herzens beim Chloroformkollaps. Zbl f Chir 1903; 30: 588-590

[3] Langenbuch K: Discussion remarks. Verhandlungen der Deutschen Gesellschaft für Chirurgie, XVI. Congress 1887; I: 9-10

[4] Boehm R: Arbeiten aus dem pharmakologischen Institut der Universität Dorpat. 13. Ueber Wiederbelebung nach Vergiftungen und Asphyxie. Arch exp Path Pharmakol 1878; 8: 68-101

[5] Koenig F: Lehrbuch der allgemeinen Chirurgie, Erste Abtheilung. Berlin, August Hirschwald, 1883, p 64

[6] Kraske P: Über künstliche Athmung und künstliche Herzbewegung. Verhandlungen der Deutschen Gesellschaft für Chirurgie, XVI. Congress 1887; II: 279-290

[7] Maass F: Die Methode der Wiederbelebung bei Herztod nach Chloroformeinathmung. Berliner Klinische Wochenschrift 1892; 29: 265-268

[8] Kouwenhoven WB, Jude JR: Knickerbocker GG. Closed-chest cardiac massage. JAMA 1960; 173: 1064-1067

[9] Keen WW: A case of total laryngectomy (unsuccessful) and a case of abdominal hysterectomy (successful), in both of which massage of the heart for chloroform collapse was employed, with notes of 25 other cases of cardiac massage. Therapeutic Gazette 1904; 20 (third series): 217-230

[10] Cheever D: Cardiac collapse during examination of a post-pharyngeal abscess; incision; circulation re-established and maintained for four hours by massage of the heart; death. Boston Medical and Surgical Journal 1905; 152: 10-13

[11] Tillmanns H: Lehrbuch der Allgemeinen Chirurgie, 4th edition. Leipzig, Veit & Comp, 1895, p 39

[12] Gurlt E: Zur Narkotisirungs-Statistik (Sechster Bericht 1895-96, 1896-97). Arch Klin Chir 1897; 55: 473-519

[13] Sick P: Zur operativen Herzmassage. Zbl f Chir 1903; 30: 981-982

[14] Rehn E: Die unmittelbare Herzmassage bei Narkosentod. Münch Med Wochenschr 1909; 56: 2462-2464

[15] Jurasz AT: Erfolgreiche direkte Herzmassage bei Narkosenscheintod. Münch Med Wochenschr 1911; 58: 83-85

[16] Von Cackovic M: Ueber directe Massage des Herzens als Mittel zur Wiederbelebung. Arch Klin Chir 1909; 88: 917-984

[17] von Mikulicz J: 1. Vorlesung. Ueber die Narkose. Deutsche Klinik 1905; 8: 23-36

[18] von Brunn M: Die Allgemeinnarkose. Stuttgart, Ferdinand Enke, 1913, pp 98-99

[19] Heydloff E: Über Wiederbelebungsversuche durch Herzinjektion bei Narkosezufällen. Monatschrift für Geburtshilfe und Gynäkologie 1920; 51: 318-330

[20] Guthmann H: Intrakardiale Einspritzung von Adrenalin-Strophantin bei akuten Herzlähmungen. Münch Med Wochenschr 1921; 68: 729-730

[21] Urban G: Lehrbuch der kleinen Chirurgie. Leipzig, Veit & Comp. 1896

Historical Remarks on Drug Therapy in Emergency Medicine

U. v. Hintzenstern*, M. Goerig**
* Department of Anaesthesiology, Municipal Hospital Forchheim, Germany
** Department of Anaesthesiology, University Hospital Hamburg, Hamburg, Germany

Today a lot of drugs are used by physicians participating in emergency medicine [11,21]. The aim of this brief report is not to give a thorough survey of the history of emergency drugs but to make a few historical remarks on drug therapy in emergency medicine and to highlight some interesting points in this matter.

When did physicians start to use drugs in order to take care of acute medical complications? A growing popularity of injectable drugs in emergency medicine began around 1900. Before this was possible some odds had to be eliminated:

- Suitable infusion cannula and hypodermic syringes had to be available for effective application[22].
- The introduction of the intravenous injection technique to clinical practice was important. The vein was pierced through the intact skin and not by venae sectio.
- The introduction of "Salvarsan" for treatment of syphilis by Paul Ehrlich in 1910 had a great influence on the clinical acceptance of intravenous injection techniques.
- Solutions like the one developed by Sidney Ringer in the 1880´s were necessary for volume replacement in hypovolemic-traumatic shock[18].
- The incidence of critical problems during anaesthesia had a great influence on the introduction of drugs in emergency medicine. In order to treat "narcotic paralysis and shock" effective different drug were developed[3,20].
- A growing understanding in chemistry with the possibility of synthesization and industrial production of new drugs in emergency medicine was e.g. "Suprarenin", which has been produced by Hoechst since 1905.

We will now move on to discuss some drugs which marked the beginning of the era of emergency drugs.

Excitants acting on the central nervous system (analeptic agents)

Camphor-group:
– **Camphor**

Camphor[1,7,14] is extracted from the camphor-tree. It stimulates respiration and lowers blood pressure by peripheral vasodilatation in small doses. Apnoe and stimulation of the vasomotor centre occur at higher doses. Natural camphor can only be dissolved in oil, hence intravenous injection was too dangerous because of possible fat embolism. Therefore, it was only applied subcutaneously resulting in a delayed and uncertain resorption in states of shock leading to natural camphor not being used in critical situations. That could be changed when water-soluble camphor was developed which could be injected intravenously in high doses, like Camphogen-Ingelheim, Camphemol-Ciba and Campherlösung-Hoechst. However, these drugs could not make their way into daily clinical use because other drugs were discovered at the same time which showed the same characteristics as camphor but had the advantage of being water soluble in their pure form and were superior to camphor regarding pharmacological properties

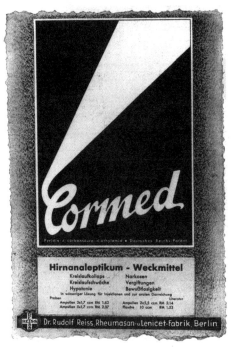

Fig. 1: Coramin (Cormed).
Manufacturer Dr. Rudolf Reiss, Berlin

– **Hexeton**

Hexeton[19,23] is an isomer of camphor. It was discovered in 1894 but it was not introduced until 1920. Primary solubility was as low as that of camphor. Any quantity of water could be added after dissolving hexeton in natrium-salicylate. Hexeton is similar to camphor regarding pharmacological pro-

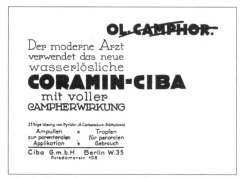

Fig. 2: Coramin (Coramin-Ciba). Manufacturer Ciba, Berlin

perties but its potency is 2 to 4 times higher. Its fast and certain onset due to its water-solubility, its fast resorption and the possibility of exact dosage led to clinical popularity.

– **Coramin (Fig. 1, 2)**

Coramin[23] was synthetized from amides of pyridine-carboxylic acid. It was considered to be a potent analeptic with an effect resembling that of camphor. The pharmacological properties were very similar to those of hexeton. Its therapeutic range has to be emphasized.

– **Cardiazol**

Cardiazol[2,10,12,17,23] is a tetrazolium which is very water-soluble. Solutions of 50% could be made without problems, had no limited storage period and were to be sterilised without dissolution. A very fast resorption and a wide therapeutic range like that of Coramin made Cardiazol into an outstanding drug.

Others:

– **Lobeline (Fig. 3, 4, 5)**

Lobeline[9,13] is an alkaloid of Lobelia inflata. It's not a remedy of newer times. It had already been used at the beginning of the 19th century in cases of bronchial asthma. It was named after Mathieu de L'Obel (1538-1616), a botanist and personal physician to Wilhelm von Oranien and King Jakob I of England. The preparation of the crystallized alkaloid could be applied systematically in pure form in a precise amount with a rapid onset. Circulatory interference is minimal, whereas stimulation of respiration is its main effect. Therefore, the application of lobeline was limited to respiratory depression caused by drugs like morphine, prussic acid or asphyxia of anaesthetized patients or newborns.

– **Strychnine**

Strychnine[20] is an alkaloid of the Indian tree Strychnos nux vomica. It is used in the form of nitrous salt. It was a strong stimulant of the respiratory and vasomotor centre in therapeutic doses and induced seizures when overdosed. Its long-lasting effect has to be emphasized. It was rarely used in Germany - unlike other countries - due to an overestimation of its dangerousness, which is, however, minimal when it is applied carefully.

– **Caffein**

Caffein[20] was not introduced into clinical use due to its limited therapeutic range. Additionally, its effect on the peripheral circulation was less than that of substances of the camphor-group.

Excitants acting on the peripheral nervous system

– **Adrenaline**

Adrenaline[6,16] was considered to be an unsurpassable drug in all cases of acute circulatory insufficiency due to its action on heart and vessels, which is still true today. Due to its strong action on the circulation, it was injected subcutaneously only, except in cases of cardiocirculatory arrest.

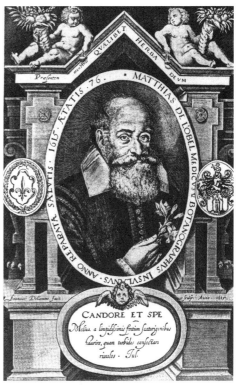

Fig. 3: Mathieu de L'Obel (1538-1616)

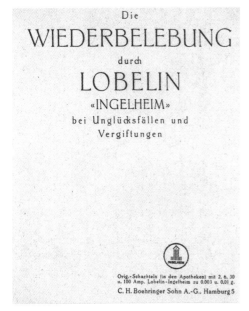

Fig. 4: Coverpage of a booklet "Die Wiederbelebung durch Lobelin Ingelheim", 1932

– **Ephedrine**

Ephedrine[23] is an alkaloid of Ephedra vulgaris, a plant that grows in Switzerland. The synthetic form is called ephetonin. Ephedrine was used as an antiasthmatic drug in folk medicine for a long time. That points out its broncho-dilating properties. Chemically it has a close relationship to adrenaline. Its potency is less but its action is longer-lasting. Oral and rectal application is possible, as cmopared to adrenaline. Therefore, it is not indicated in life-threatening situations of vasomotor collapse or asthmatic problems.

– **Pituitary extracts**

Pituitary extracts[20] were extracted from the posterior pituitary lobe and when injected they had a fast onset of action which lasted 2-3 hours like "Hypophysin" or "Pituglandol". Indications were heart and vascular collapse.

- **Strophanthin**

Strophanthin[20] was the only digitalis preparation which was used in emergency medicine. It was the drug of choice in life-threatening cardiac or circulatory insufficiency.

Mode of application (Fig. 6)

Drugs were usually administered subcutaneously, intramuscularly or intravenously. Intracardiac injection was also recommended, especially for cases of cardiac arrest[4,5,8,24,25]. Interesting experiments with intraspinal injection were performed with the result that lobeline, caffein and cardiazol were very effective in cases of respiratory paralysis[15].

Finally, taking a look at the range of modern emergency drugs, it is very striking that adrenaline was the only drug that is still in use. This drug is - about 100 years after its synthesization - supposed to be the standard drug for every cardiopulmonary resuscitation.

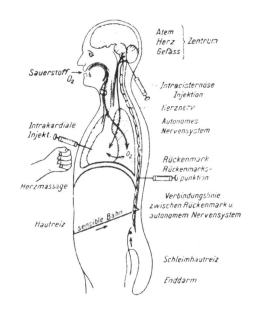

Fig. 6: Concepts of resuscitation-management in 1928

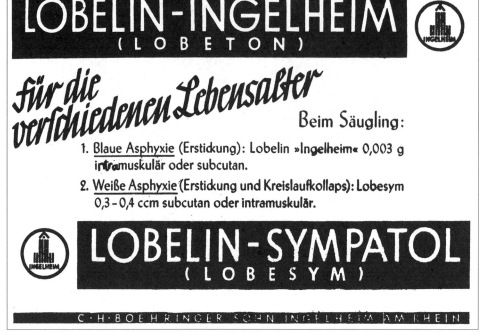

Fig. 5: Lobelin (Lobeton). Manufacturer C.H. Boehringer Sohn, Ingelheim am Rhein

References:

1. Bachem C: Zur Anwendung des synthetischen Camphers. Med Klin 1915; 73: 425-427
2. Biedermann H: Weitere klinische Erfahrungen mit dem neuen wasserlöslichen subkutan und intravenös injizierbaren Kampferpräparat "Cardiazol" (Knoll). Münch Med Wschr 1926; 1323-1324
3. Brunn Mv: Die Allgemeinnarkose. Enke, Stuttgart, 1913, pp 93-106
4. Crile DW: Resuscitation, Intracardiac Injections. Surg Gynec Obstet 1922; 35: 772-775
5. Frenzel H: Bekämpfung des Narkose-Herzstillstandes durch intrakardiale Adrenalininjektion. Münch Med Wschr 1921; 68: 730-732
6. Gottlieb R: Ueber die Wirkung der Nebennierenextracte auf Herz und Blutdruck. Arch f experiment Pathol und Pharmakol 1897; 38: 99-112
7. Guggenheimer H: Neuere klinische Erfahrungen mit Kampfer und Kampferersatzpräparaten. .Dtsch Med Wschr 1926; 20: 837-839
8. Guthmann H: Intrakardiale Einspritzung von Adrenalin-Strophantin bei akuten Herzlähmungen Münch Med Wschr 1921; 68: 729-730
9. Hellwig A: Lobelin bei Atemlähmung in der Narkose. Zbl f Chir 1921; 21: 731-732
10. Hemmerling H: Klinische Erfahrungen mit dem neuen Analeptikum "Cardiazol". Dtsch Med Wschr 1925; 39: 1618-1619
11. Hintzenstern vU: Notarztleitfaden (2nd ed). Fischer, Stuttgart 1997
12. Hippe H: Über Cardiazol. Die Therapie der Gegenwart 1926: 428-429
13. Hoechstenbach: Über "Lobelin-Ingelheim", insbesondere seine Wirkung beim Atemkollaps während der Narkose. Med Klin Nr. 29: 876-877
14. Hopmann R: Die moderne Kampfertherapie. Die Therapie der Gegenwart 1927: 293-297
15. Janossy J: Über die Wirkung intrazisternös verabreichter Medikamente. Dtsch Zschr f Nervenheilk 1926; 92: 273-279
16. Oliver G, EA Schäfer: The physiological effects of extracts of the suprarenal capsules. J Physiol (London) 1895; 18: 230-276
17. Rausche C: Klinische Erfahrungen mit "Cardiazol (Knoll)" in der Kollapstherapie. Med Klin 1926; 43: 1650-1651
18. Safar P: History of cardiopulmonary resuscitation. Anesthesia History Association Newsletter 1994; 12: 15
19. Scheid F: Über "Hexeton Bayer" und seine Bedeutung für die chirurgisch-gynäkologische Praxis. Zbl f Chir 1924; 15: 794-797
20. Schoen R: Wege zur Verminderung der Narkoseverfahren. Fortschritte der Therapie 1926; 2: 517-520
21. Sefrin P, D Blumenberg, W Otremba: Arzneimittel im Rettungsdienst. Der Notarzt 1991; 7: 44-50
22. Strauss H: Zur Methodik der intravenösen Therapie. Dtsch Med Wschr 1907;4:141-142
23. Trendelenburg P: Über die Wirkung einiger neuerer Kreislaufmittel bei Kreislaufinsuffizienz. Med Klin 1929; 41: 1573-157
24. Velden R v: Die intrakardiale Injektion Münch Med Wschr 1919; 66: 274-275
25. Vogt E: Ueber die Grundlagen und die Leistungsfähigkeit der intrakardialen Injektion zur Wiederbelebung. Münch Med Wschr 1921; 68: 732-733

We thank Mrs. Lynne Lörler very much for critically proof reading our manuscript.

Continuing Medical Education in Anesthesiology: The American Experience 1905-1940

D. Bacon,
Department of Anesthesiology, Buffalo VAMC, Buffalo, N.Y., USA

How do anesthesiologists learn new information and keep current with the expanding knowledge base within their specialty? In 1997, throughout the world there are many well established venues in which this instruction can take place. Many excellent journals publish peer reviewed papers on the latest and most interesting information generated in basic science and clinical research across the globe. Daily conversations with colleagues help refine knowledge in the flame of experience.

Today, meetings devoted to conferring new knowledge in and about anesthesiology abound. Almost every day of the calendar year there is a meeting where continuing medical education credits are awarded for studying an aspect of the specialty. This pervasive form of continuing education has a history that is fascinating to study and allows a glimpse into the origins of anesthesiology. The mere gathering of physicians interested in anesthesia is important, for it demonstrates that a community of interested practitioners exists. This is the first step in promoting learning and growth for the specialty. Further, it identifies these physicians, and others who may join, as belonging to the same community and facilitates communication and the exchange of ideas between and amongst the members of the group.

The Beginnings

The first American meeting in anesthesiology was held at the Long Island College of Medicine in Brooklyn, New York in 1905. It was the initial meeting of the Long Island Society of Anesthetists, a group founded to promote the science and art of anesthesia. This meeting set the format for the group for the next three decades. A business meeting lasting about an hour followed by two scientific papers or a paper and a demonstration of new anesthesia equipment filled the evening meeting time.[1]

In 1911, the group moved into New York City proper, and changed the name to the New York Society of Anesthetists (NYSA). The group continued to meet quarterly, and continued the format set six years before. However, the new yorkers progressively became more involved in the politics of medicine, especially within New York State and the American Medical Association (AMA). The executive committee of the NYSA met with the officers of the AMA in June of 1912 in Boston. The AMA was not interested in forming a section on anesthesia.[2]

In response to the AMA's position, the leadership of anesthesiology decided to form a national society instead. The Associated Anesthetists of America (AAA) was constructed during the 1912 AMA meeting. The group organized a the first national meeting in anesthesia for June 18, 1913 in Minneapolis, Minnesota. Held during the 1913 AMA meeting, the day long conference featured two "free paper" sessions. Thus, the latest clinical experiences in anesthesia and the newest technology where displayed for all interested to study and learn.[3] A national forum for anesthesia was established.

Adolescence

One common element between the NYSA and the AAA was Francis Hoeffer McMechan. A charter member of both organizations, he was crippled by rheumatoid arthritis and out of clinical practice by 1915. Wheelchair bound, McMechan spent his time and energy organizing anesthesia and its physician practitioners across the world.[4] As Secretary-General of the AAA, he organized the meeting and began the integration of basic sciences with clinical papers.[2] Additionally, McMechan added technical exhibits by equipment manufacturers and pharmaceutical houses as sponsors of the meeting.

By 1923, McMechan had expanded the meeting to four afternoon sessions during the AMA meeting. He had basic science researchers presenting work germane to anesthesiology, thus aiding the beginnings of an establishment of collaborative research efforts between clinicians and scientists. There was a business meeting where political issues of the day were discussed and the transactions of the association occurred. Finally, McMechan arraigned a dinner dance, where meritorious service awards were given. This helped institute a community of physicians and their spouses within anesthesiology.[5]

Three years later, in 1926, McMechan organized the first All-World Congress of Anesthetists which met in London England. Americans joined with their British and European colleagues in a meeting that featured clinical and basic science papers. Manufactures from around the world were present to show their wares.[6] The meeting foreshadowed the formation of the World Federation of Societies of Anesthesiologists.[7]

Specialty Society

Three years before the All-World Congress, in 1923, the first specialty society in anesthesia was formed. The American Society of Regional Anesthesia (ASRA) was created to honor the work of Gaston Labat. As the first president of the society, Labat devoted his efforts to popularizing regional anesthesia in America. Multi-disciplinary in origin, surgeons dominated the organization.

Meetings were held quarterly where papers were presented on the latest techniques in regional anesthesia and were published in Current Researches in Anesthesia and Analgesia. Over the next decade, these papers would shift in emphasis from surgical blocks to the management of patients with chronic pain. Eventually, as more physician specialists became involved, the ASRA took on greater importance within the national political scene in anesthesiology.[8] Being one of two societies outside of the McMechan sphere, the ASRA was critically important in the formation of the American Board of Anesthesiology.[9]

Paul Wood, the longtime secretary of the ASRA developed a unique way of insuring that all the members of the society participated in the society. He mimeographed the minutes and sent them to all members. Ralph Waters, professor and chairman of the first academic department of anesthesiology in the United States at the University of Wisconsin, commented that this method allowed him to keep up with the group despite his being almost two thousand miles away![10] The text of the papers presented was included in the minutes, allowing the members full access to the continuing medical education offered by these meetings.[11]

Striving Toward Maturity

In 1938, the Associated Anesthetists of the United States and Canada, the organization the AAA had evolved into, held its Silver Jubilee Meeting. It covered the full five days of the AMA meeting. Papers presented at the meeting covered the full gambit of topics in anesthesiology. From basic science work to the mechanics of setting up an anesthesiology service, the meeting served the needs of the physician community.

Seventeen technical exhibitors were present. This number clearly shows the emerging strength of the anesthesia market to equipment manufactures and pharmaceutical houses. The annual dinner dance, a black tie affair, cost two dollars and fifty cents a person! Indeed between the scientific program, the technical exhibits and the social program, the silver jubilee fully resembled a current anesthesiology meeting.[12]

Conclusions

In America during the 1920s and 30s, meetings of physicians interested in anesthesia became critical to the specialty for several reasons. These gatherings were important for the dissemination of new information about the specialty. The latest techniques and agents were presented and discussed by the leading experts of the day. Technical exhibits made it possible to see first hand the equipment being discussed in the lecture halls of the meeting.

The bringing together of these physicians and their spouses also developed a sense of community amongst the participants. Networking, the ability to know where to go to find solutions to everyday problems, was a feature of these meetings. Meeting colleagues who faced similar challenges in patient care made it easier to develop consensus on how to treat these concerns. Dinner dances and programs for spouses made lasting friendships possible amongst the families of these physicians.

Finally, these meetings made concerted political action by physicians for the advancement of the field possible. Brought together in one place, they could develop strategies that would carry them far in their struggle for recognition as practicing a unique field of medicine. Without these interactions, the development of anesthesiology in the United States would have been greatly retarded.

References:

1. Collected Papers and Minutes of the Long Island, New York and American Society of Anesthetists. Wood Library-Museum of Anesthesiology Collection, Park Ridge, Illinois, USA

2. Betcher AM, Ciliberti BJ, Wood PM, Wright LH: The jubilee year of organized anesthesia. Anesthesiology 1956; 17: 226-264

3. Meeting Program, Associated Anesthetists of America, Collected Papers of Albert Miller, M.D., Wood Library-Museum of Anesthesiology Collection, Park Ridge, Illinois, USA

4. Waters RM: The development of anesthesiology in the United States. Journal of the History of Medicine and J Hist Allied Sci, 1946:1:62-612

5. Program of the 10th Congress of Anesthetists. Collected Papers of Albert Miller, M.D., Wood Library-Museum Collection, Park Ridge, Illinois, USA

6. Editorial: Br J Anaesth 1926; 3:B

7. Bacon DR: The World Federation of Societies of Anesthesiologists: McMechan final legacy? Anesth&Analg 1997; 84:1130-1135

8. Bacon DR, Reddy VJ, Murphy OT: Regional anesthesia and chronic pain management in the 1920s and 30s. Regional Anesthesia 1995: 20; 185-192

9. For more information see Bacon DR, Lema MJ. To define a specialty: a brief history of the American Board of Anesthesiology's first written examination. J Clin Anesth 1992; 4: 489-497

10. Letter from Ralph Waters, M.D. to Paul Wood, M.D., March 8, 1933. The Collected Papers of Ralph M. Waters, M.D., Steenbock Library Collection, University of Wisconsin, Madison, Wisconsin, USA

11. Minutes of Meeting of the American Society of Regional Anesthesia. Wood Library-Museum Collection, Park Ridge, Illinois, USA

12. Program of the Silver Jubilee Congress of Anesthetists. Collected Papers of Albert Miller, M.D., Wood Library-Museum of Anesthesiologists Collection, Park Ridge, Illinois, USA

Eisenmengers Biomotor – Predecessor of Active-Compression-Decompression Cardiopulmonary Resuscitation

K. P. Koetter[1], W. H. Maleck[2], G. A. Petroianu[3], S. Ghisoiu[4]
[1] Neurological Intensive Care Unit, Leopoldine Hospital, Schweinfurt, Germany
[2] Neurological Intensive Anesthesiology, Klinikum, Ludwigshafen, Germany
[3] Neurological Intensive Pharmacology, Klinikum Mannheim, Germany
[4] Neurological Intensive Anaesthesiology, Spitalul Clinic Judetean, Timisoara, Romania

Introduction

In a letter to JAMA, discussing the termination of clinical trials with the Active-Compression-Decompression Cardio-Pulmonary Resuscitation (ACD-CPR), Lerman mentioned Eisenmenger's Biomotor as a possible predecessor of ACD-CPR.[1,2] He gave reference to a 1939 paper by Eisenmenger.[3]

In reply, Lurie stated that the Biomotor had been similar to other devices of its time like the Hans device.[4,5]

He argued that the Biomotor had been a cumbersome device compared to the Ambu CardioPump.

Using Eisenmenger's publication cited by Lerman, the Index Medicus, Medline and the secondary literature thereof, we tried to find further information.

Methods

1. The 1939 publication of Eisenmenger, which turned out to be an eight-part-series, was worked through. We learned from this publication that Eisenmenger was a physician in 1900 and that he had published his first paper related to the Biomotor in 1903. The Index Medicus for the years 1916-1950 was searched for his publications.
2. Medline 1966-1996 was searched for "Biomotor".
3. The "Karlsruhe Virtual Catalogue", an Internet application allowing access to the book catalogues of most libraries in Germany, was searched for the title item "Biomotor" and books of Eisenmenger.
4. Secondary literature thereof was included if either written by Eisenmenger himself or describing the Biomotor.
5. After this, two of us presented a paper at a symposium.[6] There we met Ghisoiu, who had published on the Biomotor before.[7,8] Additional information provided by him was included.
6. After the symposium, Medline was searched for further publications of Lerman, who was subsequently contacted, too.
In addition, the terms "cuirass" and "iron lung" were searched in Medline.

Results

Rudolf Eisenmenger published between 1900 and 1942:
– at least 35 papers in journals[3, 9, 42]
– at least 3 monographs[43-45]
– at least 5 patents[46-50]

Most, but not all of these publications were related to the Biomotor. Most were in German language, except for his US patent[50] and four publications in Hungarian.[10,16-18] He never had co-authors. We don't claim this list to be complete. Eisenmenger's US patent[50] mentions a further Austrian patent filed

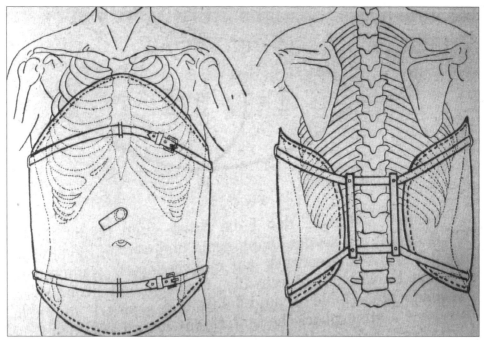

*Figure 1: Eisenmenger's 1903 diagram showing attachment of his device to the body.[11]
With kind permission of Blackwell publishers.*

August 12, 1925 and a German patent filed May 7, 1926. And there might be other publications, we don't know especially before 1916 and thus not accessible by the "Index Medicus".

We found 43 publications of other authors mentioning the Biomotor or its predecessors published between 1904 and 1996.[1,7,8,51-90]

Discussion:

Biographical data

Biographical data of Rudolf Eisenmenger can be obtained from Barth[91] and from Eisenmenger's publications. He was born in 1871 in Weißenburg (Alba Iulia). This, like all his life-stations until 1921, belonged to Siebenbürgen (Transsylvania) in the Hungarian part of the Austrian-Hungarian Monarchy and became part of Romania after World War I.

He visited the „Gymnasium" (highschool) in Broos (Orastie) and graduated from medical school in Klausenburg (Cluj) in 1896. Then he began to practice medicine in Broos. In his papers from 1900 until 1904 his address was Piski (Simeria), in 1905 and 1906 Szászváros (Orastie). In 1911 he worked in private practice as a „Kurarzt" (rehabilitation physician) in Bad Baaßen (Bazna). In 1915 he was head of a rehabilitation hospital in Hermannstadt (Sibiu).

In 1921 Eisenmenger relocated to Wien (Vienna, capital of Austria). Here he worked in private practice as a "Facharzt für Physikalische Therapie" (Specialist in physical therapy) and died in 1946.

Eisenmenger's publications

According to Eisenmenger himself, he had the idea for his resuscitation method in the winter of 1900 when his seven year old niece

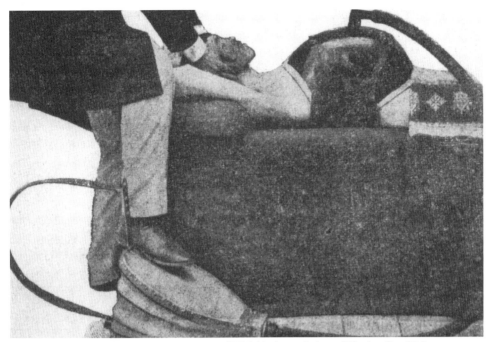

Figure 2: 1903 foto showing his device in use.[11] *With kind permission of Blackwell publishers.*

died from whooping cough complicated by pneumonia in spite of his efforts, including artificial respiration by the Silvester method.[3]

As a matter of fact, he filed his first Austrian patent the 12th of February 1900.[46] The device described herein was a chest cuirass which was sealed at the neck, the upper arms and the abdomen (Type I cuirass in the classification of Scales et al.).[92]

A second device, which was patented in Germany the 3rd of January 1901, was a box intended to seal below the axillae and at the lower abdomen (Type II cuirass).[47] In both patents only the use of external negative pressure alternating with ambient pressure is mentioned (differing from his later suction and pressure massage).

In 1900, he published his first scientific paper we know of. Herein, a device for suction on the upper thorax is proposed as a method to improve ventilation of the lung apices in tuberculosis.[9]

In 1902 he filed a patent describing an anterior cuirass sealing at the lower thorax and the pelvis (Type III cuirass) for alternating pressure and suction.[48,49]

In autumn 1903 he published this cuirass at about the same time in a Hungarian and an Austrian medical journal.[10,11]

In 1903 he proposed the use of this device not only in respiratory but also in cardiac arrest caused by drowning or intoxication.[11] As Lerman[1] pointed out, Eisenmenger was probably the first to propose the thoracic pump theory:

"If the pressure on (the abdominal wall) during inspiration is lowered faster than can be equalized (by air entering the trachea) ... the pressure in the abdomen and thorax will be markedly lowered; the blood vessels in these cavities will be under a lower pressure than those outside ... blood must stream from the periphery to this locus minoris resistentiae ... all organs in the thorax and abdomen

will be abundant with blood, including the right heart and the lungs. During expiration the blood will ... be expelled from thorax and abdomen ... obviously because of the valves - in the heart and the veins - it will only in one direction be able to flow."[11]

It should be noticed that Eisenmenger mentioned in 1903 the fact that ACD-CPR will work properly only if the pressure variations cannot be equalized by respiration - the very idea leading to the use of an inspiratory impedance valve with ACD-CPR in 1995![93]

In addition, Eisenmenger proposed in 1903 the use of his apparatus for non-emergency conditions like emphysema (with pressure only), atelectasis (with suction only) or support of expectoration. He wrote that the device could be applied in 1-2 minutes and that a complete device with shields of different size weighted only 10-14 kg.[11]

In 1904 he described *"more than 100"* experiments on a healthy person.[13] After extensive use of his device temporary apnoea ensued (probably caused by hypocapnia), something observed later by Drinker, too.[14,55] He also experimented on corpses, but without invasive techniques he could only show variations in the diameter of the neck veins.[13,14]

Furthermore, the device (with 5 cuirasses) was in 1904 commercially available for 350 German Marks from Hermann Straube (Dresden-Neustadt, Germany).[13,43] This is probably equivalent to several thousand German Marks in terms of 1997. The 20 Marks coin of 1904 was a gold coin, which is worth about 150 German Marks in 1997. The device for newborn children was sold for 30 German Marks.[43]

In 1911 he published a successful resuscitation after one hour of "Suction and Pressure Massage of the Abdomen" in a case of suicidal hanging in a 19-year old house maid. However, diagnosis of circulatory arrest was only clinical. In another case of hanging resuscitation was unsuccessful, probably caused by a broken neck. He also reports successful use of his device in several cases of paediatric pneumonia.[19]

The next important step was the development of a unit powered by a vacuum cleaner between 1921 and 1924.[21] In 1926 this device was patented in the United States

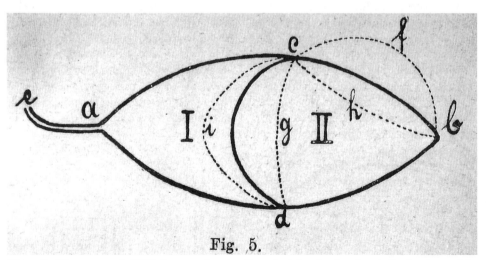

Figure 3: Eisenmenger's 1903 diagram showing the principle of action.[11] ae is the trachea, cd the diaphragm, bc the abdominal wall. With kind permission of Blackwell publishers.

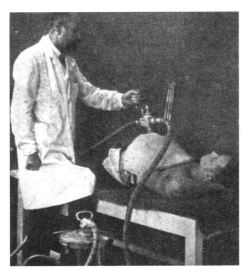

Figure 4: Eisenmenger's first electrically powered device published in 1924.[21] The standing person is Eisenmenger himself. With kind permission of Springer publishers.

and probably in Austria and Germany, too.[50] The change between the pressure and suction phases was done with a three-way-stopcock operated by a crank handle. In our abstract we misinterpreted this as a device powered by a crank handle[6].

In 1926 Eisenmenger performed trials on corpses.[22] As in 1904 he described variations of the diameter in the neck veins by using the device. Furthermore he observed that fluid could be infused only during operation of the apparatus. The paleness of the face of the corpse - who had died four hours before - disappeared and the wounds began to bleed. For this trial he used suction and pressure of 40 to 60 mm Hg each. Unfortunately the frequency of pressure changes is not stated.

In 1927 he gave a lecture at the Physiological Society in Berlin which was published in 1928.[24] Here he described an improved device weighing about 25 kg which could generate up to 100 mm Hg pressure and suction. Although the crank handle switch was retained, Eisenmenger stated that it could be replaced by a small motor or clockwork.

1929 he published trials in large dogs killed with chloroform or carbon monoxide.[26] With the methods available at this time not only normal tidal volumes and blood pressure, but also gas exchange (i.e. CO_2-exhalation) and transport of intravenously injected dye to all parts of the body were shown. In this dog model the optimum pressure and suction turned out to be 35 mm Hg. The frequency with which the device was operated seems to have been 28 min^{-1}.

In this publication for the first time the name "Biomotor" was used for the apparatus.[26]

In 1931 and 1932 he described successful treatment of heart valve diseases, "myodegeneratio cordis", asthma bronchiale and hypertension with the "Biomotor".[27-29] In the 1931 publication an automated device is shown which allowed preselection of pressure, suction, frequency and the relative duration of inspiration and exspiration.[27] Furthermore, a case of successful treatment of carbon monoxide intoxication is described where the patient was hyperventilated for 4 hours and fully recovered.[28,29]

In a lecture[29] at the Society of physicians in Vienna in 1932 he demonstrated the use of the Biomotor in a mannequin model.

For asphyctic neonates a manually operated device was recommended.

It is not quite clear in which year the Biomotor became commercially available. In his 1934 publications, however, the address of a producer named Lautenschläger in München (Munich, Germany) is given.[31,45]

With the help of this company a book was published.[45] Here practical recommendations for resuscitation with the Biomotor are given. Eisenmenger recommended the use

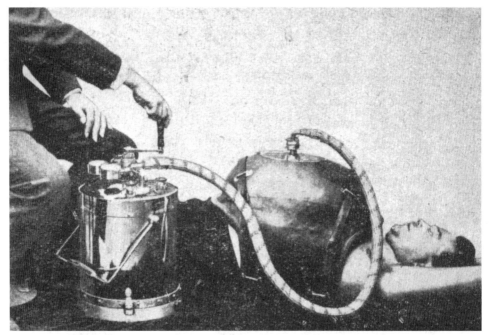

Figure 5: Eisenmenger's 1928 device with the crank handle control on the motor unit.[24]
With kind permission of Blackwell publishers.

of backward head tilt for free airways. If this maneuver failed, he recommended immediate intubation or tracheotomy. He gave detailed instructions for the changeover from initial manual resuscitation to the Biomotor without interruption of ventilation. For artificial ventilation he recommended a frequency of 15 min^{-1}, a suction of 30-40 cm H_2O and a pressure of 20-30 cm H_2O. To avoid hypocapnia he recommended the addition of CO_2 to the inspired air. In circulatory arrest he proposed an initial frequency of 20 min^{-1}. In asphyctic newborns a frequency of 80-100 min^{-1} was recommended.

In 1936 he reported successful use of the Biomotor for prolonged ventilation up to 10 days in cases of polio.[33]

In 1939 an 8-part series was published, describing use of the device in several hospitals in Europe. It was mainly used as a ventilator in cases of polio, intoxication and subarachnoid hemorrhage.[3]

In one of his last papers in 1941, he recommended in cases of circulatory arrest to alternate a pressure of 40 cm H_2O with a suction of 50-60 cm H_2O.[41]

In 1942 Eisenmenger reported the availability of manually operated devices for mine rescue.[42]

Secondary literature on the Biomotor

The first mention of Eisenmenger's device, not written by himself, is in the new inventions section of the Lancet of February 1904.[51]

Gradenwitz reported in 1905 about Eisenmenger's apparatus, its effect on respiration and circulation which was shown by experiments with fresh corpses.[52] This provoked an answer by Cox, the secretary of Alexander Graham Bell, who argued that

Eisenmenger's idea was substantially the same as Bell's in 1882.[53]

1915 Kirchberg referred to the influence of abdominal pressure changes during physical therapy on the circulation. He mentioned Eisenmenger's device and his own similar device.[54]

Drinker, while developing the iron lung, tested the Biomotor in 1929. He reported that the Biomotor was able to produce vacuum and pressure of up to 400 cm of H_2O.[55]

Roemheld mentioned in 1931 the Biomotor as an aid for his aortic physical therapy.[56]

Hassencamp evaluated in 1934 and 1936 the effect of the Biomotor on circulatory parameters in healthy volunteers, patients with circulatory and with respiratory illness.[57,58]

Hellich reported 3 cases of Biomotor application in 1935. One patient suffering from Polio could be saved, two patients died from brain death.[59] She showed that the Biomotor did not cause hyperventilation in healthy volunteers.[60]

In 1935 a case report about the life-saving use of the Biomotor for a child with polio was published by Hamburger. He mentioned that the Biomotor was much cheaper than the American Drinker respirator and recommended purchase of a Biomotor for all paediatric hospitals.[61]

Koeppen showed 1935 the circulatory and respiratory effect of the Biomotor in dogs in asphyctic circulatory arrest verified by zero invasive blood pressure. However, at the time the Biomotor was started, the animals showed a "still normal" ECG, i.e. pulseless electrical activity in terms of 1997. He successfully resuscitated 5 out of 8 dogs.[62-64]

In the same year, Scholtz mentioned the Biomotor in a review on physical therapy.[65]

Keller in 1935 and Thieme in 1936 each published a medical doctor's thesis on the Biomotor.[66,67]

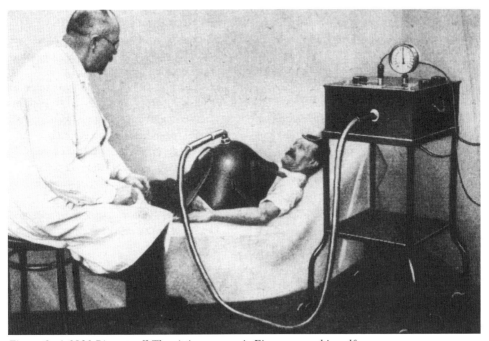

Figure 6: A 1931 Biomotor.[27] The sitting person is Eisenmenger himself.
With kind permission of Blackwell publishers.

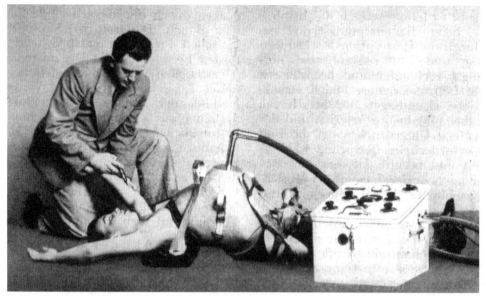

Figure 7: Biomotor for prehospital use in 1939.³ With kind permission of Blackwell publishers.

Hohberg reported 1936 two cases of respiratory arrest following intoxication with barbiturate and morphine, ventilated with the Biomotor. One patient could be saved, the other died from cardiac problems.[68]

In 1936 Nobel described a child with postdiphtheric paralysis of the diaphragm treated with the Biomotor.[69]

Fischer and Engeser compared in 1938 different methods of artificial respiration. They showed both the Biomotor and the Hans suction cups to be superior to the manual respiration with either the Silvester or the Howard method.[5,70,94] Compared to the Hans suction cups, the Biomotor was superior.

Seyfried in 1940 reported on successful treatment with the Biomotor in cases of intoxication.[71] He saw artificial circulation with the device „even in corpses", but gives no details how he diagnosed artificial circulation.

Kahn in 1940 made extensive measurements on the Biomotor's influence on respiration in healthy persons.[72]

In 1941 Weltz stated that he confirmed in animal experiments Eisenmenger's thesis that blood can be moved by changing-pressure respiration, but no details are given.[73]

Zeus measured in 1941 venous pressure after application of the Biomotor.[74]

Blumencron and Guttmann used the Biomotor in 1947 with success for the treatment of circulatory diseases.[75]

Blackwell in 1949 reported the Biomotor to be unsatisfactory as it pressed so hard on the sternum and hips that no patient had endured it for more than three hours.[76]

Doetsch described in 1950 successful treatment of hypertension with the Biomotor.[77]

Measuring cardiac output in healthy probands Fruhmann showed in 1951 an increase in systemic vascular resistance and an decrease in cardiac output with the Biomotor.[78]

Oehmig in 1954 modified a Biomotor so that it could be used for Intermittent Positive Pressure Ventilation.[79] As he also reports that this Biomotor had been unused for years, it probably indicates the beginning of the time when the Biomotor was regarded as an obsolete part of medical history.

Henderson reported in 1972 that Alexander Graham Bell worked between 1868 and 1905 repeatedly on tank- and cuirass-type devices for negative pressure ventilation. Henderson also mentioned the Gradenwitz paper on the Biomotor.[80]

In 1976 Woollam, in his extensive review on the development of tank and cuirass respirators, mentioned both the Biomotor and the mechanical predecessors. He reported unpublished experiments of Sir Robert Macintosh with the Biomotor in 1939.[81, 82]

In 1987, Lin et al. simulated different methods of external chest and abdominal compression for CPR in a computer model. They came to the conclusion that „the dramatic improvement in coronary and carotid perfusion predicted warrants an experimental investigation ... in using alternating compression and decompression as a CPR strategy" and cited the trials of Eisenmenger as the only experiments done hereon.[83]

Lerman in 1989 patented a "Cardiac Assist Cuirass", similar to Eisenmenger's Biomotor. He tested the device successfully in dogs. In several publications he regarded the Biomotor as the precursor of his device. Unfortunately his device is not commercially available.[1, 84-86]

In 1990 the first description of the device which became the Ambu Cardio-Pump was published by Lurie et al.[2]

Based on Lerman's research, 1994 Smithline et al. reevaluated Eisenmenger's method of treatment in circulatory arrest with intermittent abdominal pressure and suction.[87] They used not Lerman's device but the Hayek Oscillator (Breasy Medical Equipment, London NW4 4AU, UK).[95]

In 5 patients after failed conventional resuscitation the Hayek Oscillator was compared to mechanically optimized external chest compressions provided by the Thumper (Michigan Instruments, Grand Rapids, MI 49512-5409, US). The patients had aortic and right atrial catheters. In all 5 patients the coronary perfusion pressure was higher with the Hayek Oscillator compared with the Thumper.

It should be noted that Smithline et al. used only one set of variables on the Hayek Oscillator (rate 80 min-1, pressure and suction both 80 cm H2O, I:E=1:1) that might not necessarily represent the optimum settings. Furthermore, they used the Hayek Oscillator always after the Thumper, which probably biased the results against the Hayek Oscillator.

Tucker in 1994 in a historical review on cardiopulmonary resuscitation mentioned both the Biomotor and the Lerman device.[88]

In 1995 a Biomotor postmark was issued on the occasion of the Annual Symposium of the Romanian Society for Anaesthesia and Intensive Care.[8, 89]

Leveau, in a review on the history of respiratory care for nearly-drowned persons, includes a figure from a French book published by Cot in 1932 showing a Biomotor.[90] The only other mentioning of a French publication on the Biomotor is in the 1931 paper of Eisenmenger where he cites a presentation by a Prof. Portier at the Institut Oceanographique in 1930.[27]

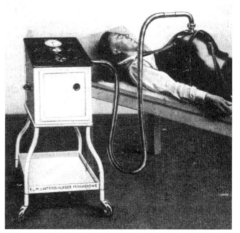

Figure 8: Another Biomotor design in 1939.[3] With kind permission of Blackwell publishers.

The evolution of tank and cuirass ventilators before 1900

Eisenmenger was not the first to propose ventilation by changes in external pressure. Both tank ventilators (enclosing the whole body except for head and neck) and cuirass ventilators (enclosing the trunk or parts of it only) had been described in the nineteenth century.

Dalziel was in the 1830's the first to propose negative pressure ventilation by means of an „air-tight box, large enough to contain the person to be experimented on (the head and neck excepted,) in a sitting posture, and a pair of circular bellows ... worked from without by a piston rod".[96]

Dalziel's box was tried by Lewins on a corpse. He reports „the dead body was made to breathe in such a manner as to lead the bystanders to suppose that the unfortunate individual was restored to life".[97]

According to Woollam, Jones in the 1860's was the next to describe a tank ventilator. Both the Dalziel and the Jones device were made for sitting patients and thus not very well suited for resuscitation.[81]

In the 1870's, however, Woillez described his Spirophore, a tank respirator in which the patients could be treated in supine position. Its concept came very close to the „Iron Lung" of the 1930's except that it was manually powered.[98-100]

The first to build a cuirass ventilator was Hauke, who in 1874 constructed for adult patients a „Pneumatischer Panzer" (pneumatic cuirass) and for children a „Pneumatische Wanne" (pneumatic tank). The influence of artificial respiration on the circulation is mentioned both in the lectures of Hauke and the following discussions at the „k. k. Gesellschaft der Ärzte". However, he did not propose to use his cuirass in circulatory arrest.[101-103]

As mentioned above, Alexander Graham Bell worked between 1868 and 1905 repeatedly on tank- and cuirass-type devices for negative pressure ventilation. Bell presented this idea publicly in 1882, one year after the death of his son at the age of 3 days.[7,53,80,104]

Doe in 1889 reported „a wooden box ... airtight, except for an opening ... intended to be filled by the nose and mouth of the child", invented by Braun in Vienna.[105]

Resuscitation in cardiac arrest before 1903

According to Husveti and Ellis, Thangam et al., and Böhrer and Goerig both external chest compressions and direct cardiac massage had been described in the nineteenth century.[106-108] The first to use closed chest compressions (in a patient) was probably Balassa in 1858. The first to use open chest cardiac massage (in animals) was Schiff in 1874. However, neither attempts at ACD-CPR nor the use of a mechanical device for cardiac resuscitation before 1903 are known to us.

It can thus be stated that although Eisenmenger was neither the first to construct a device for external artificial respiration nor the first to try resuscitation in cardiac arrest, he probably was the first to propose ACD-CPR and a device to do this.

Limitations

As our review is mainly based on publications written or referenced by Eisenmenger, it is probably incomplete and biased in favour of his device.

Conclusion

The Biomotor combined active decompression as in ACD-CPR with the circumferential pressure used in vest CPR and pressure on the abdomen as in abdominal counterpulsation CPR.[109]

The Biomotor was, however, different to these techniques:

- Unlike ACD-CPR, it acted on thorax and abdomen
- Unlike Vest-CPR, it used pressure and suction and this on thorax and abdomen
- Unlike asynchronuous abdominal counterpulsation CPR, action on thorax and abdomen was synchronous with the Biomotor.

As it is, Eisenmenger seems to have been far ahead of his time. The Biomotor was obviously used in the 1930's in several European hospitals for artificial respiration. But there were very few publications of contemporaries taking the idea of ACD-CPR seriously. The only exceptions are Gradenwitz, Koeppen, Seyfried and Weltz. Of those, only Koeppen performed well documented trials on animals.[52, 62-64, 71, 73]

After Eisenmenger's death in 1946, the idea of ACD-CPR lay dormant for 40 years until Lerman and Lin et al. rediscovered it. In the 1990's the Cardio-Pump was introduced by Lurie et al., which, in spite of major differences in design and a slightly different point of action, uses the ACD-CPR principle described by Eisenmenger in 1903.

The final proof that Eisenmenger was correct came with the experiments of Smithline et al. published in 1994.[87]

As mentioned above they showed higher coronary perfusion pressures with the Hayek Oscillator (used as a substitute for the Biomotor) than with optimized conventional CPR.

Several questions are to be solved by future work.

Firstly, if a functionable Biomotor could be found or a replica be constructed, an experimental reevaluation of the original device would be warranted as the Hayek Oscillator used by Smithline et al. is only an approximation.

Secondly, both from the historical and modern viewpoint, the technique of Eisenmenger needs further study in the animal laboratory and in patients after failed conventional CPR to clarify the optimum settings for pressure, suction, frequency, and I:E ratio. This could be done with a reconstructed Biomotor, the Hayek Oscillator, Lerman's Cardiac Assist Cuirass, or a customized device.

Thirdly, an optimized Eisenmenger technique should be compared both in animals and in patients to „conventional" CPR and „new" CPR with the Ambu Cardio-Pump, the pneumatic vest and interposed abdominal counterpulsation CPR. As the Eisenmenger technique, like vest CPR, requires a comparatively bulky and probably costly device, its clinical use would probably only be justified if superior to simpler techniques.

Finally, further archival efforts should clarify why Eisenmenger, in spite of his best efforts over a period of about 40 years, failed to convince his contemporaries. Possible causes of his failure include:
- The fact that he published almost exclusively in German.
- The fact that most of his life he worked in private practice without much opportunity to do actual resuscitations (except the two cases published in 1911)
- The fact that other key component of successful cardiac resuscitation (especially defibrillation)where not yet available.

Footnotes:

The citations from Eisenmenger's publications have been translated into English by the first and second author.

It might be of interest to the reader that Rudolf Eisenmenger was a cousin of Viktor Eisenmenger (1864-1932), famous i. a. for being a pioneer of endotracheal intubation (Wien Med Wschr 1893;43:199-201) as well as being the name-giver of the Eisenmenger-syndrome.

Acknowledgments:

We thank Prof. Dr. E. Eisenmenger (a grand-son of Rudolf Eisenmenger) and S. Eisenmenger in Vienna for identifying the physician in figures 4 and 6 as Rudolf Eisenmenger and for information on the family history.

We thank Dr. S. Lerman in Southfield for information on his Cardiac Assist Cuirass.

We thank Dr. W. Rathjen of the German Museum in Munich, Dr. Dr. S. Hahn of the German Hygiene Museum in Dresden, M. Kowalski of the Medical Historical Museum in Ingolstadt, Dr. G. Göbl of the Kresz Géza Rescue Museum in Budapest and Dr. M. Skopec of the Medical Historical Museum in Vienna for an (unsuccessful) search for a Biomotor in their collections.

Dr. G. Göbl also provided copies of publications not accessible in the German library system.

We would finally like to thank Dr. K. Szöcs and G. Szöcs for translating the Hungarian publications of Eisenmenger.

References:

1. Lerman SI: Compression-Decompression CPR: The Biomotor. JAMA 1994;272:1477
2. Lurie KG, Lindo C, Chin J: CPR: The P Stands for plumber's helper. JAMA 1990;264:1661
3. Eisenmenger R: Saug- und Druckluft über dem Bauch, deren Wirkung und Anwendung. Wien Med Wschr 1939;89:807-1036
4. Lurie KG: In Reply. JAMA 1994;272:1477-1478
5. Hans H: Device for promoting respiration. US patent 2,067,268 Filed March 20, 1935; patented January 12, 1937
6. Koetter KP, Maleck WH: Eisenmenger's Biomotor - Predecessor of Active-compression-decompression resuscitation? 4th International Symposium on the History of Anaesthesia, Hamburg/Germany, April 1997. Book of Abstracts, p. 109
7. Ghisoiu S, Gunescu G: Alexander Graham Bell (1847-1922) si Rudolf Eisenmenger (1871-1946). Timisoara Medicala 1991;36:77-82
8. Ghisoiu S: Rudolf Eisenmenger (1871-1946) si "Biomoturul" sau. Medifila 1995;22/2:16-18
9. Eisenmenger R: Beitrag zur Behandlung der Lungentuberculose. Wien Med Wschr 1900; 50:2372-2375
10. Eisenmenger R: Mosterséges légzésro szolgáló készülék. Orvosi Hetilap 1903;44:725-727
11. Eisenmenger R: Ein Apparat zur künstlichen Atmung. Wien Med Wschr 1903; 53:1730-1733
12. Eisenmenger R: Ein neuer Respirationsapparat. Zeitschrift für Diätetische und Physikalische Therapie 1903/04;7:567-570
13. Eisenmenger R: Vorrichtung zur Erzielung künstlicher Atmung und gleichzeitig künstlicher Blutzirkulation. Ärztliche Polytechnik 1904;14:113-118
14. Eisenmenger R: Künstliche Atmung und gleichzeitige "künstliche Blutzirkulation". Archiv für physikalisch-diätetische Therapie 1904;6:257-259
15. Eisenmenger R: Über eine neuartige Herzmassage. Zeitschrift für diätetische und physikalische Therapie 1904/05;8:625-627
16. Eisenmenger R: Néhány szó eljárásom és készülékem hatásáról és alkalmazásáról. Orvosi Hetilap 1904;45:556-557
17. Eisenmenger R: Uj eljárás a bronchopneumonia gyógykezelésében. Orvosi Hetilap 1906;47:131-133
18. Eisenmenger R: Uj eljárás tetszhalottak felélesztérése. Mentök Lapja about 1905
19. Eisenmenger R: Die Bedeutung der Saug- und Druckmassage des Bauches. Zeitschrift für physikalische und diätetische Therapie 1911; 15: 737-742
20. Eisenmenger R: Die künstlich erzeugten intraabdominalen Druckschwankungen. Zeitschrift für Physikalische und Diätetische Therapie 1915; 19: 326-331
21. Eisenmenger R: Wiederbelebung durch gleichzeitige künstliche Atmung, künstliche Blutzirkulation und Herzmassage. Wien Klin Wschr 1924; 37: 364-366
22. Eisenmenger R: Künstlicher Blutkreislauf in der Leiche. Wien Klin Wschr 1927; 40: 755-756
23. Eisenmenger R: Chemo- und Elektrotherapie. Wien Klin Wschr 1927; 40: 1607-1609
24. Eisenmenger R: Wiederbelebung durch gleichzeitige künstliche Atmung, künstlichen Blutkreislauf und Herzmassage. Wien Med Wschr 1928; 78: 634-638
25. Eisenmenger R: Rheumatische Erkrankungen und die physikalische Therapie. Wien Klin Wschr 1928; 41: 853-855
26. Eisenmenger R: Tierversuche mit dem Apparat zur Erzielung künstlicher Atmung, Biomotor. Wien Klin Wschr 1929, 42: 1502-1503
27. Eisenmenger R: Die therapeutische Bedeutung der regulierbaren supraabdominalen Luftdruckschwankungen. Wien Med Wschr 1931; 81: 207-209

28 Eisenmenger R: Neuartige physikalische Therapie der Kreislaufstörungen. Wien Klin Wschr 1932; 45: 591-592

29 Eisenmenger R: Supraabdominale Saug- und Druckluftwirkungen und deren praktische Anwendung. Wien Klin Wschr 1932; 45: 1105-1108

30 Eisenmenger R: Beitrag zur Prophylaxe postoperativer Thrombose. Wien Med Wschr 1933; 83: 1018

31 Eisenmenger R: Wiederbelebung auf neuer Grundlage. Zentralblatt für Gewerbehygiene 1934; 20: 147-149

32 Eisenmenger R: Druckschwankungen in der Bauchhöhle. Zeitschrift für Kreislaufforschung 1935; 27: 73-81

33 Eisenmenger R: „Herzschlag" und seine Bekämpfung. Wien Med Wschr 1936; 86: 1229-1230

34 Eisenmenger R: Prophylaktische und therapeutische Bedeutung der Atmungsübungen. Wien Klin Wschr 1937; 50: 1419-1422

35 Eisenmenger R: Neues über den "alten" Lebertran. Wien Med Wschr 1937; 87: 683-685

36 Eisenmenger R: Aus dem Gebiete der physikalischen Heilmethoden. Atmungsübungen. Wien Med Wschr 1939; 89: 263-265

37 Eisenmenger R: Die amerikanische "Eiserne Lunge" und der deutsche "Biomotor". Zeitschrift für Ärztliche Fortbildung 1939; 36: 654-655

38 Eisenmenger R: Künstliche Atmung und Wiederbelebung. Dtsch Med Wschr 1940; 66: 1420-1422

39 Eisenmenger R: Mechanische Behandlung Geisteskranker. Psychiatrisch-Neurologische Wochenschrift 1940; 42: 26-28

40 Eisenmenger R: Soll bei Pneumonie der Biomotor angewandt werden? Wien Klin Wschr 1940; 53: 295-296

41 Eisenmenger R: Rhythmisch-mechanische Druckschwankungen in der Bauch- und Brusthöhle und deren Bedeutung für das Leben und für die Organfunktion. Münch Med Wschr 1941; 88: 223-226

42 Eisenmenger R: Anwendungsgebiete und Erfolge der künstlichen Atmung mittels Biomotor. Therapie der Gegenwart 1942; 83: 363-368

43 Eisenmenger R: Ein neues Wiederbelebungsverfahren. Selbstverlag, Szaszvaros about 1905

44 Eisenmenger R: Das physikalisch-diätetische Heilverfahren. Selbstverlag, Hermannstadt about 1918; p. 167-170

45 Eisenmenger R: Supraabdominale Saug- und Druckluftherapie mit dem "Biomotor". Lautenschläger, München 1934

46 Eisenmenger R: Athmungsvorrichtung. Austrian Patent 4458 Filed February 12, 1900; patented January 15, 1901

47 Eisenmenger R: Tragbare Vorrichtung zur Erzielung künstlicher Athmung. German Patent 124,277 Patented January 3, 1901

48 Eisenmenger R: Apparat zur Erzielung künstlicher Atmung. Austrian Patent 14,664 Filed October 8, 1902; patented August 15, 1903

49 Eisenmenger R: Vorrichtung zur Erzielung künstlicher Atmung. German Patent 152,145 Patented May 3, 1903

50 Eisenmenger R: Apparatus for producing or promoting artificial breathing or respiration. US Patent 1,670,301 Filed July 7, 1926; patented May 22, 1928

51 Anonym / New inventions: Apparatus for maintaining artificial respiration. Lancet 904; i: 515

52 Gradenwitz A: A novel process of reanimation. Scientific American 1905; 93: 276-277

53 Cox CR: The new process of resuscitation proves to be old. Scientific American 1905; 93: 339

54 Kirchberg F: Wirkung der mechanischen Beeinflussung des Abdomens auf die Zirkulation. Therapeutische Monatshefte 1915; 29: 92-103

55 Drinker P, Shaw LA: An apparatus for prolonged administration of artificial respiration. I: designs for adults and children. J Clin Invest 1929; 7: 229-247

56. Roemheld L: Passive Aortengymnastik als Prophylaxe und Therapie bei Aorten- und Koronarerkrankungen. Münch Med Wschr 1931; 78: 611-613
57. Hassencamp E: Über die Wirkung der künstlichen Beatmung auf den Kreislauf. Münch Med Wschr 1934; 81:557-560
58. Hassencamp E: Erkennung und Behandlung der rechtsseitigen Herzschwäche. Medizinische Welt 1936; 10:1324-1327
59. Hellich I: Künstliche Atmung mit dem Biomotor. Münch Med Wschr 1935; 82: 421-423
60. Hellich I: Tritt bei künstlicher Beatmung mit dem Biomotor Hyperventilation ein? Med Klin 1935; 31: 780-782
61. Hamburger F: Lebensrettung bei poliomyelitischer Atemlähmung mit dem Biomotor. Med Klin 1935; 31: 1132-1133
62. Koeppen S: Untersuchungen über die Wirksamkeit von Wiederbelebungsmassnahmen bei experimenteller Erstickung. Klin Wschr 1935; 14: 1131-1133
63. Koeppen S: Wiederbelebung bei Kreislaufstillstand? Münch Med Wschr 1935; 82: 2048
64. Koeppen S: Wiederbelebung mit dem Biomotor. Zentralblatt für Gewerbehygiene 1935; 12: 100
65. Scholtz HG: Physikalische Therapie. Med Klin 1935; 31: 1407-1409
66. Keller E: Klinische Erfahrungen über die Anwendung des Biomotor. Thesis, University Würzburg 1935
67. Thieme W: Anwendung und Wirkung des Biomotors bei Lungenerkrankungen. Thesis, University Leipzig 1936
68. Hohberg B: Über zentrale Atemlähmung (durch Narkotica) und ihre Behandlung mittels "Biomotor". Deutsche Zeitschrift für Nervenheilkunde 1936; 139: 294-299
69. Nobel E: Postdiphtherische Zwerchfellähmung. Wien Med Wschr 1936; 86: 1251
70. Fischer L, Engeser J: Pneumotachographische Untersuchungen bei künstlicher Atmung. Med Welt 1938; 12: 1664-1667
71. Seyfried H: Behandlungserfolge und Aussichten bei Vergiftungen in Selbstmordabsicht. Wien Klin Wschr 1940; 53: 04-606
72. Kahn A: Untersuchungen über die Änderung des Atemtypus durch den Biomotor beim Gesunden. Trapp, Bonn 1940
73. Weltz GA: Atmungseinflüsse auf Füllung und Schlagzahl des Herzens. Archiv für Kreislaufforschung 1941; 8: 1-16
74. Zeus L: Beeinflußbarkeit des Venen-Druckes durch intraabdominale Drucksteigerung. Archiv für Kreislaufforschung 1941; 8: 330-348
75. Blumencron W, Guttmann O: Zur Wirkungsweise der Biomotoratmung auf den Kreislauf. Wiener Zeitschrift für Innere Medizin 1947; 12: 534-547
76. Blackwell U: Mechanical respiration. Lancet 1949; II: 99-101
77. Doetsch H: Der Biomotor in der Herz-und Kreislaufpraxis. Münch Med Wschr 1950; 92: 295-298
78. Fruhmann G: Kreislauf und Biomotoratmung. Münch Med Wschr 1951; 93:1849-1851
79. Oehmig H: Automatische Beatmung im halbgeschlossenen System. Anaesthesist 1954; 3: 211-212
80. Henderson AR: Resuscitation experiments and breathing apparatus of Alexander Graham Bell. Chest 1972; 62: 311-316
81. Woollam CHM: The development of apparatus for intermittent negative pressure respiration (1) 1832-1918. Anaesthesia 1976; 31: 537-547
82. Woollam CHM: The development of apparatus for intermittent negative pressure respiration (2) 1919-1976, with special reference to the development and use of cuirass respirators. Anaesthesia 1976; 31: 666-685
83. Lin CH, Levenson H, Yamashiro SM: Optimization of coronary blood blow during cardiopulmonary resuscitation (CPR). IEEE Transactions Biomedical Engineering 1987; 34: 473-481

[84] Lerman SI: Cardiac Assist Cuirass: US Patent 4,881.527 Filed November 14, 1988; patented November 21, 1989

[85] Lerman SI: Negative-pressure ventilation A historical note. Chest 1992; 101: 1480

[86] Lerman SI: The Hayek Oscillator. Anaesthesia 1996; 51: 606

[87] Smithline HA, Rivers EP, Rady MY, Blake HC, Nowak RN: Biphasic extrathoracic pressure CPR. Chest 1994; 105: 842-84

[88] Tucker KJ, Savitt MA, Idris A, Redberg RF: Cardiopulmonary resuscitation historical perspectives, physiology, and future directions. Arch Intern Med 1994;154:2141-2150

[89] Rugendorff EW: Rudolf Eisenmenger (1871-1946) und sein „Biomotor". Philatelia Medica 1995; 25/September:6

[90] Leveau P: Histoire de la réanimation respiratoire vue à travers celle des noyés. Annales Francaises de Anesthesiologie et Réanimation 1996; 15: 86-100

[91] Barth H: Von Honterus zu Oberth. Kriterion, Bukarest 1980, pp 173-174 and pp 365-371

[92] Scales JT, Wilson ABK, Sellors TH, Stevenson FT, Stott FD: Cuirass respirators. Lancet 1953; I: 671-674

[93] Lurie KG, Coffeen P, Shultz J, McKnite S, Detloff B, Mulligan K: Improving active compression decompression cardiopulmonary resuscitation with an inspiratory impedance valve. Circulation 1995;91:1629-1632

[94] Hans H: Ein neues, sehr einfaches und doch sehr wirksames Verfahren zur künstlichen Beatmung. Verhandlungen der Deutschen Gesellschaft für Innere Medizin 1934; 46: 228-229

[95] Hayek Z, Peliowski A, Ryan CA, Jones R, Finer NN: External high frequency oscillation in cats. Am Rev Resp Dis 1986; 133:630-634

[96] Dalziel J: On sleep and an apparatus for promoting artificial respiration. In: Notices and Abstracts of Communications to the British Association for the Advancement of Science at the Newcastle Meeting August 1838, Seite 127-128

[97] Lewins: Apparatus for promoting respiration in cases of suspended animation. Edinb Med and Surg J 1840; 54: 255-256

[98] Woillez N, Gosselin M: Sur le Spirophore, appareil de sauvetage pour les asphyxiés, principalement pour les noyés et les enfantsnouveau-nés. Comptes Rendus Hebdomadaires des Séances de l'Académie des Sciences Paris 1876; 90: 1447-1448

[99] Woillez EJ: Du Spirophore, appareil de sauvetage pour le traitement d l'asphyxie, et principalement pour les noyés et des nouveau-nés. Bulletin de l'Académie de Médecine Paris 1876: (2nd Ser)5:611-627 and 754-789 and 837-839

[100] Woillez M: Le Spirophore, Inventé en 1876. Bulletin de l'Académie de Médecine Paris 1939; 119: 82-85

[101] Hauke I: Der pneumatische Panzer. Wien Med Presse 1874;15:785-788 and 836-837

[102] Hauke I: Über pneumatische Therapie mit Demonstration neuer Apparate. Anzeiger der K.K. Gesellschaft der Ärzte in Wien 1876;:83-90

[103] Hauke I: Nachträgliche Bemerkungen zu der Discussion über die Wirkung der pneumatischen Wanne und Demonstration eines neuen pneumatischen Apparates. Anzeiger der K.K. Gesellschaft der Ärzte in Wien 1876;:113-115

[104] Bruce RV, Block I: Alexander Graham Bell. National Geographic 1988;174:358-385

[105] Doe OW: Apparatus for ruscitating asphyxiated children. Boston Medical and Surgical Journal 1889;120:9

[106] Husveti S, Ellis H: Janos Balassa, pioneer of cardiac resuscitation. Anaesthesia 1969; 24: 113-115

[107] Thangam S, Weil MH, Rackow EC: Cardiopulmonary resuscitation: a historical review. Acute Care 1986; 12: 63-94

[108] Böhrer H, Goerig M: Early proponents of cardiac massage. Anaesthesia 1995; 50: 969-971

[109] Halperin HR, Chandra NC, Levin HR, Rayburn BK, Tsitlik JE: Newer methods of improving blood flow during CPR. Annals of Emergency Medicine 1996;27:553-562

Alternative Analgesic and Anaesthetic Techniques The Use of Australian Plants for Pain Relief and Anaesthesia

R. Westhorpe, Department of Anaesthesie, Royal Children's Hospital, Parkville Victoria, Australia

For thousands of years before European settlement in Australia, the Aborigines had a wealth of natural resources from which to obtain medicines. The Aborigines were nomadic tribes living in widely different natural environments throughout the continent of Australia. Much of their medicine was based on magic and although the use of plants as soporifics appears to be rare amongst records of Aboriginal practices, many plants were used for relief of pain. They were generally used without elaborate preparation, and were crushed, pounded, boiled with water, or just applied or eaten in the natural state. There was little application of animal products to aboriginal medicine, apart from the use of bleached and ground kangaroo bone for the treatment of rheumatism, which appears to have been a common ailment.

Examples of pain management by Aborigines include the principle of "counter-irritation" or treatment of pain by causing continuous painful stimulation in the skin of the overlying part. They used stinging nettles or plants such as *Dendrocnide excelsa* or "the stinging tree", fine hairs of which break off on touch, injecting a small amount of very irritating liquid resulting in pain which can recur for weeks. Normally people would carefully avoid these trees, but those Aborigines with rheumatism or other chronic pain, and who lived in areas where these trees flourished, would apply the leaves over the affected area. In some tribes, lacerations were made over painful joints in a similar attempt to cure pain. This differed from the usual ceremonial scars produced by rubbing ash into an open wound.

Various parts of plants were used, sometimes the seed, the leaves, the roots, stems or bark. The bark of the Cooktown Ironwood *(Erythrophleum chlorostadis)* was boiled by the North Queensland Aborigines to make a poultice to be applied over sprains, bruises and other pains. Ligatures made of the bark of the Mallee Riceflower *(Pimela microcephala)* were wound around painful limbs.

The aromatic oils of the eucalyptus were used for headaches as well as for respiratory illnesses, and the bark of the Ironbark *(Eucalyptus pruinosa)* was stripped, soaked and wound tightly around the chest and body for pain and rheumatism.

There were many plant extracts used for headaches, toothache or sore eyes. One rainforest tree, the *Euodia vitiflora,* which has leaves with oil glands exuding an aromatic juice was known as the "toothache tree". A curious cure for headache was practiced by the medicine men of a tribe near the Murray River. A clump of grass was pulled out and the patient's head placed in the hole. The clump would then be placed on top of the patient's head and the doctor would sit on it until the headache disappeared!

When the earliest white settlers came in 1788, their own medicine was also primitive and so they either used traditional remedies from home or learned from the Aborigines how to use local plants. Of course a whole new range of diseases were presented to the Aborigines and many died of contagious diseases to which they had never previously been exposed.

At the time of the discovery of anaesthesia in 1846, Australia was a small colony of Great Britain with a population of less than 400,000. There were no medical schools until the first in Melbourne in 1863 and new developments in anaesthetic equipment and techniques were brought by surgeons returning from their travels to Europe and America (they being the only ones who could afford such journeys!)

Early Australian anaesthesia thus followed developments elsewhere, primarily those in Great Britain, although Australian doctors were quick to take on and modify overseas techniques and to devise new apparatus. They developed some innovative uses of anaesthetic agents, including the use of chloroform to treat strychnine poisoning and ether for snakebite. A Doctor Wilmott prescribed topical cocaine as a treatment for vaginismus, said to have been successful as the outcome was pregnancy! An interesting dental case is described in 1889 where the anaesthesia sequence for extraction of a painful lower molar began unsuccessfully with ether and was followed by Cocaine in increasing amounts until toxicity occurred. The resultant convulsions were treated with chloroform, and the still painful procedure was then attempted the next day with nitrous oxide, again unsuccessfully!

In the latter part of the 18th century there was considerable research into the medicinal properties of Australian plants. In a landmark presentation in 1889 to the Intercolonial Medical Congress of Australasia, Baron Sir Ferdinand von Mueller, Government Botanist for Victoria, described the then current state of knowledge of native plants and their potential use in medicine. He was particularly interested in the potential development of anaesthetic agents. Regrettably for anaesthesia, there had been little reward. Dr John Reid of South Australia had introduced "Drumine" an extract of the milk sap of *Euphorbia drummondii* as a safer local anaesthetic alternative to cocaine. There are many species of *Euphorbia* around the world and similar members can be found around the Mediterranean and in China. It was mentioned in the writings of Dioscorides and Pliny and used in Chinese domestic medicines. Others had introduced "Tonga" a similar plant extract from Fiji. von Mueller also referred to reports that an extract produced from *Erythrophleum laboucherii* produced local anaesthesia lasting as long as two days. This is a close relative of the Cooktown Ironwood. None of these were to be confirmed as useful agents, however von Mueller did make a plea for continuing research and for standardisation of terminology and measurement in pharmacology

The most prolific investigation occurred in Queensland, undertaken by Dr Joseph Bancroft who was particularly interested in a report by Dr Woolls, a naturalist clergyman who had recorded in about 1860 that "The Aborigines make holes in the trunk (of *Duboisia myoporoides*) and put some fluid in them, which when drunk on the following morning, produces stupor." In 1872, Bancroft obtained some of the plant material from which the aborigines made their potion, known to them as "pituri". He made an infusion and injected it into a cat and a puppy, both of which died rapidly. He experimented with *Duboisia myoporoides* and *D. leichhardtii* extracts on frogs and rats, noting the stupefying effect and watching the effect on the circulation by placing the web of the frog's foot under a microscope. He noted that in larger doses, excitement was followed by irregular muscle action, leading to respiratory paralysis and death. Bancroft also used an extract of *Duboisia hopwoodii* leaves, causing his cat to rush around the room blindly with dilated pupils. He was encouraged by Baron von Mueller, who suggested in a letter that he "could easily, for a little payment, get a black fellow to administer small doses of that plant". Bancroft, however used his pet cat and dog first before trying it on some of his patients, remarking "thanks to the beneficent rule of this colony, where no laws prevent professional men from experimenting..."   Of course the extract was hyoscyamine and the *Duboisia* of Northern Australia remain the largest natural sources of this important drug.

It is probably time to again investigate the potential benefits of the many plant species which are unique to Australia. Baron Sir Ferdinand von Mueller conducted an enormous volume of research over 100 years ago, but without the sophisticated resources to which we now have access.

Alternative Patients

B.M.Q. Weaver, Winscombe, North Somerset, UK

Alternative patients are any that arise from the Animal Kingdom who are not human beings and for simplification all patients may be referred to as either humans or animals. The Animal Kingdom is a very large one indeed comprising vertebrates (those with a backbone) and invertebrates (those which do not have a backbone) and an infinite variety of creatures as diverse in appearance as a butterfly, an earthworm or an elephant.

They are classified from the simplest, lowest or least complicated e.g. unicellular organisms such as the amoeba to the highest or most complicated i.e. Homo Sapiens (humans). They all recoil from noxious or unpleasant stimuli and the higher up the taxonomy of the Kingdom an individual is, the more highly developed is its nervous system. It can be said therefore, that all animals can experience pain and are sentient beings. Moreover, members of the highest class i.e. the mammals experience pain and have memory and apprehension of it in an exactly comparable manner to ourselves. For example, a dog with abdominal pain may rest on its elbows with its hind end raised, a dog in severe pain may show a facial expression of pain and a horse that has an infected facial or maxillary sinus may refuse to jump because it has memory of acute pain it experienced on landing after a jump.

Historical records clearly show that man made attempts to relieve or numb pain for many centuries before the discovery of anaesthesia.

The Roman writer Pliny (circa A.D. 61 - 113) for example, recommended the use of the boiled root of the Mandragora plant before operations and dogs were used to pull up the plant because the "Legend of the Mandrake" stated that anyone pulling it up would be sure to die. If dogs pulled it up it did not seem to matter if they died.

Furthermore, of course, many bizarre methods were used to relieve pain, especially the pain of surgery, for example, pressure to numb an area, compression of the carotid arteries to induce unconsciousness and near strangulation.

But it was not until 16th October 1846 that Surgical Anaesthesia was recognised i.e. the possibility of induced reversible unconsciousnes by inhaling a vapour. In all of time before the 16th October 1846, how were the alternative patients faring? Were their painful experiences ignored by man? The answer it seems is probably yes.

Roman records of the 4th Century describe a 'pain relief concept' - but not for the lesser animals, even though operations were performed on them, mainly neutering, castration of horses and bullocks, spaying of camels and dogs all without any pain relief! Quite apart from 'clinical operations' performed on our alternative patients, they were used extensively in experiments designed to help towards the discovery of anaesthesia.

For example:

In 1665 Sir Christopher Wren carried out the first intravenous injection; with a bladder attached to a sharpened quill, he injected tincture of opium into the vein of a dog.

In 1733 Stephen Hales measured blood pressure by cannulating veins and arteries and is well known for his measurement of arterial pressure in the horse.

In 1824 Henry Hill Hickman used carbon dioxide as an 'alternative method of anaesthesia'. He rendered various animals unconscious with this gas (not realising that he was making them hypoxic and hypercarbic) and he wrote a letter entitled "Suspended Animation".

William Thomas Green Morton, famous for that first successful demonstration of anaesthesia - carried out experiments with ether on dogs prior to the demonstration.

Since 1846, animals have continued to be used to improve techniques and develop new agents and also, to develop alternative methods of analgesia and anaesthesia. It was not long, however, after that notable event in 1846 that a humanitarian concern for pain experienced by the lesser animals became apparent (Weaver, 1987/88)[1]. In January 1847, the Times recorded the earliest use of Veterinary Anaesthesia, the Successful use of Ether on a Horse at the Royal Veterinary College, London. Then, later that year (14th August), the Athenaeum recorded experiments carried out in France to etherize bees so as to be able to take their honey without necessarily destroying their hives.

The humanitarian concern for animals soon received enforcement by legislation in the United Kingdom.

In 1887, Augustus Desire Waller (FRS) became noted for his work on chloroform, he considered that its dangers depended on the percentage of vapour in the inhaled air. He is also noted, for obtaining the first electrocardiogram using his dogs. He had several but in particular, he used his bulldog, Jimmie (Sykes,1987)[2,3]. In demonstrating this, it is recorded that 'Jimmie stood in a state of voluntary immobility with his legs in glass vessels containing saline while the electrocardiographs were made'.

Awareness of the legislation concerning experiments on animals led to the question of cruelty being raised in the House of Commons, London. In response, it is reported in the Times of the 9th July 1909 that the then Prime Minister, Mr. Gladstone had stated "I have made the acquaintance of the dog who is well accustomed to these exhibitions and LIKES standing in the water".

For the animals in the early 1900's, chloroform and ether were the main agents used, supplemented with morphine on occasions and an interesting reference to this with regard to the horse appeared in the Veterinary Record of 1900 and 1901.

The pioneer of modern Veterinary Anaesthesia was Professor John George Wright and the appearance of his book on the subject in 1941 is significant (Wright,1941)[4]. He said of the semi-open method of administering chloroform to a horse, that partial asphyxiation could easily occur and the 'good results' obtained spoke well of the horse rather than of the method. He issued a critical warning, stating that in his opinion 'Chloroform is a dangerous anaesthetic, the use of which should be avoided wherever possible'.

Through the 1940's and 1950's Professor Wright strongly supported the use of chloral hydrate (Wright, 1958)[5], but he stated that 'it remained the best narcotic at our command for the horse - at the same time, it is far from ideal'.

For small animals i.e. dogs and cats, Professor Wright revolutionised anaesthesia for them by introducing the barbiturates into clinical practice in the middle of the 1930's (Wright and Oyler,1935, Wright, 1937)[6,7].

In 1860, John Snow first recognised the potential value of rebreathing, doing so through potash in his vaporiser. Closed circuit anaesthesia, however, was slow to come into clinical use, although it was described in about 1920 by a pharmacologist, Dennis Jackson (Jackson,1927)[8]. He had obtained good results with it and, in addition, with artificial respiration, in experiments on dogs.

In the 1920's, Ralph M. Waters and Arthur Guedel developed the cuffed endotracheal tube (Guedel and Waters, 1928)[9] and, to demonstrate its safety, Guedel anaesthetised and intubated his own dog, which was called 'Airway', inflated the cuff of the tube and then immersed the dog totally in water. This was the so called 'Dunked dog Demonstration' Airway came to no harm, he apparently recovered from the anaesthetic, shook off the water and settled down for a sleep.

In the 1930's, nerve transmission and the mode of action of local anaesthetics was studied using the Giant Squid, a marine cephalopod mollusc. This creature has singularly large axons enabling research workers to study nerve impulse transmission.

In 1935 a veterinary surgeon, Geoffrey Brook introduced epidural analgesia for the ox, primarily to assist with distocia in cows (Brook, 1935)[10]. Another useful technique of local anaesthesia, particularly in cattle practice is that of paravertebral analgesia (Farquharson, 1940)[11]. For this, the dorsal and ventral branches of the last thoracic and first three lumbar spinal nerves are desensitised with local anaesthetic as they branch out from the vertebral column. The whole abdominal wall of the flank including the parietal peritoneum is then anaesthetised and a laparotomy for caesarian section or a rumenotomy can then be carried out with the animal standing.

In general practice, local or regional analgesia is used wherever possible in preference to general anaesthesia for the ox and other ruminant species, primarily because of their complicated stomach arrangement. They are herbivores and have four stomachs to aid digestion, with fermentation taking place in the rumen which is the first and largest stomach. The rumen cannot be emptied by a reasonable period of food withdrawal so that regurgitation of its content is always liable to happen once these alternative patients are anaesthetised and inhalation pneumonia can become a life threatening hazard. When general anaesthesia is needed for ruminants therefore, protection of the airway is of paramount importance and can be achieved by inserting a cuffed endotracheal tube into the trachea and, in addition, a similar tube into the oesophagus.

Some captive feral alternative patients are ruminants. For example the giraffe and also, the only known relative to the giraffe, namely the okapi.

In the 1950's, it was realised that no single agent existed that would fulfill the needs of general anaesthesia for animals, as with humans, and so called 'Balanced Anaesthesia' was introduced (Hall & Weaver, 1954)[12] whereby anaesthesia was divided into the three phases of Premedication, Induction and Maintenance. A carefully selected number of agents were used with the following objectives: A quiet induction, free of struggling or excitement, maintenance with controlled inhalation plus ancillary agents such as analgesics and muscle relaxants as required and a recovery, quiet and free of pain.

Following premedication, small animals such as dogs and cats could be held comfortably for induction of anaesthesia with an intravenous agent, notably thiopentone sodium. Endotracheal intubation was then carried out and the individuals connected to a suitable breathing system for maintenance by inhalation.

In the 1960's it was possible for this balanced approach to anaesthesia to be extended to large animals i.e. adult horses and cattle. Special breathing systems were developed to minimise resistance to breathing and to cope with the respiratory volumes involved e.g. minute volumes of around 50 litres (Weaver, 1960)[13]. Imperial Chemical Industries Limited in the early 1960's photographed what was novel in those days i.e. a horse anaesthetised with fluothane (halothane) and relaxed on an operating table without the need for hobbles or ropes to prevent dangerous leg movement.

Some of the larger captive feral animals apart from the giraffe and okapi already mentioned need to be anaesthetised from time to time and the introduction of extremely powerful sedative agents, administered via the use of a crush cage or a projectile syringe made it possible to approach such powerful and extremely dangerous animals as lions, tigers and bears. Sometimes, however, it can be difficult to judge that sedation is sufficient for it to be safe to enter the enclosure of these animals. This happened one time when a polar bear, seemingly fast asleep after being injected with etorphine by projectile syringe, came round and chased everyone out except for the keeper who took refuge up a pole in the middle of the enclosure.

Phencyclidine, the first of the cyclohexylamine derivatives was said to induce a state of 'Dissociative Anaesthesia' which was found useful, for example when it was necessary to relocate an adult gorilla.

It is apparent that there is an enormous variation between animals and this is most obvious with regard to size as for example the difference in size between a rat and an elephant. Thus, although much of the equipment that has been designed for humans can be used for a range of creatures there had to be some adjustment[5], as with the endotracheal tubes, extending the range of the Magill sizes.

The work of Stahl (1967)[14] illustrates the fact that as animals get larger as from a mouse to an elephant, the respiratory resistance decreases and the compliance increases. Professor Mapleson applied geometric scaling as a scientific approach to differences in size. He scaled parameters measured in adult humans down to the size of an infant (Mapleson, 1997)[15] and he reversed the procedure, scaling up from a 'Standard Adult Human' to an individual weighing 560 kg which a reasonable weight for an adult horse. For this large individual, the height was calculated to be twice that of Standard Man, i.e. 12 feet which would be the height of a horse if it stood up on its hind legs, the body surface area was 2 squared or 4 times that of Standard Man and the weight (volume) was 8 times that of Standard Man or 2 cubed. Such comparisons led to the realisation that 'pressure' is largely independant of size i.e. blood pressures and airway pressures are comparable.

Another feature of the Alternative Patients is that they vary considerably in SHAPE and this might be related to their lifestyle. For example, the elephant is very large and, accordingly, has a large body surface area but one which is small for its weight so that it does not need to have a high Basal Metabolic Rate (BMR) to maintain its body heat. The snake, on the other hand, is long and thin and has a very large Body Surface Area for its weight. Thus, it would need to have a high BMR to maintain body heat. It does not do so, however, and is poikilothermic, its BMR being dependant upon the environmental temperature. The Power Law Factor has enabled a number of comparisons to be made between individuals of the animal kingdom. Comparisons in a scientific manner including responses to anaesthetic and ancillary agents has been rewarding in anaesthetic research and will no doubt continue to be so for both the animal and the human patients.

In the 1960's, Professor John Clutton-Brock became interested in Electrical Anaesthesia (Clutton-Brock, 1966)[16] using a machine devised by an American veterinarian Charles Short. It became possible to anaesthetise sheep using frontal and occipital electrodes but during the anaesthetic period, the body temperature rose steadily and there was no relaxation of the skeletal muscles. Studies were therefore discontinued but some electrical analgesia remains as transcutaneous electrical nerve stimulation ot TENS.

Acupuncture is a recognised method of 'alternative analgesia' in humans and this is the case also for the animals for whom there is a Veterinary Acupuncture Society.

Perhaps related to acupuncture is the use of the TWITCH for horses. It has been known for many years that twisting a soft rope around the muzzle of a horse has a calming effect on it. This is not done in a manner that would hurt the horse which, it had been thought, was merely distracted by the procedure. However, in 1988, research workers at the Utrecht University Veterinary School discovered that use of the Twitch stimulates the release of β enkephalin which could be detected in the plasma.

Professor Clutton-Brock, apart from studying electrical anaesthesia, also investigated the analgesic effect of hypocarbia resulting from hyperventilation (1957)[17]. In addition, he considered that WHITE NOISE might be analgesic (1962)[18]. He found that this was the case but the effect was not a reliable one in all individuals. In relation to that, it is interesting to note that noise, in the form of music, has long been known to have a beneficial effect on many alternative patients. It is, for example, used to relax cows in milking parlours helping them to 'let down' their milk and, likewise, it is used in batteries of laying hens, increasing their egg production.

Non-steroidal anti-inflammatory agents have been used for many years in animals but increasingly so, in recent times and further alternative methods of analgesia for animals can include physiotherapy and homeopathy.

Finally, no consideration of alternative methods of analgesia would be complete without mentioning TENDER LOVING CARE (TLC). For the alternative patients, this is especially important for the domesticated species and particularly so for the companion animals i.e. those that have a close association with humans.

Dr. Derek Cadle, anaesthetises human patients but for a long time he has been interested in veterinary anaesthesia. He says that we owe an enormous debt to the alternative patients for their contribution to our knowledge, one that can be paid in part by ensuring that they can have the standard of care in anaesthesia and pain relief that we expect ourselves to be given.

References:

1. Weaver BMQ: The history of veterinary anaesthesia. In Veterinary History 1987/88; 5: 43-57

2. Sykes AH: A.D. Waller and Jimmie - a centenary contribution. St. Mary's Gazette 1987; 93: 23-26

3. Sykes AH: AD Waller and the electrocardiogram. Br Med J 1887; 294: 1396-1398

4. Wright JG : Veterinary Anaesthesia. 1st Edition. Bailliere, Tyndall & Cox 1941

5. Wright JG: Anaesthesia and narcosis in the horse. Veterinary Record 1958; 70: 329-336

6. Wright JG, Oyler M: Some aspects of general anaesthesia in animals. Veterinary Record 1935; 15: 1223-1233

7. Wright JG: The use of a new short acting barbiturate - pentothal sodium as a general anaesthetic in canine surgery. Veterinary Record 1937; 49: 27-29

8. Jackson DE: A universal artificial respiration and closed anaesthesia machine. J Lab Clin Med 1927; 12: 998

9. Guedel AE, Waters RM: A new intratracheal catheter. Anaesth and Analg 1928; 7: 238

10. Brook GB: Spinal (epidural) anaesthesia in the domestic animals: epidural anaesthesia in the ox. Veterinary Record 1935; 15: 597-608

11. Farquharson J: Paravertebral lumbar anesthesia in the bovine species J Am Vet Med Ass 1940; 97: 54-57

12. Hall LW, Weaver BMQ: Some notes on balanced anaesthesia for the dog and cat. Veterinary Record 1954; 66: 289-293

13. Weaver BMQ: An apparatus for inhalation anaesthesia in large animals. Veterinary Record 1960; 72: 1121-1125

14. Stahl WR: Scaling of respiratory variables in mammals. J Appl Physiol 1967; 22: 453-460

15. Mapleson WW: Dos Aspectos Fisicos Relacionados aos Aparelhos e Circuitosa Nestesicos, in Anestesiologia Pediatrica dos Fundamentos a Practica Clinica. Editors Delfino J Vale, N. Pereira E. Rio de Janeiro 1997 Revinter, Pp 93 - 103

16. Clutton-Brock J: The present position of electrical anaesthesia. Anaesthesia 1962; 21: 101-102

17. Clutton-Brock J: The cerebral effects of overventilation. Br J Anaesth 1957; 29: 111-113

18. Clutton-Brock J: Analgesia produced by white sound. Anaesthesia 1962; 17: 87 - 88

The Technique of Thermoetherization of Dr. Antonio Morales

J.C. Diz, A. Franco,
Servicio de Anestesiología y Reanimación Hospital General de Galicia – Clínico Universitario, Spain

In the first years of introduction of surgical anesthesia, there were several devices which had systems for warming up ether before its administration. Examples of these are the devices of Snow (1847) with a mechanism to keep ether in a high temperature, or preventing excessive cooling. In 1876, Lawson Tait developed a device for warming ether, and in 1877 Joseph Clover included in his apparatus a mechanism that prevented excessive cooling of ether. In XXth century, the same principle was applied by Gwathmey (1914), Shipway (1916) and Bernard Pinson and Stanley Rawson Wilson, in 1921 [1].

The Spanish surgeon Antonio Morales Pérez, chairman of surgery in the University of Barcelona, started in the last quarter of XIXth century a series of interesting experiences with hot ether, initially in dogs and finally in patients. He used hot ether almost in every operation he performed, with a method he called "Thermic etherization", and he and his disciples performed about 10,000 etherizations with this method [2]. We want to outline in this paper the experience and clinical studies of this surgeon and of his collaborators, pioneers of this special way of inhalatory anesthesia.

With this purpose, we made an analysis of direct sources, mainly the papers published by Dr. Morales and his disciples, and second-hand sources that have studied previously the work of Dr. Morales, specially the researches of Dr. Hervás from Barcelona. Additionally, we could find several interesting documents related to the investigations of Dr. Morales, as the finding in the Library of the School of Medicine of Madrid of two handwritten Doctoral Thesis written by pupils of Dr. Morales, and several papers published in medical journals of Madrid of those years.

When Dr. Morales started his experiences, there was in Spain an important change in anesthetic techniques: the use of chloroform, the most important and almost sole anesthetic during forty years, was questionable to many surgeons, and there was a progressive return to ether. Also, the antiseptic methods of Lister are introduced in Spain in the same period, and then the surgeons dare to operate organic cavities, specially abdomen. Muscle relaxation provided by ether favored this kind of surgery, without the dangers of the deep stages of chloroformic anesthesia. These two conditions played a significant role in the decision of Dr. Morales of using ether, since during the first years of his professional life he only used chloroform. Another event that influenced his decission of using ether was that when he got the chair of surgery in Barcelona he had a period devoid of clinical activity; then the only possibility for practising surgery was in animals in the laboratories of the School of Medicine, and for anesthetize animals he chose ether because it was cheaper. This allowed him to make experiments about the safety and secondary effects of ether.

Dr. Morales prepared an apparatus for thermic etherization, in which he made several modifications during his long professional life, specially trying to simplify the apparatus and the method. Díaz de Liaño, one of his disciples, designed a new device, which included electric batteries, and he called it "Electric thermic ether inhaler." The clinical experience of Dr. Morales includes about 9,000 anesthesias with hot ether, during a period of thirty years. His disciples performed about a thousand anesthesias with the electric inhaler.

Dr. Morales and his collaborators (Dr. Mut, Dr. Carreras and Dr. Díaz de Liaño were the most active) left evidence of their investigations and clinical experience in many papers: communications to the Academy of Medicine and Surgery of Barcelona, to medical congresses, in publications in medical journals and in Doctoral Thesis, which allowed us to follow in detail their works on thermic etherization. But despite the goods results they reported with this technique, it had a very little influence on Spanish surgeons.

During the last years of last century, there was an outstanding change in anesthetic techniques in Spain. In that moment chloroform was the dominant anesthetic, and ether was almost completely forgotten since the end of 1847. Nevertheless, with the introduction of Lister's antiseptic techniques the situation changed abruptly, since with them surgeons dared to operate in organic cavities, especially laparotomy, and the deepening of chloroformic anesthesia caused many accidents, threatening the life of the patient and distracting the attention of the surgeon. This was the main reason that led many surgeons to discuss the safety of chloroform and started experiences with ether, a more manageable anesthetic, without the inconvenients of chloroform and with a greater relaxing activity, which was so important for abdominal surgery.

Dr. Antonio Morales was one of the Spanish surgeons that by this time of the final quarter of XIXth century returned to ether. This physician had used ether only once during the firsts years of his professional life (1873-1886), and in the remaining chloroform [3], but, as he had some complications with this anesthetic, he decided to study ether. In this sense he did a series of experiments in dogs, more than fifty animals, in which he compared the effects of ether, chloroform and methyl dichloride. He did these experiments in the School of Medicine of Barcelona in 1886, he realized how animals died of chloroform syncope when he deepened chloroformic and methyl dichloride anesthesia, and this did not occur with ether, and besides animals were easily reanimated with oxygen during deep stages of ether anesthesia. In another series of experiments he observed that he could take the animals to deeper stages of anesthesia with hot ether, recovering very easily with the administration of oxygen [2, 4-9].

After these experiments with animals and in face of the goods results obtained, he tested thermic etherization in a patient on February the 25th 1887 [2]. For the administration of hot ether he made a device in which he made several modifications during his professional life. The apparatus, made in Germany by Hartmann, had a cylindrical deposit of brass and an alcohol lamp for warming up water. From the deposit the hot water went to a waterbath, in which there was a bottle with 250 g. of ether, and a thermometer to display the temperature, which should not go beyond 40 centigrades during the operation. From the waterbath water went to a drainage cube, as it cooled, to maintain the same warmth. The small bottle that contains ether, had a safety tube with mercury, useful to measure the tension of ethereal vapor, mixed with air that enters the bottle by an ordinary pulveriser. Air with ethereal vapor left the small bottle through a tube, going to a metallic face mask, applied to the mouth and noses of the patient [4-9].

The Dr. Morales classified the periods of thermic etherization in six stages and he used different stages in distinct kinds of surgery:
a. Light excitation.
b. Quick anesthetic stage.
c. Excitation of senses and intelligence.
d. Muscle relaxation.
e. Vegetative life.
f. Return to sensibility or "conscious anesthesia".

Indications of thermic etherization
a. Short operations: first stage.
b. Surgical procedures in which he needed general analgesia but with the patient awake.
c. Anesthesia for trauma patients.
d. Anemic patients.
e. Surgery of hysterical and epileptic patients.
f. Patients with diseases of the heart and great vessels.
g. Obstetric analgesia.

After his experiments in more than fifty dogs, Dr. Morales used hot ether for the first time on February 1887, as stated above, in a nurse who suffered a necrosis of middle third of right femur, operation performed in the Hospital of the Holy Cross in Barcelona. The surgery and anesthesia were successful [2], and so he was encouraged to continue with his clinical tests, getting very quickly a casuistry of fourteen patients, which he presented, as a memory, to the Academy of Medicine and Surgery of Madrid, but he could not attract the attention of the Academy. Then he removed the memory and presented it, now with 115 cases, to the Academy of Medicine and Surgery of Barcelona [4]. During 1887 he did 174 subjects, and in 1919 he collected the important number of 8,945 [2]. Later, in the last phase of his life, when he was already out of the University, he used hot ether in some patients of his private practice.

According to his papers, it seems that Dr. Morales had very few problems with his technique of thermic etherization. The major difficulties were of the apparatus, which suffered several modifications, especially the thermic part, since due to the danger of burst, he preferred warming ether in a distant place [8]. In this sense he published a situation of a burst in the operating room with hot ether, but the patient suffered no serious injuries [2].

The experience of this Spanish surgeon with thermic etherization is very large, as we stated previously, with no mortality attributable to ether. Only in a few instances he saw signs of respiratory palsy, difficulties to anesthetize alcoholics and certain complications in hysterical and epileptic patients. Usually he did not contraindicate his technique in any situation, except in those patients with acute diseases of the respiratory system. He even recommended hot ether in patients with cardiac disease, infants and old aged. In one of his papers he stated [2]: "I have performed every kind of operation in patients of all ages and in all the regions that enter the surgical field, finding no more contraindications that the ones I stated."

Patients with severe trauma and hypothermia were a major indication of thermic etherization according to Dr. Morales. He anesthetized these patients while he warmed them up, since hot ether worked as a thermogen, and for this he increased the temperature of the waterbath up to 41° [2]. He also made use of this effect of warming the patient as an index of the vital forces of some patients before surgery, and if he failed to raise the body temperature with waterbath at 41°, he desisted from operating, since he considered the outcome will be fatal and it was useless to practice the operation.

Dr. Morales observed some phenomenons of euphoria at the beginning of the anesthesia, which he considered as suggestions [10].

The reason of administering hot ether was that heat favored the evaporation of the anesthetic, which has its boiling point around

35°, and also that warming ether diminished the toxicity of this anesthetic. He found a lower incidence of pulmonary complications, as airway spasms, decrease of pre- and postoperative vomiting, prevention of shock and of warmth loss. He recommended the temperature of the waterbath should not exceed 40°, beginning the operation at 36°, decreasing the temperature in patients with fever, and increasing it in the hypothermic ones [9].

The idea of warming ether is not original of Dr. Morales since, as we previously mentioned, several devices before him had dispositives for regulating the temperature of the anesthetic. So the firsts ether inhalers, as those of Snow in 1847, Lawson Tait in 1876 and Clover in 1877, had such a temperature control system [1]. The apparatus of Dr. Morales has a certain similarity with that of the gynecologist of Birmingham Robert Lawson Tait (1845-1899). Dr. Morales knew that device, but he considered it imperfect in several aspects, mainly because it did not manage oxygen, and because the English surgeon only recommended temperatures between 31 and 33°, which were insufficient, according to Morales, for warming up a hypothermic patient [9, 11, 12]. Actually, the Spanish surgeon recommended the highest temperatures of all surgeons who warmed up ether.

Besides his clinical and investigative work, Dr. Morales tried to give broad diffusion to his method of thermic etherization: in communications to the Academy of Medicine and Surgery of Barcelona [4], in Medical Congresses [13], and through publications in medical journals of Madrid and Barcelona [4-9]. Furthermore, surgeons of different places of Spain went to Barcelona to study the technique of Dr. Morales [14]; however, thermic etherization had scant repercussion in Spanish surgery, and its diffusion was reduced to his collaborators [11, 12]. Two of these, Drs. Carreras Gavieso [15] and Mur Estaña [16], wrote their Doctoral Thesis about thermic etherization. Another disciple, Dr. Alfredo Díaz de Liaño, makes in March 1892 important modifications in the apparatus of Dr. Morales, using electric batteries as the source of driving and thermic energy, thus replacing the Richardson belows, and the waterbath for warming ether [17, 18].

The apparatus of Dr. Díaz de Liaño had two portable boxes; one of them had a battery, and the other had an engine or dynamo that with a wheel put in motion a little bellows, which impelled air into a small bottle with ether. A thermogenic device (probably an electric resistance) raised the temperature up to 41°, so warming the vapors of ether. A long metallic tube carried the vapors to a metallic face mask. Several wires connected the battery with the elements of the second box. On modifying the intensity of the electric current, they could control the temperature of the flow and the speed of air that carried the anesthetic vapors. This apparatus, the "electric thermic ether inhaler", was used only by his author, while Dr. Morales continued using his own method; but at the beginning of this century, in 1903, he also began using this electric device, although he recognized the merit of his collaborator in the invention of the apparatus. Dr. Díaz de Liaño did more than 1,000 electric thermic etherizations with his apparatus in the Hospital of the Holy Cross in Barcelona.

The "hot ether" was used very soon in Spain (1889) and Dr. Antonio Morales Pérez de Barcelona was the leader of a significant experience in this field. Although they obtained an important statistic and they gave large diffusion to their technique,

In summary, we pointed out how the surgical school of the Spanish surgeon Antonio Morales Pérez performed important investigations and clinical work with their method of hot ether, which they called thermic etherization, in an early era of the modern surgical anesthesia.

He and his disciples joined an important statistic, about 10,000 etherizations, without important complications, and conceived several devices for the administration of hot ether. He indicated his technique in every kind of patients and surgery, preferably in trauma patients, patients with hypothermia, with cardiac diseases, anemia, and hysterical and epileptic patients. The only formal contraindication he mentioned was in patients with acute disease of the respiratory system.

The method of warming ether is not original of Dr. Morales, and it is based on the same principles of previous (Snow, Lawson Tait and Clover), and of subsequent authors (Gwathmey, Shipway, Pinson ...). The overall result was similar in most of them, this is, they did not arouse interest among surgeons and anesthesiologists of their time.

References:

[1] Bryan Thomas K: The Development of Anaesthetic Apparatus. Blackwell Scientific Publications, London, Melbourne, 1975

[2] Morales Pérez A: La termoeterización en sus distintas formas; experimental y clínica. Consecuencias que se han podido deducir. El Siglo Médico, 1927; 80: 493-498; 521-526

[3] Morales Pérez A: Tratado de operatoria quirúrgica. N. Ramírez, Barcelona, 1881

[4] Morales Pérez A: Indicaciones especiales que puede cumplir la termoeterización como método general de anestesia quirúrgica. Real Academia de Medicina y Cirugía de Barcelona, Discurso Inaugural, 30.1.1889

[5] Morales Pérez A: Indicaciones especiales que puede cumplir la termoeterización como método general de anestesia quirúrgica. La Independencia Médica, 1888-1889; 19:285, 294, 301, 309, 318

[6] Morales Pérez A: Apuntes referentes a la Termoeterización. Boletín Clínico de la Casa de Salud de Nuestra Señora del Pilar, 1889; 3: 252-260

[7] Morales Pérez A: Indicaciones especiales que puede cumplir la termoeterización como método general de anestesia quirúrgica. La Medicina Práctica, 1889; 1:685-690, 705-709; 2:1-4, 19-22

[8] Morales Pérez A: Apéndice al discurso sobre las indicaciones de la Termoeterización. Gaceta Médica Catalana, 1890; 13: 136-138, 171-174

[9] Morales Pérez A: Indicaciones especiales que puede cumplir la termoeterización como método general de anestesia quirúrgica. Gaceta Médica Catalana, 1890; 13: 5-8, 33-36, 71-74, 101-105, 134-136

[10] Morales Pérez A: Hechos curiosos de orden sugestivo por medio de la Termoeterización. Gaceta Médica Catalana, 1889; 12: 453-454

[11] Hervás Pujal C: La anestesia en Cataluña. Historia y evolución (1847-1901). Tesis Doctoral. Barcelona, 1986

[12] Hervás Pujal C: Cahisa Mur, M. Antonio Morales y la Termoeterización. Rev esp anestesial reanim. 1990; 37: 278-283

[13] Morales Pérez A: La Electrotermoeterización. XIV Congrés International de Medicine. Compte Rendus. Section de Chirurgie Generale. 222-228 pp. Imp. J. Sastre, Madrid, 1904

[14] Martínez Suárez F: La anestesia quirúrgica y los anestésicos. Eter caliente. Rev esp med. 1906; 9: 335-342

15 Carreras Gaiviso A: La Termoeterización como método de anestesia quirúrgica. Tesis Doctoral. 136 pp. MS. Facultad de Medicina, Madrid, 1889

[16] Mur Estaña A: La Termoeterización. Tesis Doctoral. 115 pp. MS. Facultad de Medicina, Madrid, 1899

[17] Mur Estaña A: La Termoeterización como nuevo método de anestesia según el procedimiento del Dr. A. Díaz de Liaño, de Barcelona. La Oto-Rino-Laringología Española. Revista de Especialidades, 1898-1899; 1: 54-56

[18] Díaz de Liaño A: Electro-Termo-Eterizador. Nuevo aparato inventado por el Dr... La Independencia Médica, 1891-1892; 23: 296, 297

Alternative Analgesic and Anaesthetic Techniques

H. Baar, Hamburg, Germany

At all times it has been a dream of every anaesthesiologist to participate in diagnostics and therapy. As a result my teacher, Professor Rudolf Frey, perceived as early as in the late sixties that paintherapy and anaesthesiology could be complementary to one another. To make his idea come true he sent to Hans-Ulrich Gerbershagen to the USA and me to Sweden. At that time we both already had received a profound education in anaesthesiologic pain treatment. In the early seventies German doctors interpreted pain view as a symptom of disease. In addition they pointed out that it is the very own duty of a medical doctor to treat pain. They believed - and a lot of modern doctors continue to do so - that there is no need of a pain specialist or special institution for pain treatment in Germany. At that time medical doctors in Germany did not distinguish between acute pain and chronic pain syndromes being some kind of disease on their own.

Nevertheless, our teacher Rudolf Frey thought of all of the seven million patients in Germany who were suffering from chronic pain. So we were able to inaugurate the first German Pain Clinic at the Institute of Anaesthesiology at the University of Mainz as early as 1971.

After having studied John Bonica's textbook "The Management of Pain" we felt strong enough to fight chronic pain syndromes. Nevertheless, I have to concede that our knowledge about pain was very poor. We saw the problem with the eyes of an anaesthesiologist. At that time pain treatment in Germany was performed in a monodisciplinary way and mainly applying drugs. As a result our aim was to find alternative anaesthesiologic methods and techniques.

Methods like local anaesthesia as well as nerve blocks for surgical procedures as described by Bonica are closely related to those techniques that were called „Therapeutic Local Anaesthesia" and „Therapeutic Nerve Blocks". We started pain treatment by performing methods utilizing modern local anaesthetics of the amide type.

Somatic methods:

1. Weal Therapy

After injecting small amounts - about 0.05ml of a local anaesthetic intracutaneously weals do appear. By applying this method we take advantage the cutaneo-visceral reflex. Thus leads to an increased blood circulation and has a spasmolytic effect on the unstriated muscles of the internal organs related to the region where the injection has been made (Head zones)

2. Infiltration of Triggerpoint

By examining a patient who is suffering from a tension headache or from chronic cervical spine syndromes you often will find pressure sensitive points in the muscles of the neck. These small regions called "Trigger points" are surrounded by a metabolic barrier which prevents an exchange of pain producing substances like Histamine, Substance P,

Prostaglandin a. o.. Chronic pain results. Injecting 1ml of local anaesthetic into each trigger point penetrates this barrier and enables the accumulated substances are able to diffuse into the tissue of their origin.

With this method even long lasting pain syndromes may be treated successfully.

3. Scar Subinjection

Each lesion of the integument is followed by the formation of a scar. These scars may be responsible for the so called „scar pain". We do not know if small neurinoms which occur after the destruction of the skin trigger the nerve system along with irritating impulses. This leads often to chronic pain syndromes. Repeated injections of local anaesthetics under the scar, subcutaneously, results a disconnection of the irritated region from the central nerve system. I believe that the brain does not recognize pain any longer after this treatment.

4. Contralateral Therapeutic Local Anaesthesia

There is another phenomenon worth mentioning. It was described by Dieter Gross, who was one of the founders of the International Association for the Study of Pain. In patients with chronic pain of their extremities one can detect hyperalgesic points in the contralateral region i.e. the healthy uneffected extremity. After repeated injection of small quantities of local anaesthetics the pain on the affected extremity disappears. Nevertheless, Gross was able to detect this phenomenon in phantom-limb pain, too. We really have no idea, how it works. With the help of proper equipment and experience anyone is able to block any nerve or nerve plexus. Methods like peripheral nerve blocking, plexus anaesthesia, peridural anaesthesia and spinal anaesthesia are well known for surgical indications. The same techniques are applied in pain therapy.

A method that we performed in the early seventies, with good results was the neurolysis of the dorsal sensory root of the spinal nerve.

To perform this neurolysis we applied dehydrated alcohol. The specific gravity of absolute alcohol is lower than the specific gravity of cerebrospinal fluid. By placing the patient in a very special way we were able to position the patient in a way that the root of that segment that was to be destroyed, was the highest point of this arrangement. With an insulin syringe we injected - very slowly - an amount of 0.1-0.3 ml of absolute alcohol into the spinal space. With this method we were able to perform an aimed destruction of 1 to 3 dorsal spinal nerve roots by protein denaturation. It is quite obvious that the patient was not allowed to cough.

Now back to today and the methods of therapeutic local anaesthesia and nerve blocks. As mentioned above we usually repeat these injections every second day up to an amount of 9 injections within one series. We try to obtain a hang over of the pain reducing effect, that lasts longer than the effect of the local anaesthetic. If this effect does not appear after a maximum of 5 injections we exspect that this method will not work, and we either have to revise our diagnosis or change the method. Unfortunately, the desired result is obtained in 70 per cent of these cases only. For the remaining pain syndromes we have to find alternative methods: e.g. be in sympathetic nerve blocks.

In cases of disorders of the autonomic nerve system like phantom limb pain, causalgia and sympathetic reflex dystrophy for example, sympathetic nerve blocks may be helpful. With some experience it is not difficult to reach the sympathetic trunk or the sympathetic trunk ganglia. A lot of diiferent techniques for the application local anaesthetics, repeated injections or neurolytic drugs in order to destroy the sympathetic nerve tissue, are described in the literature.

The amount of positive results of repeated blocks of the autonomic nerve system are nearly the same as in blocking somatic nerves. While it is strictly forbidden to perform neurolytic, i.e. destroying blocks of somatic nerves this kind of nerve block is basically allowed in the autonomic nerve system and may be appreciated as an advantage in certain pain problems. The effect of this chemical disconnection is as effective as the surgical sympathetic trunkotomy and can be performed in high risk patients, too. The effect of both methods may last for two months to two years, but the benefit of the chemical block is: it can be repeated twice. What can be done in case none of these methods leads to sufficient pain relief? In those cases we are forced to either to revive our diagnosis or to find additional methods for the treatment of pain. This puts up the question whether these methods can be found in anaesthesiology!?

We have to realize that pain is as well a feeling, a sensation as an experience and that there is only a multi-disciplinary approach to treat its effectively. As Bonica has outlined repeatedly we often have to look for alternative methods in other medical specialities, even in psychology.

Who Introduced the Rebreathing Systems into Clinical Practice?

J. A. Baum
Department of Anaesthesia and Intensive Care
Hospital St. Elisabeth-Stift, Damme, Germany

As early as in 1850 - only 4 years after the first successful clinical performance of ether anaesthesia by William T. G. Morton (1819-1868) - the ingenious John Snow (1813-1853) recognized that ether and chloroform partially were exhaled unchanged with the expired air. To reuse these unchanged vapours in the following inspiration and thereby prolonging the narcotic effect of a given amount of anaesthetic vapour, he converted his ether inhaler into a to and fro rebreathing system (Fig. 1): The apparatus was equipped with a facemask without in- or expiratory valves and a large reservoir bag containing pure oxygen attached to the air inlet; the spiral chamber was partially filled with an aqueous solution of caustic potash which was used as carbon dioxide absorbent. In several experiments, performed on himself, Snow succeeded to demonstrate that rebreathing of the exhaled vapours was possible following carbon dioxide absorption, and that it resulted in a pronounced prolongation of the narcotic effects of the volatile anaesthetics[1].

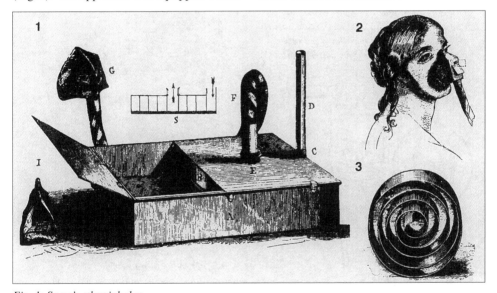

Fig. 1: Snow's ether inhaler.
1: Overall view of the apparatus (A: metal box serving as a water bath; B: spiral ether chamber; C: opening for filling in ether; D: brass tube by which the air enters which the patient inhales; F: elastic tube; G: face piece; S: section of spiral ether chamber)
2: Face piece with in- and expiratory valve.
3: Ether chamber with the bottom removed, showing the volute from Snow[1]

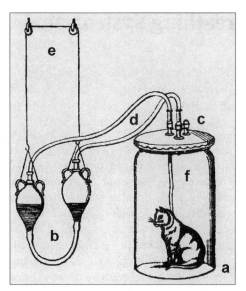

Fig. 2: Snow's closed system for experimental determination of the amount of carbon dioxide excreted during ether and chloroform anaesthesia. (a: glass jar; b: two glass vessels, filled with an aqueous solution of potash, connected together by an elastic tube; c: air tight lid with an opening for filling in the volatile anaesthetic; d: rubber tubes connecting the jar with the potash apparatus; e: mechanism to move up and down the glass vessels.) If the glass vessels were moved up and down they alternately filled with the fluid, resulting in a constant circulation of the air within the jar and the vessels and, thus, leading to absorption of the exhaled carbon dioxide by the solution of potash (from Snow[2]).

Fig. 3: Hales' closed rebreathing system. a: mouthpiece: e: unidirectional expiratory valve, i: unidirectional inspiratory valve, n: four linen diaphragms clamped into the breathing gas reservoir, soaked with calcinated potassium bitartrate for carbon dioxide absorption, o: flexible breathing gas reservoir, s: inspiratory hose (from Hales[3]).

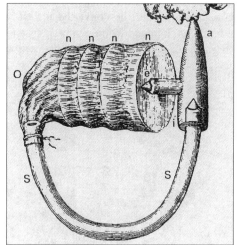

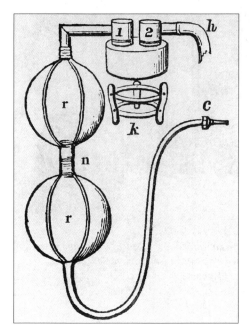

Fig. 4: Coleman's "economising apparatus". c: adapter to the nitrous oxide cylinder; r: reservoir bags; n: unidirectional valve; 1/2: metal box (economiser), filled with small pieces of slaked lime; 1: connector to the reservoir bags; 2: connector to the patient; h: tubing to the face piece; k: frame which supports the economiser on the top of the gas cylinder (from Duncum[6]).

Furthermore, Snow performed experiments on animals using a completely closed system (Fig. 2) for evaluating the carbon dioxide production during anaesthesia[2].

And yet, the principle of rebreathing exhaled air via a breathing system after elimination of "noxious vapours" had long since been known. In 1727, Stephen Hales (1677- 1761) described a rebreathing circle system by means of which „sulphureous steams" could be absorbed, destroing the „elasticity of the air" and thus rendering impossible free ventilation[3]. His circle system, which he recommended for rescue purposes, consisted of a gas reservoir made of a bladder into which four diaphragms of flannel were placed, soaked with a solution of highly calcinated tartar, a wide- bore syphon, and unidirectional in- and expiratory valves (Fig. 3).

Alfred Coleman (1828-1902) was the first to use a rebreathing system with carbon dioxide absorption in clinical practice. Nitrous oxide was delivered to a pair of reservoir bags connected with an unidirectional valve. From the proximal reservoir the patient inhaled the gas, which had to pass a tin box filled with slaked lime, via a wide-bore tubing leading to a face mask (Fig. 4). During expiration the air was expired back into the proximal reservior bag, again passing the metal box where the carbon dioxide was absorbed. By the use of his to-and-fro system Coleman wanted to decrease nitrous oxide consumption, as the usual use of high amounts of this expensive anaesthetic was a serious impediment in the spread of nitrous oxide anaesthesia[4,5]. As the patients got pure nitrous oxide, this rebreathing technique could only be used in very short lasting surgical procedures. Although Coleman commitedly advocated the use of his „economising apparatus", this technique was not generally adopted.

It is nearly unknown that at that time 1868/1869, a German dentist, Carl Sauer (1835 - 1892), described the clinical use of a quite similar to-and-fro system. Unfortunately there is no figure depicting this device[7].

In 1906, Franz Kuhn (1866-1929) was the first to publish constructive details on a concept for an anaesthetic circle system which incorporated an unidirectional valve and two canisters filled with alkalihydroxides for carbon dioxide absorption (Fig. 5). This canisters, called "Kalipatronen", were already commercially available and manufactured by Drägerwerk in Lübeck as a part of the mining rescue rebreathing apparatus. It was also Kuhn's intention to lead back unused anaesthetic gases, contained in the expired air, to the patient during the following inhalation. The amount of oxygen to be fed into the system then merely had to replenish the volume which had been consumed or got lost as a result of leaks. However, this system has never been put to clinical use since the flow resistance and the dead space of the breathing system were too big. In addition, Kuhn feared that the chemical reaction of chloroform with the absorbing material (caustic soda) might possibly do harm to the patient[8].

In 1915, Dennis E. Jackson (1879-1980) introduced a closed anaesthetic circle system

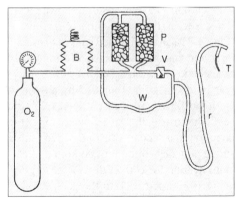

Fig. 5: Concept of a circle rebreathing system designed by Franz Kuhn, 1906.
B: bellows, P: carbon dioxide absorber,
V: unidirectional inspiratory valve,
W: breathing system, T: airway,
r: breathing tube (from Rendell-Baker[9]).

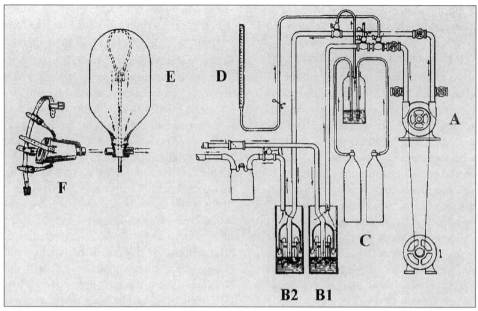

Fig. 6: Jackson's circle absorption system.
The animal inhales gas out of the gas reservoir (E) via the face piece (F). Continuously anaesthetic gas is sucked out of this reservoir by an air pump (A), passes the wash jar (B1), filled with concentrated sulphuric acid, leaves the pump in the direction to the wash jar (B2), filled with a strong aqueous solution of sodium and calcium hydrate, passes a Woulff bottle and then is returned back to the gas reservoir (E). Nitrous oxide and oxigen, obtained from the gas cylinders (C), are fed into the system in just such an amount to keep constant the gas filling of the rubber bag serving as the reservoir (E). Fluid ether or chloroform is delivered into the system from the burette (D) (from Jackson[10]).

with carbon dioxide absorption which he tested successfully in animal experiments (Fig. 6). The animal inhaled gas out of the gas reservoir via the face piece. Continuously anaesthetic gas was sucked out of this reservoir by an air pump, purified by passing a wash jar, filled with concentrated sulphuric acid. The anaesthetic gas left the pump in the direction to a second wash jar, filled with a strong aqueous solution of sodium and calcium hydrate for carbon dioxide absorption and was returned back to the gas reservoir. Nitrous oxide and oxygen, obtained from the gas cylinders, were fed into the system in just such an amount to keep constant the gas filling of the reservoir bag. Fluid ether or chloroform was delivered directly into the system from a burette. Neither the apparatus nor the method, however, met with any interest, although the use of this technology saved considerable amounts of anaesthetic gas and the apparatus itself worked reliably[10].

It is really amazing that this device exeedingly resembles the most modern electronically controlled closed circle system Physio-Flex (Fig. 7). Similar to Jackson's apparatus, the gas is kept moving continuously by a blower, oxygen and nitrous oxide are delivered into the system to keep constant the required oxigen concentration and the circulating gas volume, and the anaesthetic agent is delivered directly into the system in liquid form[11].

In 1916 Jackson described a wonderfully simple and cheap to-and-fro system for experimental anaesthesia (Fig. 8), in which a cake

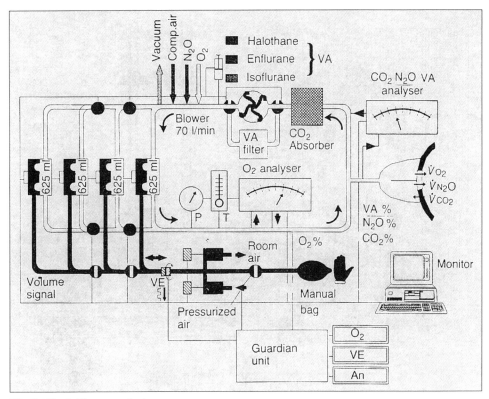

Fig. 7: PhysioFlex anaesthetic apparatus:
Closed loop feedback control of the gas composition and the gas volume within the breathing system. Driven by a blower the anaesthetic gas circulates continuously with a flow of 70 l/min. The liquid volatile agent is directly injected into the system by a motor syringe in just that amount to keep constant the preset expired concentration. Oxygen is delivered into the system in just that amount to keep constant the nominal inspired concentration, and nitrous oxide in just that amount to keep constant the circulating gas volume. The anaesthetic concentration can be decreased nearly without any time delay by bypassing the anaesthetic gas to a canister filled with charcoal (v. A. Ads.). The exact performance of the closed loop feedback control is supervised by the guardian unit (from Baum [11]).

pan covered by a shower cap, partially filled with an aqueous solution of soda lime, was used for absorption of the exhaled carbon dioxide[12].

It was Ralph M. Waters (1883-1979), who introduced the technique of anaesthesia with closed rebreathing system in routine clinical practice in 1924[13]. In his to-and-fro system, it was a metal canister filled with sodium hydroxide granules that served as a carbon dioxide absorber (Fig. 9). The patient inhaled anaesthetic gas from the reservoir bag into which he exhaled again. Adequate oxygenation was achieved by intermittent oxygen supply, whenever the patient turned slightly blue. Hans Killian (1892-1982) paid a visit to Waters in Madison (USA) in 1928 and was greatly impressed by his work with the to-and-fro system: *"...After the patient had been slightly anaesthetised in an anteroom, he (Waters) filled a large 10 litre balloon with an ethylene and oxygen mixture from the Foregger machine, at a ratio of about 80:20%. Then he switched off the machine*

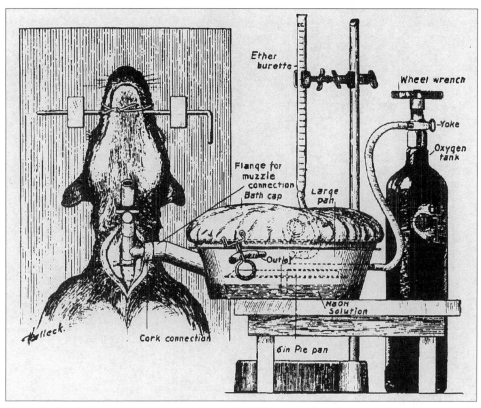

Fig. 8: Jackson's to-and-fro system. Very simple to-and-fro system built from parts bought in a ten cent store: the absorber, simultaneously serving as a vaporizer and a gas reservoir, consists of a cake and a pie pan and a bath cap (from Jackson[12]).

completely, closed the filling tap of the large rubber bag, attached a soda cartridge to it, and to the other end fitted an anaesthetic mask, which was placed onto the patient's face. The patient inhaled the gas mixture from the rubber bag only and expired back into the balloon. This was in accordance with his to-and-fro system and absorption of carbon dioxide... He (the patient) remained sleeping, although he did not receive a continuous flow of fresh gas, ethylene-oxygen. This balloon technique did not appear surprising as long as it lasted only 5 to 10 minutes for transport from the induction room to the operating theatre. But in this case it lasted much longer, 20 to 30 minutes. I noticed that Waters administered oxygen without ethylene into the bag only once, when the patient turned slightly blue. I was somewhat puzzled. Right in front of our eyes, a most remarkable event had taken place, much to my amazement. Though most of the others had not noticed it. Waters had proved that there was something wrong about our pharmacological assumptions that maintenance of the depth of sleep solely depends on the concentration of the inhalational anaesthetic... One can hardly imagine how this whole story embarrassed me. I lay awake late the following night, thinking and trying with all my might to get behind the secret and to come up with an idea about our anaesthetic methods..... We were really on the verge of an outstanding progress in the field of anaesthesia..."[14].

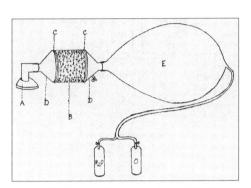

Fig. 9: The To-and-Fro system from R.W. Waters (from Waters[13]).

The gynaecologist Carl J. Gauss (1875-1957) and the chemist H. Wieland (1877-1957) were protagonists in the use of purified acetylene, called narcylene, as an inhalation anaesthetic. In cooperation with the German engineer Bernhard Dräger (1870-1928), the first anaesthetic apparatus equipped with an anaesthetic circle rebreathing system was developed and put into operation in clinical practice in 1924[15, 16]. After carbon dioxide absorption the exhaled gas, still containing unspent anaesthetic gases, was blended with fresh gas and routed back to the patient. This first aesthetic circle system (Fig. 10) already featured low resistance in- and expiratory valves, a canister filled with carbon dioxide absorbent and an overflow valve. By introducing the rebreathing technique into anaesthetic practice it was not only possible to reduce the consumption of expensive anaesthetic gases, but also to significantly reduce the discharge of this strange smelling and highly explosive agent.

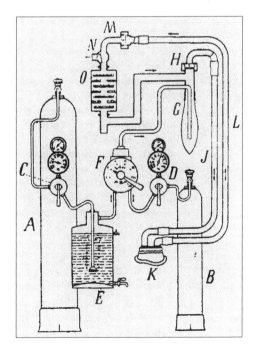

Fig. 10: Narcylene apparatus from Gauss and Wieland.
A: Gas cylinder containing narcylene,
B: gas cylinder containing oxygen,
C and D: pressure regulators and gas flow metering devices,
E: wash jar filled with water to purify narcylene from acetone,
F: gas blender,
G: reservoir bag (Sparbeutel),
H: inspiratory valve,
J: inspiratory limb,
K: face mask,
L: expiratory limb,
M: expiratory valve,
N: spill valve,
O: carbon dioxide absorber (Kalipatrone) (from Gauss[15]).

Bernhard Dräger applied for a German patent for an anaesthetic circle system (Fig. 11) on October 2nd, 1925, which was granted on January 26th, 1927[17].

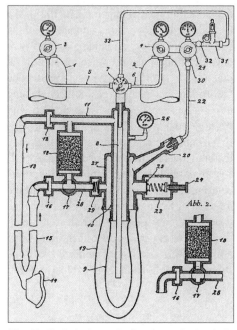

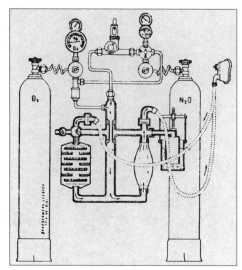

Fig. 12: Flow diagram of the circle absorption system of the Dräger Lachgas Narkose Apparat Model A (from Haupt[20]).

Fig. 11: Technical scetch of an anaesthetic circle system as submitted to the German patent office by Bernhard Dräger on 2nd October, 1925. Legend: 7: gas blender, 9: reservoir bag, 12: inspiratory valve, 13: inspiratory limb, 14: face mask, 15: expiratory limb, 16: expiratory valve, 18: carbon dioxide absorber, 17: three-way tap (in Abb. 2 the absorber canister is switched off by turning this tap and the whole expired gas leaves the breathing system via the spill valve: non-rebreathing mode), 29: spill valve. The second bag (19), the injector (20) and the pressure limit valve (23) are needed to generate and transmit a continuous positive pressure, shown at the manometer (26), to the breathing system (from Dräger[17]).

Together with Paul Sudeck (1866-1945) and Helmut Schmidt (1895-1979) Dräger developed another anaesthetic apparatus, as well equipped with this circle system (Fig. 12), for application of oxygen and nitrous-

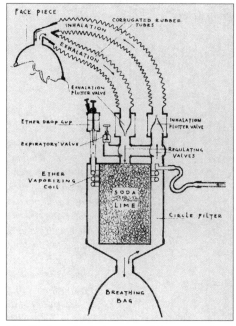

Fig. 13: Sword's circle system. The technical scetch shows the principle of the Sword circle system in an improved design (from: Anesthesia and respiration appliances, Catalog No. 9, Foregger Company, New York, 1949).

oxide, which became commericially available as the "Lachgas- Narkose-Apparat Modell A" from 1926 onwards[18, 19, 20].

As it was just recently revealed and published by Richard Foregger[21], the son of the famous engineer Richard von Foregger (1872-1960), not until a few years later, between 1928 and 1930, Foregger and Brian C. Sword (1889-1956) constructed a similar circle absorption system (Fig. 13) in the United States of America[22], following corresponding recommendations from Hans Killian and Helmut Schmidt.

Thus, not Waters but Coleman in 1869 was the first to introduce the to-and-fro system into clinical practice. Furthermore, neither Sudeck and Schmidt nor Sword but Gauss, Wieland and Draeger in 1924 were the first to use a circle system in anaesthesia.

References:

[1] Snow J: On Narcotism by the Inhalation of Vapours. Part XV. The effects of Chloroform and Ether Prolonged by Causing the Exhaled Vapour to be reinspired. London Medical Gazette 1850; 11: 749-754

[2] Snow J: On Narcotism by the Inhalation of Vapours. Part XVI. Experiments on determine the amount of carbonic acid gas excreted under the influence of chloroform. London Medical Gazette 1851; 12: 622-627

[3] Hales S: Analysis of the air. Experiment CXVI. In: Statical Essays: Containing vegetable staticks; or, an account of some statical experiments on the sap in vegetables & also, a specimen of an attempt to analyse the air, by a great variety of chymio-statical experiments, which were read at several meetings before the Royal Society. Vol I. Second Edition, W. Innys, London, 1731, 264- 273

[4] Coleman A: Action of nitrous oxide. Br med J, April 25, 1868: 410

[5] Coleman A: Re-inhalation of nitrous oxide. Br med J, August 1, 1868: 114-115

[6] Duncum BM: The Development of Inhalation Anaesthesia. Oxford University Press, London 1947. Reprint edited on behalf of the History of Anaesthesia Society by the Royal Society of Medicine Press, London 1994. pp. 287- 289

[7] Sauer C: Vorläufige Mittheilung der weiteren Versuche, mit Stickstoffoxydul-Gemischen zu anästhesieren. Ber Klin Wochenschr 1869; 6: 366-367

[8] Kuhn F: Die perorale Intubation mit und ohne Druck. III. Teil. Apparat zur Lieferung des Druckes für die Überdrucknarkose. Deutsche Zeitschrift für Chirurgie 1906; 81: 63-70

[9] Rendell-Baker L: History of Thoracic Anaesthesia. In Mushin W. W. (Edit.): Thoracic Anaesthesia. Blackwell Scientific Publications, Oxford 1963

[10] Jackson DE: A new method for the production of general analgesia and anaesthesia with a description of the apparatus Used J Lab. Clin. Med. 1915; 1: 1-12

[11] Baum JA: Low Flow Anaesthesia. The Theory and Practice of Low Flow, Minimal Flow and Closed System Anaesthesia. Butterworth Heinemann, Oxford 1996: pp. 125-127

[12] Jackson DE: The employment of closed ether anesthesia for ordinary laboratory experiments. J. Lab. Clin. Med. 1916; 2: 94-102

[13] Waters RM: Clinical scope and utility of carbon dioxid filtration in inhalation anaesthesia. Anesth. Analg. 1924; 3: 20-22

[14] Killian H: 40 Jahre Narkoseforschung. Verlag der Deutschen Hochschullehrerzeitung, Tübingen 1964: S. 75-76

[15] Gauss CJ: Die Narcylenbetäubung mit dem Kreisatmer. Zbl f Gyn 1925; 23: 1218-1226

[16] Foregger R: A question of priority: who introduced the CO_2 absorption method with the circle breathing into anaesthesia practice? Anaesthesist 1995; 44: 917-918

[17] Dräger AB: Vorrichtung zum Einatmen von Gasen unter Überdruck, insbesondere für Betäubungszwecke. Patentschrift Nr. 439657, Reichsdruckerei, Berlin, 1927

[18] Sudeck P, Schmidt H: Über Gasnarkosen. Zbl f Chir 1926; 20: 1271-1275

[19] Drägerwerk (ed.): Dräger-Stickoxydul-Narkose-Apparat nach Prof. Dr. Sudeck und Dr. Helmut Schmidt. Modell A. Gebrauchsanweisung Nr. 35, Lübeck, 1927

[20] Haupt J: Die Geschichte der Dräger-Narkoseapparate. 1. überarbeitete Version. Drägerwerk AG, Lübeck, 1996: S. 31-33

[21] Foregger R: Richard von Foregger, Ph.D., 1872-1960. Manufacturer of anesthesia equipment. Anesthesiology 1996; 84: 190-200

[22] Sword BC: The closed circle method of administration of gas anesthesia. Current Researches in Anesthesia & Analgesia 1930; 9: 198-202

The Closed System:
1946 – 1996. A 50 Years Perspective.

C. Parsloe
Hospital Samaritano, São Paulo, SP, Brasil

I first saw cyclopropane To and Fro Closed System in the hands of Ralph Waters on October, 1946. Shortly after I used it extensively during my residency and learned to admire its inherent simplicity. All that was needed was to use the metabolic flow of oxygen and the correct amount of cyclopropane, both easily measured in water flowmeters, and to keep the rebreathing bag from overfilling or emptying. Once familiar with the handling of the canister and its proper position over the patient's pillow it became quite easy to master the technique. It was possible to use it with the patient in the lateral or the prone position. The rationale for the closed system with a potent gas was simply stated by Harold Griffith : "the bag is full of oxygen and enough cyclopropane is administered according to the desired level of anesthesia".

Until 1924, when Waters introduced the to and fro closed technique, closed system meant rebreathing of expired air in order to conserve carbon dioxide as a respiratory stimulant. Yandell Henderson's widely held concept on the acapnic theory of shock offered a basis for rebreathing carbon dioxide. Waters conceptual change meant that now carbon dioxide was rightfully considered a waste product needing adequate pulmonary excretion. and absorption by soda lime within the closed anesthesia system.

Waters original rebreathing bags were quite large, with a volume greater than the functional residual capacity, acting like a spirometer.

At first, ether and nitrous oxide were used. Later, in the 30s cyclopropane was introduced clinically by Waters. Because or its limited availability at the time of introduction, its cost and explosiveness, it proved to be the ideal agent for the closed system. It seemed as though cyclopropane and the closed system were made for one another. In fact, the closed system saw its apogee during the 30s and the 40s, after the introduction and widely spread use of cyclpropane.

The canister used for adults had a 450 gr. capacity for soda lime. At the patient end of the canister a 90 degree curved elbow served both as the mask connecting piece and the gas inlet. The rebreathing bag in the 40s had a 5 liter capacity and its tail could be closed with a clamp or partially or fully opened if so desired.

Endotracheal intubation greatly facilitated the manual control of ventilation. No ventilators were used and the "educated hand" reigned supreme. When a facial mask was used it had to be properly applied in order to avoid leaks. If the operation required a nasogastric tube the handling of the system needed to be meticulous to preserve its closed characteristic.

Several size canisters with a capacity for 350, 180 and 90 gr. were introduced for use in different size children.

Shortly after its introduction the closed circle system became widely used and in fact supplanted the to and fro canister on account of its easier handling. The drawback in the first models was the too small canister used with a 450 gr. capacity. In order to extend the useful life of the system a two canister circle was developed by Adriani offering the possibility of using one or the other canister or by-passing both. In 1953 Kapesser substituted the small canisters in the Adriani filter with two 750 gr. capacity canisters. Still they could be used singly. Morris used one 750 gr. canister in a simple circle arrangement, called the Universal filter, in which it was easier to change the canister when needed.

The jumbo double, large capacity, canister arrangement was the forerunner of present day highly efficient circle systems. Elam, Brown and Ten Pass made the first modern studies of carbon dioxide absorption in circle absorption systems working with a Liston Becker capnograph in the 1950s.

Bloomquist introduced a small canister circle system for pediatric use. The original model had an Elam type two one way valves placed at the patient end of the circle. It was simple to assemble, to clean and to use. Later models placed the usual adult type one way valves at the filter end of the circle.

The Revell circulator and later Neff's and Takaoka's Venturi circulating devices served to decrease the mechanical dead space under the mask and to increase the effficiency of carbon dioxide absorption.

In 1952, Lucien Morris introduced the copper kettle vaporizer. It grew out of Waters request for a precision vaporizer for chloroform. Since this agent proved unworthy of re-introduction, the kettle was used as a precision vaporizer for ether. It made a distinct difference in the administration of ether permitting small increments of vapor concentration without irritating the airway.

Soon after Halothane was introduced and with it the perceived need for a calibrated vaporizer allowing precise control of the vapor output. It was then realized that with a diluent flow of 5 liters per minute the kettle Halothane vapor output was linear. Thus, 100 ml vaporizing flow into the kettle originated a 1 % Halothane vapor output. This finding, together with the development of the Fluotec Mark 2 calibrated vaporizers, which required a 5 liters per minute inflow for a stable vapor output concentration decreed the demise of the closed system. The use of 5 liters inflow into the circle system became the common practice and the era of the semi-closed absorption system was ushered in. By now, the to and fro canisters were a thing of the past and the circle filters were in common use.

In 1954, Severinghaus described the square root of time absorption of nitrous oxide and later Lowe applied the concept to the absorption of volatile agents, originally with metoxyflurane and halothane.

The new quantitative era of closed anesthesia system was introduced with a simple periodical syringe injection in pre-determined times of the required doses of the liquid volatile agent.

The next development consisted in the introduction of anesthetic agent monitors with digital read outs and graphical display of the inspired and the end tidal concentrations. Thus, pharmacokinetics was brought into daily use in the operating room. Now, the anesthesiologist could follow in real time the increase or the decrease of the alveolar anesthetic agent concentration thereby anticipating the resulting pharmacodynamic effects rather than having to wait for circulatory or respiratory signs as indicators of the level of anesthesia. The original inherent simplicity of measuring a gas in a flowmeter could now be emulated by reading the inspired and the expired concentrations of the agents in a monitor.

The next logical step was to build a micro-processed, calibrated or kettle type, vaporizer with a display to indicate the effluent vapor per minute as well as the liquid agent consumption. This already exists and together with agent monitors is giving new impetus to the closed system anesthesia with volatile agents.

Next came the last generation of anesthesia machines dedicated to the closed system of which the Physioflex is an example. Computer control and a pharmacokinetic model allows for deciding on a given end tidal concentration which the machine provides for in a metabolic oxygen environment.

The ultimate step could be the introduction of a potent, non explosive anesthesic gas which could again be easily measured in a flowmeter. This would cause a veritable revolution in the administration of closed system inhalation anesthesia since the volatile agents would disappear and with them the need for vaporizers. The anesthesiologist could then fill the system with oxygen and simply administer the adequate amount of the gaseous agent.

Nathan Zuntz (1847-1920) and his Contributions to the History of Anaesthesia

H. C. Gunga
Department Physiology, Freie Universität Berlin, Klinikum Benjamin Franklin, Berlin, Germany

Abstract

Nathan Zuntz (1847-1920), working as a professor of animal physiology at the "Landwirtschaftliche Hochschule" (Agricultural University) in Berlin from 1881 until 1918, was a key person in the history of physiology. Since 1881 he studied in his laboratory the change of metabolism at rest and during exercise. At the beginning of the 90's, Zuntz started research in the field of high altitude physiology. In view of the variety of questions and the considerable methodological problems Zuntz first studied the effects of lowered PO_2 on the human body in a hypobaric chamber. In addition, Zuntz conducted several expeditions to the Monte Rosa. In 1902 Zuntz and the Austrian Hermann von Schroetter (1870-1928) conducted two balloon ascents up to 5 000 m in Berlin and performed studies in airships and planes. Zuntz retired in 1916 and died soon after on March 22 1920 in Berlin. Zuntz was the author of one of the most productive physiological works in the German-speaking countries and especially his research in metabolism, respiration and blood gases could be considered as fundamental contributions to the history of anaesthesia.

Nathan Zuntz (1847-1920) (Fig. 1) was working as a professor of animal physiology at the "Landwirtschaftliche Hochschule" (Agricultural University) in Berlin from 1881 until 1918.1 He started his career with a thesis written under the guidance of the famous German physiologist Pflüger (1829-1910) about contributions to blood physiology,

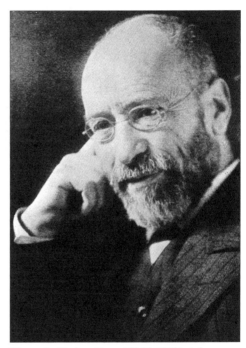

Figure 1: Nathan Zuntz (1847-1920) at the age of about 65 years

proving thereby that erythrocytes are involved in the binding of carbondioxide in the blood. From 1870-1881 Zuntz worked as a professor in Bonn and moved then to the Agricultural Academy in Berlin (Fig. 2) to take the chair for animal physiology. During the first years there he developed together with Geppert the famous „Zuntz-Geppert' respiration apparatus" (Fig. 3). With this apparatus Zuntz was able to measure the metabolic rate during rest and excercise. The apparatus was composed of a mouthpiece, a

455

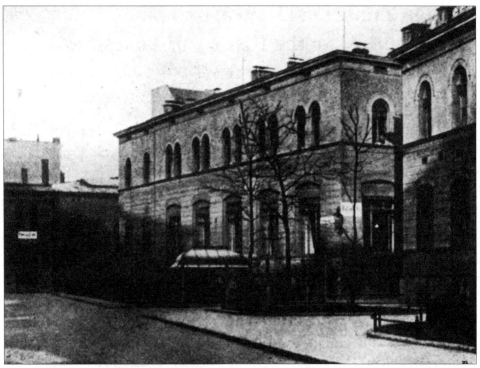

Figure 2: The Department of Animal Physiology guided by Zuntz at the Agricultural Academy in Berlin

valve mechanism which separated the exspiratory and inspiratory air, a gasmeter which measured the respiratory volumes and the analysis appliance itself which measured the volumes of carbon-dioxide and oxygen from a sample of exspiratory air. At the end of the 1880's the range of his works stretched from blood, circulation and muscular physiology to nutrition and digestion physiology, animal breeding and even embryology. Together with Adolf Loewy (1862-1936) Zuntz started studies on excercise physiology and high altitude physiology in the early 90's, especially on the physiology of marching. This topic was ordered to Zuntz by the Ministery of War. He should try to determine the limits of tolerable load for marching soldiers. For this kind of studies he invented the treadmill (Fig. 4) which later was combined with a x-ray apparatus to study circulation under physical exercise. Zuntz noticed from the beginning that such a physiological research in the laboratory (i.e. respiration chamber, Fig. 5) had to be supplemented with physiological field

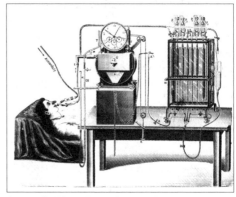

Figure 3: The „Zuntz-Geppert Respirationsapparat" in a typical experimental setup (resting position)

data, especially for studies on exercise at high altitude. Therefore in addition, Zuntz first analyzed the effects of lowered PO_2 on the human body in a "Pneumatischen Kammer" (hypobaric chamber) and after the completion of the international research station Capanna Regina Margherita on the top of the Monte Rosa (4500 m, Italy) in 1893 he began to study exercise physiology in the field. Together with Adolf Loewy (1862-1936), the Italian Angelo Mosso (1846-1910), and the Austrian Arnold Durig (1872-1961) Zuntz conducted several expeditions to the Monte Rosa. As a synopsis of these high altitude studies Zuntz published in 1906 his famous book on high altitude climate and mountain trekking. For this special kind of field studies in the Alps Zuntz invented a respiration apparatus, the "transportable Gasuhr" (transportable gas exchange measuring device,

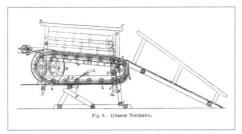

Figure 4: The "Zuntz-Lehmann'sche Laufband" (treadmill) invented in 1889

Fig. 6). In 1902 Zuntz and the Austrian Hermann von Schroetter (1870-1928) conducted two balloon ascents up to 5 000 m in Berlin. For these ascents Zuntz and v. Schroetter constructed an oxygen supply system which was later successfully used by balloon flyers and aviators (Fig. 7). Besides that they planned a pressure cabin for extreme altitudes above 10 000 m which has to be

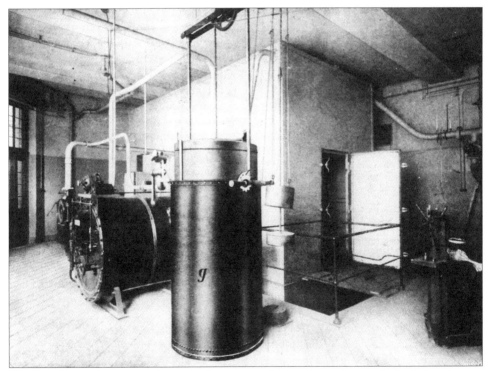

Figure 5: The respiratory chamber at the Department of Animal Physiology at the Agricultural Academy in Berlin

considered to be the forerunner of the modern systems in aviation and astronautics and published independent papers on aviation which are international unique concerning their style and extent. In 1910 Zuntz, Durig, and v. Schroetter participated alltogether with Barcroft (Cambridge) and Douglas (Oxford) at the famous "International Teneriffa Expedition" (Canary Islands) which was guided by Pannwitz. With the beginning of World War I (1914) the civil research in high altitude and aviation medicine was paralysed in Germany. Because of the war the food supply of the German population went down

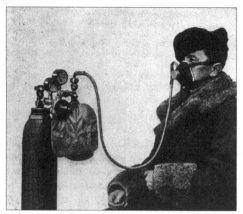

Figure 7: *An oxygen supply system invented by Zuntz and v. Schroetter in 1902 which was later successfully used by balloon flyers and aviators.*

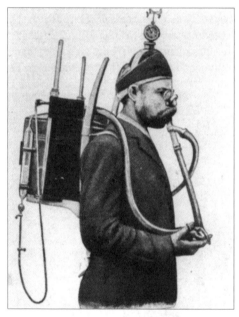

Figure 6: *Adolf Loewy (1862-1936) is wearing for field studies the transportable gas measuring device invented by Zuntz and an anemometer to measure air velocity on the top of his head*

and Zuntz was asked by the German government due to his outstanding knowledge in nutritional physiology to work with high priority in this field again. Zuntz recognized soon that the extensive stock farming was one of the main reasons for the food shortage in Germany. He proposed the slaughter of 8-9 millions hogs which was carried out as Zuntz had demanded it. This massive slaughter in the spring of 1915 became history as the "Schweinemord" (pig murder). Zuntz retired in 1916 and died 1920 in Berlin.

In summary, Zuntz invented several fundamental methods to quantify gas exchange and metabolism under resting conditions and during physical exercise. These methods are in the textbooks of physiology and anaesthesia still today. He must be regarded a one of the most productive German physiologist who developed a unique style of research in the laboratory and in the field.

References:

1. This article is based on three articles published earlier, mainly:
a) Gunga HC: Leben und Werk des Berliner Physiologen Nathan Zuntz 1847-1920). Abhandlungen zur Geschichte der Medizin und der Naturwissenschaften. 1989; 58: 1-343
b) Gunga HC, Kirsch K: Nathan Zuntz (1847-1920) - A German pioneer in high altitude physiology and aviation medicine, Part I: Biography. Aviation Space and Environmental Medicine 1995; 66: 168-171
c) Gunga HC, Kirsch K: Nathan Zuntz (1847-1920) - A German pioneer in high altitude physiology and aviation medicine, Part II: Scientific work. Aviation Space Environmental Medicine 1995; 66: 172-176

Construction Faults in Anaesthetic Equipment and Ventilators

J. Stoffregen,
Husterstraße Hagen, Hagen, Germany

Errare humanum est – obviously this is true for people designing and making anaesthetic equipment and ventilators. The author offers a report on a number of hazards he has encountered during his working life.

1 ~ an insecure connection between gas supply and circle breathing system
2 ~ a dangerous 3-way tap
3 ~ a projecting oxygen control knob
4 ~ a halothane vaporiser with the filling system on the top
5 ~ confusing connections on an ether bottle
6 ~ absent back-flow valves in flowmeters
7 ~ an adhesive label obscuring the upper part of a CO_2 flowmeter
8 ~ O_2 leakage due to a broken thread on an ether bottle
9 ~ a misplaced warning sign on a halothane vaporiser
10 ~ a wrongly sited ether dropper in a circle system
11 ~ potentially jamming breathing system valves
12 ~ N_2O and O_2 pipeline outlet confusion
13 ~ failure of in-line volumeter due to water condensation
14 ~ mini-repirators jamming during the inspiratory phase etc.

I have personally experienced all these problems and tried to correct or avoid them in subsequent equipment - more or less successfully. Some of these mal-functions will be described; n.b. the „rat" symbol in the illustrations has been used for teaching students.

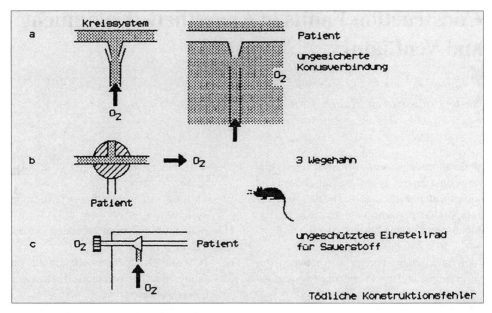

Figure 1: (a) In the left-hand upper quadrant, an unsecured connection between gas supply and the circle system caused the worn rubber tube to detach itself from the metal cone and oxygen flowed into the theatre instead of into the lungs of the paralysed patient. At (b), a potentially lethal 3-way valve, allows semi-closed as well as circle-system usage. In the wrong position the entire gas supply to the patient would be cut off. The unprotected projecting oxygen control knob in (c) was vulnerable to accidental misuse. I convinced the suppliers of the need to add a protective frame.

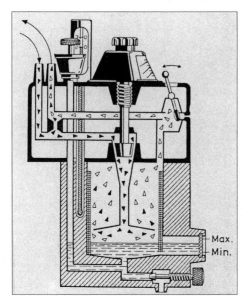

Figure 2 shows a halothane vaporiser with the filling device aperture on the upper surface producing overfilling, which would allow delivery of 15% or more. This actually took place.

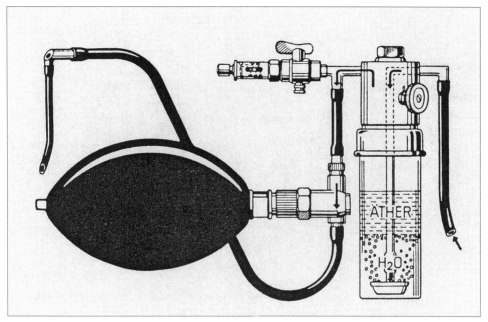

Figures 3: The ether bubble-through bottle had identical cones on the inlet and outlet sides. If wrongly connected, the patient received liquid ether with fatal results.

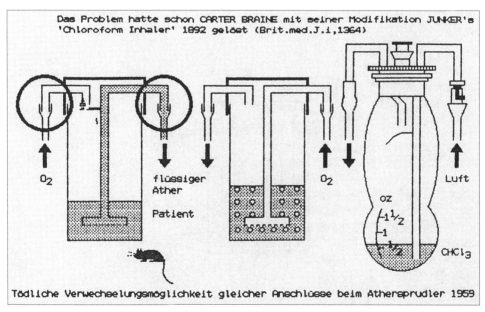

Figure 4: The same problem occurred over a century ago with Junker chloroform bottles for which Carter Braine produced a modification with differing inlet and outlet connections. He wrote that "Changing the tube is impossible as one (inlet) has a bayonet catch, the other (outlet) being plain". [Carter Braine. A safety Junker inhaler. British Medical Journal 1892; 1, 1364.]

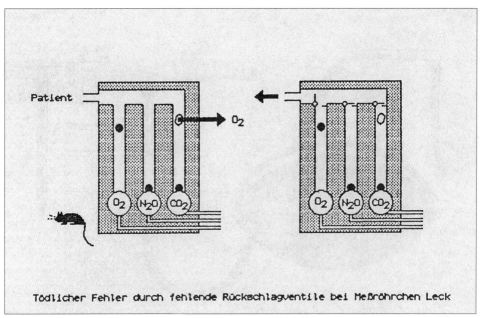

Figure 5: shows the result of omitting the back-flow valve in a flowmeter block. In this case the patient died because of unrepaired damage to an unused CO_2 flowmeter. The oxygen supply passed into the theatre atmosphere.

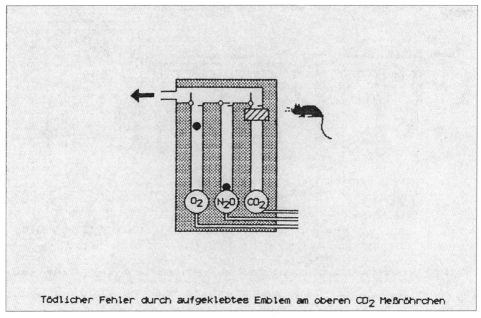

Figure 6: A firm's negligence is shown in Figure 6; an adhesive label was stuck over the upper part of the CO_2 flowmeter; the flow was fully on but was concealed from the anaesthetist's view.

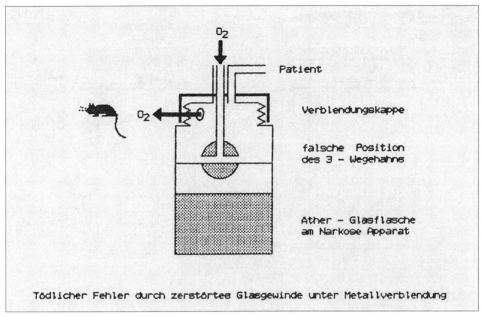

Figure 7: The result of an un-noticed breakage of the glass thread of an ether bottle is shown. Concealed by the metal cover it was undetectable during use and allowed the oxygen flow to pass out into the theatre. I did not detect the fault, but when the patient became cyanosed I changed the machine and the colour returned to normal. Only later we discovered the damage when the apparatus was dismantled.

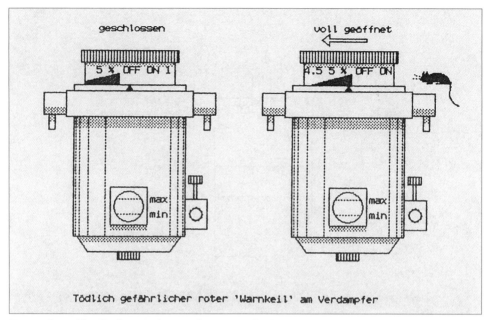

Figures 8a and b: The danger of a wrongly positioned red warning sign on a halothane vaporiser output concentration control is shown in Figures 8a and b. Even when closed the position of the triangle is misplaced by only 20mm.

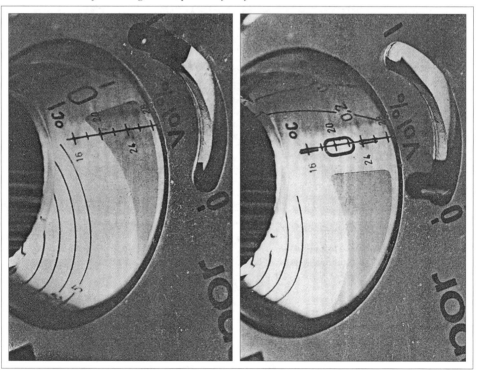

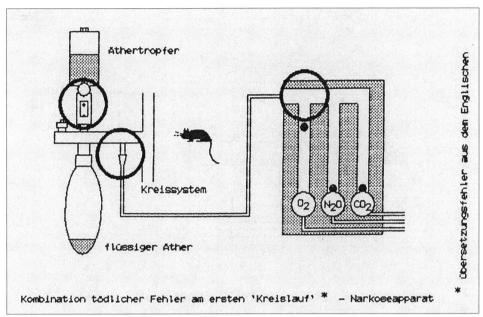

Figure 9: Here an example of unwise design in an early post-war machine is shown. On the left an ether drop-bottle, which should only be used in a non-rebreathing sysytem, may discharge into the circle-system. Rebreathing of lethal ether concentrations could occur after 10 - 15 minutes. For early detection, we used to feel the bottom of the rubber bag; when the inside became slippery we quickly closed off the dropper. The right-hand side of the illustration shows the omission of back-flow valves, while the circle on the left indicates an unbelievably careless connection between the oxygen supply and the circle -system.

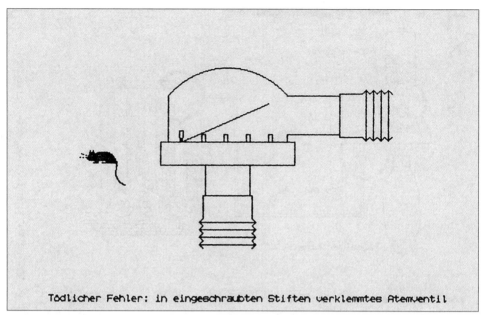

Figures 10 shows how badly placed screws could cause a breathing valve to jam open, resulting in dangerous increases in CO_2 rebreathing.

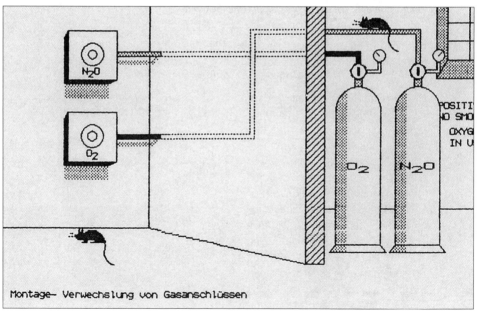

Figure11 illustrates the misconnection of gas terminals in a newly commissioned theatre.

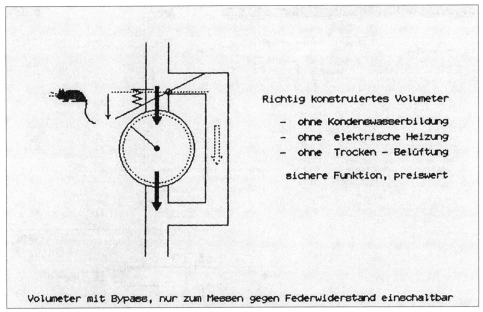

Figures 12a indicates the result of putting a volumeter on-line in a rebreathing system rather than in a by-pass. Water condensation caused mal-functioning. The correct technique is illustrated in Figure 12b.

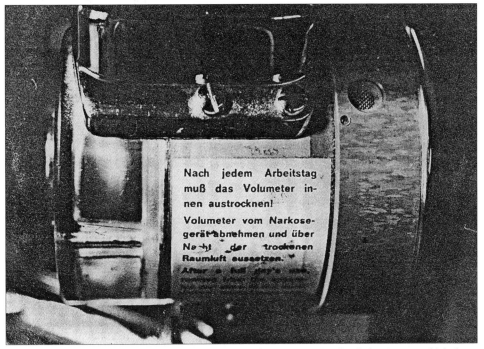

Figure 12b: To read the volumeter it should be activated against a spring-loaded resistance which closes automatically at the end of the procedure.

469

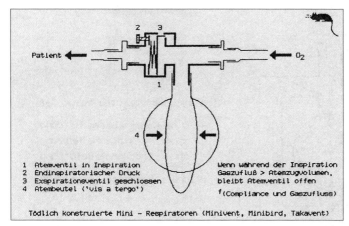

Fig. 13a

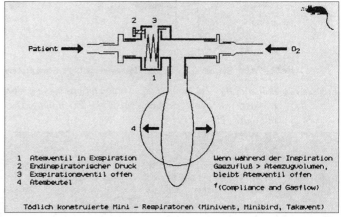

Fig. 13b

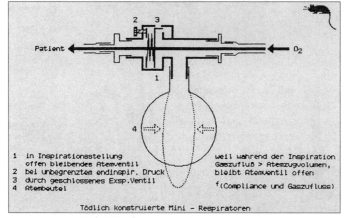

Fig. 13c

Figures 13 a,b,c: These figures show the results of construction faults in Minirespirators. Under given circumstances, eg. when the fresh gas flow is greater than the tidal volume, the inspiratory valve remains open, the lungs may become hyperinflated and the heart finally stops.

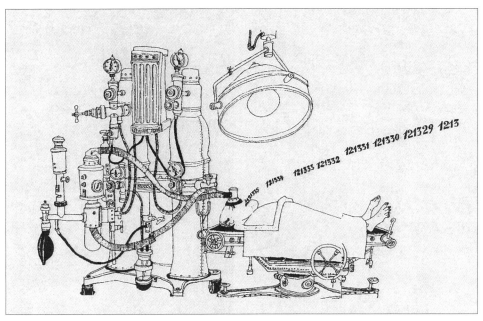

Figures 14:
A cartoon making fun of the first German-made circle system machine.

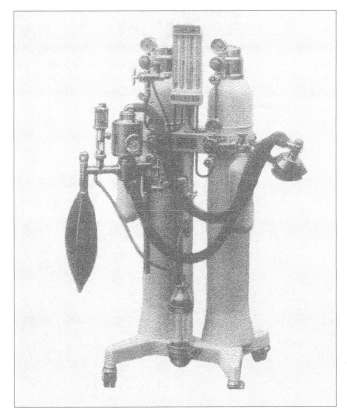

Figure 15:
A picture of the original Model F of the Dräger-Company, Lübeck, - note the ether drop-bottle.

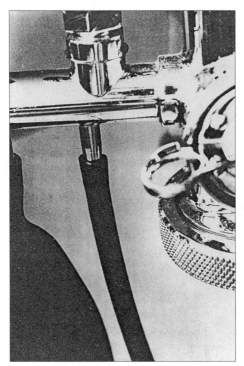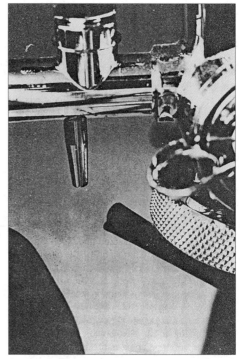

Figure 16: Worn-out by prolonged use, the rubber tubing in Figure 16 became detached frrom the metal cone and oxygen passed into the theatre rather than into the patient's lungs. You may think that these are once upon a time stories from long ago, but I assure you that each of the faults in the equipment discussed above has killed patients. In England during the war there was a famous poster: "Careless talk costs lives". On anaesthetic machines it could be said that careless construction cost lives!

Answers to Opponents of Obstetric Anaesthesia 1847-50

J. R. Maltby[1] and Ch. K. Davies[2]
[1]Foothills Hospital and [2]Rockyview Hospital, Calgary, Canada

The attitude to pain in the mid 19th century was quite different from today's attitude in highly sophisticated western medicine.[1] The demonstration by Morton in 1846 that ether could abolish the pain of surgery and by Simpson in 1847 that it could do the same for labour pains and operative obstetrics posed a new dilemma. It was now possible to abolish or prevent pain, but was it right to do so? Attempts were made to distinguish between physiological and pathological pain while others considered some pain to be ennobling and other types to be merely destructive. By the time Simpson introduced ether, and subsequently chloroform, into obstetric practice he was Professor of Midwifery in Edinburgh and internationally renowned. He was also a champion of causes in which he believed and he never flinched from controversy.[2,3]

Medical Objections

Incautious and injudicious use

Concern was expressed that the use of ether and chloroform was not always certain to be successful or safe. Over-enthusiasm for the wonders of pain relief might bring these agents into disrepute and thus consign them to oblivion.[4] Simpson responded to the safety aspect of ether by publishing mortality data on 302 amputations in 49 hospitals.[5] Mortality was 23% in etherized patients, 29-57% without anaesthetic. He then collected maternal morbidity and mortality data on 800 cases from his own and other midwifery practices in Edinburgh and from colleagues in the British Isles and Europe.[6] Maternal morbidity and mortality were due to the common causes of ruptured uterus, haemorrhage and puerperal fever. No deaths were attributed by any of his correspondents to ether or chloroform. Fearmongers suggested that ether and chloroform would cause hydrocephalus, epilepsy and idiocy. No such cases were reported although the last two conditions might not have been diagnosed within a few months of birth.

Abolition of uterine contractions

Concerns were also expressed that labour would not progress if ether and chloroform abolished uterine contractions as well as the pain they caused. However, Baron Dubois of the Academy of Medicine in Paris wrote that ether suspended the physiological pains of labour without abolishing uterine or abdominal muscle contractions, and was not unfavourable to the life or health of infants.[7]

Pain as a guide to manipulations

There were fewer objections to pain relief for operative interventions than for the physiological pains of labour. Nevertheless Meigs of Philadelphia contended that the patient's pain was an invaluable guide to correct application of forceps. He could not justify „casting away my safest and most trustworthy diagnosis, for the questionable equivalent of ten minutes exemption from a pain."[8] Simpson did not mince words in his response, "I think every man who ventures to use the forceps in any midwifery case, ought to know the anatomy of the parts implicated, a 1000 fold better than you here presuppose."[9]

Moral Objections

These were not religious objections per se although they may have been made by individuals with strong religious views. Meigs was among those who equated etherization with drunkenness,[10] whereas Channing in Boston made a clear distinction between the beneficial medicinal use of ether and chloroform and their popular social use. He considered the latter not only immoral and injurious but dangerous to the point of causing death.[11] A further objection was the possibility of the woman becoming sexual aroused during etherization. This caused one writer to state that, "having feelings of such kind excited and manifested in outward uncontrolled actions, would be more shocking even to anticipate, than the endurance of the last extremity of physical pain."[12] The equating of beneficial medical management with social frivolity was clearly inappropriate, whereas the possibility of confusion and sexual arousal had the potential to be embarrassing and legally dangerous for the unchaperoned male practitioner.

Religious Objections

The story of God's punishment for Eve, and thus of all women, for eating from the tree of life in the Garden of Eden appears in Genesis iii, 16: "Unto the woman He said, I will greatly multiply thy sorrow and thy conception; in sorrow shalt thou bring forth children..." (King James version of the Bible, 1611). Although this was the translation most commonly used by Protestants in Britain, some patients and medical men interpreted the Hebrew word translated 'sorrow' as pain. Simpson claimed that he often heard patients and others strongly object to the use of anaesthesia in labour on the ground that this was contrary to the express commands of Scripture and that some doctors, for the same reason, refused to relieve their patients from the agonies of childbirth.[3]

Edinburgh, Scotland

It appears that Simpson wrote his pamphlet *Answer to the Religious Objections Advanced Against the Employment of Anaesthetic Agents in Midwifery and Surgery*[3] in response to these individuals, rather than to any formal ecclesiastical movement or denomination of the church. Simpson was not anti-religious. He was an elder in the Free Church of Scotland and was concerned that women were suffering because of this misinterpretation of the Bible. He pointed out that the Hebrew word translated as 'sorrow' meant 'labour' or 'toil' and not 'pain', for which a completely different Hebrew word was used in other parts of the Old Testament. Furthermore, if the supposed punishment of pain during childbirth was to be accepted by women, the punishment of 'tilling the field by the sweat of their faces' must be accepted by men (Genesis iii, 17-19). Simpson quoted Calvin who had observed that God himself caused Adam to sink into a deep sleep so that removal of one of his ribs to create Eve would not cause pain.

The lack of objection from organised religion is suggested by the fact that when Dr. Thomas Chalmers, the Scottish theologian, was asked by Professor Miller, a friend of Simpson's, to write the theological part of an article on etherization for publication in the North British Review in May 1947, Chalmers replied that he did not see any theological aspect. Miller explained that some people were urging objections against the use of ether in midwifery because this improperly enabled women to avoid the primeval curse. Chalmers then added that, if some 'small theologians' really took such an improper view of the subject, he would certainly advise Mr. Miller not to 'heed them' in his article. Chalmers' could not accept the extraordinary idea that, under Christian dispensation, the God of Mercy should wish for and delight in the sacrifice of women's screams and sufferings in childbirth. Simpson suggested that Chalmers may have thought, like some other clergyman, that if God had "beneficently vouchsafed to us a means of mitigating the agonies of childbirth," it was also God's intention that we should employ these means. Simpson echoed this last comment on the title page of his pamphlet by quoting from the New Testament, James iv, 17: "Therefore to him that knoweth to do good and doeth it not, to Him it is Sin."

This lack of organised religious opposition or widespread individual opposition has led one author to conclude that there was never any formal conflict between religion and medicine, and that the whole episode was no more than artefact and extrapolation in the writing of this part of anaesthetic history.[13] He may be correct that Simpson's pamphlet was written to forestall organised objections that did not arise, and that later writers misinterpreted the pamphlet as evidence of opposition that did not occur or that rapidly evaporated. Nevertheless, a book by Bainbrigge, a Liverpool surgeon, in 1848[14] and a series of three articles by De Sola, Lecturer in Hebrew in Montreal in 1850[15] suggest that concerns may have been more widespread.

Liverpool, England

Bainbrigge's experience in Liverpool confirms Simpson's experience that objections arose mainly in the minds of women themselves on religious grounds, whereas his professional colleagues hesitated or opposed anaesthesia in childbirth because of the supposed danger. He used many of Simpson's arguments, quoting the parable of the Good Samaritan and arguing that we cannot preach the relief of one type of suffering and not another. He claimed that most medical men who objected to the administration of chloroform had little practical experience of its effects. He argued that it would be wrong to abandon its use from vague ideas of danger, but that its use should be regulated with judgement and caution.

Montreal, Canada

The series of articles by the Rev. Abraham De Sola, Lecturer on Hebrew Language and Literature at the University of McGill College, Montreal agreed with Simpson that the word translated 'sorrow' in Genesis iii, 16 meant physical labour, toil or effort without any reference to pain. He used similar arguments to those of Bainbrigge and Simpson and believed that the use of anaesthetics in labour was good and proper. He could not understand the denunciations against women unless the same denunciations were made against men, the ground and the serpent. According to the literal impact of v.17-19, those who ate the products of the earth without experiencing 'sorrow' in procuring them, and those who used cattle to plough, were transgressors of the word of Scripture. He supported "many logical and convincing arguments in refutation of the actual and imaginary objections of the literalists" and agreed with those who believed" that the whole science and whole art and practice of midwifery is . . . one continuous effort to mitigate and remove the effects of that curse."

Conclusion

The objections to the use of ether and chloroform following their introduction into midwifery practice were, by and large, overcome by convincing arguments from Simpson himself and others. The beliefs of objectors, though conscientiously held, appear to have been built on false premises that led to erroneous conclusions. Abolition of pain during labour and delivery did not prove to be as dangerous as feared by the more conservative members of the medical profession. Indeed, it encouraged the use of instrumental deliveries in difficult cases and led to other advances in obstetric practice. In answer to the moralists, the distinction had to be made between legitimate medical use of anaesthetics and the social frivolity of inhaling such agents. The religious objections appear to have been the beliefs of individual members of the public, mostly women, and individual members of the medical profession. Simpson's forceful personality and his willingness to fight for what he believed to be right were largely responsible for winning the battle for women's rights to painless childbirth. His strong humanitarian arguments prevailed and patients demanded anaesthesia. The objections are also believed to have been finally laid to rest when Queen Victoria, temporal head of the Church of England, accepted chloroform from John Snow for the birth of her seventh child, Prince Leopold in 1853,[12] although it seems likely that, by then, most of the doubters were convinced of its value and acceptability.

References:

[1] Caton D: "The poem in the pain." The social significance of pain in western civilization. Anesthesiology 1994; 81: 1044-1052

[2] Shepherd JA: Simpson and Syme of Edinburgh. Edinburgh: Livingstone, 1969

[3] Simpson JY: Answer to the Religious Objections Advanced Against the Employment of Anaesthetic Agents in Midwifery and Surgery. Edinburgh: Sutherland and Knox, 1847

[4] Wintle FT: Etherization. Lancet 1847; i: 162-163

[5] Simpson JY: Etherization in surgery, Part 2. Does it increase or decrease the mortality attendant upon surgical operations? Monthly Journal of Medical Sciences 1847-8; 8: 697-710

[6] Simpson JY: Anaesthetic midwifery. Report on its early history and progress. Edinburgh: Sutherland and Knox, 1848

[7] Dubois P (Reported by Campbell C): On the inhalation of ether applied to cases of midwifery. Lancet 1847; 1: 246-249

[8] Meigs CD: Letter to Prof. J.Y. Simpson. Dated 18th February 1848. In: Meigs CD. Obstetrics

[9] Simpson JY: The propriety and morality of using anaesthetics in instrumental and natural parturition. Association Medical Journal 1853; 582-589

[10] Meigs CD: Obstetrics: the Science and the Art. 4th ed. Philadelphia: Blanchard and Lea, 1863: 353

[11] Channing W: A Treatise on Etherization in Childbirth. Boston: Ticknor 1848: 153

[12] Smith WT: The inhalation of ether in obstetric practice. Lancet 1847; i: 321-323

[13] Farr AD: Early opposition to obstetric anaesthesia. Anaesthesia 1980; 35: 896-907

[14] Bainbrigge WH: Remarks on Chloroform in Alleviating Human Suffering Addressed Particularly to the Female Sex. London: Highley, 1848

[15] De Sola A: Critical examination of Genesis III, 16, having reference to the employment of anaesthetics in cases of labour. British American Journal of Medical and Physical Science 1850; 5: 227-9, 259-62, 290-293

[16] Ellis RH (Ed): The Case Books of Dr. John Snow. London: Wellcome Institute for the History of Medicine, 1994: 271

Anaesthesia in Gynaecology and Obstetrics from the Turn of the Century until 1935 – Documents of the Women's Hospital of Upper Austria

H. Eiblmayr,
Department of Anaesthesiology, Landesfrauenklinik OÖ, Linz, Austria

Searching for data concerning the historical development of anaesthesia in obstetrics and gynaecology, I read about five thousand hospital reports to write this paper, as there are no known statistical reports! "The present-day Womens Hospital of Upper Austria in Linz" was constituted as a "Hospital for Women in Labour and Foundlings" (Fig. 1) in "Pruners foundation" in

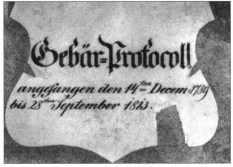

Fig. 2

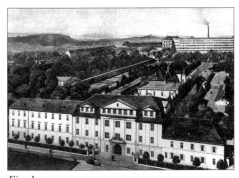

Fig. 1

1789 and was then turned into a social institution for the poor or anonymous wealthy pregnant women. There was a medical high school, a "Lyceum" and the education in obstetrics was served at this hospital.

At times poorly caused by war and famine it was necessary to find a larger place to meet the growing social and medical problems and the new institution was born out of an expansion of the original facilities. (Fig. 2, 3) ... despite the dreadful obstetric problems, testified in the hospital reports, from 1789 onwards, there were no known analgetic concepts until 1890 except an alcoholic solution of opium. Mortality of mothers ranged between 20 and 25 % due to puerperal sepsis, severe haemorrhage, rheumatic fever and cardiac failure or other infectious diseases meningitis, tuberculosis or typhoid fever. Around mid 19th century, only 10 % of the newborns delivered at the hospital, or the foundlings were registered still being alive a year later!

In 1890 Prof. Dr. Ludwig Piskacek was appointed director of the "Hospital for Women in Labour" and of the "Educational Establishment for Midwives" in Linz. Born on the 16th of November 1854 in Karcsag, Hungary and having completed medical education at the University of Vienna – (the director at that time being Prof. Dr. Eduard Albert) – he obtained a diploma in surgery in 1884; he commenced studies and work at the Clinic for Obstetrics and Gynaecology at the University (the director being Prof. Dr. Joseph Spaeth) organizing for and achieving precise asepsis there. As he had previously seen so many women, dying from septic

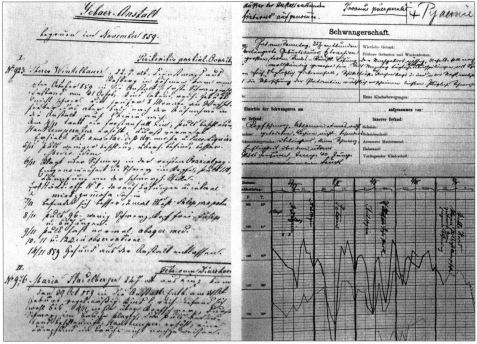

Fig. 3

infections, he was renown as a campaigner for antisepsis in obstetrics and surgery during his whole lifetime.

Prof. Dr. Piskacek (Fig. 4) resided in Linz between 1890 and 1901. Among various innovations in his life he managed to establish a peculiar operating theatre and gas and water supply in the hospital. In 1890, 304 women in labour were registered in the hospital. (Fig. 5) Ten years later, 486 obstetric and 89 gynaecology patients attended the hospital. Preoperative disinfection was performed by bathing and wrapping the patient in sterile clothes the night before the operation, followed by thorough iodoform and mercury sublimate disinfection of the operating site and the surgeon's hands the next day. For anaesthesia the "Billroth - mixture" (Fig. 6) - an alcoholic solution of ether and chloroform or chloroform was administered for laparatomy; ether only was

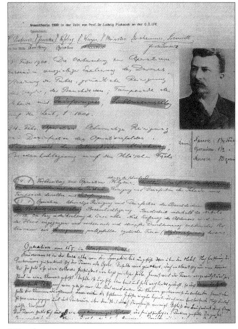

Fig. 4

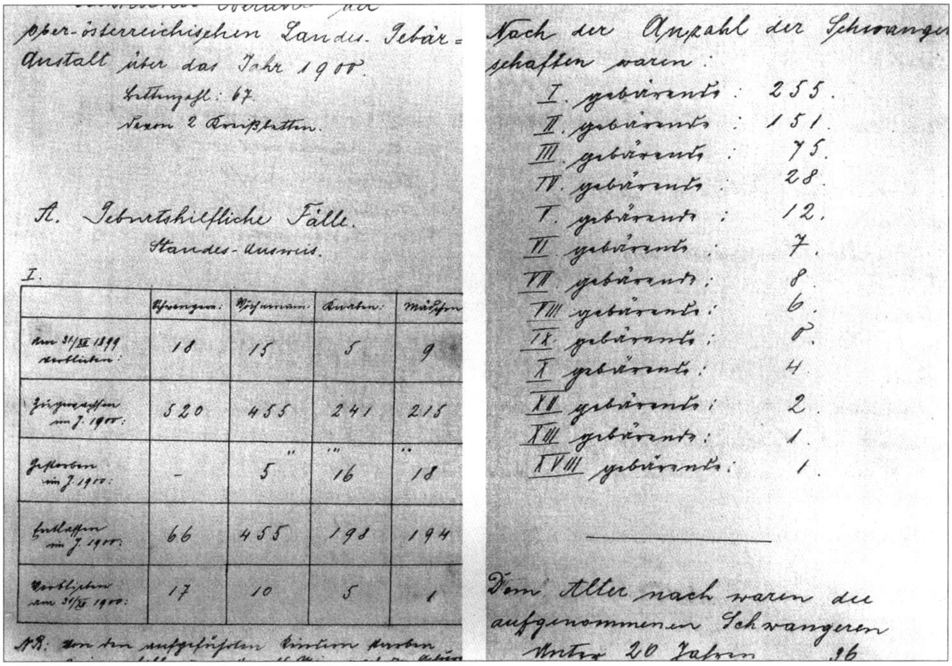

ober-österreichischen Landes-Gebär-Anstalt über das Jahr 1900.
Bettenzahl: 67.
davon 2 Kreißbetten.

A. Geburtshilfliche Fälle.
Standes-Ausweis.

I.

	Schwangere	Wöchnerinnen	Knaben	Mädchen
Am 31/XII 1899 verblieben:	18	15	5	9
Zugewachsen im J. 1900:	520	455	241	215
Gestorben im J. 1900:	-	5	16	18
Entlassen im J. 1900:	66	455	198	194
Verblieben am 31/XII 1900:	17	10	5	1

NB: Von den aufgeführten Kindern starben ...

Nach der Anzahl der Schwangerschaften waren:
I. gebärende: 255.
II. gebärende: 151.
III. gebärende: 75.
IV. gebärende: 28.
V. gebärende: 12.
VI. gebärende: 7.
VII. gebärende: 8.
VIII. gebärende: 6.
IX. gebärende: 0.
X. gebärende: 4.
XII. gebärende: 2.
XIII. gebärende: 1.
XVIII. gebärende: 1.

Dem Alter nach waren die aufgenommenen Schwangeren
unter 20 Jahren 96

Fig. 5

Anaesthesia 1890 - 1910

...... in gynaecology:

"Billroth - mixture" ... alcoholic solution of ether and chloroform

or **Chloroform** used at laparotomy

Ether for short interventions, e.g. curettage

...... in obstetrics:

Ether administered for

...fetal evisceration and craniotomy on impending uterine rupture

...intrauterine shifting of the prolapsed umbilical cord prior to vaginal delivery

...turning the malpositioned fetus to a footling presentation in a persistent oblique position

...alleviation of pain and suffering of the dying mother following uterine rupture

Chloroform and **Morphia treatment** for eclamptic convulsions

mortality rate: 1890: mothers 6% newborns?

1900 - 1910: mothers 1,64% newborns 8%

Fig. 6

used for short interventions in gynaecology.

In obstetrics ether was used mainly, besides chloroform, to terminate eclamptic convulsions; the therapy in eclampsia included morphine and chloralhydrate-enemas and lukewarm to warm baths (Fig.7). Management in obstetrics sometimes appears to be cruel, especially if the baby has to die in order to save the mother's life. Mortality rate changed from 1890 to 1910: 1890 8% of the mothers died during labour due to uterine rupture caused by an uncommon birth malformation and rachitic pelvic deformity, from bleeding disorders and uterine atony or from a septic infection during labour; the statistical data concerning newborns is unknown. In 1910 the mortality rate could be reduced to 1,64 % for the mothers and came to 8 % for the newborns.

Prof. Dr. Piskacek was nominated the new director of the Clinic for Gynaecology and Obstetrics in Vienna in 1901. His successor at the womens hospital in Linz was Prof. Dr. Heinrich Schmit (Fig. 8). Born on the 2nd of July 1866 in St. Poelten, Lower Austria, he studied medicine in Vienna, was educated as a surgeon at the clinic of Prof. Dr. Albert and remained at the University of Vienna for 6 years as a gynaecologist under Prof. Dr. Schauta.

Soon after his moving to Linz he introduced many innovations. Gynaecology was separated from Obstetrics - a modern wing with high ceilings and bright rooms for the patients was built within the following two years. In 1921 two new stories were added to the central building and a balcony was placed on top of one wing to be used for solar-therapy by mothers and babies.

Nuns attended to the gynaecological patients, worked in the kitchen, the garden and the chapel, while midwives took care of the women in labour.

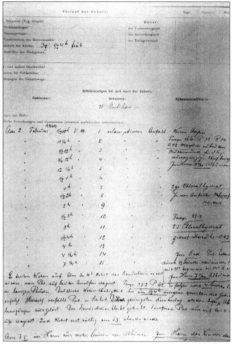

Fig. 7

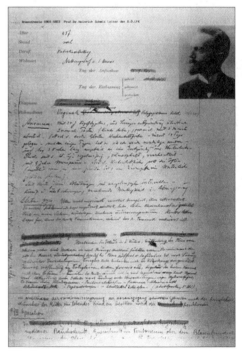

Fig. 8

The number of patients increased as the growing number of social assurances encouraged them to enter a hospital, and affluent patients confided more in modern medicine at a hospital than in private nursing. The surgical program in gynaecology was extended to cancer management, also hysterectomy for myomatous uterus or cystic tumours.

Obstetrics expanded due to the use of anaesthesia for forceps delivery to save the life of the mother in cases of malpositioning; many of the babies still died. Complications - like a rupture of the uterus occurred and often led to hysterectomy. Caesarean section is mentioned as Sectio classica or Sectio vaginalis Duerksen.

What was new in Anaesthesia? (Fig. 9)
Pre-medication was introduced
"Schleich-Narkose" replaced the
"Billroth-mixture"

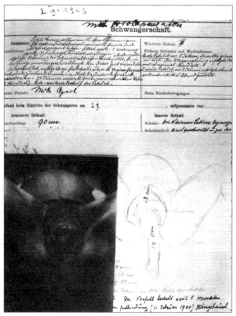

Fig. 10a

```
Anaesthesia 1910 - 1927

Premedication: Scopolamin and Morphine s.c.
"Schleich - Narkose"
"Schimmelbusch - mask"
Induction of anaesthesia with Pernocton
Tropacocain 2% for lumbar anaesthesia
Venesection for phlebotomy and i.v. infusion of saline

..... news in gynaecology and obstetrics:
extended cancer surgery
increasing number of forceps deliveries and caesarean section
mortality rate: mothers 1,6%    newborns 8-10%
```

Fig. 9

Incision of the uterine orifice before forceps delivery, the rate of caesarean section reached 7,8 %, one being performed on a dying mother, suffering from terminal cancer.

What was new in anaesthesiology? (Fig.13)
A new kind of pre-medication was applied. Evipan, a new barbiturate was introduced.

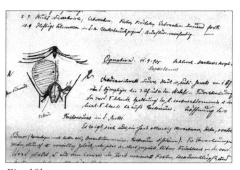

Fig. 10b

Fig. 11

481

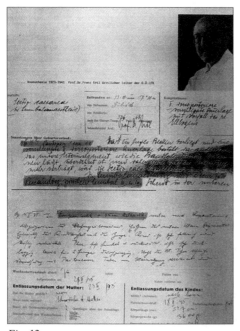

Fig. 12

Ether was applied by dripping technique or the Ombrédanne apparatus. (Fig. 14). An increasing number of lumbar anaesthesia, besides local infiltration anaesthesia and mesenteric or splanchnic blockade - was widely applied for major surgery. Intravenous saline was regularly administered during surgery. Since 1923 blood pressure (measured by use of Riva-Rocci apparatus) was noted on the chart, as well as pulse, respiration rate and temperature. Until 1927 anaesthesia was administered by physicians only; when the hospital lacked physicians, nurses dripped the ether. Between 1935 and the first years after the World War II, we can find minor development in anaesthesia in our hospital only.

```
Anaesthesia 1927 - 1935

Premedication: Pantopon s.c., Scopolamin

Anaesthesia induction: Evipan

"Ombredanne" anaesthesia apparatus

increasing number of lumbar anaesthesia with Percain 0,5%

local infiltration, mesenteric and splanchnic anaesthesia with Novocain

i.v. infusions during surgery

blood pressure (measurement began in 1923 by the use of "Riva-Rocci" apparatus)
was noted as well as pulse and respiration rate and temperature on the chart

.... news in gynaecology:

increasing carcinoma surgery (up to 10% of the total operations in one year!)

x-ray therapy in cancer since 1932

.... news in obstetrics:

caesarean section rate 6,5 - 7,8%

mortality rate: mothers 0,7%  newborns 4-5%
```

Fig. 13

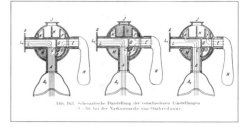

Fig. 14

References:

Oberoesterreichisches Landesarchiv:
   HS Nr. 67: Gebaerprotokolle 14. Dez. 1789 -28. Sept. 1813
   HS Nr. 68 - 74: Gebaerprotokolle 1791 -1848
   HS Nr. 222: Protokoll über die in das geburtshilfliche Ambulatorium aufgenommenen Gebrenden 1879-1890

   HS Nr. 310 - 346: Protokolle der Frauenklinik 1900-1934

Guggenberger Ed, Piskacek, L : Univ. Prof. Dr. Heinrich, Univ. Prof. Dr. Franz Ertl - biographic dates in: Obersterreichische Ärztechronik 1962

Pain relief for childbirth in 1930s Britain

A. S. Williams
Institut of Education, University of London, UK

At the end of the 20th century, women in Britain generally expect to be offered pain relief for childbirth. But in the late 1920s, chloroform and twilight sleep were the only methods available, and only to those women who could afford the care of a doctor. This situation was considered intolerable by a voluntary organisation called the National Birthday Trust Fund (NBTF), which conducted a vigorous campaign in the 1930s to bring pain relief in labour to mothers who were poor. The nature of this pioneering work and its contribution to the development of obstetric anaesthesia is the subject of this paper. Such a focus on a lay organisation provides an unusual approach to the history of anaesthesia, which tends to limit its subject to the work of the service provider and medical institutions.

The NBTF was set up in 1928 as a way of helping to reduce the high rate of maternal mortality.[1] At that time, nearly one in 200 women in England and Wales were losing their lives in childbirth and the rate was steadily rising.[2] The founder of the Trust was Ina, Lady George Cholmondeley, who was assisted by the wealthy and powerful Marchioness of Londonderry; the chief leaders of the organisation in the 1930s were Lucy Baldwin, wife of the Conservative Prime Minister, and Lady Rhys Williams. Several vast committees were set up, boasting prominent members of the social and political elite, most of whom were women. The organisation aimed 'to secure for the poorer mother the same relief from suffering as is invariably offered to her well-to-do sister'[3] – and since poor mothers gave birth at home under the care of a midwife, the priority of the Trust was the improvement of midwifery care. It therefore created the Joint Council of Midwifery to influence the development of maternity policy relating to midwives and established a national headquarters for midwives in London. It also set up the first human milk bank in Britain and organised a supplementary feeding programme for impoverished pregnant women. The work with the highest profile, however, was the crusade to bring pain relief to mothers in childbirth, which was led with passionate commitment by Lucy Baldwin.

Attitudes to pain relief in labour

Over the centuries in Western culture, the agony of childbirth has been regarded as woman's punishment for her natural sinfulness and has been sanctioned by the Bible: 'In sorrow,' states Genesis, 'thou shalt bring forth children.'[4] The common view, observed the London Count Council (LCC) Public Health Committee in 1933, was that a woman was doing 'something morally wrong' in evading the pain of labour.[5] 'How can a woman have that motherly affection for her offspring,' wrote Mr G. to the Minister of Health, 'if she bares [sic] it without any pain?'[6] Mrs Baldwin had contempt for men with such opinions. 'When a man shewing prejudice talks to me on this subject,' she said briskly, 'I have very great difficulty in preventing myself from telling him what I think.' She then added, 'And it is rather a tremendous thing if a man once hears what a woman thinks of him, because he so rarely does.'[7]

The problem of public opinion was compounded by ignorance since, as one mother wrote to the Birthday Trust in 1938, 'the mothers don't know such a thing [pain relief] exists'.[8] This was particularly true of poor mothers: the LCC Public Health Committee reported that 'Anaesthesia in labour is still outside the experience of the class of women coming into municipal hospitals.'[9] Spreading information about the possibility of pain relief, advised Louis Rivett, an obstetrician who was involved with the work of the NBTF, had to be done carefully. 'We shall have to go slowly,' he warned in 1930, 'as in a conservative country like this it must take some time to get everyone used to such an innovation.'[10]

Because childbirth was a shared experience of women that discounted social rank, pain relief was identified by some feminists as linked to the struggle for women's suffrage. 'In Finland, that little progressive nation which was the first in Europe to give the franchise to women,' commented Mrs Baldwin, 'they always give anaesthetics to women in childbirth.'[11] A similar connection was made in the USA in 1910-20 by the National Twilight Sleep Association, which regarded the availability of analgesia as a fundamental right and was led by suffragists.[12] Virginia Woolf argued in Three Guineas that if rich women were as common as rich men, 'You could provide every mother with chloroform when her child is born.'[13]

The NBTF wanted to make analgesia available to all women, 'regardless of income'.[14] Poor women were even more likely to suffer severe pain than their wealthier sisters, as a result of pelvic disorder caused by inadequate nutrition in childhood.[15] However, the LCC's Public Health Committee found that there was some suspicion among working class women about the idea of pain relief;[16] it attributed this to the fact that anaesthesia in labour was 'associated with obstetrical disasters. The suggestion of its use arouses a fear that the doctor anticipates an abnormal labour.'[17] For this reason, reported a District Nurse, 'they all dread chloroform and beg me not to call the doctor in.'[18] In any case, the lives of working class women -- short of money and food for their families and without running water -- were so difficult and exhausting in this period, that relief of pain in labour was not likely to have been a priority.

However, a number of letters sent to the Trust reveal that some poor women were desperate for help. 'I have had to have all my children in the horrible pangs of childbirth,' complained a 'Mother in York' to the Trust, 'because I never have had money, not even to pay for a doctor.' Pregnant again, she felt that 'after what I have gone through year after year I cannot go through with it. My nerves are terrible.' A woman expecting her third baby lay awake at night dreading the delivery: 'I can of course only afford a Midwife. She is very good, and very kind and very efficient, but oh for the knowledge that the last hellish pains could be lost in an anaesthetic.' Yet another woman begged for £2 to pay a doctor's bill so that she could have some pain relief: 'I am a coward and cannot sleep at night,' she explained, 'for thinking of the time to come.'[19] A mother of seven children wrote to Mrs Baldwin: 'I am looking forward with dread to another confinement next month.... I'm sure God will bless your efforts to bring this merciful thing [of chloroform] nearer to poor creatures. Then childbirth will not be dreaded nearly so much.'[20]

Chloroform capsules – 'Brisettes' and 'Zombs'

Since most British women delivered their babies at home under the care of a midwife, promoting the use of analgesia in hospitals would make little difference to the majority of mothers. The only way forward, realised the Birthday Trust, was to develop a method of relief that was suitable for use by midwives in the home environment. Dame Janet Campbell, Senior Medical Officer in the Department of Maternal and Child Welfare at the Ministry of Health, fully approved of this plan. Not only was she concerned about the suffering of mothers in labour, but she also believed that putting analgesia into the hands of midwives would lower the rate of maternal death. She explained that because the death rate of mothers was nearly 3 per 1,000 higher for doctors' cases than for midwives' cases, as a result of their readiness to intervene with forceps, it was important for midwives to be able to offer the services women wanted. She believed that lower middle class women, who suffered most from unnecessary forceps, only chose a doctor's attendance because he could give them chloroform.[21]

The Trust's first initiative was the development of crushable chloroform capsules, which were thought up by the President of the Midwives Institute.[22] They were intended chiefly for use during the second stage of labour, by a midwife acting alone. In order to overcome the risk of a midwife applying too much chloroform from the drop bottle, Rivett had 20 minims of chloroform put into crushable glass capsules.'[23] The midwife put these capsules into rolls of gauze, crushed one of them, then tucked the gauze roll container into a mask. The patient was allowed to sniff the mask at the onset of a pain, and the dose was sufficient to produce analgesia for seven to ten minutes.[24] The capsules were manufactured under the name of 'Brisettes' and 'Chloroform Zombs' and were tried out in various hospitals. One doctor wrote gratefully to Lady Rhys Williams: 'We still continue to use thousands of capsules without any ill-effects.'[25] At this stage, the Central Midwives Board (CMB) sanctioned the use of capsules by midwives, though only under the direction and personal supervision of a doctor; this ruling was reiterated in the Board's 1934 Annual Report.

There were many enthusiastic verdicts on the performance of the capsules: five of the six patients at Oldswinfond who used capsules 'received wonderful relief and can scarcely find words to express gratification.'[26] Even 'nervous primipara' were grateful.'[27] Often, mothers 'Did not know the baby was born' and did 'not remember birth of child; or the manual removal of placenta and membranes.' But not all health workers were happy. The Medical Officer of Health (MOH) for Greenwich complained they made women wave their arms about and turn over, while a Wolverhampton hospital said that the capsules made women 'very hysterical and difficult to manage.'[28] The MOH for Wareham and Purbeck Rural District Council said that his midwives flatly refused to use the capsules any more.[29] There were technical problems, too. 'The capsules were anything but crushable, observed one doctor,[30] while the Matron at Alexandra Maternity Home reported that some of her capsules had exploded.[31] Another doctor reported 'the horrifying experience of entering a house and finding a capsule between a patient's clenched teeth, only a small part showing. She was, of course, semiconscious.'[32]

As part of its Empire Crusade for Mothers, the Birthday Trust sent capsules to all corners of the empire: to the Gold Coast, Nigeria and Bombay in 1932, Gibraltar and Burma in 1933, Nigeria in 1932, Canada in 1933, and Calcutta in 1935[33]. Some British health workers took the capsules with them when they went abroad, such as nurse working with poor women in India who had watched the use of chloroform capsules in the Rotunda Hospital in Dublin.[34]

In November 1933, the Trust asked the British College of Obstetricians and Gynaecologists (BCOG) to investigate the safety of chloroform capsules and their administration by midwives in the home.[35] The Trust hoped to discover new information that would persuade the CMB to rescind its requirement that midwives should only use capsules under medical supervision. The College agreed to carry out the study, but insisted that it would have to look into other methods of pain relief as well, since chloroform can be dangerous.[36] It developed the following terms of reference: 'to investigate the use of analgesics in labour with special reference to the use of chloroform capsules and the employment of any analgesic by midwives.'[37] Thirty six hospitals attached to teaching schools and the large maternity hospitals throughout England, Wales, Scotland, Northern Ireland and Eire co-operated in the study. It was conducted in institutions, rather than domiciliary practice, on the grounds that results would be recorded more accurately there.[38] Consequently, the very reason for initiating the study -- to investigate analgesia suitable for use by midwives in a home environment -- was neglected.

In all, nearly 10,000 cases were investigated.[39] Almost 4,000 women were given nitrous oxide and air administered with the Minnitt Gas and Air Apparatus, which had been developed in 1933 by Dr R. J. Minnitt, an anaesthetist in the Liverpool hospitals. Five thousand women were given chloroform (2,500 by capsules, 1,500 by the Mennell inhaler, and the rest by the Christie Brown inhaler); and nearly 1,000 women were administered paraldehyde per rectum. There is no record of the basis on which women were allocated the different methods of pain relief.

The BCOG's eventual report in 1936 concluded that chloroform should not be used by midwives acting alone, because immediate and delayed dangers had occurred in the investigation. Paraldehyde per rectum was not recommended, either, on the grounds that it did not provide adequate analgesia at the time of the actual birth. The only method that received full approval was the Minnitt Gas and Air apparatus, which was described as a safe and satisfactory method of producing analgesia for use by midwives, so long as they had been specially trained. It was important 'to press forward the use of the Minnitt Gas and Air apparatus,' argued the report, 'rather than to continue the supply of chloroform capsules.'[40] All interest in chloroform capsules was promptly abandoned and the Trust shifted its allegiance to the Minnitt Gas and Air machine.

Gas and Air

Dr Minnitt's machine developed out of a meeting he attended at the Royal Society of Medicine to discuss the use of nitrous oxide and oxygen for obstetric pain relief.[41] The disadvantages of this seemed clear and the suggestion was made of substituting air for oxygen; this had already been tried in America by McKesson, but it had failed because he had given too high a concentration of the gas. Minnitt resolved to make an attempt himself. He consulted his friend, A. Charles King, a well known medical instrument maker, with whom he produced an apparatus that was used for the first time at the Liverpool Maternity Hospital on 16 October 1933. The concentrations of the Minnitt machine were originally 45 per cent nitrous oxide and 55 per cent air, but this was later altered to 50 per cent of each. The apparatus consisted of a reduced pressure regulator attached to a small rubber bag in a metal drum, with an automatic valve shutting off the flow of gas when the patient did not inhale.[42] Dr Minnitt showed his machine to the Association of Anaesthetists in October 1933, after which a similar machine was made for Wellhouse Hospital, Barnet, where an anaesthetist called John Elam embarked on a study of its use. A paper on the two studies was read to the Liverpool Medical Institute on 22 February 1934.

The Trust supported this early work of Dr Minnitt, after Dr Elam had drawn its attention to the new machine in December 1933,[43] and paid for the method to be tested at the Liverpool Maternity Hospital.[44] While Elam became very friendly with the Trust, Minnitt appears to have kept his distance and Lady Rhys Williams described his letters as 'cryptic'.[45] Following a telephone call in 1934 from the Trust, in which he was urged to consider the suitability of his apparatus for midwives, he said it should not be used in hospitals without trained staff and that it should 'not [sic] be used by midwives acting alone.'[46] Only when he was completely sure of its safety did he advocate its use by midwives.

Immediately after the BCOG report of 1936, the CMB set up a committee to advise midwives on the use of Gas and Air. It recognized the administration of this analgesia as treatment within the province of the midwife, so long as the conditions recommended by the BCOG were met. These conditions were: that the midwife had been properly trained; that the patient had been examined within the month before confinement by a medical practitioner, who had handed the midwife a certificate stating that the mother was in a fit condition to receive Gas and Air; and that an additional person – a state registered midwife, state registered nurse, senior medical student, or pupil midwife – was present.

The need for the presence of a second trained person seriously limited its use, since in many areas it was difficult to find one trained midwife, let alone two. In country districts, observed the <u>News Chronicle</u>, 'it is the exception for a village to have more than one nurse, and when there are two the poorer homes cannot afford to pay a double fee.'[47] In 1938, the CMB asked for the BCOG's opinion on the rescinding of this regulation, but the earlier recommendation was reaffirmed.[48] In 1945, following sustained pressure from organizations like the National Federation of Women's Institutes and the NBTF, the regulation was altered to allow members of St. John or the Red Cross, or similarly qualified people, to be the second person present.[49]

Despite the CMB's restrictions, the Trust embarked on an energetic campaign to distribute Gas and Air machines. The models selected for distribution were the Minnitt-Walton apparatus, made by Messrs. A Charles King, and the Queen Charlotte's Model B, made by the British Oxygen Company (BOC); in 1939, the Autogesia Self-Administered apparatus, made by the Dental Manufacturing Company, was also approved by the Trust.[50] The Queen Charlotte's Apparatus produced by BOC was based on Louis Rivett's 'design of a modification of the Minnitt and Davies Gas and Air machines.'[51] Minnitt would 'not allow his name to be associated with this model',[52] probably out of a sense of loyalty to his friend Charles King, who had used his design to build the first Gas and Air apparatus in 1933. Eventually, however, his name was given to a Gas and Air machine by BOC. In September 1939, BOC took over Messrs Coxeter and Son, which had supplied Charles King with the Minnitt apparatus.[53] Then, in 1943, the BOC produced a new machine based on the Minnitt principle, but with the advantages of the Queen Charlotte's model -- and called it a Minnitt Gas/Air Apparatus.

Machines were sent to hospitals, District Nursing Associations (DNAs) and County Nursing Associations (CNAs), either free or at a nominal cost of five pounds. The manufacturers offered discounts to the Trust[54] and by the mid-1940s, 119 machines had been supplied to hospitals, both voluntary and municipal, and 160 machines had been supplied to 124 DNAs and CNAs.[55] Gas and Air machines were also sent to far flung parts of the world -- to Athens,[56] Hong Kong[57] Calcutta,[58] Mexico[59] Singapore,[60] Honolulu[61] and Colombo.[62]

'We are very proud of the Gas and Air apparatus you gave us,' wrote two midwives in the Rhondda in South Wales,' and hope to do good work with it.'[63] The West Hampstead DNA said it wanted to 'give our patients the benefit of this new boon.'[64] However, the machines could not always be used. 'Having to send two nurses to these cases certainly restricts its usefulness,' complained the Hampstead DNA. The Kilburn and West Hampstead DNA reported that, 'This year we are facing the difficulty other Associations have in securing the attendance of the second midwife at the time she is needed.'[65] Another obstacle was the heavy weight of the machines. Even when cylinders of nitrous oxide were delivered to a mother's home by BOC, a service provided by BOC throughout the nation for a minimal charge,[66] the midwife still had to carry the actual apparatus.

The training of midwives to administer Gas and Air was regarded as a priority by the Birthday Trust Analgesics Sub-Committee,[67] but opportunities for this were disappointing. British Oxygen reported that it had received 'an increasing number of enquiries from bewildered Midwives and Medical Officers of Health on this subject.'[68] 'Very few hospitals,' observed the Trust in dismay, 'appeared to be holding courses of instruction for outside midwives.'[69] John Elam reported to the Manchester Evening News, 'I have seen gas apparatus provided free of charge by the National Birthday Trust standing in the corner of the labour ward, covered with rust and dust.'[70]

In the middle of 1937, the Birthday Trust sought information from hospitals and Nursing Associations about the kind of Gas and Air training that was available. A few said they held courses, which midwives from outside the hospital were invited to attend[71]; some said they could only offer places on their courses to their own midwives[72]; others had not yet been approved by the CMB as a teaching hospital in the administration of Gas and Air[73]; yet others regretted that the teaching resources and in anaesthetics were already taken by up medical students.[74] There were several reasons for this slow progress. One was simple resistance to the idea of midwives providing pain relief, which led the Honorary Secretary of a Berkshire NA to turn down the Trust's offer of a Minnitt machine.[75] Another reason was the CMB's requirement that two trained people be involved in the administration of Gas and Air – as their nurses were always on their own, said some Nursing Associations, they could not see the point of sending anyone on a course.[76] As a result of all these problems, only 29 out of 188 local authorities had provided their domiciliary midwives with training by 1939.[77]

Opposition by GPs

On the whole, general practitioners (GPs) opposed the idea of midwives using Gas and Air, and the British Medical Association (BMA) passed a Resolution to this effect at its 1939 Annual Meeting. This Resolution had no official bearing on the work of midwives, since the Central Midwives Board, and not the BMA, was their statutory body, but it angered many of those who supported the analgesia campaign. Shortly after the BMA meeting, the Independent MP Eleanor Rathbone referred in Parliament to 'the selfish attitude of a certain portion of the medical profession who expressed their views the other day,'[78] and a letter to the Trust said that it was only because of the 'inarticulacy ... of thousands of working class women', that the strength of the resentment against the 'recent decision of the B.M.A. has not been realised.'[79] The Department of Health for Scotland anticipated similar opposition from Scottish doctors when it considered giving midwives the authority to use Gas and Air. When it wrote in 1937 to the Ministry of

Health asking for information on the practice in England, it was especially interested in finding out 'whether there has been any opposition by the medical profession.'[80]

At this time, argues Frank Honigsbaum, an historian of British medicine, the GP was being squeezed out of midwifery by a pincer movement: pressure from obstetricians trying to consolidate their role as experts and to create a need for women to give birth in hospital; and pressure from midwives, 'who, aided by the revolutionary Minnitt machine and the backing they received from public health officers under the 1936 Midwives Act, took over an ever-increasing share of home confinements.'[81] During the debate that preceded the passing of the Resolution at the 1939 meeting of the BMA, a number of doctors said they 'wanted to stop midwives controlling the midwifery of the country'.[82] The GPs' struggle to maintain a central role in childbirth failed. By the end of the Second World War, only about one out of three GPs still practised midwifery.[83] They succeeded in sabotaging midwives' use of analgesia, however. According to Maternity in Great Britain, the report of the 1946 national birth survey into the economic and social aspects of pregnancy and childbirth, the negative attitude of GPs was 'the deciding factor' in the delay to develop and provide analgesia for childbirth.[84] Honigsbaum agrees with this, stating that doctors managed to prevent such use in any extensive way until after the war.[85]

The end of the decade

Whereas in 1930, only one hospital in Britain (Queen Charlotte's Hospital in London) had given pain relief on a regular basis to mothers in 'normal' labour, by 1936 few voluntary hospitals did not do so; many municipal hospitals, too, including all those under the control of the LCC, had adopted the policy of providing relief to every mother in labour.[86] By 1939, the administration of analgesics by midwives was included in the Ministry of Health Returns made by each local authority.[87] All this represented a major development in the provision of pain relief in labour. But the Birthday Trust's goal of bringing pain relief to all women, regardless of income, was still a distant dream by the end of the Second World War. Just 20 per cent of women delivering at home in 1946 were given any sort of pain relief, and only eight per cent of those attended by midwives, reported Maternity in Great Britain. The most common analgesic was chloroform, which was used in 14 per cent of domiciliary confinements. Only one in five practising midwives was qualified to administer Gas and Air, which was used in 5 per cent of cases. Moreover, the use of Gas and Air was practically limited to England, where 7 per cent received it as compared with only one mother out of 433 women in Wales and none in Scotland.[88]

However, the Birthday Trust had achieved a major success in the shifting of attitudes about pain relief in childbirth. Since the late 1920s, said Lady Baldwin, 'one by one I have seen the old arguments against [pain relief] go down.'[89] Indeed, the 1946 national birth survey found that the most commonly stated reason for dissatisfaction with treatment during labour was the lack of analgesia.[90] In 1946, for the first time, the Women's Cooperative Guild called for pain relief to be made available for normal labour; then, the following year, it demanded that all midwives be trained and equipped to provide this.[91] A building labourer's wife, who delivered her baby at home with the assistance of a midwife, complained that, 'Something should be given. I was tired out before I started. People with plenty of money don't have to suffer pain.'[92] The Mass-Observation report, Britain and her Birth-Rate (1945), quoted one woman as asking, 'Rich people don't suffer, why should we?' Another complained, 'if you have money you can have the best anaesthetics and everything. That's not right is it?'[93] The disparity between rich and poor in the provision of pain relief had not, after all, been removed. A letter to The Lady in 1942 complained that, 'this is not democracy. One of the most cruel class divisions yet remaining in this country is that rich mothers need not suffer in childbirth as though we were still in the Stone Age, while poorer ones far too often do.'[94]

This inequality between rich and poor started to come to an end following the Second World War, as a result of the health service established by the National Health Service (NHS) Act of 1946. The NHS took responsibility for the provision of adequate and safe methods of pain relief to all mothers who required it, although it took some time to develop sufficient resources to deliver a universal service. A remarkable distance had been travelled since the 1930s, when few working class women had expected or demanded any relief from the pain of childbirth. Mrs Baldwin and the Birthday Trust had taken a leading role in a revolution that not only transformed the experience of childbirth, but also narrowed the gulf between the lives and the expectations of poor women and rich women.

References:

[1] A full history of the organisation is given in Women and Childbirth in the Twentieth Century. A history of the National Birthday Trust Fund, 1928-1993 (Sutton, 1997). Initially the charity was called the National Birthday Fund, but changed its name to National Birthday Trust Fund in 1930, when it became a Trust Fund. For the sake of simplicity, it will be referred to as a Trust Fund throughout this paper.

[2] These figures are based on the classification in use from 1911 onwards and do not include associated causes. A. Macfarlane and M. Mugford, Birth Counts (HMSO, 1984), p. 271

[3] 'Safer Motherhood' (n.d.[1936]) [National Birthday Trust Fund archives held by the Contemporary Medical Archives Centre at the Wellcome Institute for the History of Medicine in London (hereafter NBTF)/G4(1)]

[4] Genesis 2:21

[5] Report of LCC Central Public Health Committee (CPHC), October 1933 [NBTF/H1/5]

[6] G. to Bevan, n.d. [1949] [Public Record Office (hereafter PRO)/ MH134/145]

[7] Report of Dinner at Goldsmith's Hall, 8 May 1934 [NBTF/G7/4(1)]

[8] Oatley to 'Lucy Baldwin's Birthday Trust Fund', 19 January 1938 [NBTF/ H3/2/1]

[9] Report of LCC CPHC, October 1933

[10] Rivett to Williams, 21 June 1930 [NBTF/ F2/5/1(1)]

[11] Draft of Mrs Baldwin's speech at the Mansion House, 11 December 1929 [NBTF/ G1/2(2)]

[12] Judith Walzer Leavitt, 'Birthing and Anaesthesia: The Debate over Twilight Sleep', Signs 6, 1 (Autumn 1980), p. 154

13 Virginia Woolf, Three Guineas (1938; rpt. The Hogarth Press, p. 79
14 Suggested draft for Middle Part of Letter to the NFWI [NBTF/ H1/1]
15 Jacques Gelis, History of Childbirth (Polity Press, 1991), p. 152
16 Laetitia Fairfield, 'Anaesthesia in Normal Labour' [c. 1933] [Greater London Record Office (hereafter GLRO)/ Ph/Gen/3/6]. I am grateful to Lara Marks for drawing my attention to this trial.
17 Report of LCC CPHC, October 1933
18 Margery Spring Rice, Working-Class Wives (1939; rpt. Virago, 1989), p. 67
19 Letters received as a result of the press appeal, 1930 [NBTF/ F3/2/2(1)]
20 From 'A Mother in Stockton-on-Tees', 17 June 1931 [NBTF/ F3/2/2(1)]
21 'Suggestions Concerning the Future Policy of the N.B.T.F.' (5 December 1932) [NBTF/F2/5/1(1)]
22 Williams to Manningham-Buller, 18 March 1931 [NBTF/ F2/5/1(1)]
23 L.C. Rivett, 'Chloroform capsules during labour', BMJ (29 October 1933)
24 National Birthday Trust Fund, Maternal Welfare (1936), p. 27
25 Fairfield to Williams, 30 June [1934] [NBTF/ F7/4]
26 Elgood to NBTF, 16 August 1933 [NBTF/ H1/1]
27 Thierens to NBTF, 7 February 1934 [NBTF/ H1/1(1)]
28 Completed forms from Springfield Maternity Home, Greenwich and Wolverhampton on the Effectiveness of the Capsules are contained in file [NBTF/ H1/6(10)]
29 Elgood to NBTF, 16 August 1933 [NBTF/ H1/1]
30 Elder to NBTF, 21 June 1933 [NBTF/H1/1]
31 Mentioned in reply by NBTF to Matron, 4 November 1932 [NBTF/ H1/1]
32 Elder to NBTF, 27 June 1933 [NBTF/ H1/1]
33 Letters to NBTF [NBTF/ H1/1]
34 Ennis to NBTF, n.d. [NBTF/ H1/1]
35 Meeting of NBTF Medical Committee, 13 October 193[3] [NBTF/ H1/1]
36 Fletcher Shaw to Cahn, 19 December 1933 [NBTF/ H4/1/1(1)]
37 Maternal Welfare, pp.27-8
38 BCOG, Investigation into the use of Analgesia suitable for administration by midwives [1936] [NBTF/ H4/1/1(1)]
39 For further details of this study see minutes of meetings of BCOG Analgesics Sub-Committee [Royal College of Obstetricians and Gynaecologists (hereafter RCOG)/T4]
40 Investigation into the Use of Analgesia
41 For a discussion of this, see D. J. Wilkinson, 'Nitrous Oxide in the 1920s and 1930s', in History of Anaesthesia Society Proceedings, 16 (Proceedings of the Joint Meeting with the Section of Anaesthetics, RSM, London, 10 December 1994), pp 81-84
42 Ellen P. O'Sullivan, Dr Robert James Minnitt 1889-1974: a pioneer of inhalational analgesia, in Journal of the Royal Society of Medicine 82 (April 1989), p. 221
43 Elam to NBTF, 28 December 1933 [NBTF/ F10/1/1]
44 Garry to NBTF, 19 April 1934 [NBTF/ H2/1]
45 Williams to Rivett, 22 September 1934 [NBTF/ F5/1/11]
46 Account of telephone call between Dr Minnitt and NBTF, 30 June 1934 NBTF/ H2/1]
47 'The Countrywoman Now Thinks for Herself', News Chronicle (2 June 1938)
48 Farrer Brown to BCOG, 7 June 1938 and 12 December 1938 [RCOG/ B2/26]
49 Meeting of BCOG Analgesics Sub-Committee, 15 April 1942 [RCOG/ T4/ J26]. Regarding pressure from the organisations mentioned, see correspondence in file [RCOG/B2/27].
50 Meeting of NBTF Analgesics Sub-Committee, 3 July 1939 [NBTF/ A1/15/1]
51 Rivett to Secretary, BCOG, 17 September 1936 [RCOG/ B2/26]
52 Mennell [to Fairbairn], 5 October 1936 [RCOG/ B2/26]

53 King to Meyer, 12 March 1937 [NBTF/ H3/1(4)]
54 King to Meyer, 16 November 1936 [NBTF/ H2/1]
55 NBTF 'Report on Gas/Air Analgesia' (1948) [NBTF/H2/5]
56 King to NBTF, 12 November 1934 [NBTF/ F2/2/2(1)]
57 King to NBTF, 10 July 1935 [NBTF/ H2/1]
58 King to NBTF, 25 September 1935 [NBTF/ H2/1]
59 NBTF to King, 18 December 1935 [NBTF/ H2/1]
60 Wren to Meyer, 10 April 1936 [NBTF/ F2/2/2(3)]
61 King to Meyer, 16 April 1936 [NBTF/ H2/1]
62 S. Shavaratman, Medical Superintendent, DeSoysa Lying-In Home, Colombo, 'Report on use of Queen Charlotte's Gas/Air Apparatus', 14 April 1937 [NBTF/ F2/2/3]
63 Jones to Williams, 8 March 1937 [NBTF/ H3/2/1]
64 West Hampstead DNA to NBTF, 27 May 1937 [NBTF/ H3/3(1)]
65 'With regard to difficulties arising from C.M.B. Rule, quotations from Nursing Associations, collected by Lady Rhys Williams' [NBTF/ H3/2/3(2)]
66 Extract from the Report of the BCOG into the use of Analgesics [NBTF/ H3/1(1)]
67 Meeting of Analgesics Sub-Committee, 10 March 1937 [NBTF/ A1/15/1]
68 Chapman to O'Reilly, 12 November 1937 [NBTF/ H3/1(1)]
69 Meeting of NBTF Analgesics Sub-Committee, 29 March 1938 [NBTF/ A1/15/1]
70 'Report on Gas/Air Analgesia'
71 For example, the Liverpool Maternity Hospital: see letter to NBTF, 10 July 1937 [NBTF/ H3/2/1]
72 London Hospital: see letter to NBTF, 15 March 1937 [NBTF/ H3/2/1]
73 Leeds Maternity Hospital: see letter to NBTF, 12 July 1937 [NBTF/ H3/2/1]
74 for example, St Thomas's Hospital: see letter to NBTF, 18 March 1937 [NBTF/ H3/2/1]
75 Reported in Minutes of NBTF Executive Committee, April 6 1937 [NBTF/ A1/3]
76 Northamptonshire NA: see letter to NBTF, 19 November 1937 [NBTF/ H3/2/1]
77 Diana Palmer, 'Women, Health and Politics, 1919-1939: Professional and Lay Involvement in the Women's Health Campaign' (PhD thesis, University of Warwick, 1986), p. 268.
78 'Medical Notes in Parliament', BMJ (5 August 1939)
79 Camp to NBTF, 10 August 1939 [NBTF/ H3/1/1]
80 Department of Health for Scotland to Ministry of Health, 29 October 1937 [PRO/ MH55/625]
81 Frank Honigsbaum, The Division in British Medicine. A History of the Separation of General Practice from Hospital Care 1911-1968 (Kogan Page, 1979), pp. 158-9
82 'The Midwife as Anaesthetist', Lancet (29 July 1939)
83 The Division in British Medicine, p. 159
84 Joint Committee of the Royal College of Obstetricians and Gynaecologists and Population Investigation Committee, Maternity in Great Britain (Oxford University Press, 1948), p. 78
85 The Division in British Medicine, p. 158, footnote b
86 'Suggested Draft for Middle Part of Letter'
87 Information given to secretary of NBTF by secretary of Midwives' Institute, Meeting of NBTF Analgesics Sub-Committee, 13 December 1939 [NBTF/ A1/15/1]
88 Maternity in Great Britain pp. 82-83
89 'Anaesthetics for Mothers', p. 9
90 Maternity in Great Britain, p. 86
91 Women's Cooperative Guild Annual Report for 1946, p. 46; Annual Report for 1947, p. 49 (Women's Cooperative Guild papers, Bishopsgate Institute, London)
92 Maternity in Great Britain, p. 80
93 Britain and her Birth-Rate, p. 113
94 Letter to The Lady (21 May 1942)

Joseph Sebrechts and Spinal Anesthesia in Belgium.

P. Desbarax,
Anesthesia Museum Verantare, Antwerp, Belgium

In 1928, the French Association of Surgery asked Professors Forgues and Basset to prepare a report on spinal anesthesia for its annual meeting (11). These rapporteurs collected 104 datasets including 222,467 cases treated with spinal anesthesia. This remarkable report was a landmark in the history of spinal anesthesia. At the meeting, 38 speakers out of 49 were clearly in favour of this technique of anesthesia while 7 accepted it for specific indications and only 5 were against it (12). Amongst the datasets collected, that of Dr. Joseph Sebrechts was the largest with 25,000 cases, all performed by himself and his colleagues. As this was the largest series of cases ever produced, it incited the organisers of the meeting to ask Dr. Sebrechts why he remained attracted to this mode of anesthesia.

To better understand the successive developments of this anesthesia technique, some historical background is necessary. In 1895, James Leonard Corning (USA) performed his first perilumbar injection. This neurologist from New York experimented with the action of cocaine on the spinal nerves of dogs. By injecting cocaine hydrochloride between the spinous processes of dorsal vertebrae in a patient, he performed the first epidural anesthesia for treatment of sciatalgia. In 1894, a similar injection performed intrathecally induced a "spinal anesthesia" and this became the name he gave to this procedure. Heinrich Quincke had already introduced lumbar puncture as a diagnostic procedure in 1891. Applying the techniques of these two pioneers, August Bier from Kiel performed in 1898 a spinal anesthesia in a patient to whom he did not dare to give chloroform. Encouraged by this result, Bier experimented on himself a cocaine spinal anesthesia with a two ml solution of cocaine at 1 percent. This convinced him to perform a similar anesthesia on one of his assistants and the technique was completely successful. Joseph Sebrechts started to use spinal anesthesia in 1910 and progressively applied it to 67 percent of his surgical cases. At that time, he did not publish his results but demonstrated this technique to many Belgian and foreign surgeons who were interested in the practice of spinal anesthesia. However, the enthusiasm of the surgeons for this mode of anesthesia rapidly decreased due to frequent failures, dramatic incidents and accidents and long-term sequellae including headaches and paralyses. Most of these drawbacks were due to lack of preciseness and technical failures when performing this technique.

During World War I (1914-1918), interest in spinal anesthesia resurged as many eminent surgeons treated often younger and healthier patients. However, after the war, spinal anesthesia was again forsaken because many patients, exhausted by the living conditions during the war, were less able to tolerate the technique, while the medicines used were also of poorer quality. Sebrechts, however, remained committed to the technique of spinal anesthesia and pursued his studies despite many reserves. One of his eminent tutors wrote to him: "I do not understand how

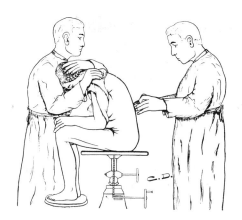

Fig.1 : The position of the patient

spinal anesthesia can improve the surgery".

At the meeting of surgery in 1928 in Paris, Joseph Sebrechts was asked to give his opinion and to describe his technique of spinal anesthesia. After a first article published in 1929 in the Flemish Journal of Medicine (2), this surgeon from Bruges decided to publish a more extensive study on 28,000 cases (5). In this remarkably clear and precise document Sebrechts displayed great objectivity and teaching skills. He did not underestimate the real dangers due to imprudence or superficiality and urged respect for the slightest details. Most of his recommendations are still actual : "Today, a good surgeon should not only be skillful and have manual dexterity, he must be first of all a good physician with intellectual gifts, moral qualities and professional competence. He must continuously improve his technique, asepsis and anesthesia. No surgeon will contest that anesthesia is of primary importance for the success of the surgical procedure. Anesthesia should, for a sufficiently long period,

a) suppress the anxiety of the patient, suppress his sensory modalities,

b) offer to the surgeon perfect muscular relaxation, maximal retraction of internal organs and an operating field without blood oozing,

c) all this, without intoxicating the patient, without impeding his vital functions or inducing postoperative complications.

I am convinced that the progress of science will, one day, offer this ideal anesthetic to the surgeon" (7).

In his research endeavour, Sebrechts used and studied all available methods to realise this goal : general inhalational anesthesia (1,2), local, rectal, intravenous, peridural and spinal anesthesia (3). The latter technique was the one he preferred.

Dr. Sebrechts stated the following: "For successfully practising spinal anesthesia, the surgeon most choose a single well-known technique, excluding all others, and he must try to understand the curious events that may disorient him in the beginning. We are convinced that all experienced spinal anesthetists will obtain excellent results with different techniques. Fully conscious of our responsibility, we recommend beginners to use our technique that is simple and efficacious and that will not give bad results".

Joseph Sebrechts did not want to impose an exclusive method, but simply explained and defended his procedure :

1) He had little experience with the spinal anesthesia techniques of Jonnesco and Le Filiâtre and was not in favor of supradiaphragmatic spinal anesthesia.

2) Locoregional anesthesia is an established technique and should, if possible, be preferred to spinal anesthesia.

3) If subumbilical surgery requires important muscle relaxation, spinal anesthesia is the method of choice.

4) If the anesthetist is experienced, spinal anesthesia can also be practiced for supraumbilical surgery.

5) If general anesthesia is contra-indicated due to the general health status of the patient, spinal anesthesia is indicated.

This last reason was the most important one for Joseph Sebrechts. He stated: "Spinal anesthesia has made major abdominal surgery better and less murderous, firstly, because of the paralysis of the abdominal wall and visceral contractions yielding a silent abdomen, which greatly facilitates the technical execution of surgery and avoids an excessive Trendelenburg position ; secondly, by decreasing hemorrhage due to the lowered blood pressure ; thirdly, by the remarkably benign postoperative course". One also avoids the excitation of the awakening period frequently seen following general anesthesia. The danger of this excitation phase for the stability of osteosyntheses is well known.

That the patient maintained his consciousness was considered as an inconvenience. Anxiety and the presence of many spectators (!) could trouble the patient. Administration of a narcotic agent (today we call it premedication) was considered for decreasing excitability. A screen separated the head of the patient from the operative field. Other useful methods were blocking visual and auditory stimuli to the patient.

Sebrechts considered that there were only few contra-indications for spinal anesthesia since the technique could be modulated and administered to all types of patients, including children. Diseases of the central nervous system and infection of the dorsolumbar region were obvious contra-indications for this technique.

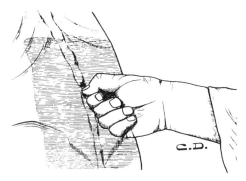

Fig.2: Identification of the L3-L4 intervertebral space

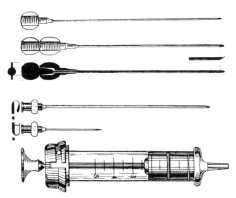

Fig.3 : The instruments used : the needle of Gentile in nickel, a large needle for drug aspiration, a fine needle for skin anesthesia, a glass Record syringe (from left to right).

The technical aspects of the spinal anesthesia practiced by Joseph Sebrechts will gradually evolve (6). Not only he explained the reasons why he selected a particular drug or technique, but, most importantly, he funded his arguments on precise and well-explained physiological considerations. During the initial years he deplored the lack of interest manifested by physiologists for spinal anesthesia, and he wished that more thorough studies should be undertaken. Awaiting further confirmations of his clinical observations, Sebrechts displayed a remarkable knowledge of human physiology. Let us remind that he always pretended to be a humanist and physician first, before being a surgeon.

Cocaine was not used very often at that time although Le Filiâtre still used this drug for "generalized anesthesias" because it provided less muscle paralysis and stimulated the orthosympathetic system. Stovaïne induced a perfect muscle relaxation by its strong action at the spinal motoneurones but was accompanied by meningeal irritation. Novocaïne, specially the french brand, was more active than the original drug (allocaïne, syncaïne, neurocaïne, neocaïne, etc.) and was an excellent drug that Sebrechts used for a long time. In 1926, he discovered tutocaine

495

(soluble para-aminobenzoate from Bayer) that was used by Alessandri from Rome. This anesthetic gave more prolonged anesthesia with good muscle relaxation. If tutocaine was more toxic than novocaine, its advantages overrided its inconveniences because Sebrechts believed that the general toxicity of the drug was not the cause of spinal anesthesia accidents. It was sufficient to avoid too large concentrations of tutocaine, and a 2 % solution with 0.25 mg adrenaline seemed to be an adequate anesthetic for Sebrechts. He mentioned as inconveniences related to this drug its difficult solubilisation of the powder in the cerebrospinal fluid (CSF) and a more frequent occurrence of nausea than with novocaïne (30 % of patients vs. 20 %). He also used percaine as will be explained later.

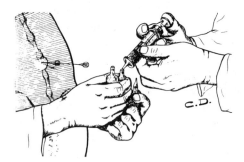

Fig.5 : *Solubilisation of the local anesthetic with CSF*

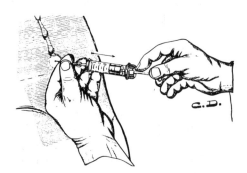

Fig.4 : *The technique of CSF aspiration*

Physiological aspects of spinal anesthesia.

Sebrechts explained that spinal anesthesia was not a physiological transsection of the spinal cord, but an anesthesia that was radicular and not segmental. The anesthetic impregnation of the spinal roots was more rapid than that of the peripheral nerves. Indeed, the latter are covered with a sheet that is less permeable to the anesthetic. At a specified level, the alcaloid acts first on the posterior roots with segmental disappearance of pain and heat sensitivities followed by loss of tactile sensitivity and muscular inputs. The anterior roots are impregnated, in turn, after the dorsal roots, often to a lesser degree, as if they were more resistant or as if the anesthetic drug was already less concentrated. Then, muscular paralysis occurs but to a lesser extent than the abolition of sensitivity and muscular inputs. Still later one observes paralysis of the sympathetic fibres that regulate visceral activity and vasomotor control. This phenomenon induces increased peristalsis and vasodilatation, that is one of the major causes for circulatory hypotension appearing usually after 10 - 15 minutes. This hypotension was often designated as "the storm of the 20th minute".

All these effects of root impregnation disappear in inverse order. The sympathetic nervous system paralysis disappears very quickly, often after 15 minutes, and one observes a reduction of the hypotension with blood pressure becoming normal before the end of surgery. Muscle paralysis disappears next and the "silent abdomen" retroceeds at a time that the patient has not yet recovered tactile and painful sensitivities.

In the clinical practice, one must wait for surgery till the blood pressure increases, i.e. about 15 minutes, to avoid accidents due to hypotension. If one starts too early, the blood pressure will decrease further and violent tractions on the viscera may elicit considerable, even catastrophic hypotensive reflexes.

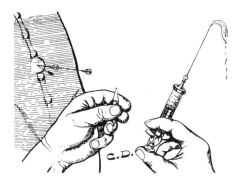

Fig.6 : Discarding excess anesthetic solution before mixing with adrenalin (glass vial in left hand)

The injected alcaloid does not behave as an inert substance : once injected into the spinal fluid, the drug progressively dilutes in the totality of the cerebrospinal fluid following the laws of gravity and, to a lesser degree, the natural diffusion of two miscible liquids. Thus, the density of the solution is most important. The cerebro-spinal fluid has a density of 1,107 (today this value ranges from 1,001 to 1,009). If one injects in the sitting position a solution with higher density (a hyperbaric solution), this solution will have a tendency to "descend", while a solution with a lower density (hypobaric solution) will have the tendency to "ascent". It thus is the position of the patient on the operating table that will condition the level of anesthesia.

For anesthesia of the lower part of the body with a heavy solution, it will suffice to put the patient in horizontal position. For anesthesia of the upper part of the body the patient will remain in Trendelenburg position. With a light solution (hypobaric) the movements of the surgical table are inversed : head down for anesthesia of the lower body, horizontal for anesthesia of the upper part of the body.

The technique of spinal anesthesia.

So far for the basic physiological concepts. We will now observe the evolution of the reasoning of Joseph Sebrechts and the successive modifications to his technique (4). The patient received a premedication with morphine and atropine to be calm and at ease. An intravenous serum infusion was installed to have permanent and rapid access to the circulation. After skin disinfection with iodine, a lumbar puncture was practised in sitting position at the level of L3-L4 ,which was easier to perform by non-experimented practitioners (Fig.1). The patient curved his back, the head was flexed, his feet on a small bench and he was kept in this position by an assistant. The nail of the surgeon indicated where the puncture was to be done (Fig.2). A local anesthesia (1 - 2 ml of novocaïne - adrenalin) allowed easy and non-painful punction. The fine nickel needle of Gentile was preferred for the spinal puncture because it would not break (Fig.3). Adequate depth of needle insertion was obtained when cerebrospinal fluid flowed through the needle when the stylet was removed. Sebrechts then advanced the needle 1 - 2 mm further to ensure that the bevel was entirely inside the spinal subarachnoid space. Then, 4 ml of cerebro-spinal fluid was aspirated with a 5 ml glass syringe (Fig.4) and one or two ampoules of tutocaïne, containing 0.04 g per ampoule, were dissolved in this volume (Fig.5). One thus obtained solutions of 1 or 2 % depending on the needs. The normal dose for an "average" patient was 0.06 g tutocaine and this dosage was most often used by Sebrechts. He obtained this dosage by discarding 1 ml of the mixture contained in the syringe (Fig.6) and adding 0.25 mg adrenalin in one ml. The syringe was then connected to the needle and filled by aspiration with cerebrospinal fluid to a volume of 5 ml. This mixture was slowly injected. The obtained anesthesia was sufficient for the lower abdomen and lower limbs with exception for the appendix and the descending colon. To obtain a more extended level of anesthesia a barbotage of the solution was performed twice (Fig. 7). Then anesthesia

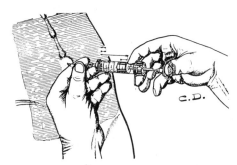

Fig.7 : The technique of barbotage

was adequate for the appendix, the descending colon and the umbilical region. For surgery on the stomach, gall bladder, spleen and kidneys a triple barbotage was recommended. Dr. Sebrechts was not in favor of spinal anesthesia for supradiaphragmatic surgery, as already mentioned.

The patient was then put horizontally on the surgical table with head and shoulders resting on a pillow (Fig.8). After 15 minutes the tutocaïne was "fixed", the table was set in slight Trendelenburg position and surgery could start. In case of alert, intravenous lobeline and adrenalin (0.5 mg) stabilized the condition of the patient. After surgery the patient was transported in slight Trendelenburg and put in his bed. He would remain in this position for 1-2 days with pillows under the head and the knees. After 2 days the bed was placed horizontally and the patient's head raised with one or more pillows.

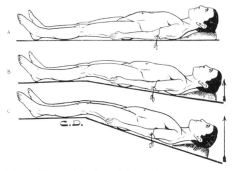

Fig.8 : The positioning of the patient

With his practice increasing, J. Sebrechts noticed in 1920 that some patients showed no loss of sensitivity, no muscle relaxation nor sympathetic block despite the fact they had received spinal anesthesia in perfect technical conditions. At that time, he used low concentrations of novocaïne and observed this lack of anesthesia in about 1/400 cases. He initially thought this was due to technical errors. However, he discovered such totally absent anesthesia in five patients belonging to the same family, all operated by him at different times. Each of these patients had received spinal anesthesia with successively modified but always technically correct procedures. All needed considerable amounts of general anesthetics for their surgery (5). These four men and their mother all had the same physical appearance, were calm, reasonable and strong.

"Since this time, we have the distinct impression that, in a given family, all the children that have the same physical appearance as one of the parents behave as their parent with regard to spinal anesthesia. This new concept of individual resistance (or sensitivity) of familial origin is indisputable. We have the impression that those resistant to spinal anesthesia are subjects with very active sympathetic nervous system : they will need 0,08 g of tutocaïne. But this 'special resistance or sensitivity", which has nothing to do with nervosity, can vary with physiological or pathological conditions. For instance, pregnancy increases sensitivity to spinal anesthesia, and drug intoxications, bowel ileus, uremia in prostatic patients, icterus, the ascites accompanying cancer all should incite to the greatest caution and impose the use of lesser doses (i.e. 0,04 g tutocaine when the ordinary dosage is 0.06 g). The ascitic peritonitis of tuberculosis, on the contrary, makes patients resistant to spinal anesthesia. There also exists a racial factor: the Anglosaxons are more resistant and the Italians more sensitive than we are".

How can one detect these hypersensitive or hyperresistant patients ? Some situations already described give an indication. In these patients a premedication with morphine and scopolamine given one hour before surgery will induce not only quietness but even somnolence and sleep. This sign, which is easy to interpret, will indicate sensitivity to spinal anesthesia (as well as to other forms of anesthesia). On the contrary, if the patient is fully awake and can even stand up and walk, he will be resistant to spinal anesthesia.

If during the installation of a spinal block, the given dose would be too high, one should administer intravenous stimulants, digalene, coffeine, even adrenalin. In case of resistance to spinal anesthesia, and rather than to switch to general anesthesia and its complications, it seemed logical and innocuous to Sebrechts to administer a new dose of tutocaïne, identical to the first but without adrenalin, or even a third spinal dose in very rare cases.

After this long digression on sensitivity and resistance to spinal anesthesia, Joseph Sebrechts underscored the advantages of the spinal method : the abdominal silence, the reduced bleeding. The contraction of the uterus also greatly facilitates cesarean section. The postoperative course is much simpler : there is less intoxication, less vomiting, heart, kidneys, liver and lungs are spared and resumption of feeding occurs earlier. Although infrequent, thromboembolism is a severe complication and cephalea a non-negligible nuisance.

The occurrence of cephalea merits some attention (5). Sebrechts acknowledged that until 1928 he witnessed a 5 % incidence of light cephalea and 1 % of persisting cephalea. One can distinguish headaches due to hyperpressure of the CSF, possibly due to a meningeal reaction, and headaches resulting from hypopressure of the CSF, due to persistant leakage of fluid through the hole in the dura mater according to Leriche. Sebrechts confirmed that the hyperpressure cephalea was indeed due to a meningeal reaction : a simple lumbar punction, and thus also the punction followed by injection of any solution, induces a meningeal reaction, by the presence of blood in the CSF, by the introduction of cells charged with iodine, by infection of the solution. Thus develops a real meningitis with hyperpressure of the CSF from which the patient usually recovers. If one performs the punction in a skilled way with a fine needle, and if asepsis of the needle, the syringes and the solutions are perfect, cephalea will occur very unfrequently.

Sebrechts attributed the pathogenesis of the hypopressure cephalea to different mechanisms. If one withdraws brutally 10 ml CSF in the lumbar region, the orthostatic pressure of the spinal fluid column is dramatically reduced and the medulla oblungata will obstruct the occipital aperture, thereby producing a "primary bulbar accident".

Moreover, the injection of the anesthetic, a foreign solution, can cause headache. If 5 ml of a percaine solution of 1/1500 is injected spinally, the pressure of the CSF will, instead of increasing by the amount of fluid injected, almost instantaneously decrease, and as one injects more and anesthesia progresses, the pressure decrease of the CSF will become more important (8). This drop in pressure is likely the result of changes of blood perfusion in the extradural space eliciting the same effects as the brutal substraction of CSF during lumbar puncture, i.e. an obstruction of the occipital aperture by the medulla oblungata.

Other changes occur as well. The choroid plexus will secrete a more abundant quantity of fluid to compensate for the pressure drop of the CSF by reflex activation. Blocked by the descent of the medulla oblungata, this fluid cannot leave the cranium to reach the perimedullar space and will increase the intracranial pressure. One can thus understand why the intravenous injection of distilled water, that diminishes the secretion of the chloroid plexus, can in some patients relieve the symptoms.

Professor Sebrechts, applying all these concepts, then concluded : "We do not substract fluid, we inject fluid ; we do not use concentrated solutions of anesthetic but, on the contrary, very dilute solutions. The puncture needle is very thin, the equipment well sterilised. The head-down position during the injection and after surgery avoids the herniation of the bulbus and the rise in intracranial pressure. In practice, one can say that cephalea have disappeared with exception in those patients in whom reactional intracranial hypertension followed a circulatory depression that has to be treated with ephedrine".

Objections to the use of spinal anesthesia.
"One has blamed spinal anesthesia for a high mortality as indicate the first published results. It has to be said that in the beginning surgeons choose spinal anesthesia for the bad cases that would not tolerate general anesthesia. This led to incidences of 6-8 deaths/10,000 cases, considered related to spinal anesthesia. Nevertheless, with experience, technical progress and respect for details, the mortality rate is 1/5000 cases in a department that is organized for spinal anesthesia. Some surgeons are against spinal anesthesia. Having witnessed the major catastrophies of the past, they fear the responsibility they could be blamed for. These accidents are the result of technical failures, inactive drugs, resistance (or sensitivity) to spinal anesthesia of familial origin, or sequellae such as cephalea or paralysis of cranial nerve VI.

Those who practise spinal anesthesia must know the physiological and pathological consequences that result from this anesthesia to better control the technique."

Joseph Sebrechts then gives an interpretation of observed clinical events. "After a spinal anesthesia with tutocaine 2 %, the patient lying in horizontal position with the head supported by a pillow, one will observe the following.

1) A faint and slow pulse : the hypotension is due to the paralysis of the anterior roots (from T1 to L3) ; the orthosympathetic paralysis causes bradycardia because the vagus nerve can exert its function unimpeded ; this bradycardia in turn will decrease blood pressure. The paralysis of the abdominal and thoracic muscles decreases the aspiration of venous blood by the vena cava ; the heart, receiving less blood, is thus deprived of a physiological stimulant for its contraction (Bainbridge reflex).

2) Breathing becomes more superficial and slower. This can be explained by the loss of action of the abdominal and the six last intercostal muscles innervated by the same roots. The diaphragm ensures sufficient ventilation but there is nevertheless a slight cyanosis and a state of sleepiness. If the anesthetic solution reaches the second cervical root all ventilation is arrested. This "bulbar alert" is not brutal : it is preceded by hypotension, then slowing of the breathing followed by a progressive decrease of consciousness and finally by intense cyanosis. The intracardiac injection of adrenalin and artificial breathing can still save the patient.

3) Nausea and vomiting : they are always announced by the hypotension. Their explanation by vagotonia, due to the paralysis of the orthosympathetic and the predominance of the vagal systems, is incorrect as a preoperative or peroperative injection of atropine has no inhibitory influence on vomiting after spinal anesthesia. It could be more related to a moderate bulbar anemia that excites the pneumogastric nerve. Other reasons for vomiting are reflexes caused by traction on the viscera when the sympathetic block is not yet or no more present. The preoperative injection of opiates, psychical trauma and an uncompensated state of shock are other cau-

ses of vomiting. For all these reasons the incidence of nausea and vomiting occurs in 30 % of patients treated with tutocaine - adrenalin which is not negligible. But nausea and vomiting do practically not occur following surgery.
4) Rectal evacuation : this is due to the activity of the vagus nerve increasing peristalsis. Here, atropine is efficacious".

Spinal anesthesia with percaine.

In the beginning of the 1930's, percaine (Ciba) appeared in clinical practice. This was the occasion for Sebrechts, who was always looking for a better or the ideal drug, to experiment with different concentrations, including the hypobaric percaine solution of Jones (8). This solution will show great benefits for supraumbilical spinal anesthesia. This hypobaric solution 1/1500 (ampoules of 20 ml with NaCl 0.5 %) had a density of 1.003 and provided a longer anesthesia and muscle relaxation with preservation of the orthosympathetic functions. Thus, sympathetic block was no more the main concern, which shifted to impairment of breathing. For this reason, progressively increasing amounts of the percaine hypobaric solution had to be administered to ensure safety in use. Joseph Sebrechts knew the objections of his colleagues with regard to spinal anesthesia. He considered that it was possible to obtain with this solution a successful and absolutely safe spinal anesthesia specifically tailored to the needs of each patient. He described this technique in minute details in 1934 (7,9). At that time he had experience of 35,000 cases, all performed under his supervision.

A premedication with morphine-scopolamine is given one hour before the procedure. This premedication already gives some indication on the sensitivity of the patient for spinal anesthesia, as previously explained. A midline lumbar puncture is practised between L3 and L4 after rigourous desinfection of the skin with iodine and local anesthesia of the needle trajectory with 1-2 ml of novocaine 1 % or percaine 2% with adrenalin, which makes the puncture totally pain-free. The positioning of the patient may vary : the sitting position, the easiest for the beginner, with curved back, head flexed on the thorax and feet resting on a bench, or a lateral position which is more comfortable for the patient. The correct placement of the needle is indicated by the flow of CSF and the needle is then pushed further for 1-2 mm to ensure that its bevel is inside the subarachnoid space. The patient is then prudently turned into a ventral position, the needle staying in place. The operating table is kept horizontally for a "high" spinal block or in slight Trendelenburg for a "low" spinal anesthesia. Five ml of the Jones' solution (1/1500) are slowly injected and the pulse is observed (6). If hypotension is precocious and profound, this results from a mild syncopal reaction due to anxiety, and nausea may occur. This type of hypotension should not be of concern as it suffices to reassure the patient, refresh his face, urge him to breathe deeply and to give oxygen if needed. Preventive administration of ephedrine is not warranted, except in fragile patients, because ephedrine will impair the quality of the anesthesia and increase blood oozing. If the alert is however serious, ephedrine or adrenalin may be indicated. If the pulse slows down progressively, it indicates that the spinal block reaches the sixth thoracic segment and the accelerating orthosympathetic fibres of the heart. After 5 minutes the extension of the spinal block is verified by pinching the skin of the upper body with a Kocher clamp, without informing the patient but observing changes in facial expression. If anesthesia is insufficient in the tested area (the upper borders of the surgical field), if the pulse beholds its frequency or its slowing disappears, a second injection of 5 ml is given. This is repeated every five minutes till skin clamping in the surgical field is no longer percieved by the patient.

Thus, Professor Sebrechts insisted on feeling the pulse. He thought it was not necessary to measure blood pressure ! Pulse frequency and amplitude provided sufficient information on the circulatory status and the beating of the aorta during surgery was an unquestionable sign of adequate circulation.

The dose to be administered was variable and related to the condition of the patient. A person sensitive to spinal anesthesia would be treated with 10 ml, while someone resistant to spinal block might receive more than 90 ml, and, between these extremes, a normal patient would be treated with about 20 ml.

Unilateral anesthesia for surgeries on the appendix and kidney was obtained with a lumbar punction in the lateral position, the patient lying on the healthy side (10). Once the spinal block was "fixed", the patient was cautiously turned on the back in slight Trendelenburg, the spinal needle having been removed. It was imperative to wait 30 to 35 minutes after the puncture to avoid "the storm of the 20th minute", the time of maximal hypotension that required all the vigilance of the practitioner. The maximal hypotension occurred later with percaine than with novocaine or tutocaine and appeared at 30-35 minutes. Only then could surgery start. One could object to this long delay before starting the surgical incision. But Sebrechts used this time for correct installation of the patient with adequate protection of pressure points (heels, elbows, arms) and placing pillows underneath the patient for avoiding decubitus lesions and paralysis. Furthermore, the perfect surgical conditions obtained shortened duration of surgery and avoided troubles and delays due to an inadequate anesthesia.

In conclusion, the originality of Joseph Sebrechts' method lies in the adaptation of the dose of the anesthetic injected to the sensitivity of the patient : "A standardisation of the dose for a given anesthesia level is an illusion". Some of his colleagues had previously fixed the dose of the anesthetic to be administered as a function of the weight of the patient. Others, like Howard Jones (London), measured precisely the length of the spinal canal befor substracting a certain amount of CSF and administering as a single injection the volume of the anesthetic solution that carries his name. The technique of Jones did not find wide acceptance in the surgical practice.

Sebrechts tested the sensitivity of each patient in three different ways: the response to the premedication, the notion of resistance or sensitivity to spinal anesthesia and the adaptation of the dose of anesthetic administered. The lack of adhering to this imperative evaluation was the probable reason why many surgeons abandoned spinal anesthesia.

Is this method an ideal method of anesthesia ? Sebrechts stated that all methods can be improved, and that all drugs elicit adverse events, but he was convinced that one day drugs and methods would approach perfection. Do we not have the same search and hope today? Sebrechts already envisioned our speciality: "We believe that the time has passed that the surgeon's conscience could accept to entrust any patient to any anesthesia from the hands of occasional helpers" (8). A great reflexion of an eminent surgeon who was a pionier of our speciality.

References:

[1] Sebrechts J: Techniek na de nephrectomie. Vlaamsch Gen. Tijdschrift n° 10, 1928
[2] Sebrechts J: De techniek van de Rachianesthesie. Vlaamsch Gen. Tijdschrift n° 37, 1929.
[3] Sebrechts J: Ce que j'ai vu dans les Hôpitaux américains. L'Assistance Hospit. n° 5, Sept-Oct 1929
[4] Sebrechts J: Quelques faits observés au cours de l'anesthésie rachidienne. (Essais d'interprétation). Comptes rendus du Congrès National des Sciences, 29 June 1930
[5] Sebrechts J: Note au sujet de la Rachianesthésie. Rapport du Dr De Beule. Bulletin de l'Académie Royale de Belgique, 1930; 10 : 480 - 490 and 543 - 638
[6] Sebrechts J: Modifications de notre technique de la Rachianesthésie depuis la note publiée le 28/9/1930. Bulletin de l'Académie Royale de Belgique, 11: 1931
[7] Sebrechts J: [Conference given at the Société Royale de Médecine of Ghent] Revue Belge des Sciences Médicales 6 : n°4 : 1934
[8] Sebrechts J: Bulletin de la Société Royale Belge de Gynécologie et d'Obstétrique 15 : n°4 : 1934
[9] Sebrechts J: Spinal Anaesthesia, Brit Med J Anaesth 12: n°1: Oct 1934
[10] Sebrechts J, Derom F: L'Anesthésie en urologie, J Belg Urol n°3 : June 1937
[11] Forgues E et Basset A: Rapport du Congrès de Chirurgie, Paris. 1928, 199
[12] Deniker M: La Rachianesthésie d'après le rapport présenté par Mrs. Forgues et Basset pour le 37e Congrès de Chirurgie. Journal de Chirurgie 32 : n°4 :1928

Additional reading references.

Sebrechts J: Anesthésies Rachidiennes, 31.000 cas personnels. 9th Congress of the International Society of Surgery, 1932
Sebrechts J: Over Rachianesthesie. Lecture given at Brugge. Flemish Assoc. Surgery and Gynecology, 24/9/1933
Sebrechts J: Greffes Osseuses. Intern. Soc. Surgery 10th Congress Sept 1938
Sebrechts J: Quelques facteurs de progrès chirurgical. Le Scalpel 1934
De Winter L, Sebrechts J: Le collapsus électif et l'apicolyse dans la tuberculose pulmonaire. Archives Médicochirurgicales de l'Appareil Respiratoire. 7 : n°5 : 1932
Chalier A: La Rachianesthésie . G. Douin et Cie 1929
Forgues E, Basset A: La Rachianesthésie; sa valeur et sa place actuelle dans la pratique. Masson et Cie 1930
Forgues E: Précis d'Anesthésie Chirurgicale, Anesthésie Générale, Rachidienne, Locale. G. Douin et Cie 1934
Adriani J: The Chemistry and Physics of Anesthesia. Charles C. Thomas Publ. Springfield, 1962
Moore D: Regional Block. Charles C. Thomas Publ. Springfield, 1981
Desbarax: Heelkunde in Vlaanderen. Gemeentekr. 1990, 225-235

Flavio Kroeff-Pires and his Contribution to Intravenous Regional Anaesthesia

H. Nolte†
Department of Anaesthesiology, Klinikum Minden, Germany

When looking at the publications in scientific journals of textbooks of the past 30 years dealing with intravenous regional anaesthesia, the historical survey mostly begins with a short sentence. This could be something like: "Intravenous regional anaesthesia was described by Bier in 1908. After initial enthusiasm the method was soon forgotten, until it became more popular again due to the report by Holmes in The Lancet in 1963."

Holmes himself writes in his classical article: "Although some present-day textbooks of local analgesia mention the method in passing, it seems to have been largely forgotten since the time of Bier".

Holmes summarizes the article as follows: "A safe simple method of producing analgesia of the limbs, which does not require special training or extensive experience, is described. The method is a modification of Bier's "venous anaesthesia" described fifty-five years ago".

In 1969 a symposium on intravenous regional anaesthesia took place in Worcester, Massachusetts. Holmes held the introductory entitled "The history and development of intravenous regional anaesthesia". In this lecture he also makes the following statement:

"Of Bier's technique, however, very little was heard apart from isolated reports by Morrison and Herreros and passing reference in some textbooks".

Some sentences later he says:

"In 1963 I described a series of cases using this method, unaware that there had been a report from Czechoslovakia published the year before by Riha. This worker used a curious mixture of Panthesin® (p-Aminobenzoyl-N-diethyl-leucinol), asorbic acid, penicillin and streptomycin."

Riha's article was published in 1962 in the German journal "Der Anästhesist" without describing the technique in detail. The only striking fact, however, was the failure rate of 18% in 32 patients!

In spring 1990, after opening of frontiers between West and East Germany, I was invited to give a guest lecture at the Medical Academy of Erfurt, Thuringia, on the subject of intravenous regional anaesthesia. Following the lecture I met Dr. Ursula Müller, a specialist in anaesthesiology from Erfurt. She told me to have written her doctoral thesis on intravenous regional anaesthesia in 1977. She drew my attention to the fact that as early as in 1954 a modification of Bier's technique had been described in Brazil - which means in Portuguese language - which was comparable to that reported on by Holmes in 1963.

The following citation can be taken from the thesis:

"The merit of rediscovering intravenous regional anaesthesia is attributed to Holmes, who reported on the application of venous anaesthesia in 30 patients. But prior to Holmes, whose report was published in the Anglo-American literature, Flavio Kroeff-Pires, a Braziilian from Porto Alegre, had published a detailed article on the modernized, modified Bier's technique in "Revista Brasileira de Anestesiologia" in 1954. He had been introduced to the method an assistant of

Professor Bado, head of the Department of Traumatology and Orthopedics in Montevideo/Uruguay, who was visiting the Hospital de Pronto Socorro upon invitation of the city of Porto Alegre, Brazil.

Between 1946 and 1954 Kroeff-Pires performed hundreds of anaesthetic procedures after Bier. Possibly, Holmes did not know the Brazilian literature because he did not - speak Portuguese. The techniques described by Kroeff-Pires and Holmes are very similar."

The difference between both techniques consisted in the application of the local anaesthetic. Kroeff-Pires applied procaine 0,5%, and Holmes recommends lidocaine 0.5%. While Holmes applies 40 ml lidocaine to block the upper extremity, Kroeff-Pires reports on a volume of 80 ml for the upper and 150 ml for the lower extremity. From today's experience it can be maintained that by applying the less toxic agent procaine Kroeff-Pires could increase dosage and volume. At present, intravenous regional anaesthesia is performed using 0.25% lidocaine or prilocaine with a dosage of 1 ml/kg body weight for the arm and 1.5 ml/kg body weight for the leg. As early as in 1954 Kroeff-Pires also recommended the double tourniquet and the elevation of the arm instead of using an Esmarch bandage.

Thus it was nine years prior to Holmes that Kroeff-Pires described the modification of Bier's "venous anaesthesia", which is widely used today. Kroeff-Pires published his report in Portuguese. In contrast, Holmes' article was published in English and could therefore be understood worldwide without major difficulties.

Nevertheless, it is regrettable that apart from English hardly any other language is taken into consideration particularly in science. We should not forget that e.g. Portuguese is the mother tongue of more than 100 million people.

Particularly in the field of medicine, historians and librarians should be able to find possibilities of allowing the access to scientific information from all languages into all languages.

References:

[1] Kroeff-Pires F: Metodo de "Bier" para anaesthesia regional de membros. Revista Brasileira de Anestesiologia 1954; 4:21-24

[2] Holmes C: Mck. Intravenous Regional Anaesthesia. Lancet I 1963, 245

[3] Müller U: Die intravenöse Regionalanästhesie als Betäubungsmethode bei der ambulanten Extremitätenchirurgie. Dissertation. Medizinische Akademie Erfurt (Germany) 1977

Reconstruction of the Ancient Egyptian Mouth-Opening Instrument – the Practice of Artificial Respiration 5000 Years ago

A Ocklitz, Department of Anaesthesiology
St. Gertrauden Krankenhaus Berlin, Germany

There is an astonishing relief in the Abu Simbel Temple, showing the famous battle of Kadesh in 1275 BC. A medical act is depicted in the turmoil of that scene. A badly wounded Hittite prince is being treated by a helper. The rescuer, obviously skilled in medicine, is using the head-tilt-chin-lift-method to keep the respiratory tract free[1]. This proves that the principle of freeing the respiratory tract was common at that time.

This finding relates to the achievements of a group of emergency doctors in ancient Egypt. The members of this organisation called themselves exorcists of Serqet named after the goddess Serqet, and they adhered to specialist standards. They been able to treat life-threatening conditions caused by snake bites or scorpion stings for example. The activities of this group are well documented, for example in the sitting statue of the rescuer Djet-Hor in the Egyptian Museum in Cairo. Engelmann and Hallof translated the inscription on the statue as follows: This is the doctor who prepares the way to revive the dead, who puts air into the closed nose (!) of he who is without breath, to resuscitate him by moving his arms by making use of all the methods of the exorcists of Serqet.[2]

It is not sure whether all these methods form a system of cardio-pulmonary resuscitation as we would define it. However further hints on this knowledge may be written down in the Cult of the Dead. Approximately at the time when the pyramids were built, a ritual was added to the Cult of the Dead. It is not clear whether this so-called Opening of the Mouth ceremony originally duplicated a funeral procedure or whether it was more a medical process. Here you can see the Opening of the Mouth ceremony as it is depicted in the 3300-year-old Hunefer Papyrus (Fig.1).

This ritual was of extraordinary significance because it fulfilled the main purpose of the pharaonic Cult of the Dead. The aim was to resuscitate the Pharaoh after mummification for eternal life in the hereafter. Wallis Budge, a legend among Egyptologists, noticed that the procedures carried out in this ritual were performed on the fresh corpse in very ancient times. This leads to the conclusion that the Egyptians did have experience of resuscitation-like procedures using those obscure instruments.

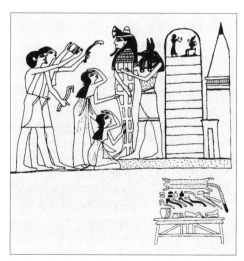

Fig.1: Papyrus Hunefer: The Opening of the Mouth ceremony.

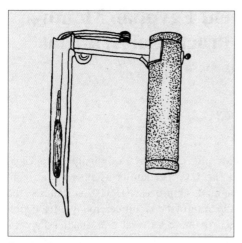 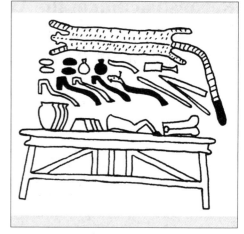

Fig. 2: The U-shaped laryngoscope designet by Magill. *Fig. 3: Side table, papyrus Hunefer.*

Real or symbolic opening of the mummys mouth with an iron device was central to the opening of the mouth ceremony. However all that were part of the ritual have astonishing parallels in modern emergency procedures, as I was able to demonstrate in the 1/96 issue of the German medical journal Der Anaesthesist[3]. Apart from opening the mouth, the eyes were also opened with a so-called eye-opening device that might be comparable today's pupillary function tests. Even teeth were extracted symbolically just like false teeth are removed before artificial respiration today. So-called Horus fingers in the form of gold tubes were held to the mouth, and possibly symbolized intubation. Intubation with gold tubes should not be considered hypothetical. The first tubes used this century were also made of metal, and Avicenna described on an "Arabic method of intubation" with finger-shaped gold tubes a thousand years ago[4].

Numerous other parallels seem unimportant compared with the astonishing characteristics of this mouth-opening device, which was described as a Chisel of Iron in the Pyramid texts. It was very similar to the u-shaped laryngoscope designed by Magill (Fig.2) and it had apparently been made of meteoric nickel iron since the earliest times.

According to Wainright, the meteoric iron used in the ancient Egyptian mouth-opening device may have contained 10% nickel[5]. An actual mouth-opening could be performed with this device without stability problems. The German palaeontologist, Pahl, proved that mouth-opening was indeed performed, althoug later only in symbolic Form[6].

The methods used by the ancient Egyptians in the Opening of the Mouth Ceremony can be seen particularly clearly in the side table in the Hunefer Papyrus (Fig.3). Its similarity to modern anaesthetic tables is amazing. Like today, mouth-opening devices of various shapes and sizes, according to the size and form of the mouth, are prepared to be used arranged from left to right.

The best way to show that this astounding correlation is more than coincidental is to reconstruct the device according to what is shown in the Hunefer papyrus, and to test its functional characteristics on an intubation phantom. I did this early last year and wrote a paper on it, which was accepted in autumn 1996 by Der Anaesthesist and will be published in July 1997[7]. Hunefer's mouth-opening chisel shows the following characteristics:

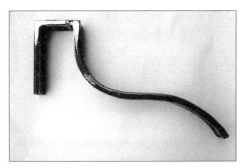

Fig. 4: The Mouth-Opening Device.

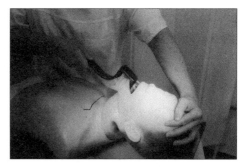

Fig. 6: The mouth-Opening with the reconstructed chisel using the ancient method.

1. It is a full-metal or all-wood instrument.
2. It has 2 perfect right-angles at its head.
3. Its tongue depressor is perfectly straight.
4. Comparison with the figure shown in the Hunefer Papyrus a metal profile of almost l0mm can be found.

The instrument I reconstructed is an exact, and I emphasise exact, replica of the one shown in the Hunefer Papyrus (Fig.4). It is 22mm wide, nearly 10mm thick, 40mm deep between the angles, and has an 80mm long depressor. It also corresponds to the full-metal instrument to be seen in the 3300 year-old tomb painting of Ank-Her-Kha and the wallpainting in the tomb of Tut-Ank-Amun. In these pictures, the mummy is in upright position, symbolising the beginning of resuscitation.

For the device to function in the sense of emergency medicine, the subject must be in

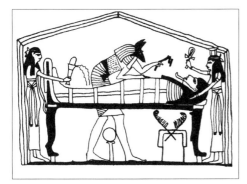

Fig. 5: Tomb of Nekhtamun, 19. Dyn.; Deir el-Medineh, Thebes.

a supine position. There is a painting showing this position in the tomb of Nakht-Amun from Deir el-Medina (Fig.5). The mortuary priest, holding the iron device in his hand, assumes a position known as inverse intubation in polytrauma management today[8]. This painting from Medina shows how the ancient Egyptians actually used the mouth-opening device. Deir el Medina plays an important role in this context. The desert settlement near the kings' tombs was the so-called 'Secret Place', where the decorators of the kings' tombs were forced to live interned and shielded from the world. These tomb decorators were the only ones in Egypt who knew the sense and purpose of the pharaonic Cult of the Dead. They called themselves 'Doctors at the Place of Truth'. They saw their work as medical because it involved the resuscitation of the dead pharaoh for the afterlife.

I will now show you my reconstructed mouth-opening chisel, used in exactly the same position as shown in the tomb painting in Deir el-Medina (Fig.6). As you can see, this device, which looks so angular and awkward, is very easy to manipulate. This can be seen very well in the video documentation which I showed on March 1st this year at a plenary lecture at the Vienna Intensive Care meeting and at the Deutscher Anästhesiekongress International last week[9] (the film will be shown also after this lecture). The ergonomics of the long handle are particularly effective on the CLA-phantom. Even without a light source, a depressor of this shape opens the larynx entrance in such way as to allow easy and safe/secure intubation. However an assistant is needed to insert the tube. In my opinion, this is the only way intubation could have worked in ancient Egypt. The method of intubation we know could never hardly have worked because the devices would have needed the described thickness because of the material used. Numerous wooden models of the mouth-opening device found in tombs prove this. Rolled steel, which would have allowed a flatter profile, was not known then and is not shown in any painting. There are no paintings showing our laryngoscope handling method today, therefore it is unlikely that it was used this way.

The ergonomically favourable power transmission with the ancient Egyptian mouth-opening instrument is only possible when the depressor is held in like this. Because of its material and functional characteristics, the device, which I reconstructed, makes us suppose that it was developed for more than just symbolic purposes.

All reproductions were made by F. Knolle.

References:

[1] Felkai P: Az jralesztsi kisrletek els nyoma az kori Egyiptomban. Orvosi Hetilap 1986; 28: 1709-1712

[2] Engelmann H, Hallof J: Medizinische Nothilfe und Unfallversorgung auf staatlichen Arbeitsplätzen im alten Ägypten. Zeitschr ägypt. Sprache und Altertumskunde 1995; 122/2:119-120

[3] Ocklitz A: Künstliche Beatmung mit technischen Hilfsmitteln schon vor 5000 Jahren?. Anaesthesist 1996; 1: 19-21

[4] Shehata MA: History of laryngeal intubation. M.E.J. Anaesth. 1981; 6/1:49-55

[5] Wainwright GA: Iron in Egypt J Egypt Archeol 1931; 18:3-15

[6] Pahl WM: The ritual of opening the mouth: arguments for an actual body-ritual from the viewpoint of mummy research. In: Science in Egyptology. Manchester Univ Press, Manchester 1986, P 211-217

[7] Ocklitz A: Rekonstruktion des altägyptischen Mundöffnungsgerätes. Anaesthesist 1997; 7:599-603

[8] Ocklitz A: Deir el-Medina und das Totenritual der Alten Ägypter: Kemet 1996; 5/3: 25-27

[9] Ocklitz A: Kardio-pulmonale Reanimation in Ägypten schon vor 5000 Jahren? Wiener Klin Wschr 1997; 109/11:406-412

Experiments with the "Laryngoscope" from Papyrus Hunefer on a Mannequin

K. P. Koetter[1], W. H. Maleck[2]

[1] Department of Neurological Intensive Care Unit, Leopoldina-Hospital, Schweinfurt, Germany
[2] Department Anaesthesiology, Klinikum, Ludwigshafen, Germany

Introduction:

In 1995 Ocklitz published a new interpretation of the Ancient Egyptian funeral ritual of the "Opening of the Mouth". His hypothesis is that knowledge about pulmonary resuscitation existed in the earliest times of Ancient Egypt (i.e. about 3,000 BC) but declined later, leaving a funeral ritual[1-4]. Although the ritual is mentioned in texts from the Old Kingdom dating about 2,500 BC, there are no pictures of it. However, papyri and murals from the New Kingdom (about 1,550-1,100 BC) show the device for the ritual[5-10]. Presumably the best picture of the ritual is preserved in the Papyrus Hunefer (New Kingdom, about 1300 BC)[1,3,4,5,6]. The persons depicted have a very "professional" attitude, so they were used recently for Cerebyx[R] advertisement[11]. One mouth-opening instrument is shown in the hand of a priest. Four more are depicted on a table showing assorted funary devices that can be interpreted as resuscitation equipment[12]. The mouth-opening instruments are similar to the U-shaped laryngoscopes of Jackson and Magill in the first half of the 20th century[13-16]. Ancient Egyptian texts emphasize that the instrument used was made from (meteoritic) iron.[6]

The "orthodox" egyptologist consider this ritual to be a statue ritual later performed on (bandaged) mummies.[6] Pahl, however, proved that manipulation of the mouth had been performed on actual bodies.[17] Roth published an interpretation of the opening of the mouth ritual which, although different from Ocklitz, is medical in nature. She believed that it was a symbol of cutting the umbilical cord and cleaning the mouth of the (reborn) mummy[18-20].

Methods:

We wanted to verify the medical implications of Ocklitz hypothesis by reconstructing the Opening of the Mouth instrument as depicted on the papyrus Hunefer and using it on a mannequin. We tried to build it to scale. We assumed a height of the priest of 160 cm. This yields a length of the blade of about 8 cm, a length of the handle of about 30 cm and a distance of blade and handle of about 5 cm. The thickness of the handle is about 2 cm. Thickness of the blade is about 1.5 cm at its base and 1 cm at its tip. The width of the blade can not be determined as all pictures show the instrument in profile.

Based on this, a first prototype has been manufactured by RFQ Medizintechnik (Tuttlingen, Germany) in August 1995. It was a steel abdominal retractor reshaped according to the picture from papyrus Hunefer (Fig. 1). It allowed the intubation of a mannequin, but the procedure was painful because of the thin handle. Ocklitz was informed of our experiment in February 1996, when the lectures for the One-Day-Meeting of the Ancient Astronaut Society were submitted[21-23]. Later the instrument was equipped with a wooden handle by joiner's workshop Herrmann (Mannheim, Germany). Now intubation was comfortable, and the thickness of the handle that of the original in papyrus Hunefer. Still, the blade is thinner than 1 to 1.5 cm of the original (Fig. 2).

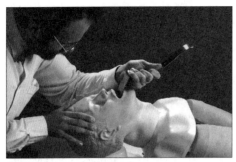

Figure 1:
The first replica of the Mouth-Opening instrument consisted of a steel abdominal retractor.
It is shown in use on a Laerdal Airway Management Trainer.

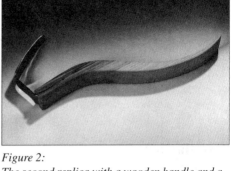

Figure 2:
The second replica with a wooden handle and a steel blade.

In September 1996 a pilot study was undertaken with this new blade on a Laerdal Megacode Trainer (Laerdal, Stavanger, Norway). This is a whole-body resuscitation trainer with airways similar to the head-and-thorax-only Laerdal Airway Management Trainer, which has been used by several groups for evaluation of training, laryngoscopes or operator positions[24-34]. Assuming that the Ancient Egyptians practiced intubation for resuscitation in the same setting as we do today in the prehospital setting, the mannequin was placed on the floor of a classroom with its head to the window. The only light source was diffuse natural daylight, which provided just enough light for direct vision of the glottis. After a short training for four persons (both the authors and two medical students) intubation of the Laerdal Megacode Trainer without help was possible three times each. The following positions were used by each intubator:
- sitting at the head of the mannequin[29] (Fig. 3)
- straddling over the thorax[29,35] (Fig. 4)
- kneeling beside the mannequin (Fig. 5).

Results:

The mean time to intubate was 9.3 seconds; maximum time was 14.4 seconds. All intubations were performed without complications (no oesophageal malposition, no "clicks" representing possible tooth damage).

Discussion:

For the medical lay audience at the One-Day-Meeting a video was shot in October 1996. It presented the intubation with a modern laryngoscope and the "Hunefer-blade" on a Laerdal Airway Management Trainer. The video was shown in a session including a lecture of Ocklitz, including discussion for the audience[21-23].

At the German Anaesthesia Congress 1997 and the Fourth International Symposium on the History of Anaesthesia our replica was presented as well as one made by Ocklitz.[36-40] He used a comparatively unknown CLA-mannequin for his trial. Here, as well as in a recent publication, Ocklitz criticized our replica[41].

His first objection was directed towards the material we used. We admit that an iron-nickel alloy simulating meteoritic might have been better. However, our aim was not to build an exact copy. We wanted to show that an instrument with the shape like that in the hand of the priest in Papyrus Hunefer allowed intu-

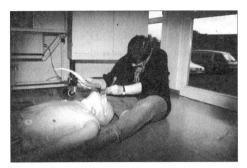

Figure 3:
Intubation at the head of the mannequin (Laerdal Megacode Trainer). The room was so dark, that the flash was activated automatically. Nevertheless, natural light was sufficient to intubate without artificial light.

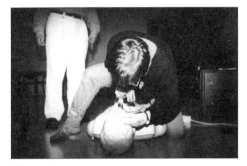

Figure 4:
Intubation straddling above the thorax.

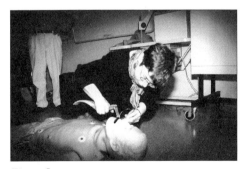

Figure 5:
Intubation kneeling at the side of the mannequin

bation without artificial light. Beside this, Ocklitz used steel, too.

The second was that, Ocklitz believed that our blade was too thin (its thickness comes to about 2 mm); his 8 mm thick instrument would resemble the original. A close look at the instrument in the hand of the priest reveals, that it has to be at least 10 mm thick. Intubation with such a thick instrument (given that it is not profiled) would probably be impossible. The instrument of Ocklitz requires excessive strenght, counteraction at the forehead and a second person to introduce the tube. But the artist creating the papyrus might have exaggerated the thickness of the blade for clarity as the height of the priest in the original is only about 20 cm. So the use of a blade thinner than 10 mm seems justified. Trials with a "meteoritic" alloy would be needed to clarify minimum thickness.

The third reason, Ocklitz mentions that the instrument must have been made from a single block, i.e. forbidding the use of a wooden handle with a separate blade. Again, we do not agree. As mentioned above, there seems to be a thinner tip of the blade in the Hunefer papyrus. The scene in the tomb of Nachet-Amun clearly shows a straight blade attached to a J-shaped handle[6]. Finally, in the tomb of Ken-Amun there is a millimeter-thin blade attached to a thick J-shaped handle (the only doubt is that we only know drawings of the damaged original)[6,7].

Ocklitz`s fourth complaint concerns the construction of the device. He demands exact 90 degree angles for religious and technical reasons. As to "religious" reasons see below. Technically there is no reason why (meteoritic) iron should not have differing angles, and some of the instruments on the table in papyrus Hunefer as well as the instrument in the tomb of Onuris-Cha show bigger angles[5,6].

Interestingly, the shape of Ocklitz' instrument follows the instruments on the table in papyrus Hunefer rather than the instrument in

513

the hand of the priest (as ours does). For the instruments on the table, however, no scale is available.

Finally, one should consider that according to the hypothesis of Ocklitz intubation as a medical procedure was known in the earliest times of Ancient Egypt and later declined to a religious ritual. The pictures from the New Kingdom, nearly 2,000 years later, show ritual instruments that might be different from the original medical instruments. This makes a "original" reconstruction unlikely anyway.

Conclusion:

Both the trials of Ocklitz and our group renders intubation with a replica of the Egyptian mouth-opening instrument to be feasible. Differences in detail (exact form of the replica, type of mannequin) do not seem to make a difference.

The egyptologists, however, disapprove Ocklitz' ideas[42]. To convince them, new sources on the origins of the Opening of the Mouth ritual or Ancient Egyptian medicine would be needed. Otherwise Ocklitz' hypothesis probably can neither be proven nor refused.

References:

[1] Ocklitz A: Das Mundöffnungsritual der alten Ägypter. Ancient Skies 1995; 19/1:8-11

[2] Ocklitz A: Die Pyramiden - Reanimationskapseln? Ancient Skies 1995; 19/6:7-9

[3] Ocklitz A: Das altägyptische Mundöffnungsritual im Licht der modernen Wiederbelebungsmedizin. Kemet 1995; 4/4:31-33

[4] Ocklitz A: Künstliche Beatmung mit technischen Hilfsmitteln schon vor 5.000 Jahren? Anaesthesist 1996; 45:19-21

[5] Faulkner RO, Andrews C: The Ancient Egyptian Book of the Dead. Paperback, British Museum, London 1993, Cover and p.53-54

[6] Otto E: Das ägyptische Mundöffnungsritual. Vol. II: Kommentar. Harrassowitz, Wiesbaden 1960.

[7] de Garis Davies N: The Tomb of Ken-Amun at Thebes. Vol. 1, Metropolitan Museum, New York 1930, Plate 61

[8] Carter H: Das Grab des Tut-Ench-Amun. Brockhaus, Wiesbaden 1981, p.81

[9] Martin GT: The Hidden Tombs of Memphis. Paperback Ed., Thames and Hudson, London 1992, p. 128-129

[10] Forman W, Quirke S: Die Macht der Hieroglyphen. Kohlhammer, Stuttgart 1996, p. 123

[11] Parke-Davis, Division of Warner Lambert Co.: The last time I used i.v. Phenytoin was 1996 B.C. Academic Emergency Medicine 1997; 4/5:Inside of Cover

[12] Maleck W, Kötter K, Petroianu G: Die Katze auf dem heiligen Blechtisch oder Kannten die Ägypter das "Oesophageal Detector Device"? Ancient Skies 1995;19/5:10-12

[13] Jackson C: The technique of insertion of intratracheal insufflation tubes. Surg, Gynec and Obstet 1913;17:507-509

[14] Cooper SD: The evolution of upper airway retraction: new and old laryngoscopy blades. In: Benumof JL: Airway Management. Principles and Practice. Mosby, St.Louis 1995, p. 374-411

[15] Magill IW: An improved laryngoscope for anaesthetists. Lancet 1926;i:500

[16] Westhorpe R: Magill's laryngoscopes. Anaesthesia and Intensive Care 1992;20:133

[17] Pahl WM: The ritual of opening the mouth: arguments for an actual-body-ritual from the viewpoint of mummy-research. In: David RA (Ed.) Science in Egyptology. Manchester University Press, Manchester 1986, p. 211-217

[18] Roth AM: The pss-kf and the "opening of the mouth" ceremony: A ritual of birth and rebirth. Journal of Egyptian Archaeology 1992; 78:113-147

[19] Roth AM: Fingers, stars, and the "opening of the mouth": The nature and function of the ntrwj-blades. Journal of Egyptian Archaeology 1993; 79:57-79

[20] Harer WB: Peseshkef: The first special-purpose surgical instrument. Obstetrics & Gynecology 1994; 83:1053-1055

[21] Kötter K: Experimente mit dem Intubationsspatel von Papyrus Hunefer am Simulator. Lecture, One-Day-Meeting of the Ancient Astronaut Society, Mannheim, November 2nd, 1996

[22] Maleck W: Notfallmedizin im Alten Ägypten. Lecture, One-Day-Meeting of the Ancient Astronaut Society, Mannheim, November 2nd, 1996

[23] Ocklitz A: Medizintechnologie bei den Pharaonen. Lecture, One-Day-Meeting of the Ancient Astronaut Society, Mannheim, November 2nd, 1996

[24] Bishop M J, Harrington R M, Tencer A F: Force applied during tracheal intubation. Anesth & Analg 1992; 74:411-414.

[25] Bucx M J L, van Geel R T M, Wegener J T, Robers C, Stijnen T: Does experience influence the forces exerted on maxillary incisors during laryngoscopy? A manikin study using the Macintosh laryngoscope. Can J Anaesth 1995; 42:144-149.

[26] From R P, Pearson K S, Albanese M A, Moyers J R, Sigurdsson S S, Dull D L: Assessment of an interactive learning system with "sensorized" manikin head for airway management instruction. Anesth & Analg 1994; 79:136-142

[27] Gough JE, Thomas SH, Brown LH, Reese JE, Stone CK: Does the ambulance environment adversely affect the ability to perform oral endotracheal intubation? Prehospital and Disaster Medicine 1996; 11:141-143

[28] Hodges U M, O'Flaherty D, Adams A P: Tracheal intubation in a mannikin: Comparison of the Belscope with the Macintosh Laryngoscope. Br J Anaesth 1993; 71:905-907.

[29] Koetter KP, Hilker T, Genzwuerker HV, Lenz M, Maleck WH, Petroianu GA, Fisher JA: A randomized comparison of rescuer positions for intubation on the ground. Prehospital Emergency Care 1997; 1:96-99

[30] Maleck WH, Kötter KP, Bauer M, Weber M, Herchet J, Petroianu GA: Geknickt oder aufrichtbar? Fünf Laryngoskopspatel im Test. Anästhesiologie & Intensivmedizin 1996; 37:621-624

[31] Nathanson M H, Gajraj N M, Newson C D: Tracheal intubation in a manikin: Comparison of supine and left lateral positions. Br J Anaesth 1994; 73:690-691.

[32] Petroianu GA, Maleck WH, Jatzko A, Altmannsberger S, Bergler WF: Intubation mit Transillumination. Unterweisung von Unerfahrenen am Modell. Anästhesiologie & Intensivmedizin 1996; 37:511-514

[33] Rubens A J, Stoy W, Piane G: Using interactive videodisc to test advanced airway management skills. Prehospital and Disaster Medicine 1995; 10:251-255.

[34] Stratton SJ, Kane G, Gunter CS, Wheeler NC, Ableson-Ward C, Reich E, Pratt FD, Ogata G, Gallagher C: Prospective study of manikin-only versus manikin and human subject endotracheal intubation training of paramedics. Annals of Emergency Medicine 1991; 20:1314-1318.

[35] Gürtner I, Kanz K-G, Lackner C, Schweiberer L: Inverse Intubation beim Polytrauma. Indikation, Technik, Erfahrungen. Intensivmedizin und Notfallmedizin 1993;30:426-427

[36] Kötter KP, Maleck WH: Versuche mit dem "Intubationsspatel" aus Papyrus Hunefer am Simulator. Anästhesiologie Intensivmedizin Notfallmedizin Schmerztherapie 1997; 32:S60

[37] Kötter KP, Maleck WH: Experiments with the "laryngoscope" from Papyrus Hunefer in a mannequin. Fourth International Symposium on the History of Anaesthesia, Book of Abstracts. p.123

[38] Ocklitz A: Künstliche Beatmung im alten Ägypten? Anästhesiologie Intensivmedizin Notfallmedizin Schmerztherapie 1997; 32:S60

[39] Ocklitz A: Reconstruction of the ancient Egyptian mouth-opening instrument - the practice of artificial respiration 5000 Years Ago. Fourth International Symposium on the History of Anaesthesia, Book of Abstracts. p.122

[40] Ocklitz A: Video-film-documentation on the experimental use of the reconstructed Egyptian mouth-opening instrument. Fourth International Symposium on the History of Anaesthesia, Book of Abstracts. p.187

[41] Ocklitz A: Rekonstruktion des altägyptischen Mundöffnungsgeräts. Anaesthesist 1997; 46:599-603

[42] Anonym: Haken im Hals. Der Spiegel 1997; 51/17:256-258

The History of Separation of the Airways

K. Wiedemann, E. Fleischer, P. Dressler
Department of Anaesthesiology
Thorax-Klinik Heidelberg, Heidelberg, Germany

The history of separation of the airways has been amply documented in reviews and textbooks[37,43]. The present communication attempts to review the thought processes that lay behind the evolution of events concerned with the subject. The necessity to separate the main airways arose in the physiological laboratories of the nineteenth century, primarily to resolve the question of whether the lung actively secretes carbon dioxide[41,45].

In our century, the process of airway separation served to answer a number of questions such as energy metabolism in man[25], blood circulation in the non-ventilated lung[18,26] - a puzzling issue still under the contemporary term, hypoxic pulmonary vasoconstriction - and the more troublesome process of trying to substantiate Ferdinand Sauerbruch's contention on the beneficial influence on the circulation of his differential pressure method[38]. The simplest means of obtaining gas for analysis, for introducing different gases or for simply excluding the lung from ventilation was to catheterise one main bronchus (Table 1).

Siegfried Wolffberg is reputed to be the first to introduce a catheter into a main bronchus[45] as suggested by his teacher, the famous physiologist Eduard Pflüger (1829-1910). This grisly instrument consisted of a small rubber tube as the bronchial catheter proper, wich was housed inside an abortion catheter as used by the French obstetrician Stéphan Tarniér. The inflatable distal portion of this device served to obtain an airtight seal inside the main bronchus. The

Respiratory Physiology: Endobronchial Catheters

Author	Year	Species	Features	Reference
Pflüger EFW	1871			45
Wolffberg S	1871	dog	Tarnier's cannula	45
Bernard C	1875	dog		1
Loewy A	1905	man	left	25
v. Schrötter, H				
Hess R	1912	rabbit	left, hook	18
v. Rohden F	1913	rabbit	left, hook	38

Table 1

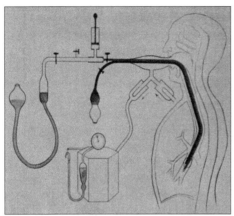

Fig. 1: Silver catheter for intubation of the bronchus intermedius by Loewy and von Schrötter. A smaller silver catheter is aligned for feeding air to the endobronchial cuff. Attached devices are one way valves for respiration, spirometry and gas analysis[25].

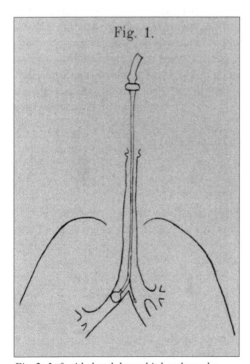

Fig. 2: Left-sided endobronchial catheter by R. Hess[18] *used in rabbits.*
A carinal hook is reported for the first time.

inflatable distal portion of this device served to obtain an airtight seal inside the main bronchus. Claude Bernard (1813-1878) in his "Leçons sur l'Asphyxie"[1] mentions airway separation in a dog breathing carbon dioxide into one of its lungs and ambient air into the other. However, technical details were not given. An account of the first use of endobronchial catheterisation in man was published in 1905 by Adolf Loewy (1862-1936) and Hermann von Schroetter (1870-1928) after successful work on the metabolism of the horse with a semilar device.[25] (Fig.1). A thin-walled silver tube was deliberately placed in the right main bronchus because it was felt that access there was easiest. A second small silver catheter served for inflation of the endobronchial rubber cuff. The more detailed description, however, reveals considerable difficulties in keeping the device in its proper place (Fig.1,2).

The much debated carinal hook made its appearance on the catheter used by Rudolf Hess[18] for experiments on the pulmonary circulation in non-ventilated lung regions (Fig.2). Despite the unfamiliar way of presentation Hess strongly advised keeping strictly to the left main bronchus for intubation. The previously mentioned experimental problems in respiratory physiology were tackled by some workers by the introduction of two separate airways into the tracheobronchial tree (Table 2). In their simplest form these consisted of two tubes of differing length, shaped to match the tracheobronchial anatomy. The earliest mentioned device is Head's combination of a tracheal cannula and an endobronchial catheter[17]. While this design can be easily traced up to contemporary devices, the technique of exteriorising the endobronchial section in a similar way to a chest tube, as suggested by Kuma[23], was never used in human subjects. A more sophisticated design in 1892 by the physiologist B.

Respiratory Physiology: Double Lumen Devices

Author	Year	Species	Features	Reference
Head H	1889	rabbit	2 tubes, right	17
Werigo B	1892	rabbit	coaxial tubes, left	41
Maar V	1902	turtle	2 tubes, left	26
Mathieu P Hermann H	1925	dog	DL, carinal separator	30
Kuma S	1925	dog	left, transthoracic + tracheostomy	24
Churchill ED	1927	dog	2 tubes, left	10
Moore RC	1927	dog	2 tubes, left	32
Tørning K	1933	rabbit	coaxial, right	5

Table 2

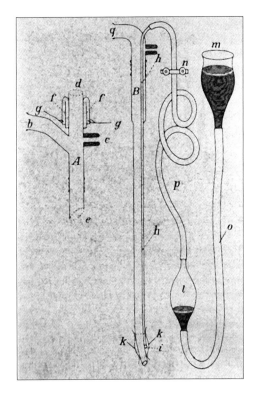

Werigo of St Petersburg[41] (Fig. 3) was a coaxial double-lumen tracheostomy cannula for rabbits. The principle involved may have had some bearing on the first attempts to separate the airways in man and may well have been on Liljestrand's mind[5] when advising Paul Frenckner (1896-1967) on the constrtion of a double-lumen bronchoscope[13] (Fig. 3,4).

The French physiologists Mathieu and Hermann[30] in the 1920s, in dogs obtained gas for analysis and pressure tracings from each lung by a double lumen airway which termi-

Fig. 3: Coaxial double lumen tracheal cnnula for use in rabbits.
A: Tracheal (outer) cannula with side arms (b) for ventilation and gas sampling (c).
B: The left endobronchial (inner) cannula (B) with the lumen (q) for ventilation and side arm for gas sampling to be introduced through cannula A. For airtight seal the bronchial cuff (k) was filled with water from reservoire l under pressure regulated by varying the height of mercury reservoir m [41].

519

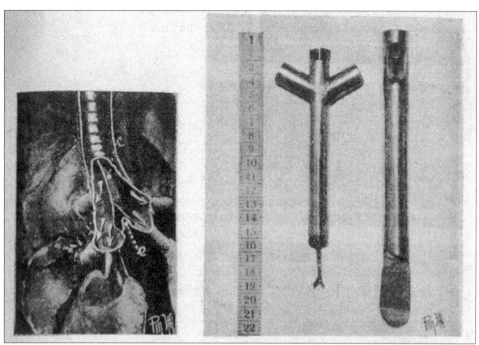

Fig. 4: Airway seperator in dogs[30]. Left: The double-lumen device is shown in situ. The seperator blade ("eperon") with its double rim rests firmly in the carina ("cloison"). Right: details of the device.

```
                    From Blocker to Univent


   Author            Year   Tube                  Technique    Refer.
  ---------------------------------------------------------------------
  | Magill I        |1934| catheter/cuff        | r-scope   |  29  |
  | Crafoord C      |1938| tampon               | r-scope   |  12  |
  | Rusby LN        |1943| cuff/mesh            | r-scope   |  39  |
  | Thompson VC     |    |                      |           |      |
  | Moody J         |1948| cuff/beryllium       | blind     |  31  |
  |                 |    | hooks                |           |      |
  | Stürztbecher,F  |1953| TT/blocker           | stylette  |  40  |
  | Macintosh R     |1955| TT/blocker           | blind     |  28  |
  | Leatherdale RAL |    |                      |           |      |
  | Inoue H         |1982| TT/movable blocker   | f-scope   |  19  |
  | Nazari S        |1986| TT/M. blocker,hook   | f-scope   |  33  |
  ---------------------------------------------------------------------

   1: TT      = endobronchial tube
   2: r-scope = rigid bronchoscope
   3: f-scope = fibreoptic bronchoscope
```

Table 3

nated in a separation blade resting on the carina (Fig.4). This feature may have given rise to ideas about double-lumen tubes in industrial designers who have never had to face the daily struggle for the crucial position of an airway separator!

The development of pulmonary surgery for the treatment of tuberculosis and bronchiectasis called for practical techniques and for some means to clear the bronchial tree of the affected lung of pus an secretions. Varying endobronchial blockers were constructed (Table 3) and were improved to withstand the surgical assault on the delicate cuff structures, for example by shielding with nylon mesh as in the Vernon-Thompson blocker [39]. In order to keep them more securely in position, beryllium hooks were incorporated, as in Moody's version [31] (Fig.5) (Table 3).

Clarence Crafoord (1899-1984) of Sabbatsberg hospital, Stockholm, one of the most active thoracic surgeons of his period, insisted on a tampon soaked with a local anaesthetic, being pushed into the main bronchus of the affected side [12]. He maintained that this procedure served the double purpose of sealing off the diseased lung and of obtunding, by the local anaesthetic, dangerous cardiovascular reflex activity. As it had become desirable to introduce a blocker and a tracheal tube, Ivan Magill resorted to passing both an endobronchial blocker and an endotracheal tube down his - or as we now learn, Wade's - tracheoscope [44]. He elaborated on that technique in his comprehensive lecture to the Royal Society of Medicine in 1936 [29] (Fig.6). The desire to do away with broncho- and tra-

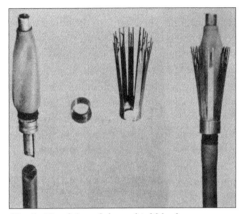

Fig. 5: Moody's endobronchial blocker featuring array of berrylium hooks wich upon inflation of the cuff were supposed to engage to the bronchial wall [31].

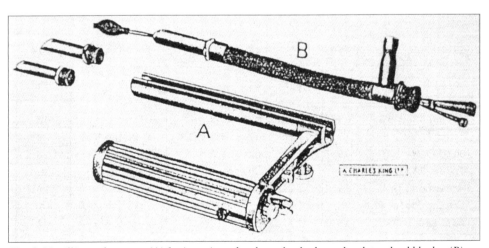

Fig. 6: Magill's tracheoscope (A) for insertion od endotracheal tube and endotracheal blocker (B) under cocaine local anaesthesia prior to induction of general anaesthesia. Manufactured by Charles King [29].

cheoscopes for the simultaneous introduction of tracheal tubes and endobronchial blockers led Fritz Stürtzbecher (1917-) [40] (Fig.7) and later Sir Robert Macintosh(1897-1989) and Leatherdale [28] to produce a fixed combination of the two devices.

The one with the shorter endobronchial catheter was intended for pneumonectomy. The logical next step of having a movable blocker housed inside an endotracheal tube did not come until 30 years later, when Hiroshi Inoue[19] in a letter to the editor of the Journal of Thoracic and Cardiovascular Surgery described what was later called the "Univent Tube"[9]. More obviously than the Univent in the combination of endotracheal tube and endobronchial catheter designed by Nazari et al[33], placement of the latter requires a fibrebronchoscope to securely position the catheter tip and to engage the attached carinal hook in the entrance either to the right upper lobe bronchus or to the left main bronchus.

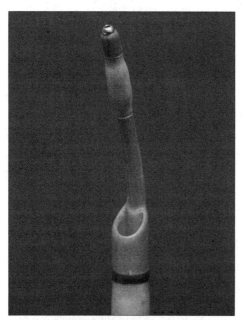

Fig. 7: Combined endotracheal tube and endotracheal blocker by Stürtzbecher. This model featuring a short blocker tube was intended for pneumonectomy [40].

```
Prevention of Spread: Endobronchial Tubes


Author            Year   Features              Technique        Refer.

Gale JW           1932   L/R  1 cuff           blind              14
Waters RM
Rovenstine EA     1936   L/R  2 cuffs          blind              43
Magill I          1936   L/R  1 cuff,spiral    r-scope*           29
Gordon W          1955   R    hook, slot       (blind)            16
Green RA                      2 cuffs          r-scope
Macintosh R       1955   L    2 cuffs          blind              28
Leatherdale RAL                                stylette
Pallister WK      1959   L    3 cuffs          r-scope *          34


L = left       R = right         * r-scope = rigid bronchoscope
```

Table 4

An alternative to sealing off the main bronchus of the diseased side was intubation of the opposite main bronchus. This was suggested as early as 1932 by Gale and Waters [18] (Table 4). Ivan Magill (1888-1986) described a pair of armoured tubes 1936. The side intended for the right main bronchus featured a length of spiral bare wire at the tip to allow adequate ventilation of the right upper lobe. However, according to Machray, writing in 1958, anaesthesia had not developed sufficiently for the successful use of these tubes in the 1930s.

Devices which had a wider application only came into being after the general adoption of controlled ventilation and muscle relaxants for thoracic surgery [27]. To be positioned properly, most required the use of a bronchoscope. The Gordon-Green tube [16] was designed for intubation of the right main bronchus; here, for the first time, a slot in the endobronchial cuff is encountered in combination with a carinal hook. The Pallister tube [34], better known as the Brompton tube, was intended for more conservative forms of lung surgery for malignancies, that is e.d. the sleeve resection described by Price-Thomas [36], Johnston and Jones [22]. If the endobronchial cuff was pricked by the surgeon's needle, the tube had an inner spare inflatable cuff.

During the late 1920s the famous Swedish physician Hans Christian Jacobaeus (1879-1937) of the Sabbatsberg Hospital in Stockholm [20], became interested in the problem of how to obtain spirometric data from a single lung in order to decide on treatment methods such as thoracoplasty (Table 5). The widely known physiologist Gunnar Liljestrand suggested to him endobronchial catheterisation, similar to Pflüger and

From Bronchospirometry to Double Lumen Tube

Author	Year	Device	Features	Ref.
Liljestrand G	1930	Pflüger catheter		21
Jacobaeus HC, Frenckner P, Björkman S	1932	Jackson scope	cuff	20
Jacobaeus et al (s.a.)	1932	coaxial DL* scope	2 cuffs	5
Frenckner P	1934	parallel DL scope	2 cuffs	13
Frenckner P	1934	flexible DL scope	(discarded)	13
Gebauer PW	1939	rubber DL tube	left	15
Zavod WA	1940	rubber DL tube	steel-inforced	
Carlens E	1949	rubber DL tube	left, hook	9

* DL = double-lumen

Table 5

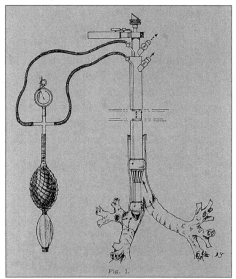

Fig. 8a: Coaxial double lumen rigid bronchoscope designed by P. Frenckner [13] and used by the group of Jacobaeus [5,20] for bronchospirometry. Note intubation of the right main bronchus.

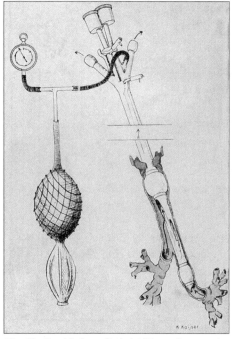

Fig. 8b: Double barrelled rigid bronchoscope by P. Frenckner [13] in clinical use for many years at Sabbatsberg Hospital, Stockholm [21,5].

Wolffberg's procedure [21]. He head a Jackson bronchoscope equipped with a rubber cuff an endobronchial seal and modified for spirometry. Sequential intubation of both main bronchi with this instrument proved too cumbersome and time-consuming and it never left the animal laboratory [5].

Due to the technical ingenuity of Paul Frenckner (1897-1967), the ENT member of the group, and again on the suggestion of Liljestrand, a double-lumen bronchoscope was constructed, clearly featuring two ideas put forward by the physiologists: two co-axial tubes - as in Werigo's cannula - and intubation of the right main bronchus as advocated

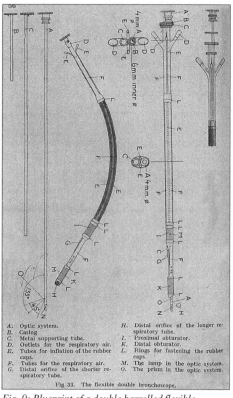

Fig. 9: Blueprint of a double barrelled flexible bronchoscope intended for spirometry, and optical system for placement and control of position, designed by P. Frenckner. The device was never used clinically [13]. For details see blueprint legend.

by Loewy and von Schrötter[13,21,25,41]. In contrast to theoretical calculations, a change from laminar to turbulent flow occurred in this device and poorly tolerated increases of resistance were found, even during quiet breathing. A double-barrelled bronchoscope was then made by Frenckner and was used in patients for more than four years[13] (Fig.8a,8b). Separate tracings from each lung could now be obtained for tidal volume, oxygen consumption and carbon dioxide production. The respiratory function of diseased lungs could be assessed and decisions taken on surgical treatment. Concerned about the bulk of the instrument, Frenckner developed a flexible double-lumen device consisting of two semi-elastic, silk-woven catheters contained in a rubber tube (Fig.9). It was introduced under the guidance of an urethroscope-like optical system. Unfortunately the device was discarded due to problems with kinking tubes. The question still remains; why was the obvious next step - construction of a rubber double-lumen catheter - not undertaken? It is particularly puzzling as Paul Gebauer [15]published a description of his device almost at the same time (Fig.10,11).

This is still more strange since from the beginning, Frenckner was involved in thoracic surgery with Clarence Crafoord (1899-1984)[12] for whose patients he used controlled ventilation by means of the so-called spiropulsator[13], a pressure-cycled ventilator he had designed. The potentially enormous advantage of a double lumen tube for that kind of surgery must have escaped everybody's attention in that team since it still relied on endotracheal intubation with a single-lumen tube of Crafoord's own design with the previously mentioned tamponade of the main bronchus of the diseased lung by a cotton swab soaked in local anaesthetic. To make things more strange, the ultimate design of the left endobronchial tube with

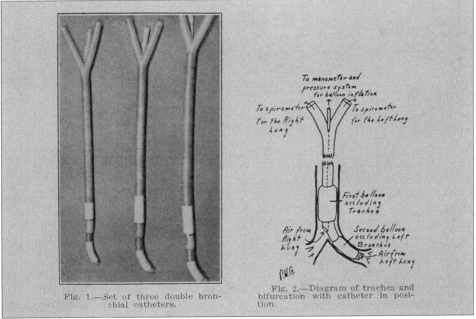

Fig. 10: Rubber double lumen tubes designed for bronchospirometry by P. Gebauer. Note similarity to the later Carlens tube, save the carinal hook.

525

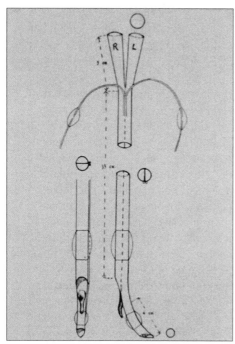

Fig. 11: Construction details of the Carlens double lumen tube [9]. Compare to diagram of Gebauer's tube in Fig. 10.

the carinal hook, put forward by Eric Carlens (1908-1990) in 1949[9], was also primarily intended for bronchospirometry (Fig.11). For this indication the carinal hook certainly served its purpose, for it reliably prevented the tube from being inserted too far down the left main bronchus and jeopardising spirometry. (The more frequent event in thoracic surgery - expulsion of the tube into the trachea during surgical activity near the hilum - is not prevented by the hook.) The annoying tendency of the hook to engage in laryngeal structures during intubation was be prevented by tying it down on to the shaft with a slipknot which was released once the tip of the tube was safely in the trachea. The influence of the ENT department may be deduced from the long preserved method of insertion recommended - by guidance of a laryngeal mirror [4]. This tube seemed virtually to have been taken out of the hands of its inventor. All publications on the use of the double-lumen tube in surgical and anaesthetic practice were under the name of the surgeon, Viking Björk [2,3]. Even in a paper published in 1953 in Anesthesiology, Carlens ranked as second author only [4]. For left pneumonectomies, the tube, of course, had to be pulled back into the trachea before the main bronchus could be clamped [4]. This disadvantage brought about the development of right endobronchial tubes by Roger Bryce-Smith and Salt[7], and White[42] (Table 6).

It is undeniable that double-lumen tubes for right endobronchial intubation were more difficult to place and to maintain in position with the lateral eye in the endobronchial section facing the entrance to the right upper lobe. The required position could only be checked, and then only imprecisely, by auscultation, by relying on the correct placement of the carinal hook in the case of the White tube, or by chest X-ray. For this reason, Clarke [11] observed in 1962: it would be wise to have a regular and happy acquaintance with the use of the Carlens catheter before the use of the White tube is begun. The advent of fibreoptic bronchoscopy and new construction materials contributed much to the popularity of double lumen tubes today. Already a survey among British anaesthetists published by Pappin in 1979[35] showed that the double-lumen tubes designed by Frank Robertshaw (1918-1991)in 1962, with greater internal diameters and without carinal hooks, were used predominantly. Of tubes with carinal hooks, only the Carlens type retained some popularity. Endobronchial single-lumen tubes had fallen into disfavour, as was the case with endobronchial blockers. Only one institution was still inserting a tampon (Tampax[R])into the main bronchus of the diseased lung.

Double Lumen Tubes in Thoracic Surgery			
Author	Year	Features	Refer.
Björk VO Carlens E	1950	left, hook	2
Bryce-Smith R	1959	left	6
Bryce-Smith R Salt R	1960	right, slot	7
White GMJ	1960	right, slot, hook	42
Robertshaw FL	1962	right, slot, left	37
Burton NA Watson DC	1983	right /left PVC*	8

* PVC = Polyvinylchloride

Table 6

The history of airway separation may be summarised best in the words of one of its pioneers, Frank W Robertshaw: Much of the early lung surgery was concerned with the treatment of tuberculosis and bronchiectasis. Its aim was to remove or collapse those parts of the lung which, by producing quantities of infected secretions, gave rise to chronic cough and the risk of spreading infection. The problems encountered in these wet lung cases played an important part in the development of thoracic anaesthesia and led to the development of a variety of techniques which have in turn made better surgery possible [37].

References:

1. Bernard MC: Leçon sur les anesthésique et sur l'asphyxie. In: Cours le Médicine du College de France. Paris 1875, Librairie J B Bailliere, Londres
2. Björk VO, Carlens E: The prevention of spread during pulmonary resection by the use of a double-lumen catheter. J Thorac Surg 1950; 20: 151-157
3. Björk VO, Carlens E, Crafoord C: The open Closure of the bronchus and the resection of the carina and of the tracheal wall. J Thorac Surg 1952; 23: 419-4284
4. Björk VO, Carlens E, Friberg O:Endobronchial anesthesia. Anesthesiology 1953; 14: 60-72
5. Björkman S: Bronchospirometrie. Eine klinische Methode, die Funktion der menschlichen Lungen getrennt und gleichteitig zu untersuchen. Acta Med Scand 1934, Suppl 56: 1-199
6. Bryce-Smith R: A double-lumen endobronchial tube. Br J Anaesth 1959; 31: 274.75
7. Bryce-Smith R, Salt R: A right-sided double lumen tube. Br J Anaesth 1960; 32: 230-31
8. Burton NA, Watson DC, Brodsky JB, Mark JB: Advantages of a new polyvinylchloride double lumen tube in thoracic surgery. Ann Thorag Surg 1983; 35: 78-84
9. Carlens E: A news flexible double-lumen catheter for bronchospirometry. J Thorac Surg 1949;18: 742-46
10. Churchill ED, Agassiz A: A method for separating the air breathed by the right and left lungs, together with the effect of pulmonary circulatory changes on this divided breathing. Am J Physiol 1926;76: 6-19
11. Clark AD: The White doublelumen tube: A report on its use in fifty cases. Br J Anaesth 1962; 34: 822-24
12. Crafoord C: On the technique of pneumonectomy in man. Acta Chir Scand 1938-1939, Suppl 53-57; p 1-142
13. Frenckner P: Bronchial and tracheal catheterization and its clinical applicability. Acta Oto-Laryngologica. 1934; Suppl XX: 1-134
14. Gale JW, Waters RM: Closed endobronchial anesthesia in thoracic surgary. J Thorag surg 1932; 1: 432-437
15. Gebauer PW: A catheter for bronchospirometry. J Thorac Surg 1939; 8: 674-82
16. Gordon WR, Green RA: A new right endobronchial tube. Lancet 1955; 1: 185
17. Head H: On the regulation of respiration. Part 1. Experimental. J Physiol 1889; 10: 1-70
18. Hess R: Über die Durchblutung nicht atmender Lungengebiete. Dtsch Arch Klin Med 1912; 106:478-88
19. Inoue H, Shohtzu A, Ogawa J, Kawada Sh, Koide Sh: New device for one-lung anesthesia: Endotracheal tube with movable blocker. J Thorac Cardiovasc Surg 1982; 83:940-41
20. Jacobaeus Hc, Frenckner P, Björkman S: Some attempts at determining the volume andfunction of each lung separately. Acta Med Scand 1932; 79:174-218
21. Jacobaeus HC: Bronchospiometry - a review of present experiences and some further investigations. J. Thorac Surg 1938; 7: 235-261
22. Johnstone JB: Jones PH: The treatment of bronchial carcinoma by lobectomy and resection of the main bronchus. Thorax 1959; 14: 48-54
23. Kuma S: Experimentelle Untersuchungen über Respiration und Zirkulation der Pneumothoraxlunge. Mitt. Aus d. Med. Fakult. d. Kais. Kyushu-Univ. 1925;10: 117-143
24. Kuma S: Experimentelle Untersuchungen über die operative Lungenkollapstherapie Mitt. Aus Med. Fakult. d. Kais. Kyushu-Univ. 1925; 10: 145-159
25. Loewy A, v. Schrötter H: Untersuchungen über die Blutcirculation beim Menschen. Zschr f exp Path u Ther 1905; 1: 197-311
26. Maar V: Experimentelle Untersuchungen über den Einfluss des Nervus vagus und des Nervussympathicus auf den Gaswechsel der Lungen. Scand Arch f Physiol 1902; 13: 269-315
27. Machray R: Anaesthesia for the surgical treatment of chest disease.Turberc Index Includ Chest Diseases 1958; 13: 172-178

28. Macintosh R, Leatherdale RAL: Bronchus tube and brochus blocker. Br J Anaesth 1955; 27: 556-57

29. Magill IW: Anaesthesia in thoracic surgery with special reference to lobectomy. Proc R Soc Med 1936; 29: 643-53

30. Mathieu P, Hermann H: Recherches sur la fonctionpulmonaire par l'emploi d'un diviseur d'air tracheal. Physiol Path Gen, 1925; 23: 39-46

31. Moody JD; Durham NC: A method of broncial occlusion for the prevention of tracheobronchial spread during lobectomy and pneumonectomy: clinical application. J Thorag Surg 1948; 17: 681-89

32. Moore RL: A Study of the Hering-Breuer-Reflex. J Exp Med 1927; 46: 819 ff

33. Nazari St, Moncalvo F, Bellizona G, Scaroni MT, Mapielli A: A new method of separate lung ventilation. J Thorac Cardiovasc Surg 1988; 95: 133-45

34. Pallister WK. A new endobronchial tube for left lung anaesthesia, with specific reference to reconstructive pulmonary surgery. Thorax 1959;14: 55-57

35. Pappin JC: The current practice of endobronchial intubation. Anaesthesia 1979; 57-64

36. Price Th C: Conservative resection of the bronchial tree. J R Coll Surg Edinb 1956; 1: 169-186

37. Robertshaw FL: Anaesthesia for pulmonary Surgary. In: General Anaesthesia. Eds: Gray TC, Nunn JF, Utting JE. 1980, Vol 2, 4th Ed. P 1325-1349

38. v Rohden F: Zur Blutzirkulation in der Lunge bei geschlossenem und offenem Thorax und deren Beeinflussung durch Über- und Unterdruck. Inauguraldissertation. F.C.W. Vogel, Leipzig 1913

39. Rusby LN, Thompson VC: Carcinoma of the lung: diagnosis and surgical treatment. Postgrad Med J 1943; 19: 44-46

40. Stürtzbecher F: Die Blockade feuchter Lungen mit einem Spezialkatheter. Anaesthesist 1953; 2:151-52

41. Werigo B: Zur Frage über die Wirkung des Sauerstoffs auf die Kohlensäureausscheidung in den Lungen. Pflügers Arch Physiol 1892; 51: 321-361

42. White G M J: A new double lumen tube. Br J Anaesth 1960; 32: 232-34

43. White G M J: Evolution of endotracheal and endobronchial intubation. Br J Anaesth 1960; 32: 235 246

44. Wilkinson D J: Who was Dr. Reuben Wade? In: Volume of Abstracts; Anaesthesia. 4th International Symposium of Anaestessia. Hamburg, FP 2, 3

45. Wolffberg S: Über die Spannung der Blutgase in den Lungencappilaren. Pflügers Arch f Physiol 1871; 4: 465 ff

The Story of the Wendl-Tube and its Use

H.K. Wendl
Wedel-Hospital, Wedel, Germany

In the fifties the Swiss anaesthetist Werner Hügin said that most physicians are capable of the most difficult diagnostical considerations, but are unable and helpless when faced with a case of acute suffocation. In 1955 I was confronted with an eclamptic patient suffering from multiple convulsions, followed by death of suffocation. Standard procedure at that time was the insertion of an oropharyngeal airway tube (Guedel - tube) having opened the patient's mouth.

Regarding this dramatic case, I thought of establishing a nasopharyngeal airway by means of a rubber tube - per vias naturalis, i.e. through the nose. In the Merck Manual 1961, no nasopharyngeal airway device is mentioned[1]. A special tube for this purpose was not available.

After having carried out some research, i.e. anatomical measurements in dead corpses and anaesthetized patients, I developed a standard tube made of soft red rubber manufactured by the Rüsch Company, known as Wendl-Tube which was mentioned in the Pschyrembel Medical Dictionary in 1986 for the first time[2].

Standard diameteres of tubes available for adults are Charrière 28-32 mm with a total length of 17 cm. In 1958 Dibold made some recommendations for children with a special scale[3].

Charrière 28 is a universal size that usually fits and can easily be put through the nose to the hypopharynx. The medium distance from the nostril to the hypopharynx comes to about 14 - 15 cm. The tubes are neither supposed to reach the trachea nor the esophagus. This is the reason why they are kept relatively short with a maximum lenght of 17 cm. The cone-shaped enlarged end sticks out of the nostril about 3 cm. Small adjustments can be made to improve ventilation by varying the depth of the tube. The movable rubber flange must be adjusted to lie on the nostril after the tube has been placed because it keeps the tube in situ[4,5]. To confirm that the tube is located correctly, one has to ensure that expired air is felt over the opening of tube. To be on the safe side in case shallow, ventilation it may be necessary to keep the lips and the other nostril closed (Fig. 1). If there is no breathing at all, mouth to nose breathing must be established via the tube. This we demonstrated in a film in which a fully curarized volunteer was kept oxygenized for 10 minutes without any difficulties[6].

This method does not compete with endotracheal intubation. Experience shows that even laymen are capable of inserting the tube successfully after quick instructions only. According to Werner Hossli it became part of the first aid kit of the Swiss Army in 1957[7].

Compared to the old oropharyngeal airway devices the nasal-tube provides a number of distinct advantages in emergency and first aid medicine:
- it can be put in place much more easily
- it is much more readily tolerated by restless patients
- it can be applied widely

On top of this, the tube has also been helpful when applied as an outer tube for the in-

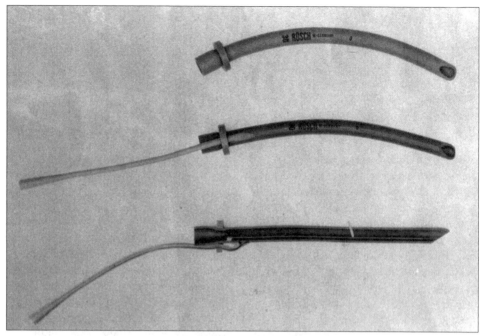

Fig. 1: Wendl's nasopharyngeal tubes. Above, the prototype with adjustable flange. Below, double-barreled tube. This type allows the application of oxygen or the insertion of a line for capnometry.

sertation of a thinner inner tube to facilitate suction. In cases of nose bleeding, it can be used as a tamponade as well as in cases of maxillo facial and jaw fractures. Its main function is to keep the upper airway clear in unconscious patients. According to Friedrich Ahnefeld, Wendl's tube is the device of choice to keep the upper airway open if the intubation of the tracheal is not intended or cannot be performed (8). Cardiopulmonary resuscitation became very popular in the mid-fifties, which favoured the invention of the tube, since free airways are mandatory for a successful procedure. The original prototype of the Wendl tube has been accepted. In 1965, ten years after the invention, about in 10 000 and 1992 more than 300 000 (!) of it were sold by the Rüsch-Company.

The patent was valid only until 1980, so that copies of the original could be manufactured, but not all of them met the neccessary specifications. The soft red rubber is by far the best material for the Wendl tube, because it is less traumatic as compared to polyethylen and other plastics which I do not generally approve of. Red soft rubber is slightly more expensive but a good value for little money. Apart from the prototype, there is a double barrelled tube that can be used for oxygen insufflation in cases of a reduced breathing volume. The standard length of this tube does not allows its insertion into the esophagus and thereby possible damage to the stomach (Fig. 3). Therefore the reported stomach ruptures, as mentioned by S. Geroulanos in a case report, are not likely to happen with an original Wendl tube [9].

If - on the other hand - the tubes are too short they may not reach the hypopharynx and fail to keep the airway open. The oxygen tube looks like the prototype with an oxygen pipeline inserting 3 cm from the cone shaped end. From this point down to the flute shaped end of the tube must be double barrelled inside.

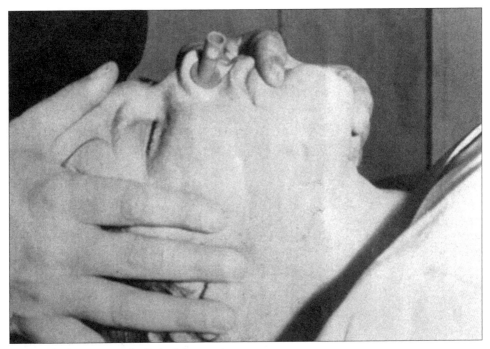

Fig. 2: The nasoparyngeal tube in daily practice

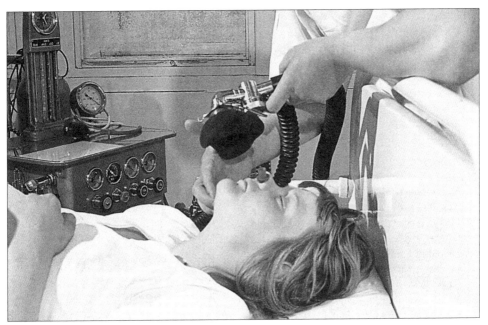

Fig. 3: The nasopharyngeal-tube in place by the flange. The cone-shaped end sticks out bout 2 cm. The tube can be used as a mouth piece for mouth to nose breathing, while left nostril and lips are held closed by the left hand thumb and indexfiger.

In any case, apart from more theoretical considerations, the advantages in the practical management for the unconscious or comatous shallow breathing patients are obvious. If the device seem to be too simple, give a thought to the fact that every idea, once fully developed, will seem thoroughly simple when in use. However, from the initial idea to the final product there are many steps, such as choosing the components of the product (soft red rubber in this case) and measuring lenght, width etc. The Rüsch-Company applied its know-how to provide these nasopharyngeal airways at reasonable costs. In times of expensive high-tech-medicine this has to be mentioned.

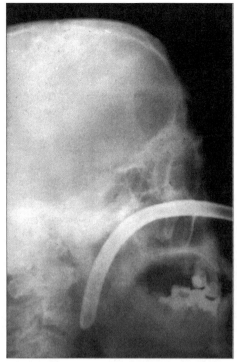

Fig. 4: An Y-ray to demonstrate the lenght of the tube in an anaesthetized patient.

References :

[1] Merck-Manual: MSD, 10 th Edition, Rahway, New Jersey 1961
[2] Pschyrembel W: Klinisches Wörterbuch. de Gruyter, Berlin 1986
[3] Dibold E: Freihaltung der oberen Atemwege in der Kiefer- und Gesichtschirurgie. Anaesthesist 1958; 100 : 298
[4] Wendl HK: Einfache Methode zur Freihaltung der oberen Luftwege. Hamburger Ärzteblatt 1958; 11 : 380-381
[5] Wendl HK: Nasopharyngeal tube. Disaster Medicine, Vol. II. Springer, Berlin-Heidelberg 1980
[6] Wendl HK: The naso-pharyngeal airway. Demonstration on a curarized patient.The film was produced in 1965. and is available by the author.
[7] Hossli W: personal communication
[8] Ahnefeld FW: Notfallmedizin, Springer, Berlin-Heidelberg 1980
[9] Geroulianos S: Magenruptur nach Sauerstoffinsufflation mit einem Nasen-Rachen-Katheter. Schweizer Medizinische Wochenschrift 1972; 102

Captain G.T. Smith-Clarke: Automobile and Medical Engineer

Chief Engineer: Alvis Car & Engineering Company 1922-1950

A. Padfield
Royal Hallamshire Hospital Sheffield S10 2RX, UK

George Thomas Smith-Clarke was born in Bewdley on 23rd December 1884 into a family whose roots lay in the Industrial Revolution. His full time education ended at the age of 13 but he went to evening classes whilst working as a bus conductor and in a pharmacy (an early contact with the medical profession). In 1902 he joined the Great Western Railway and was transferred to the Road Motor Department, Coventry in 1905. Here he was involved in the servicing & repair of both steam & petrol engined lorries and he attended evening classes at the Regent Street Polytechnic in 1910-12 for the City & Guilds Course in auto-mobile engineering. He was injured in a boiler explosion in 1912 and needed surgery to his nose and mouth; consequently he could not take the City & Guilds final examination. Nevertheless he was promoted to Chief Draughtsman in 1913 and in 1915 he became Captain in the Royal Flying Corps at the Aeronautical Inspection Directorate for Coventry. He was responsible for the testing of all the aero engines made by many famous motor engineers in Coventry and other cities. In his spare time he built a cyclecar and a motorscooter.

T.G.John, who founded the Alvis Car & Engineering Company in 1920, had met Smith-Clarke during the Great War. In 1922 John invited him to visit the works and see the Alvis 10/30 car. Even though it was superior in speed and handling to similar cars of that period, Smith-Clarke described it as 'a very poor car, very badly built'! He was promptly asked to join the firm and he created the famous Alvis 12/50 which in late 1923 won the 200 mile race at Brooklands at an average speed of over 93 mph. The basic design remained in production for 10 years and several hundred survive to-day (one is owned by the author). Smith-Clarke, however, was not satisfied and decided that front wheel drive (FWD) was better for competition. He reversed the 12/50 engine and in 1925 a FWD Alvis was winning sprints and hillclimbs. In 1926 Alvis FWD cars with redesigned engines went on sale to the public and at Le Mans in 1928, FWD Alvises were 6th & 9th winning their class.

* * *

In 1935 Smith-Clarke became Chairman of Coventry and Warwickshire Hospital (Fig. 1). His early contact with medicine both in a chemist's shop and as a patient had made him sympathetic and interested in medical problems - a parallel may be drawn here with William Morris, Lord Nuffield. For 25 years until his death in 1960 he was involved in medical bodies but also in very practical ways; designing, making and modifying medical equipment from the Iron Lung to surgical scissors. He himself designed and made an automatic angiocardiograph in 1949, an electrically driven trepanning cutter for neurosurgery and a tool for removing broken femoral pins. He also designed a foot operated suction unit, a stretcher and hoist for lifting patients into a tank for hydrotherapy he had planned for a Coventry hospital and a stroboscope for eye

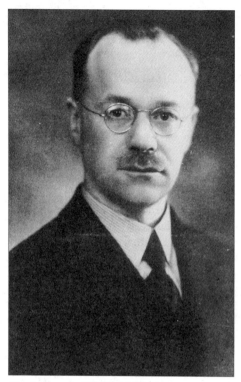

Fig. 1: Captain G.T. Smith-Clarke

tests. However, Smith-Clarke should be best known for his modifications and then complete redesign of the Both 'Iron Lung'. His James Clayton Lecture to the Institution of Mechanical Engineers in 1956 gives the full details of this work. In 1938/9 Lord Nuffield had paid for several thousand iron lungs and they were distributed throughout Britain and the Empire becoming the most commonly used device for respiratory failure following bulbar poliomyelitis. When Smith-Clarke retired from Alvis in 1950 polio was epidemic and much feared; the iron lungs (actually made of wood) were decaying and they were not 'user friendly'.

Smith-Clarke on one of his hospital visits had been horrified at the distress of a woman taken out of an iron lung to be washed and tidied up. He redesigned the cabinet with better access ports and windows, lighting and heating, a pressure alarm, better wheels and balance for mobility, improved tilting and sliding devices and a split collar for more comfort. The Both pump was modified to make it less noisy with more useful respiratory rates, variable inspiratory/expiratory ratios and finer adjustment of positive and negative pressures. The pump unit had been designed for hand operation in case of electricity failure but it required a strong man to do it even for a short time. By changing to a lever action with a better mechanical advantage it was possible for a nurse to operate the pump for some time without fatigue. Modifications had been carried out by August 1952 on an iron lung in Coventry and were accepted by the Birmingham Regional Hospital Board and by the Ministry of Health soon after. Kits of parts were needed to modify iron lungs around the country and were manufactured by a new company: Cape Engineering of Warwick. Smith-Clarke also made an adaptor so that the modified Both pump would power 'Cuirasse' ventilators and he redesigned the Rocking Bed so that it could be actuated by the pump motor.

With Smith-Clarke's encouragement two Alvis ex-employees had founded Cape Engineering and he was able to help them in various ways. When he completely redesigned the iron lung, Cape Engineering produced the prototype to his instructions in March 1954. The Coventry Cabinet Breathing Machine Mark I was not wholly successful as various design details were unsatisfactory, notably the use of fibreglass for the top cover. After about eight had been made, a Mark II Coventry was constructed of metal and put into production. A large number of Mark II machines were delivered to hospitals both at home and abroad.

When Smith-Clarke heard of the use of intermittent positive pressure ventilation during the severe polio epidemic in Copenhagen in 1952 and he set to work to design a machine to provide this. He spent some time trying to perfect an automatic inspiratory/expiratory valve but decided that mechanically operated valves were more reliable and efficient. The machine he designed, which Cape Engineering produced, had cam operated poppet valves like a automobile engine and in fact the prototype used Morris car inlet valves! Many electrically driven ventilators were produced and used in anaesthesia but were superseded by a combined anaesthetic machine and ventilator manufactured by Cape and designed in conjunction with Dr Waine; anaesthetist at Coventry.

Smith-Clarke died at home on 28th February 1960 having been in failing health for several years. He was not honoured by his country for diverse activities in automobile and aero engineering for over fifty years, for his help in the design of the Jodrell Bank radiotelescope (he was a keen amateur astronomer) and, not least, for his altruistic services for mankind. The author hopes that he has redressed this lack of recognition to a small extent.

Louis Ombrédanne and his Ether Inhaler. The Man and his Contribution to Anaesthesia in Central Europe viewed Today and in his Time.

J. Plötz, Department of Anaesthesia, Klinikum Bamberg, Germany

Louis Ombrédanne was a Paris surgeon of international distinction, but possibly his ether inhaler was more responsible than his surgical accomplishments for his place in posterity. Born in 1871, he began his professional career in the hospital of the Paris suburb of Saint-Antoine where his father, shining example to the son, worked for 45 years as general practitioner. In 1920, Ombrédanne became the chief-of-staff of the Hôpital des Enfants-Malades, in 1925, full professor; he retired in 1941 and in 1956, broken-hearted, he followed his beloved wife who had died several months earlier. His clinical and scientific work is quite diverse with pediatric surgery dominating. Functioning as author and editor, he left behind a publication catalogue of 200 titles, six of which are of anaesthesiological relevance.

Prof. Louise Delègue, the first director and present Chef Honoraire of the Département d'Anesthésie of the Hôpital des Enfants-Malades, recalls the year 1938 and the man who was at that time already 67 years old: "His stately figure, his moustache à la Napoleon III, his elegant appearance impressed me as a young student. His heigth, his firm voice, his direct glance all underscored the authority of his position as chairman and clinical director of the most distinguished pediatric surgery in Paris and France..." His former students extol his inventive spirit, the soundness and lucidity of his research and teaching; they admire his independence, sincerity, and indisputable self-assurance and recall his friendly attitude toward the sick but also his sensitivity and dejection when he suffered setbacks[1,2]. The small patients would call to him: "Monsieur, donnez-nous nos billes!" (give us our marbles), and he would treat them - using his own operation and anaesthesiological techniques. Ombrédanne was patriotic, loved military pomp, always carried his Képi de Colonel with him and signalled his chauffeur by clairon de cavalerie to tell him to make ready to go. His private sector was composed of the family, literature, music and country life outside of the metropolis on his estate in Septeuil, but also to a great part of handicraft and tinkering. In retirement he even became an apprentice to a book-binder and described the knowledge he acquired[2].

Ombrédanne criticized the closed English inhalers in the following ways: the discontinuity of their functioning due to frequent lifting of the mask to allow influx of fresh air; application of liquid ether with only a limited evaporation surface; ensuing clinical complications. With his apparatus of 1908 he aimed at providing a more continuous course of anaesthesia whereby fresh air would be drawn in with every breath and the exhaled air would be more effectively enriched with the narcotic agent by sending it through a chamber containing sponges or felt imbibed with ether. By way of a lever the mechanism could be regulated so that the patient in position zero inhaled mainly fresh air, only a small amount of exspired gas and no ether, in the middle position 4 less fresh air but more exspired air containing ether, and in position 8 the least amount of fresh air and the most exspired air saturated with ether[3]. Sir Robert MacIntosh spoke of "a French modification and equivalent"[4], but also of an "outrageous crib of the Clover"[5]. Wawersik places the Ombrédanne between the Clover and its successors and the EMO-inhaler[6]. According to Barry, more than 25000 units of the apparatus were sold just by the Paris company of Collin alone[7].

As opposed to its native country, the inhaler made its mark in non-French publications only after a considerable delay. The gynaecologist Henkel of Jena and the surgeon Boit of Königsberg became acquainted with it at the university clinics in Buenos Aires and Kowno/Lithuania and reported on it starting in 1927[8,9]. Following this and up until the early post-war period, the use of the apparatus became extensive in all of Europe with the exception of Great Britain. The following circumstances might have encouraged its acceptance in Germany: ether, applied by auxiliary persons in an open system, had been for the most part a routine procedure, but the dose-dependent secretion and obstruction of the respiratory passage were considered substantial problems. However, the pharmacologist, Paul Trendelenburg of Berlin, was able to demonstrate here in Hamburg at the Meeting of Natural Scientists and Physicians in 1928 that a reduction of the ether dosis - in this case 50 %- can by all means occur with an accelerated saturation of arterial blood when the alveolar ventilation is incremented by CO_2 to the inspired air[10]. Involuntarily he thus promoted the Ombrédanne principle of functioning.

Advantages noted in publications from the very beginning were the facility of use by auxiliary personnel, less excitation, precision of the dosage, rarer respiratory problems and cost reduction; a Polish author wrote in 1932 that these qualities had even been recognized by the Germans who otherwise rejected any and all French accomplishments[11]. A cost comparison of anaesthesia for two similar stomach resections shows that the reduction in drugs leads to a quick amortization of the mask. The only disadvantage noted is its weight of 1.000 g, about the double of the Clover. Due to patent law, the attempt to construct the apparatus out of light-metal had to be abandoned[12]. To improve manageability, alterations in positioning were undertaken: hanging it, suspending it, altering its standing and holding position. Clinically and experimentally the apparatus was closely studied, for example, in relation to the course of respiratory, cardiovascular, and metabolic parameters, the vaporization behavior of the individual components of an ethylchloride/ether/chloroform mixture or to O_2 and CO_2 content in in- and exhaled air, in the alveoli, in arterial and venous blood[13]. These studies, aspiring towards more knowledge, were followed in World War II by only insipid repetitions of the claim that auxiliary personnel could apply Ombrédanne anaesthesia anytime under field conditions. Some rather odd memorabilia have surfaced lately: in the South Atlantic in 1982 a slightly damaged Ombrédanne inhaler with the name of its manufacturer „Industria E.L. Argentina", fell into the hands of the British; as late as 1985, a West German company was offering it to customers in eastern Europe, and in 1996 two brand-new specimens were discovered unpacked in a company ware-house in Leipzig.

Viewed today it seems justified to me to conclude that the Ombrédanne inhaler smoothed the course of anaesthesia in comparison to the drip method, allowed the controlling signals from the operating surgeon to the person performing the anaesthesia to be more precise, and reduced the danger of perioperative respiratory complications. The paradox is that its qualities presumably contributed not only to more safety in anaesthesia but also to the delay in the transfer of modern anaesthetic standards from the

Anglo-Saxon countries to central Europe. This delay is, however, the fault of others rather than Louis Ombrédanne. He who, according to his student Jacques Mialaret, followed with great interest in his retirement the development of anaesthesia, expressed his attitude succintly with the following words: "All methods are of a transitory nature, and the assumption that one of them could be definite means the anegation of progress"[14].

Acknowledgement

I thank Prof. Louise Delègue for personal communications and her permission to quote.

References:

[1] Fèvre M: Louis Ombrédanne (1871-1956). Nécrologie. La Presse Médicale 1957; 65: 99

[2] Van Doorne L: Louis Ombrédanne (1871-1956): L'homme au masque. Dissertation, Caen 1996

[3] Ombrédanne L: Un appareil pour l'anesthésie par l'éther. Gaz Hôp 1908; 81: 1095

[4] Macintosh Sir R: Saved by the flagg. In: Atkinson R S and T B Boulton (eds): The History of Anaesthesia. International Congress and Symposium Series Number 134. The Parthenon Publishing Group, 1989

[5] Macintosh R A: Ralph M Waters Memorial Lecture. Anaesthesia 1970; 25: 4

[6] Wawersik J: Entwicklung der Narkosegeräte. In: Zinganell K (ed): Anaesthesie - historisch gesehen. Anaesthesiologie und Intensivmedizin Vol 197. Springer Berlin Heidelberg New York London Paris Tokyo, 1987

[7] Barry C T: The Ombrédanne inhaler. Anaesthesia 1961; 16: 184

[8] Boit: Dreijährige Erfahrungen mit dem Äthernarkoseapparat nach Obrédanne. Arch klin Chir 1927; 148: 117

[9] Henkel M: Narkoseapparat von Ombrédanne-Collin. Z Geburtsh 1928; 41: 146

[10] Trendelenburg P: Theorie des Narkotisierens mit Gasen. Narkose u Anästhesie 1929; 2: 1

[11] Szymonowicz J: Zalety stosowania uspienia aparatem Ombrédanne'a. Polska Gaz Lek 1932; 11: 335

[12] Hauberrisser E: Narkose. Fortschr d Zahnheilk 1929; 6: 86

[13] Fohl T, Eitel H: Klinische und experimentelle Studie über die Inhalationsnarkose mit Rückatmung. Klin Wschr 1929, 32: 1487

[14] Mialaret J: Louis Ombrédanne (1871-1956). Mem Acad Chir 1969; 95: 1

The Ombrédanne Inhaler and its Modifications

C. Parsloe
Hospital Samaritano, São Paulo, SP, Brasil

Louis Ombrédanne, a French surgeon, at the suggestion of Nélaton, designed a new ether - air inhaler in 1908. It was based on the principle of rebreathing expired air in order to provide CO_2 respiratory stimulation. It took 5 years to develop the prototype. The admission of air, however limited, represented an improvement on the Clover inhaler. Ombrédanne's inhaler was known in everyday practice as the Ombrédanne apparatus or mask. It was relatively small, simple, portable and required no expertise to be handled. Consequently, it achieved much popularity in Continental Europe and in Latin America as well as in the Francophone areas of the World for more than 4 decades. When I first used it during the 1940s it was found in every operating room in Brasil.

It was manufactured in France by Collin and proved to be a resistant piece of apparatus with a long working life time. Collin had changed the original ether reservoir giving it an spherical form. *Une boite de fer blanc pour bonbons anglais.*

Ombrédanne stated that an anesthesia apparatus is not an automatic device to put patients to sleep. It is a device which allows for the continuous administration of the necessary and sufficient anesthetic dose. Improperly used it may cause cyanosis. He established 5 *propositions* or principles for the development of the new inhaler.

1st Principle - Induction with a mixture of ether vapour and fresh air is impossible; maintenance with ether - air is possible. The difficulty of ether induction was in fact one of the main reasons for developing the new inhaler.

2nd Principle - Confined air breathing to take advantage of CO_2 stimulation of breathing. Julliard large open mask to a certain extent created rebreathing conditions and it was apparent that it facilitated induction.

3rd Principle - The channels inside the inhaler should be of large diameter. He was aware of the need to prevent increased resistance to breathing through narrow channels.

4th Principle - Fresh air is necessary throughout the anesthesia; the necessary proportion need not be large. The first part of the principle concerned his witnessing of Clover's inhaler use in London which he criticised on account of the need to periodically remove it from the face of the patient in order to allow breathing of fresh air. Ombrédanne was familiar with Buxton's text-book description of the Clover inhaler.

5th Principle - The vaporizing surface should be large. Originally he used sponges and later pieces of felt in the reservoir to imbibe the liquid ether and act as vaporing surfaces.

The main advantage of the Ombrédanne inhaler was its simplicity of operation since no special skills were required and no gases were used, except air. The inhaler could be visualized as a 3 - way stop - cock allowing the patient to breathe variable mixtures of fresh air , confined air and ether vapor. A removable lid on top of the ether reservoir allowed for pouring ether to be imbibed in the felt. On the lower part, a short wide bore metallic connector received a metal mask piece which was covered with a rubber cushion. A dial on the left side of the inhaler could be moved from 0 to 8 which progressively increased the amount of expired air and ether vapor breathed while decreasing the diameter of the air intake.

On the right side of the inhaler, a pigs bladder served as the rebreathing bag. It was not possible to assist respiration, which was not a detriment to its use since such a concept did not exist at the time. The patient breathed spontaneously throughout the anesthesia. In fact, one of the anesthetic complications was apnea, called the blue syncope, which required manual methods of artificial respiration performed by the surgeon and the administration of respiratory stimulants such as lobeline by the anesthetizer.

Ombrédanne stated that carbon dioxide in small amounts is a useful adjuvant to anesthesia but it has to be kept low in order to avoid accidents, such as cyanosis.

At the time Yandell Henderson's physiological teachings were dominant and the acapnic theory of shock was widely accepted. Thus, rebreathing expired air was considered essential to maintain respiration during anesthesia and to prevent shock.

Over the years the inhaler's shortcomings became apparent and several modifications were introduced in order to overcome its perceived limitations.

The apparatus had to be used in the vertical position. Therefore, it was difficult to use it if the patient had to be in the lateral position and even worse, in the prone position. A metallic right angle piece could be placed between the short connecting piece from the inhaler and the mask for use with the patient in the lateral position. A long tube could be adapted between the short connecting piece from the inhaler and the mask when the patient was in the prone position. The narrow diameter of this tube was severely critised by Macintosh in his book Physics for the Anaesthetist.

Thalheimer used a metallic device placed between the rebreathing bladder and the inhaler in order to introduce carbon dioxide into the system. A Leclerc stop-cock in the device could be opened or closed allowing for the introduction of carbon dioxide from a rubber reservoir bag of 2 liters capacity. The carbon dioxide was provided from a commercial Sparklet containing 4 liters of gas. When deemed necessary, the same Thalheimer device could be used to administer ethyl chloride.

Desplas placed a similar device directly at the mask which seemed like a better location for immediate effect. He also used a Sparklet as the source for carbon dioxide.

Robert Monod, who was later instrumental in furthering the idea of A World Federation of Societies of Anaesthesia, used a rubber tube placed at the mask piece for addition of CO_2.

Years later in the late 40s when oxygen cylinders were brought into the operating room many anesthetizers found a simple way to administer oxygen by using a rubber tube under the mask.

Dogliotti-Giordanengo modified the Ombrédanne inhaler allowing for the administration of ethyl chloride and even nitrous oxide.

Martinez used a long, large bore, tube placed between the inhaler and the mask. Furthermore, he fixed the inhaler on a trolley with 2 large cylinders, of oxygen and nitrous oxide. In fact, this modification removed the inhaler from the patient making the handling of the apparatus considerably simpler since the anaesthetist only had to hold the face mask. Thus, operations on the head and the neck or in extreme Trendelemburgs position could be used without much difficulty. The mask could be held by a strap around the head thus effectively removing the anesthetist from the proximity of the operating field. The flow of gases or ethyl chloride vapor was delivered by means of a Thalheimer device placed directly at the mask.

In 1950, Nesi (1) from Buenos Aires, introduced the last modification and in fact the first one that was physiologically sound. The air inlet was closed and replaced by an inlet at the center of the regulating dial for the administration of small flows of oxygen; an expiratory valve was added and the pigs bladder substituted by a rubber bag which allowed for assisted or controlled respiration. A flexible connector could be adapted to an endotracheal tube. Professor Nesi used this modification in 2 patients for lobectomies.

By this time modern equipment was becoming available in most parts of the world and the Ombrédanne inhaler was being removed from every day use. Anesthesia machines with flowmeters and carbon dioxide absorbers, allowing for physiological gas exchange and for assisted or controlled respiration were commonly used. Henderson's acapnia theory was no longer accepted and Waters had proved that instead of rebreathing carbon dioxide it should be removed from the breathing systems. Untoward effects were no longer observed during anaesthesia and patients could be successfully maintained anaesthetised for any lenght of time.

During its extensive use over a period of more than 40 years, when there were no anesthesiologists available, Ombrédanne's inhaler was handled by different types of non qualified personnel and permitted the advancement of surgery. The need for controlled respiration after the introduction of curare, for the administration of oxygen and for removal of carbon dioxide from the breathing system, which was not possible, certainly were major determinants of the ubiquitous Ombrédanne inhaler demise.

References:

Ombrédanne L: Un appareil pour l'anesthesie par l'éther. Gazette des Hôpitaux Civils et Militaires. La Lancette Française 1908; 81: 1095, 1908

Forgue E: Précis d'Anesthésie Chirurgicale. G. Doin & Cie 1934

Maisonnet J: Manuel Pratique d'Anesthésie Chirurgicale. G. Doin & Cie 1936

Hesse F, Lendle L, Schoen R: Anestesia Geral e Parcial, Companhia Melhoramentos de So Paulo, 1937. Portuguese translation from the German text

Kirschner M: Tratado de Tecnica Operatoria General y Especial. Editorial Labor S. A., 1940. Spanish translation from the German text

Dogliotti AM: Tratado de Anestesia. Editorial Scientifica, 1943. Portuguese translation from the Italian text.

Martinez JM: Tratado de Anestesia. Salvat. Barcelona 1946

Macintosh RR, Mushin WW: Physics for the Anaesthetist. Charles C. Thomas, Publisher 1947

Weißer Ch: Der Ombrédanne Aether-Inhalator. Anaesthesist 1983; 32: 51-54

(1) Nesi JA: Personal communication.

Russian Modifications by Sadevenko and Gersch of Ombrédanne's Inhaler (1908)

J. W. R. McIntyre †
University of Alberta Hospital, Edmonton, Canada

Louis Ombrédanne described his inhaler in 1908[1] and French trade and cultural routes helped models to be widely distributed: South America, Indo-China, Japan, Germany and Eastern Europe. In 1933[2], Sadevenko drew attention to what may well have been the Russian point of view. Ombrédanne's inhaler was: functionally satisfactory; ergonomically too large, too heavy, with too high a centre of gravity; economically unsatisfactory because of its short life; and cost because it was an import. The claim that its life was short must surely indicate that the Russian environment for the inhaler was unusually rigorous.

Sadevenko described his own inhaler which he claimed, without evidence, to be functionally just as effective as Ombrédanne's device. The improvements were ergonomic and economic. Weight was reduced from approximately 935G to 450G. The centre of gravity was lowered and it conformed to the shape of the hand. It was Russian made, less complex and cheaper. Indeed Sadevenko's inhaler would be easier to handle, but its working diagram[2] does not indicate reduced complexity.

Gersch writing from Kineshem in 1935[3] shared that final view and had his own criticisms of Sadevenko's inhaler. Functionally, the external regulator of delivered vapour concentration was unreliable. Economically, the construction was difficult and costly. It was the product of somebody working in a favoured environment and not in an under-privileged regional hospital. (Kineshem was probably about 300 miles northeast of Moskow). Line diagrams of his own first inhaler certainly show a much simplified device that was satisfactory in clinical use. His second device, described at the same time, was even simpler and closely resembles an early prototype of Ombrédanne's described in 1908[1].

Clover's inhaler[4] was adopted around the world according to British trade and culture routes, and because of a satisfactory clinical function, merited improvement of its defects as perceived by certain anesthetists during the subsequent years. Functionally: the ether delivery was calibrated. Ergonomically: the ether reservoir was made visible; the water jacket was made accessible, the reservoir could be refilled while the mask was on the patients face, a lever control of the control tube was incorporated, the weight was reduced, it was more easily grasped, the centre of gravity was lowered, and the body-mask union was improved. From an economic point of view, the significance of changes made uncertain but a reduced verdigris formation may have saved money. The device was often sterilizable. From 1877 these modifications occurred during the subsequent 25 years[5,6]. The chronology of the improvements of the Clover inhaler and the attempted adoption and modification of Ombrédanne's inhaler in Russia, reflect the unfortunate timelag in the development of anaesthesia practice in those two countries.

References:

[1] Ombrédane L: Un appareil pour l'anesthésie per l'éther. Gaz d Hôp, Par 1908: Ixxxi: 1095-1100

[2] Sadevenko GY: Dr. Sadevenko apparatus for ether narcotisation. Sovet Khir 1933; 3:122-8

[3] Gersch LY: New simplified apparatus of Ombrédanne type. Sovet Khir 1935; 7: 154-157

[4] Clover JT: Portable regulating ether inhaler. Br Med J. 1877; i:69-70

[5] Galley AH, King AC: Modifications of the Clover's ether inhaler. Anaesthesia 1948; 3: 147-153

[6] Thomas KB: The Development of Anaesthesia Apparatus. Blackwell, Oxford 1975

The Göttinger Model - a Trichloroethylene-Vaporizer

P. Ahrens and U. Braun
Department of Anaesthesiology, Emergency- and Intensive-Care-Medicine
University of Göttingen, Germany

We would like to present to you an anaesthetic instrument, which caused some attention in the early fifties of our century, especially in obstetrics. We are referring to the Goettinger model, designed by Professor Hans Hosemann and his assistant Theodor Hickl.

These two gynaecologists from Goettingen developed in cooperation with the Draeger Company Lübeck their own vaporizer, encouraged by the positive experience of Angloamerican obstetricians with the application of Trichloroethylene (later called Trilene). They called it the Göttinger Model. They used Trilene as an analgesic, not as a hypnotic drug in the obstetrics in Germany, according to Seitz from Frankfurt.

In the beginning the main problem was to get the pure Trichorethylene. This substance was created by the German E. Fischer in 1864. It desintegrated very quickly into the explosive Dichloracythelene, hydrochloric acid, Phosgen and Carbomonoxyde. After World War 2 the German industry was able to manufacture extremely pure Trilene. In 1950 there were nearly 20 devices for Trilene delivery. The two doctors Hosemann and Hickl created their own apparatus, because they considered the existing models (narcotic and analgetic) as too difficult to handle.

This handy model with a height of only 12cm was filled with 7 ml Trilene. The strength of the used glass prevented patients of biting it into pieces. The inhalator was placed around the patients neck using a cord. The wide mouthpiece reduced negative olfactoric sensations and it prevented irritations of the mucosae. The patient's hand, which enclosed the apparatus increased the evaporation of the Trilene through its warmth. The introduction into this simple technique of using this system was mostly performed in the labour room; the application in home deliveries was seen as an advantage too. It took fifteen minutes to teach the patient

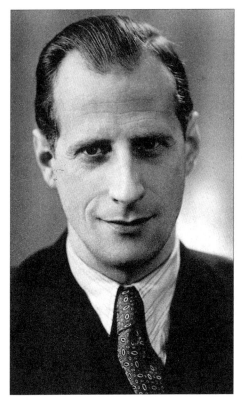

Portrait of Hans Hosemann

The clinical experience showed a pain-soothing effect without consciousness being clouded. So guidance of the patients by the midwife and the obstetrician was possible at any time. Depending on the strength of their labour pains the women could regulate the analgesia themselves individually. The pain reducing effekt through the vapour started after 15-30 minutes and lasted for about 10-15 minutes. Another advantage was the low vaporizer-price of 15 DM per piece, which was quite cheap even in those times.

In the years 1950-1952 more than 2000 births were performed by the Goettinger gynaecologists with the help of the Goettinger Model. All births were without any maternal complications and intrauterine asphyxia occured more seldom than before. The exact numbers were 4.3 % intrauterine asphyxia with using trilene, versus 5.2 % without trilene. The duration of birth and the uterine contractions were also not negatively influenced. 95 % of the women were satisfied with this treatment, of which 83 % were completely, only 17 % were partially satisfied.

Although Hosemann and Hickl predicted a glorious future for this procedure, soothing of labour pains with Trilene did not come to stay. One important reason was the relative danger of the substance, which was only realised after some time. Besides cardiac arrhythmias the potent lipophilia led to liver- and kidney damages. Apart from that paresthesia and paralysis of cerebral nerves occurred.

Today it appears to us, that the main reason for completely giving up trichloroethylene-analgesia was the wide introduction of the more harmless nitrous-oxide with even better forms of application. Hosemann himself wrote in 1951, that analgesia with nitrous oxide might play a significant role in the future.

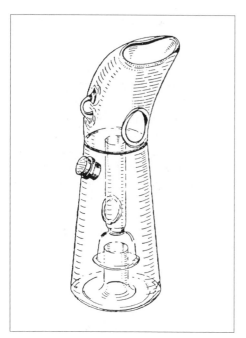
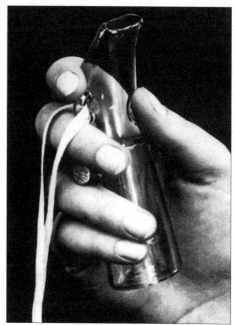

2. + 3. Figures of the Göttinger Modell

References:

Hosemann H: Die Schmerzlinderung unter der Geburt. Med Klin 1951; 46: 70-74

Hosemann H: Die Wirkung des Trichloräthylens als Analgeticum; Arch Gyn 1951; 180: 44-47

Hosemann H: Schmerzlinderung mit Trichloräthylen; Urban & Schwarzenberg Verlag, München 1952

Hosemann H, Hickel Th: Erfahrungen mit der Anwendung von Trichloräthylen zur Schmerzlinderung unter der Geburt; Dtsch Med Wschr 1951; 76: 725-727

Forgotten Jewish Pioneers of German Anaesthesia

M. Goerig and J. Schulte am Esch
Department of Anaesthesiology,
University Hospital Hamburg, Germany

The contribution of Jewish investigators to the development of anaesthesia in Germany has never been honored, although their achievement concerning pain therapy during the passed 150 years has been outstanding. We have not been able to find out what this ignorance results from, since the important role that Jewish physicians have played in other medical fields has been mentioned repeatedly. The Jewish origin of a lot of famous people involved in the medical profession has not become commonly known, because they converted to christianism, changed names, have been forgotten due to the turmoil raised through nationalism or even had to die during this time [27]. Lacking interest in or unawareness of historical events and not wanting to face the facts could be additional reasons.

The authors of this article would like to fill this gap and to illustrate the importance of Jewish physicians in the development of anaesthesia in Germany, though it certainly is impossible to go into detail and to appreciate their contribution as deeply as it deserves to be appreciated. This is going to be about innovations that have become indispensable in our daily routing and have been developed in the second half of the last century and invented by Jewish doctors of medicine. Before getting into detail of this development, the authors would like to point out some facts on the economic crisis during the thirties that led to the banishment of the Jewish.

The healing art comprised a significant number of Jewish origin in Germany, because

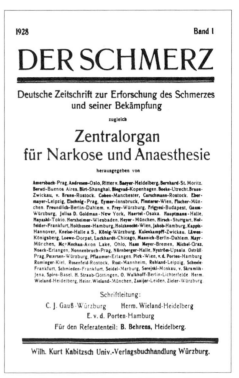

Fig. 1 Cover page of the first German Anaesthesia journal "Der Schmerz", 1928[13]

of a strong flow into different academic profession after the middle of the last century. The French Revolution in 1789 gave rise to changed attitudes and ideals that granted proper conditions for tolerance, acceptance and equality of rights even having an influence on the expulsion of Jewish in certain German states, although it took decades until were allowed to pick up a profession. In 1871 after the German Reich being founded, complete equality of rights was certified. Prejudice was still an inhibitory factor inspite of it all, as can be proved by the fact, that they were rarely employed in civil service.

If a Jew had decided to obtain an academic career he had to choose between being a lawyer or a physician in order to be socially accepted. This resulted in a proportionally high share of them in these fields. At the turn of the century about 16% of the practitioners - as compared to 1.2% of the overall population - were of Jewish origin. This was even more obvious in major cities like Berlin or Frankfurt them amounting up to 45%, which did not change for decades! Relating to the fact that they were often better off than their "German" colleagues - remember, a lot of the private clinics belonged to them - they became a favourite target for hostilities and eruptions of hatred for the nationalists [24].

Jewish people often became specialists in hospitals, worked in a private practice, kept important positions among other practitioners or in the industrial or economic field, as well as in trade unions. So it does not seem strange that Jewish doctors played an important role in publishing two of the first German journals on anaesthesiology, e.g. Co-editors of "Der Schmerz" (i.e."Pain") were Jewish specialists: Jurisprudence - Ludwig Ebermayer (?) (Leipzig), anaesthesiologist - Ernst von der Porten (1884-1940) (Hamburg), ophthalmologist - Anton Elschnig (1863-?) (Prague), otorhinolaryngologists - Karl Amersbach (1884-?) (Prague) and Cesar Hirsch (1897-1940) (Stuttgart), pathologist - Gotthold Herxheimer (1872-1936)(Wiesbaden), pediatrician - Ernst Rominger (1886-1967) (Kiel), pharmacologist - Siegfried

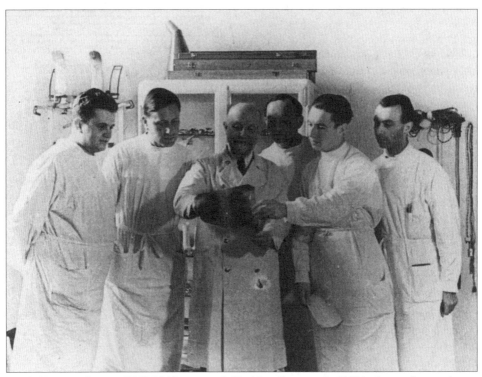

Fig. 2 Hermann Strauss (1868-1944) surrounded by his colleagues. In 1907 he invented a popular venous cannula which is still in use [13]

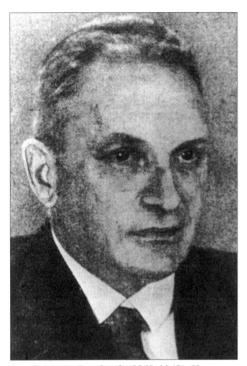

Fig. 3 Moritz Borchardt (1868-1948). He was a great supporter of intravenous anaesthesia techniques [13]

Loewe (1884-1962) (Dopart) and Pick (Vienna), physiologist - and Emil Ritter von Skramlik (1886-1970)(Jena), psychiatrist - Max Rosenfeld (1871-?), and Guido Holzknecht (1872-1931)(Vienna), urologist - Eduard Pflaumer (1872-1957)(Erlangen) (Fig. 1). All of the above mentioned specialists in Germany became unemployed after the nationalsocialist party took over. Some of them were banished or murdered, others committed suicide. In addition to the economic crisis, young consultants had great difficulties looking for jobs, since the number of students admitted to universities trippled between 1925 and 1932. As the "Law for the Reconstruction of civil service" became effective on April 7th, 1933, the conditions for working Jews worsend dramatically, since they had to leave communal and public hospitals, University- hospitals and other public institutions resulting in unemployment and poverty [2]. In 1938 the whole affair was topped by a law prohibiting Jewish physicians to treat patients other than Jews and forcing them to call themselves "Krankenbehandler" (i.e. who is treating the sick) instead of "Arzt" (i.e. doctor of medicine). Considering these circumstances it is not really suprising that the number of "non-Aryan" practitioners fell from 9.000 in April 1933 to 4.000, in July to 5.000 in January 1936, to 3.900 in January 1938, and finally only 709 non-Aryan people "treating the sick" were left. At this point in time thousands of physicians, especially the younger ones, decided to leave the country heading for other countries in Europe, Palestine or other places overseas, e.g. the United States. The elder ones though could not get themselves together to dare a step like this giving a variety of reasons, rendering them as helpless as other non-Aryans who did not find the courage to leave everything behind [24].

Looking at the development of infusion therapy and techniques in anaesthesia, we find quite a few Jewish medical doctors to have been involved, e.g. Emil Schwarz (1865-1955) who worked in Halle/Saale in 1880 can be considered a pioneer in infusion therapy. He wrote a script about his result after having carried out experiments on animals in order to become a senior lecturer (i.e. "Habilitation") at a time when this method still was believed not to be appropriate. Schwarz was born in Vienna, went to the Rudolfspital in Vienna, where he occupied an executive Position and emigrated to the United States of America in the beginning of World War II, working as a research assistant in the department of hematology until his death in 1955 [12].

A few years after his thesis on infusion therapy had been accepted there was a change in views on this method - it was antiquated not to be skilled in this regard resulting from the invention of Salvarsan. Paul Ehrlich

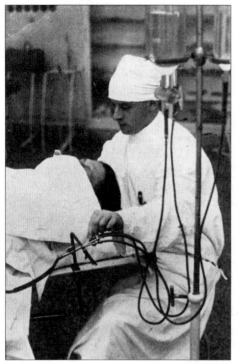

Fig. 4 Ernst Berla (1901-1962) performing an intravenous ether anaesthesia [13]

linked to an apparatus for anaesthesia for the administration of oxygen and chloroform [48]. Another forgotten pioneer in intravenous techniques was Felix Mendel (1862-1925), but we do not know whether they ever met[35].

We have not yet been able to disclose, whether Strauss knew Moritz Borchardt (Fig.3) (1868-1948), chairman of the Department of Surgery at a hospital in Moabit/ Berlin from 1919-1933, who was keen on achieving advances in the field of neurosurgery as well as anaesthesiology, e.g. he believed in intravenous administration of ether and published a lot of data about this method along with his co-worker Cohen (?) and Ernst Berla (1901-1962)[3] (Fig.4). Being Jewish, Borchardt had to retire and was able to emigrate to South America. He died in Buenos Aires in 1948 [39].

(1854-1914) and his Japanese co-worker Sachahiro Hata (1878-1938) discovered that from a toxicological point of view this substance had to be administered intravenously, initiating a widely spread desire for a training in this procedure. Unfortunately, a suitable needle for puncturing veins was lacking, giving rise to the evolution of several cannulaes, e.g. the "Strauss-cannule", that is still available. It has been created by the internist Hermann Strauss (1868-1944) (Fig.2) from Berlin, who presented it for the first time in 1905 [42]. At that time he was working in a Jewish hospital in Berlin, the place that he had to leave because he was taken to the concentration camp Theresienstadt in 1942, where he died in 1944 [39]. He definately had been in contact with the Jewish surgeon Heinz Wohlgemuth (1863-1936) who worked at the same hospital and whose name is

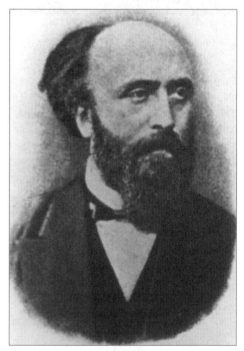

Fig. 5 Oskar Liebreich (1839-1908) who described the hypnotic qualities of chloralhydrate [23]

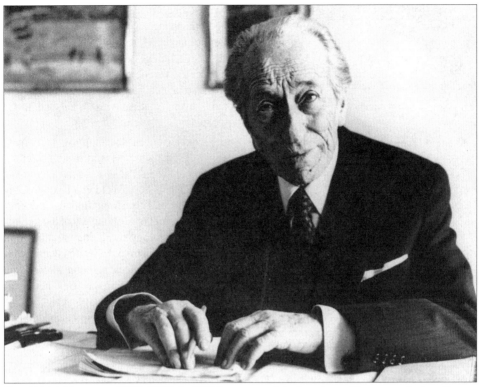

Fig. 6 Erich Simenauer (1901-1988). In 1930 he suggested the broad use of hyperosmolaric saline solution in hypovolemic situations [13]

Borchardt still lived in Germany when Hellmut Weese (1897-1954), a chemist in Wuppertal, introduced "Evipan" (hexobarbital) giving a new touch to intravenous anaesthesia. The Jewish origin of his colleague has remained veiled for a long time and unfortunately no biographic details have been revealed yet.

In this affair, another person should be mentioned as well: the pharmacologist Oskar Liebreich (1839-1908) (Fig.5) from Berlin synthesized chloralhydrate, that anaesthesiologists would not want to miss even today[23, 28,29]. The French surgeon Cyprien Oré (1828-1878) applied this compound intravenously and published his results in 1873. Liebreich was a great admirer of Carl Ludwig Schleich (1859-1922) who inaugurated anaesthesia by infiltration and supported him at times when other surgeons laughed at him.

Prof. Dr. Franz Schueck (1888-1958) was Head of the Department of Surgery at the Urban Krankenhaus in Berlin and worked with Erich Simenauer (1901-1988) (Fig.6) in the early thirties on a new technique of infusion therapy administering small amounts of concentrated sugar or saline infusion, today known as "small-volume resuscitation"[11]. After having performed experiments on animals they applied this method to patients suffering from severe blood loss, and the success was convincing. After injecting 30 ml of a 40% solution, the intravascular volume multiplied times twenty in a very short period of time, i.e. 3-5 minutes. He could convince executives of the "Chemische Fabrik Guestrow A.G." (a company manufacturing chemical products) to sell ampullaes named "Schockcalorose" containing 30 ml of a sterile solu-

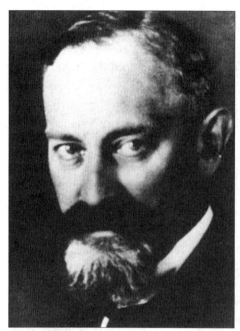

Fig. 7 *Ernst Unger (1875-1938), who already used Meltzer`s insufflation technique in 1910* [13]

tion, that could be given any time. Unemployment struck them when the Nationalsocialist Party took over in 1933 forcing them to leave the hospital and eventually the country [40,41].

Simenauer, taken into custody, managed to escape to Tansania via Cyprus, with the aid of a SA-officer whom he had operated on a few months prior to his flight. He specialized in tropical medicine later on. He returned to Berlin after the end of the war, where he became a highly regarded man and died in 1988. Schueck succeeded in leaving Germany in the middle of the thirties emigrating to the United States of America. He died in New York in 1958.

Ernst Unger (1875-1938) (Fig.7) was another Jewish physician involved in the development of infusion therapy being the first person in the German Reich to build up a blood bank in the early thirties. A few decades had passed since he had published results with Bettmann (?), an internist, on the advantages of apnoeic oxygenation according to Samuel James Meltzer (1851-1922) for head surgery and suggested to apply this technique in order to overcome paralysis of the muscles involved in breathing in 1912. In 1938 Unger had a severe accident with his car that he did not survive [1,44].

Meltzer, born in Russia, grew up in Prussia, worked with the physiologist Hugo Kronecker (1839-1911) and migrated to the United States before World War I, supposedly because of racial discrimination. In New York he became chief of a laboratory of the department of physiology still being entangeled in airway management publishing an article on an inflatable pharyngeal tube that allowed the insufflation of oxygen in the "Berliner klinische Wochenschrift" [30-34].

Ferdinand Sauerbruch (1875-1951), a leading thoracic surgeon, had a great influence on the lacking spread of Meltzer`s method. Right from the beginning it had been announced that the anaesthesiologist was the one inhaling a great deal of the anaesthetic. The discussion about this matter again came up in the middle of the twenties, initiating the analysis of the air inside the operation theatres. Julius Hirsch (1892-1963) and Adolf Kappus (1900-?) being in charge of affairs concerning hygiene at the Charité in Berlin could prove the efficacy of preventive measures [22]. Being afraid of explosive agents administered during anaesthesia carbon filters were introduced. The Nationalsocialist taking over had a massive impact on them, too. Hirsch died a few years later from a natural cause, whereas Kappus emigrated to Turkey being involved in the foundation of the University of Istanbul. After World War II he was a member of a Swiss pharmaceutical company for many years.

As for local and regional anaesthesia, Jewish physicians and scientists have made contributed over the decades. It is a com-

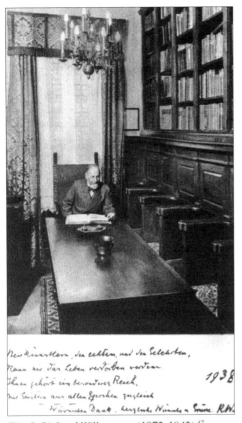

Fig. 8 Richard Willstaetter (1872-1942) [47]

monly known fact, that Carl Koller (1857-1944) who discovered the anaesthetic properties of cocain was of Jewish descent. The fact that the chemist Richard Willstaetter (1872-1942) (Fig.8) was the one to purify and to find a substitute for cocaine at the end of the last century has not been spread as far [47].

Caesar Hirsch (1897-1940) (Fig. 9), an otorhinolaryngologist tried different substitutes for cocaine on patients. After World War I he accepted the chair for ENT in the Marienkrankenhaus in Stuttgart - the department soon belonged to the largest ones in the south of Germany. He was a man with an outstanding surgical qualification and published a highly regarded book on local anaesthesia [16]. Nevertheless he had to leave Germany head over heels due to his Jewish ancestors, since he had been threatened by a SA-officer whom he had to face in court a few years previously. He reached New York via Switzerland and France, changed his name to "Hearst" and put many articles and books on techniques in local anaesthesia to press, since he was not given a working permit as an ENT-specialist[18,19]. This made him take the necessary steps to move to Seattle where he had been promised employment - unfortunately, this did not work out, making him commit suicide in 1940[9,15].

Hirsch´s contribution to anaesthesia comprises a detailed book with excellent figures and didactics on local anaesthesia and his strive that cocaine be replaced by synthetic substitutes not leading to dependence - applying "Pantocaine" and "Tutocaine" for surface anaesthesia on mucose membranes[17]. He discussed the aspects of intravenous

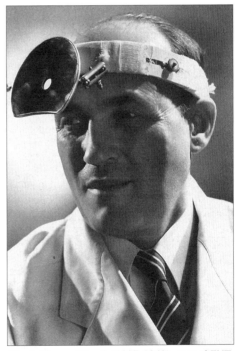

Fig. 9 Ceasar Hirsch (1897-1940) reputed ENT specialist and editor of a well-known textbook of local anaesthesia technics [13]

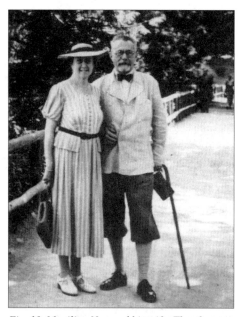

anaesthesia for ENT-surgery in German speaking countries and became co-editor of the journal "Der Schmerz" (i.e. "Pain"), that was in press after 1928 [9].

Even though all the above mentioned practitioner made significant contributions to the development of anaesthesia, they all stayed with their speciality instead of becoming anaesthesiologist.

Around the turn of the century the discussion on nitrous oxide became an important issue again. At the University of Heidelberg intense studies on this compound have been carried out utilizing so called "Rotameters". The gynocologist Maximilian Neu (1877-1940) (Fig.10) was engaged in these experiments since he applied the new technical device. Detailed facts on the bibliography of this important person have been veiled until today due to his Jewish heritage, though the author feels proud to lighten up this matter[10].

While he was studying, Neu had the

Fig. 10 Maxilian Neu and his wife. The photo was taken in summer 1938 in Heidelberg. He was the first to use "Rotameters" in anaesthesiology[13]

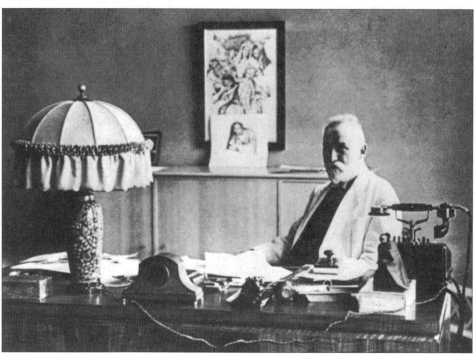

Fig. 11 Eugen Fraenkel (1854-1938) intrododuced "Strophantin" into clinical practice

opportunity to meet German speaking pioneers relating to the application of nitrous oxide, who probably inspired him to conduct further experiments on this product at the Institute of Pharmacology in Heidelberg in 1908 [8]. At that time Rudolf Gottlieb (1864-1924) was head of that institute, being a member of the well-known "Naturhistorisch-Medizinischer Verein in Heidelberg" (i.e. natural-historic medical association in Heidelberg), that was to "support natural science and medicine and report on research in every field of science including demonstrations and discussions in regularly held meetings". The internist Eugen Fraenkel (1854-1938) (Fig.11), who was involved in the intravenous application of strophantine, personally knew Neu and wished to become a gynaecologist just like Neu but could not accomplish this much to his regret, since he suffered from tuberculosis[12]. Fraenkel introduced Neu to Hans Bunte (1848-1925), an engineer at the Technical University in Karlsruhe, who was in charge of checking the reliability of rotameters. Being a member of the "Naturhistorisch-Medizinischer Verein in Heidelberg",too, Bunte informed Gottlieb about the innovation of this device. Gottlieb immediately recognized its importance and arranged with the "Deutsche Rotawerke" (i.e. German enterprise manufacturing rotameters) in Aix-la-Chapelle for the construction of an apparatus that allowed an exact admixture of nitrous oxide to oxygen in 1910[36]. After having carried out trials with it on animals the apparatus was introduced to clinical practice the same year[5,6,37,38].

Even though the apparatus proved effective in daily routine, it was not very persuading, since nitrous oxide had to be imported and thus was quite expensive. In addition gynaecologists and surgeons mastered local anaesthesia well. On top of this World War I had an influence, too, lundering further investigations. At this point in time Neu had built up his own private practice without completely retreating from his tasks at the Gynaecological Department of the Universityhospital. Yet, with the Nationalsocialists taking over in April 1933, he had to suffer from persecution (Fig.12). He and his wife took their own lives just prior to being taken to a concentration camp in the south of France in October 1940[10].

Nobody has ever been able to trace, if Neu managed to meet the owner of the "Rotawerke" in Aix-la-Chapelle, the Jewish business-man Felix Meyer (1875-1951). Meyer was full of innovating ideas having many patents even in the medical field. He was forced to sell his enterprise to somebody of Aryan descent in 1938 and luckily accomplished to escape to Belgium in 1939 before war broke out (Fig. 13a, 13b). He died in Switzerland in 1951 [12].

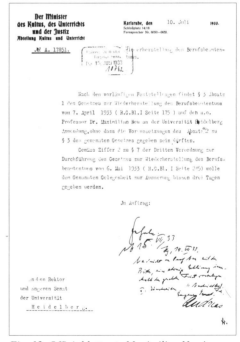

Fig. 12 Official letter to Maximilian Neu in which it was announced that the "Law for the Reconstruction of civil service" became effective on April 7th, 1933 [13]

561

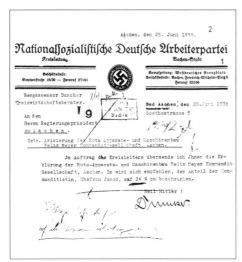

Fig. 13a Copy of a letter in which some details of the sale of the "Rotameter firm" to somebody of Aryan descent were discussed[13]

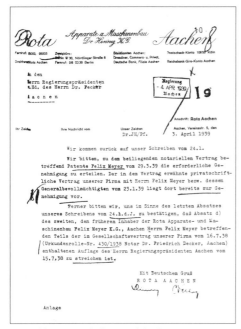

Fig. 13b Copy of a letter of the firm "Rota Apparate u. Maschinenbau" concerning some "unsolved patent problems" of the the former Jewish owner, Felix Meyer[13]

Ernst von der Porten´s (1884-1940) (Fig.14) fate, a medical doctor from Hamburg, resembles that of Maximilian Neu in many aspects. Right from the beginning of his medical career he was interested in anaesthesiology probably resulting from having had to face different aspects of this speciality while working on his thesis at the Department of Gynaecology at the University of Heidelberg - Maximilian Neu being a colleague at the same place. It has not been proved though feasable that they knew each other especially considering their Jewish religon.

After having returned to Hamburg von der Porten was employed as a medical attendant at the Department of Surgery at the general hospital St. Georg under the supervision of the head of department Paul Sudeck (1866-1945)[43]. Sudeck was very interested in unsolved problems in anaesthesiology, which probably was the reason that von der Porten exclusively played the part of an anaesthesiologist in different hospitals in Hamburg. He was deeply involved in research and published loads of articles on anaesthesiology and pleading for a professional team of anaesthesiologist to be set up[43,45]. He took part in many congresses on anaesthesiology and repeatedly visited conferences in the United Kingdom in order to obtain knowledge on their methods, e.g. the first International Congress on Anaesthesiology in Nottingham. This is where he met Maurice Cohen (1875-1929), who was Jewish as well, and was the founder of the British Journal of Anaesthesia in 1923 along with Edmund Boyle (1875-1941). He was also introduced to Francis Hoeffer McMechan (1879-1939), a pioneer in anaesthesiology in the United States of America, who was the editor of "Current researches in Anaesthesia and Analgesia" since 1922[43]. These two acquaintances definetly reassured him to publish a journal on anaesthesiology in German which he succeeded in: only two years later "Der Schmerz - Deut-

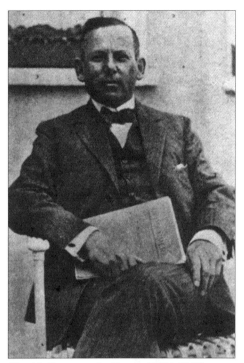

Fig. 14 Ernst von der Porten (1884-1940), the first German professional "full-time anaesthesiologist" [43]

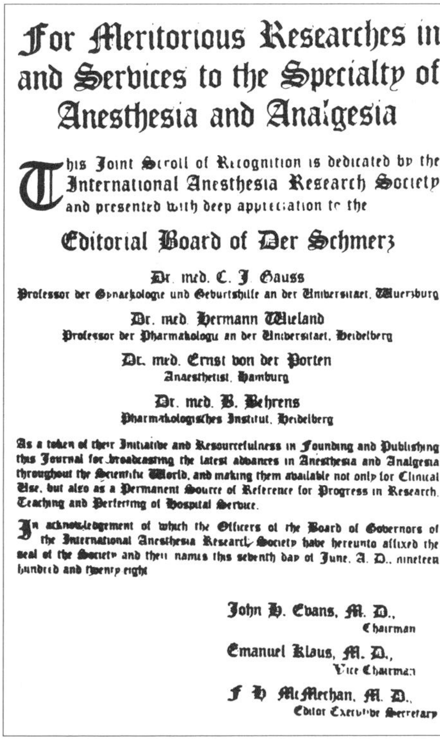

sche Zeitschrift zur Erforschung des Schmerzes und seiner Bekämpfung, zugleich Zentralorgan für Narkose und Anaesthesie" (i.e. "Pain - German Journal to investigate pain and its treatment, at the same time central organ for narcosis and anaesthesia). He was honored for his achievement at the Seventh Annual Congress of Anaesthesiologists in Canada and the United States of America in Illinois along with his co-editors Carl Joseph Gauss (1875-1957) and Hermann Wieland (1885-1929) in a scroll of recognition (Fig.15). After the unification of the two journals "Der Schmerz" (i.e. Pain) and "Narkose und Anaesthesie" (i.e. Narcosis and Anaesthesia) to "Schmerz, Narkose und Anaesthesie" (i.e. Pain, Narcosis and Anaesthesia) he was still involved in this affair, had to leave due to Nationalsocialistic power, though [12]. He emigrated to Belgium in 1938, where he was detained in 1940 after the invasion by German troups and had then been taken captive for being a Jew by Germans. He was transferred to a concentration camp in France close to the Spanish border where he committed suicide.

Only a few years had passed since the pharmacologist Julius Geppert (1856-1937) (Fig.16) who worked at the University of Bonn, had caused a sensation by presenting different apparatus that allowed to administer defined amounts of the vapor of ether, when Karl Kueppers (?), an engineer from Aix-la-Chapelle, had gotten a patent on his rotameter for the exact admixture of different

For Meritorious Researches in and Services to the Specialty of Anesthesia and Analgesia

This Joint Scroll of Recognition is dedicated by the International Anesthesia Research Society and presented with deep appreciation to the

Editorial Board of Der Schmerz

Dr. med. C. J. Gauss
Professor der Gynaekologie und Geburtshilfe an der Universitaet, Wuerzburg

Dr. med. Hermann Wieland
Professor der Pharmakologie an der Universitaet, Heidelberg

Dr. med. Ernst von der Porten
Anaesthetist, Hamburg

Dr. med. B. Behrens
Pharmakologisches Institut, Heidelberg

As a token of their Initiative and Resourcefulness in Founding and Publishing this Journal for broadcasting the latest advances in Anesthesia and Analgesia throughout the Scientific World, and making them available not only for Clinical Use, but also as a Permanent Source of Reference for Progress in Research, Teaching and Perfecting of Hospital Service.

In acknowledgement of which the Officers of the Board of Governors of the International Anesthesia Research Society have hereunto affixed the seal of the Society and their names this seventh day of June, A. D., nineteen hundred and twenty eight

John H. Evans, M. D.,
Chairman

Emanuel Klaus, M. D.,
Vice Chairman

F H McMechan, M. D.,
Editor Executive Secretary

Fig. 15 Joint Scroll of recognition for services to the speciality of anaesthesia; it was presented to the Editorial Board of "Der Schmerz" in appreciation of their founding, editing and publishing this journal during the 7th annual congress of anaesthetists in Minneapolis, Minn., june 11-15, 1928 [13]

gases [4,12,14,25,26]. Geppert's apparatus with an integrated spirometer that permitted to controll the dose of the inhaled ether according to the tidal volume was first to be seen in 1899[7]. Praising the advantages of this device, it could still be admired at the University of Gießen in 1940 with Geppert not being alive anymore. He was crushed by loneliness since he was not allowed to teach any longer rooting from him being half a Jew.

The application and the technique of epidural injection has first been reported by a French urologist, Fernand Cathélin (1873-1945). Maximilian Hirsch (1877-1944) from Vienna was a devoted supporter of this method and had a great impact on the development of the necessary equipment[20]. He also promoted the administration of ether according to Paul Sudeck and herewith influenced its spread by claiming it to be harmless [21]. Hirsch seemed to have been interested in the history of anaesthesia, too. He was displaced to the concentration camp in Theresienstadt, where he died in 1944.

As outlined above, it was the intention of the authors, to illustrate the importance of some Jewish physicians in the development of anaesthesia in Germany. However, it was impossible to go into detail and to appreciate their contribution as deeply as it deserves to be appreciated.

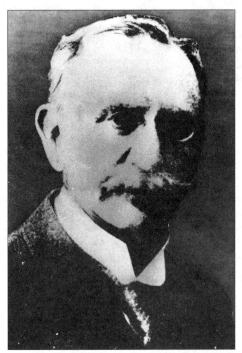

Fig. 16 Julius Geppert (1856-1937). In 1899 he invented a sophisticated anaeshetic apparatus [7]

References:

1. Ayisi K, M Goerig: The merits of Samuel James Meltzer and John Auer for the development of apneic oxygenation. In: The History of Anesthesia. Proceedings of the Third International Symposium. Publ. (ed): B R Fink, L E Morris, C R Stephen, Wood Library-Museum of Anesthesiology 1993, p. 32-40
2. Comité des Délégations Juives, Paris: Die Lage der Juden in Deutschland 1933, Paris 1934 Wiederaufgelegt 1983 bei Ullstein, Ullstein Verlag Frankfurt-Berlin-Wien 1983
3. Elkin R: Das Jüdische Krankenhaus in Berlin zwischen 1938 - und 1945. Edition Henrich, Berlin 1993
4. Fenster E: Der Aetherdampf-Narkoseapparat nach Geppert-Poppert. Schmerz-Narkose-Anaesthesie. 1940; 6: 145-147
5. Foregger R: The rotameter in anesthesia. Anesthesiology 1946; 9: 549-557
6. Foregger R: Early use of rotameter in anaesthesia. Br J Anaesth 1952; 24:187-195
7. Geppert J: Eine neue Narkosemethode. Dtsch Med Wschr 1899; 27: 433-435 and 28: 457-466
8. Goerig M: Historical use of nitrous oxide in Germany. The History of Anaesthesia Society-Proceedings. 1994; 16: 68-80
9. Goerig M: Caesar Hirsch - ein unbekannt gebliebener Protagonist lokalanästhesiologischer Techniken. Anaesthesist, Suppl 1995
10. Goerig M, J Schulte am Esch: The man behind the technique: Maximilian Neu and the introduction of flowmeter-systems in anaesthesia. Anesthesiology, Vol. 83, No. 3A, Suppl. A 1020
11. Goerig M, Th Standl, J Schulte am Esch: Small - Volume Resuscitation - eine Errungenschaft unserer Tage? Anaesthesist 1996; 45, Suppl 1 A 93
12. Goerig M, J Schulte am Esch: Der Beitrag jüdischer Ärzte für die Entwicklung der modernen Anaesthesieverfahren. AINS, in press
13. Goerig, M: collection and Nordrhein-Westfälisches Hauptstaatsarchiv, Düsseldorf
14. Gundel, H G: Julius Geppert (1856-1937) - Pharmakologe. Lebensbilder aus Hessen, Band 2, 265-266
15. Hearst P: Son of Caesar Hirsch, personal communication, December 1995
16. Hirsch C: Lehrbuch der Lokalanästhesie des Ohres und der oberen Luft - und Speisewege. Enke, Stuttgart 1925
17. Hirsch C: Die Stellung des Kocains in der Lokalanästhesie einst und jetzt. Schmerz 1928; 1: 105-113
18. Hirsch C: 50 years of local anesthesia in otolaryngology. Act Oto Laryngolica 1934; 21:256-278:
19. Hirsch C: Prolonged analgesia after tonsillectomy by nerve blocking anesthesia. Ann. Otololy, Rhinology & Laryngology 1938;12: 1035-1044
20. Hirsch M: Instrumentarium, Technik und Erfolge der epiduralen Injektionen. Zbl f Chir 1906; 21: 595-599
21. Hirsch M: Der Ätherrausch. Franz Deuticke, Leipzig-Wien 1907
22. Hirsch J, Kappus A L: Über die Mengen des Narkoseäthers in der Luft von Operationssälen. Zschr f Hyg und Infektionskrh 1928; 110 :391-398
23. Hoffmann K : Der Pharmakologe Oskar Liebreich (1839-1908). Med Mschr 1958; 7: 475-477
24. Kümmel WF: Die Ausschaltung der jüdischen Ärzte in Deutschland durch den Nationalsozialismus. 30-50. In: Pross Ch, R Winau (Ed): Nicht Mißhandeln - Das Krankenhaus Moabit. 1920-1933 - Ein Zentrum jüdischer Ärzte in Berlin, 1933-1945 Verfolgung - Widerstand -Zerstörung. Edition Hentrich, Berlin 1983
25. Küppers K: Neuer Gasmesser. Chemiker Zeitung 1910; 34:876
26. Küppers K: Gasmesser, bei dem innerhalb eines Zylinders ein Schwimmer sich entsprechend der durchströmenden Gasmenge in bestimmter Höhenlage einstellt. Patent 215225, 30.8.1908, Reichspatentamt, München 1908

[27] Kröner K: Die Emigration von Medizinern unter dem Nationalsozialismus. 78-86. In: J Bleker, N Jachertz (Ed) Medizin im Dritten Reich. Deutscher Ärzte Verlag, Köln 1993

[28] Liebreich O: Das Chloralhydrat - ein neues Hypnoticum und Anaestheticum. Bln klin Wschr 1869; 6: 325-327

[29] Liebreich O: Das Chloralhydrat und seine medizinische Anwendung. Bln klin Wschr 1874; 11: 50-52

[30] Meltzer S, Auer J: Continuous respiration without respiratory movements. J Experim Med 1909; 11: 622

[31] Kagan S A : Samuel James Meltzer (1851-1920). Med Rec 1939; 150: 243
Meltzer A: Dr. Samuel James Meltzer and intratracheal anesthesia. J Clin Anesth 1990; 2: 54

[32] Meltzer SJ: Der gegenwärtige Stand der intratrachealen Insufflation Bln klin Wschr 1914; 15: 677

[33] Meltzer SJ: Pharyngeale Insufflation, ein einfacher Apparat für künstliche Atmung am Menschen; nebst Bemerkungen über andere Methoden der künstlichen Atmung. Bln klin Wschr 1915; 17: 425

[34] Meltzer S J: Simple devices for effective artificial respiration in emergencies. JAMA 1910; 60:1407

[35] Mendel F: Der gegenwärtige Stand der intravenösen Therapie. Bln klin Wschr 1908; 49: 2187-2190 and 50: 2223-2227

[36] Menge M, M Neu: Demonstration zur Morphin-Skopolamin-Stickoxydul-Sauerstoff-Narkose beim Menschen. Dtsch Med Wschr 1910; 36: 2367-2368

[37] Neu M: Ein Verfahren zur Stickoxydul-Sauerstoffnarkose. Münch Med Wschr 1910; 36: 1873-1875

[38] Neu M: Die Stickoxydul-Sauerstoff-Narkose. Arch f klin Chir 1911; 95: 550-557

[39] Pross Chr, R Winau: Nicht Mißhandeln - Das Krankenhaus Moabit. 1920-1933 - Ein Zentrum jüdischer Ärzte in Berlin, 1933-1945 Verfolgung - Widerstand - Zerstörung. Edition Hentrich, Berlin 1984

[40] Schück F: Schockbekämpfung durch intravenöse Injektion hypertonischer Lösungen. Zbl f Chir 1932; 32: 2027-2029

[41] Simenauer E: Rasche aktive Auffüllung des Blutgefäßsystems. Beitrag zum Wasserhaushalt des Menschen. Med Klin 1930; 11: 385-388

[42] Strauss H: Zur Methodik der intravenösen Therapie. Dtsch Med Wschr 1907; 4: 141-142

[43] Tschöp M: Ernst von der Porten 1884 - 1940 - In der Geschichte der deutschen Anästhesiologie. Springer, Heidelberg-Berlin-New York 1986

[44] Unger E, Bettmann M: Beitrag zu S.J. Meltzer´s Insufflationsnarkose. Bln klin Wschr 1910; 21: 958-961

[45] von der Porten E: Narkosemaske für Operationen in Bauchlage. Zbl f Chir 1914; 29: 1214-1215

[46] von der Porten E: Zum Anaesthesisten-Kongress in Minneapolis. Schmerz 1928; 2: 263-264

[47] Willstaetter R: Aus meinem Leben. Von Arbeit, Muße und Freuden. Verlag Chemie, Weinheim 1949

[48] Wohlgemuth H: Eine neue Chloroform-Sauerstoffnarkose. Arch f klin Chir 1901; 64: 664-681

The Importance of Collaborative Research to Academic Anesthesiology: Ralph Waters and the University of Wisconsin Model

D. Bacon, Department of Anesthesiology, Buffalo VAMC, Buffalo, NY, USA

If one clinical specialty can bridge the divergence between the basic science laboratory and the bedside, it is anesthesiology. Each anesthetic is in a sense an experiment in applied pharmacology, physiology and pathophysiology. The student of the discipline applies the principles of basic science in a clinically relevant manner. Bellevue surgeon Arthur Wright thought this was one of the roles of anesthesiology in the medical school curriculum – to demonstrate this lesson to medical students.[1]

Anesthesiology, as an academic discipline, however is young. While appointments to medical school faculties in anesthesiology can be traced to the first two decades of the twentieth century[2], Ralph Milton Waters created the first academic department within the medical school in 1927 at the University of Wisconsin. Historically, Waters' accomplishment was not simply being first, nor solely evident in the number and quality of the research produced within the department, but that almost every successfully academic department for over the past seventy years has followed his model. In late twentieth century American Anesthesiology, over sixty percent of academic chairman have been trained by physicians trained by Waters or his residents and their residents.[3]

Anesthesiology may have been unique in allowing an effortless integration of basic science and clinical application. Yet, acceptance in the medical school, especially for anesthesia; a specialty thought to be below the dignity of many physicians, must have been difficult. How did Waters create this department? What was critical to his success? What role did the medical school and especially the basic scientists play in the creation of this seminal department?

Ralph Waters

Ralph Waters was uniquely suited to create an academic department. When he arrived in Madison, Wisconsin in 1927, Waters had already practiced anesthesia for fifteen years in the community. He had published extensively in the literature, including a paper with Arthur Guedel, the pioneer of the signs of ether anesthesia, that described both a cuffed endotracheal tube, and provided evidence that the tube protected the airway while anesthetized. More importantly, Waters had studied the effects of carbon dioxide on humans during anesthesia. His work had impressed Chancy Leake, a noted pharmacologist at the University of Wisconsin.

Waters' challenge upon arrival, was to create an academic department of anesthesia and intercalate it into the university community. Writing about his reasons to go to Madison twenty-three years after his arrival, Waters justified his move saying he had four primary reasons for coming to the university. First, he wanted to provide the best possible clinical service to the patients of the State of Wisconsin General Hospital. Secondly, he wanted to teach medical students and interns the fundamentals of anesthesia – in the classroom as well as the operating room. Thirdly, he aspired to start a residency training program for physicians. Finally, Waters desired to continue his work on the underlining principles of anesthesia by collaborating with the basic science faculty at the University.[4]

Collaborative Research

Without the interest and help of the basic science researchers within the medical school, Waters' ambitious residency training program would have failed. Collaboration, however, occurred almost before the post graduate program took off. Waters on arrival was a welcomed addition to the medical school faculty. Pharmacology professor Chauncy Leake wrote,

I want to tell how very happy we are to have you here with us and to express my great pleasure at the opportunity of cooperating with you...Dr. Schmidt [Chief of Surgery] mentioned that you were anxious to work up some research problem in anesthesia, and I should be happy to cooperate with you in any way.... We should be very happy to have you talk to our students at the 11 o'clock lecture, Thursday, March 8, on the general subject of practice anesthesia and post-anesthetic care of the patient..."[5]

Leake and Waters spent time together in the laboratory. They produced an elegant study on the effects of anesthetics on erythrocytes, paying careful attention to the influence of oxygen and carbon dioxide levels. The use of oxygen as a routine supplement to an anesthetic was unusual in the 1920s, carbon dioxide was often administered to help keep patients breathing. Thus the study was designed to answer questions on the interactions of red blood cells not only in the presence of anesthetics, but also in varying oxygen and carbon dioxide environments.[6]

Shortly after the study was published, Leake left Madison for California and a new chair in Pharmacology was appointed, Arthur L. Tatum. It was not long before Waters and Tatum developed an effective collaborative working relationship. One of Tatum's interests was local anesthetics. Studying the "new" local anesthetic procaine, Tatum published studies done in animals which investigated its toxicity.[7] Waters paralleled the work in humans. Waters attempted to prevent the toxic reaction to the drug by using premedication to prevent seizures.[8]

The introduction of cyclopropane was one of the most important works to come out of the Madison collaborative experience. The anesthetic properties of the gas were discovered by Velyien Hendersen and G. H. W. Lucas in 1928 in Toronto, Canada. They lacked a suitable place to trial the drug, and Waters volunteered. Over the ensuing years, the fame of the department would be assured by the research into cyclopropane.[9]

Continuing the collaborative work with the department of pharmacology and adding a member from the department of physiology, cyclopropane and its effects on the body were studied. An early paper plotted cyclopropane concentrations against cardiac and respiratory changes.[10] This paper, entitled "Cyclopropane Study with Especial Reference to Gas Concentration, Respiratory and Electrocardiographic Changes", is particularly interesting because of the authors affiliation. Seevers was from Pharmacology, Meek from Physiology, while Rovenstine and Stiles were an attending anesthetist and resident in anesthesiology respectively. Thus, the Waters' department bridged the three disciplines in a productive manner, and one in which patient care was improved.

The work with cyclopropane continued. The pharmacologists worked out cyclopropane's solubility in a variety of substances including human blood. This was a key concept in understanding the clinical observation of the rapid onset of action of the agent.[11] Another clinical observation that patients under cyclopropane anesthesia had a propensity for cardiac arrhythmias that could lead to sudden death, was investigated in the laboratory. Concentrations of sympathomimetic amines were measured in dogs under cyclopropane, ether and chloroform anesthesia.[12] Review articles outlining the pharmacology of cyclopropane were also coauthored by the clinical and basic science faculty.

Conclusions

Waters' department was critical to the development and acceptance of anesthesiology as a medical specialty. At a time when the giving of an anesthetic was thought to be below the dignity of most physicians, or work worthy of only the most junior intern or a nurse, Waters, by working with basic scientists helped create a scientific basis to anesthesia. His most famous resident, Emery Andrew Rovenstine would leave Madison for Bellevue hospital in New York City. Transplanting the Wisconsin model, Rovenstine flourished and guaranteed that academic anesthesia would not die with Waters. One of Rovenstine's residents, Emmanual Papper would be critical in securing National Institute of Health monies to support basic science inquiry in anesthesiology twenty years after Waters had left academia.

Ralph Waters believed in his mission, making a place for anesthesiology in the medical school, and demonstrated the belief held by other physicians that anesthesiology was the natural bridge between the basic science and the clinical one. Using his colleagues in the basic sciences to help establish not only a research program, but some of the scientific principles of the specialty, Waters proved the importance of collaborative research specifically to anesthesiology and to medicine in general.

References:

1. Wright AM: Teaching and anesthesia service from the viewpoint of surgery. Current Researches in Anesthesia and Analgesia 1935; 14:248-250

2. For example Thomas Drysdale Buchanan was Professor of Anesthetics at New York Medical College in 1913. John Henry Evans was appointed Assistant in Anesthetics at the University of Buffalo in 1913. Bacon DR, Yearley CK. Among the first. Anesthesia and Analgesia. 1991; 71:684-692

3. Bacon DR, Ament R: Ralph Waters and the beginnings of academic anesthesiology in the United States: The Wisconsin Template. J Clin Anesth 1995; 7:534-543

4. Waters RM: Pioneering in Anesthesiology. Post Graduate Medicine. 1948; 4:267

5. Letter from Chauncy Leake, Ph.D. to Ralph Waters, M.D., February 2, 1927. The Collected Papers of Ralph Waters, M.D., Steenbock Library Collection, University of Wisconsin, Madison, Wisconsin, USA

6. Leake CD, Lapp H, Waters RM: The effects of anesthetics on osmotic resistance of erythrocytes; carbon dioxide and oxygen. Proc Soc Exp Bio & Med. 1927; 31:464-466

7. Tatum AL: Experimental inflitrative anesthesia. J Pharmacol Exp Ther 1931; 42:276

8. Waters RM: Procaine toxicity: its prophylaxis and treatment. J Am Dent Assoc 1933; 20:2211-2215

9. A glance through the bibliography of Robbins BH. Cyclopropane Anesthesia. Baltimore: Williams & Wilkins Co 1940 pp.155-165. clearly demonstrates the importance of the work done in Madison

10. Seevers MH, Meek WJ, Rovenstine EA, Stiles JA: Cyclopropane study with especial reference to gas concentration, respiratory and electrocardiographic changes. J Pharmacol Exp Ther 1934; 51:1-17

11. Orcutt FS, Seevers MH: The solubility coefficients of cyclopropane in for water, oils and human blood. J Pharmacol Exp Ther 1937; 59:206-210

12. Orth OS, Stutzman JW, Meek WJ: Action of sympathomimetic amines in cyclopropane, ether and chloroform anesthesia. Am J Physiol 1939; 126:595

13. Seevers MH, Waters RM: Pharmacology of anesthetic gases. Physiology Review 1938; 18:447-479

14. Wright AM: Teaching and anesthesia service from the viewpoint of Surgery. Current Researches in Anesthesia and Analgesia. 1935; 14:248

Stethoscopy during Anaesthesia: Past, Present and Future

J. W. R. McIntyre †
Department of Anesthesiology, University of Alberta Hospital, Edmonton, Alberta, Canada

René Théophile Hyacinth Laennec[1-4] was born in France on 17 February 1781. His childhood was complicated by ill health, domestic disruption and, in 1793 during the Terror, the use of a guillotine in his village square. Parisian medical students lived harshly, but by 1803 he had graduated with distinctions in medicine and surgery. His subsequent enlightened professional life dedicated to scientific method and his patients welfare left him little opportunity to enjoy the horse riding, hunting, and woodworking he loved.

At the beginning of the 19th century diagnosis was largely based on a patient's medical history, and direct auscultation of a chest was thought disgusting by many physicians, unethical with female patients and occasionally impossible. The circumstances that led Laennec to auscultate indirectly with a quire of paper rolled into a cylinder was a patient whose gender and age made ear to the chest auscultation unethical or, according to an apocryphal account[5], unwise. His success led to further experiments using wood, Indian cane and other less satisfactory materials.

Laennec's treatise "De l'Auscultation Mediate" was finished on August 6, 1818,[4] and published in two volumes accompanied by a wooden stethoscope on August 15, 1819. In January, 1820, a London periodical published an anonymous 33-page review that included the statement,"those who neglect to possess themselves of the work, either in the original or in the translation, inflict a deep wound on their best interest."[6] The stethoscopes were imported to England for sale by Trentall and Wurtz, booksellers of Soho, or made locally by Alnutt of Piccadilly. In 1821, a John Forbes published a translation but reduced in length from Laennec's version and with modified nomenclature. Forbes considered physicians would appear ridiculous, transport of the device troublesome, and anyway it could not be the sole basis of a diagnosis.[2] However, by the time of Laennec's death from tuberculosis in 1826 and a second enlarged edition had been published, he had been visited by nearly 300 students, including luminaries of English medicine. Typical English academic views were those of Sir Charles Scudamore.[7] "He (Laennec) did not advocate the adoption of physical principles in physic or intend to displace established tenets. He sought merely, by the use of the stethoscope, a simple but philosophical instrument, to reduce the excessive degree of conjecture which still prevails in the diagnosis of thoracic disease."[7] Other practitioners were less enthusiastic. The new information did not alter therapy and Laennec's descriptive analogies to sounds were too obscure for verbal instruction of students. As late as 1837, stethoscopists were a minority group against which there was considerable prejudice. However, by 1846, and the advent of clinical anaesthesia, generations of students educated in the 1820's had been exposed to the stethoscopy discipline[8] and even by 1832 a stethoscope with a flexible tube of spiral wire covered by caoutouc cloth had been developed.[9] Many other designs during subsequent decades allegedly altered acoustic performance and convenience.[9] Ultimately in 1893 Solis-Cohen[10] described an oesophageal stethoscope. This modification of a previous design by Richardson included a rubber capsule containing a diaphragm of goldbeaters skin to function as a resonator and preventer of gastric fluid reaching the ears of the stethoscopist. Solis-Cohen's primary purpose for the as yet experimental instrument was cardiovascular diagnosis. Relatively recent reviews of stethoscopy exemplify the high regard in which it continues to be held in the practice of medicine.[11-16]

The purposes of the present report are to trace the arrival of praecordial and oesophageal stethoscopy into operating room anaesthesia practice; and to discuss the relevance of contemporary stethoscopic developments to future anaesthetic practice.

The first relevant journal publication discovered, dated 1896 by Kirk of Glasgow Western Infirmary, seems[5] to provide the earliest clinical account of auscultation in the operating room.[17] An ordinary binaural stethoscope sufficiently lengthened by Indianrubber tubing was first employed. Then a phonendoscope[9] was substituted and a watch added. Two hundred patients under chloroform anaesthesia were studied. In addition to comments on heart rate and rhythm, emphasis was placed on the finding that "the character of the pulse may be no index to the force of the heart". He was closely involved with the Glasgow Committee on anaesthetic agents. Clearly he saw the stethoscope as a clinical research tool, a sequel to his laboratory experiments described by Duncum.[18]

This is in contrast to Cushing's advocacy, published in 1908[19,] of routine continuous auscultation of cardiac and respiratory sounds during the entire course of anaesthesia. That idea arose from a practice in the Hunterian laboratory for experimental surgery and was employed clinically by the etheriser S Griffith Davis using a praecordial phonendoscope.[20] The next reference[21] in 1924, documents surgeon and anaesthetist monitoring simultaneously the heart and, to some extent, respirations via a praecordial stethoscope. Kane stated specifically that the anaesthetist should have both ears blocked to avoid distractions.

Three decades preceded any further publications about stethoscopy and clinical anaesthesia but eventually those concerned oesophageal stethoscopes,[22-26] breathing circuit sensing sites[27-31], detection of air embolism[32] and its value when remote patient monitoring was necessary.[33-35] Authors also described amplification of sounds to facilitate access to them[33, 35, 36-39], or video display.[40,41]

Textbooks[42-75] published between 1878 and 1955 ignored the stethoscope as a device to employ during anaesthesia. However, in 1955, Knight and Tarrow[57] included one among essential equipment, but its use was not described. Virtually every textbook since then has referred positively to stethoscopy during anaesthesia. In 1982, Gravenstein and Paulus[66] stated "auscultation is a relatively recent addition to the anaesthetist's armamentarium but it is now firmly established practice. No patient should be anaesthetised without use of a praecordial or oesophageal stethoscope." Implicitly, those opinions were presented by Blitt and Hines[75] in 1995.

Customarily, journal articles present new devices that, in due course, are no longer of interest to readers, so the paucity of publications during the first century of practice is only limited evidence that stethoscopy was little used in the operating room during that time. In contrast, textbooks provide broad evidence of current practice at the time they are published. During that time until approximately 1955, the use of human senses was often described. Not only could useful information be obtained visually and auditorally but touch and smell were also important. In general, anaesthetists seem to have been reasonably content with the sensing possibilities available to them. There were two other reasons for lack of interest in stethoscopy. One was that its use seemed undignified and to some impugned the clinical competence of the user. Another was that, in days when ether or chloroform were carried on the person in elegant bottles about 10 cm high and wire framed masks often folded for convenient stowing, an unruly flexible stethoscope seemed an encumbrance. Stethoscopy was largely ignored. Thus there is strong evidence that until post WWII only a minority of anaesthetists employed stethoscopy routinely during anaesthesia. What might account for the major change in practice at that time?

Successful entry of a monitoring device into clinical practice requires certain demands be satisfied.
1. A perceived need by the clinician for that kind and quality of information.
2. An ability to respond clinically to the new information.
3. Convenient use of the device.

Anaesthetists might have been content to continue indefinitely with their customary sensory information with perhaps an assistant to monitor the pulse or sphygmomanometry introduced around the turn of the century. Nevertheless, other developments made this difficult. Firstly, patients were not as accessible, and more people and instruments were clustered around the patient. Secondly, the advent of relaxants and manual ventilation nullified many clinical signs. Thirdly, the need for a continuous supply of vital information became increasingly apparent and anaesthetists could respond more effectively to the information they received.

Nevertheless, convenience of management with the stethoscope was a real but little documented problem. Longer operations made anaesthetists restless, as they are today[76] and though artificial ventilation by hand immobilised them at the head of the table, there were many occasions when the patient breathed spontaneously. Lengthening stethoscope tubing severely diminishes the performance and, to increase the anaesthetists mobility, short range transmitters and amplifiers [33,35,36-39] were described but failed to become popular because of noise pollution and the publicity of physiological events. More recently, in 1983, a video display of stethoscopic information during anaesthesia was described but the ergonomic problems of auscultation in the operating room remained, and during this time the increasing availability of pulse oximetry and capnography reduced anaesthetists interest in it. The limitations of heart sound changes as indicators of cardiac depression were already understood.[40,77] Nevertheless, oximetry changes demand more diagnostic data, such as that provided by auscultation, as does PETCO2 measurement lacking a waveform display. Moreover, there may be a clinically important delay if the system is multiplexed, and under other circumstances capnography may not even be possible.

The recommendations of Gravenstein and Paulus[66] as well as Blitt and Hines[75] are based on sound clinical principles. Adverse stethoscopic sounds precede the functional evidence of compromised pulmonary function and additionally complement pulse oximetry, and even capnography, for diagnostic purposes. Nevertheless, some authorities believe that except for certain clinical situations, continuous stethoscopic monitoring is largely ignored in adult anaesthetic practice. If that is so, it is probably because it is too difficult. Other activities take precedence, and amplification of sounds contributed to noise pollution. Technology that transduces stethoscopic sounds to visual displays is consistent with the unified visual displays appreciated by contemporary anaesthetists or, in its own right, supplies information from which the good clinician can predict blood gas changes.

Thus, current developments in general medicine may have implications for future anaesthesia practice.

Important historical studies of acoustics associated with stethoscopy[78-82] have been followed by contemporary publications that not only include brief histories of displays of auscultatory sounds but reveal contemporary interest in them. In 1977, Murphy et al[83] demonstrated visual lung sound characterization by time expanded wave form analysis and, in 1981, he related them to Laennec's model and current text book terms.[84] He focused on the mechanism, production, and transmission of normal and abnormal lung sounds which themselves may vary from beat to beat, in contrast to the relative uniformity of heart beats. He concludes that if the huge amount of information contained in lung sounds could be filtered and applied, like Laennec's correlation of careful observation and correlation, a powerful diagnostic tool would be created. Selig (1993)[85] detailed the clinical requirements for physicians' hearing and the development of cardiac acoustics. He concluded with reference to heart and lung sounds, that in an age of pocket computer technology, the future capabilities of electronic stethoscopes are far reaching and can also embrace compensatory devices for selective hearing defects. Thus the story of stethoscopy and anaesthesia remains incomplete [86].

Acknowledgements

I express my thanks to Professor Akitomo Matsuki of Hirosaki, Japan for access to his medical library, to Ms Jeannette Buckingham and her colleagues in the John Scott Medical Sciences Library for their constant support, as well as Marilyn Blake of the Department of Anaesthesia, University of Alberta.

References:

1. Sakula A: In Search of Laënnec. J of the Roy Coll Phys London 1981; 15:55-7
2. Sakula A: RTH Laennec 1781-1826. His life and work: a bicentenary appreciation. Thorax 1981; 36:81-90
3. Hoyle C: The life and discoveries of Rene Laennec. Br J Tuberc 1944; 38:24-35
4. Keers RY: Laennec: his medical history. Thorax 1981;36:91-4
5. Fox ERW: Mrs Laennec and the stethoscope. The Western J of Med 1981; 134:73-4
6. Jarcho S: An early review of Laennec's treatise. Am J Cardiol 1962; 9:962-9
7. Jarcho S: Scudamore on Monsieur Laennec's method (1826), Am J Cardiol.11 1963; 507-12
8. King LS: Auscultation in England 1821-1837. Bull Hist Med 1959; 33:446-453
9. Sheldon PB, Doe J: The development of the stethoscope. Bull NY Acad Med 1935; 11:608-26
10. Solis-Cohen S: Exhibition of an oesophageal stethoscope, with remarks on intrathoracic auscultation. Trans Cell Physicians Philadelphia 1893; 3.5 XV:218-21
11. Hale-White W: The history of percussion and auscultation. Lancet 1924; 1:263-5
12. Young RA: The stethoscope: past and present. Trans Cell Physicians Philadelphia 1931; 54:1-22
13. Editorial: Listening to the lungs. BMJ 1978; 2:1789-90
14. Sakula A: Laennec's influence on some British physicians in the nineteenth century. J Roy Soc Med 1981; 74:759-767
15. Andrews JL, Badger TL: Lung sounds through the ages - from Hippocrates to Osler. JAMA 1979; 241:2625-2630
16. Reiser SJ: The medical influence of the stethoscope. Sc Am 1979; 240:148-56
17. Kirk R: On auscultation of the heart during chloroform narcosis. BMJ 1896; 2:1704-6
18. Duncum BD: The development of inhalational anaesthesia, 1st ed. Oxford University Press, 1947
19. Cushing H: Technical methods of performing certain cranial operations. Surg Gynecol Obstet 1908; VI:227-34
20. Shephard DAE: Harvey Cushing and Anaesthesia. Can Anaes Soc J 1965; 12:431-442
21. Kane E ON: Wearing of branching stethoscope by surgeons and anaesthetist during operation. Surg Gynecol Obstet 1924;39:508
22. Smith C: An endo-esophageal stethoscope. Anesth 1954; 33:566
23. Pryor WJ: Oesophageal stethoscope. Anaesthesia 1964; 19:295-6
24. Cullingford DW: An endo-oesophageal stethoscope. Br J Anaesth 1964; 36:524
25. Baker AB, McLeod C: Oesophageal multipurpose monitoring probe. Anaesthesia 1983; 38:892-7
26. O'Dea J, Hall I: Oesophageal stethoscope. Anaesthesia 1987; 42:1337-8
27. Laycock, JD, Auscultation in anaesthesia. BMJ 1954; 1:151-2
28. Cole F: A new stethoscope for the anesthesiologist. Anesth Analg. 1954; 33:143-4
29. Anand JS: A simple pediatric constant monitoring device. Anesth Analg 1972; 51:387-8
30. Kainuma M, Shimada Y: A breathing circuit stethoscope for continuous monitoring of breath sounds. Anesth Analg 1987; 66:1057-8
31. Doyle JD, Teves LY, Jhwar BS: Phonocardiographic monitoring using a special endotracheal tube. Can J Anaesth 1990; 37:5105
32. Marshall BM: Air embolism in neurosurgical anaesthesia; its diagnosis and treatment. Can Anaesth Soc J 1965; 12:255-61
33. Wilson ABK, Fothergill L, Taylor S: Some applications of a new electronic stethoscope. Lancet 1956; 271:1027-8

34. Feingold A, Lowe JH, Holaday DA et al: Inhalation anesthesia and remote monitoring during radiotherapy for children. Anesth Analg 1979; 49:656-9
35. Sarnay AJ, Kemp JA: Monitoring ventilation during computed tomography scan. Anesthesiology 1985; 63:729
36. Shane SM, Ashman H: An improved device to amplify the sounds of respiration of anesthetised patients. JAMA 1957; 163:261
37. Douglass R, Doddapaneni B: Esophageal stethoscope amplifier. Anesth Analg 1985; 64:377-8
38. Ginott N: Vacuum stethoscope attached to a tape recorder (A simple device for monitoring respiration and pulse rate). Anaesthesia 1977; 32:896-7
39. Redon D: Inexpensive stethoscopic transmitter. Anesthesiology 1987; 67:283
40. Rence WG, Cullen SC, Hamilton WK: Observations on the heart sounds during anaesthesia with cyclopropane or ether. Anesthesiology 1956; 17:26-9
41. Huang KC, Kraman SS, Wright BD: Video stethoscope - a simple method for assuring continuous bilateral lung ventilation during anesthesia. Anesth Analg 1983; 62:586-9
42. Turnbull L: The advantages and accidents of artificial anaesthesia. Philadelphia: Lindsay and Blakiston 1878
43. Lyman HM: Artificial anaesthesia and anaesthetics. New York: William Wood and Coy. 1881
44. Gwathmey JT: Anesthesia. New York: Appleton and Coy 1914
45. Flagg PJ: The art of anaesthesia. Philadelphia: JB Lippincott Coy 1919
46. Blomfield J: Anaesthetics in practice and theory. London: William Heinemann Ltd 1922.
47. Hewitt Sir FW: Anaesthetics and their administration. London: Hendry Frowde and Hodder and Stoughton 1922
48. Hadfield CF: Practical Anaesthetics. London: Bailliere, Tindall, and Cox 1923
49. Maxon LH: Spinal Anesthesia. Philadelphia: JB Lippincott Coy 1938
50. Flagg PJ: The art of anaesthesia. Philadelphia: JB Lippincott Coy 1939
51. Goldman V: Aids to anaesthesia. London: Bailliere, Tindall and Cox 1941
52. Lundy JS: Clinical anesthesia. Philadelphia: WB Saunders Coy 1942
53. Minnitt RJ, Gillies J, 7th ed, Textbook of anaesthetics. Edinburgh: Livingstone 1948
54. Macintosh RR, Bannister FB, 4th ed. Essentials of general anaesthesia. Oxford: Blackwell 1952
55. Archer WH: A manual of dental anesthesia. Philadelphia: WB Saunders Coy 1952
56. American Medical Association: Fundamentals of anesthesia. 3rd ed. Philadelphia: WB Saunders Coy 1954
57. Knight RT, Tarrow AB: Management of the anesthesia. In: Hale DE (Ed) Anesthesiology. Philadelphia: FA Davis Coy 1955
58. Proctor DF: Anesthesia and Otolaryngology. Baltimore: William Wilkins Coy 1957
59. Dornette WHL: The use of monitors in anesthesia. In: Hale DE (Ed) Anesthesiology. Oxford: Blackwell 1963
60. Lee JA, Atkinson RS: A synopsis of anaesthesia. 5th ed. Bristol: John Wright and Sons Ltd 1964
61. Davenport HT: Paediatric anaesthesia. Philadelphia: Lea and Febiger 1967
62. Morrow WFK, Morrison JD: Anaesthesia for Eye, Ear, Nose, and Throat Surgery. Edinburgh: Churchill Livingstone 1975
63. Collins VJ: Principles of Anesthesiology, 2nd ed. Philadelphia: Lea and Febiger 1976
64. Saidman LJ, Tysmith N: Monitoring in Anaesthesia: New York: John Wiley and Sons 1978
65. Hug CC: Monitoring, In: Miller RD (Ed) Anesthesia. New York: Churchill Livingstone 1981
66. Gravenstein JS, Paulus DA: Monitoring practice in clinical anesthesia. Philadelphia: JB Lippencott Coy 1982
67. Gregory GA (Ed): Pediatric anesthesia. New York: Churchill Livingstone, 1983

68. Hug CC: Monitoring. In: Miller RD (Ed). Anesthesia, 2nd ed. New York: Churchill Livingstone 1986
69. Nunn JF, Utting JE, Brown BR: General Anaesthesia. 5th ed. London: Butterworths 1989
70. Taylor TH, Goldhill DR: Standards of care in anaesthesia. Butterworth Heinemann 1992
71. Calverly RK: Anesthesia as a specialty: past present and future. In: Barash PG, Cullen BF, Stoelting R. Eds. Clinical Anesthesia: Philadelphia: JB Lippencott Coy 1992
72. Maccioli GA, Calkins JM, Collins VJ: Monitoring the anesthetised patient. In: Collins V, Principles of anesthesia; 3rd ed. Philadelphia: Lea and Febiger 1993
73. Runciman WB, Ludbrook GL: Monitoring. In: Nimmo WS, Rowbotham DJ, Smith G (Eds) Anaesthesia, 2nd ed. Oxford. Blackwell Scientific Publications 1994
74. Stevens MH, White PF: In: Miller RD (Ed) Anesthesia, 4th ed. New York. Churchill Livingstone 1994
75. Blitt CD, Hines RL (Eds): Monitoring in anesthesia and critical care medicine, 3rd ed. New York: Churchill Livingstone 1995
76. McIntyre JWR†: Implication of anaesthesiologists' varying location during surgery. Int J of Clin Monit and Computing 1995; 12:33-6
77. Bosomworth PP, Dietsch JD, Hamelberg W: The effect of controlled hemorrhage on heart sounds and the magnitude of the peripheral pulse. Anesth Analg 1963; 42:131-40
78. Williams CJB: On the acoustic principles of the stethoscope. Lond M Gaz 1837; XX:349-53
79. Johnston FD, Kline EM: An acoustical study of the stethoscope. Arch Int Med 1940; 64:328-39
80. Rappaport MB, Sprague HB: Physiologic and physical laws that govern auscultation and their clinical application; acoustic stethoscope and electrical amplifying stethoscope and stethograph. Am Heart J 1941; 21:257-318
81. Ertel PY, Lawrence M, Brown RK et al: Stethoscope acoustics I. The doctor and his stethoscope. Circulation 1966; XXXIV:889-98
82. Ertel PY, Lawrence M, Brown RK et al: Stethoscope acoustics II: Transmission and filtration patterns. Circulation 1966; XXXIV:889-98
83. Murphy RLH, Holford SK, Knowler WC: Visual lung-sound characterisation by time expanded wave form analysis. New Eng J Med 1977; 296:968-971
84. Murphy RL: Auscultation of the lung: past lessons, future possibilities. Thorax 1981; 36:99-107
85. Selig MB: Stethoscope and phonoaudio devices: historical and future perspectives. Am Heart J 1993; 126:262-268
86. McIntyre JWR: Stethoscopy during anaesthesia. Can J Anaesth 1997; 535-42

Preoperative Fasting 1846-1996

J. R. Maltby
Foothills Hospital, Calgary, Canada

Thirteen years before Morton's public demonstration of ether anaesthesia in Boston, William Beaumont published *Experiments and Observations on the Gastric Juice and the Physiology of Digestion.*[1] He had treated Alexis St. Martin, a Canadian fur trapper who was shot in the stomach in Michigan territory in 1822. The wound eventually healed, leaving a gastric fistula through which Beaumont recorded his observations on the process of digestion and gastric emptying, of which the following is one example:

Experiment 33.
March 13. At 1 o'clock, P.M. – Dined on *roasted beef, bread* and *potatoes.* In half an hour, examined contents of stomach – found what he had eaten reduced to a mass, resembling thick porridge.

At 2 o'clock, examined again – nearly all chymified – a few distinct particles, still to be seen.

At 4 o'clock, 30 mins., chymification complete.

At 6 o'clock, examined stomach – found nothing but a little gastric juice, tinged with bile.

The time from ingestion to complete emptying of a variety of easily digested solids in other experiments varied from 2 to 6 hours. Beaumont also observed a marked difference between solids and clear liquids: water, ardent spirits, and most other fluids are not affected by the gastric juice, but pass from the stomach soon after they have been received. Whether or not Beaumont's book was widely read by the medical profession, fasting guidelines in most anaesthesia texts in the first hundred years of anaesthesia were consistent with his observations.

Fasting Guidelines 1847-1960

Neither of the earliest books on anaesthesia that were published in 1847 by Robinson[2] and Snow[3] mentioned preoperative fasting. Even in 1858 Snow recognized only the unpleasantness of vomiting, not its dangers:[4]

"... chloroform is very apt to cause vomiting, if inhaled while there is a quantity of food in the stomach. The sickness is not attended with any danger but it constitutes an unpleasantness and inconvenience which it is desirable to avoid. The best time of all for an operation under chloroform is before breakfast ... It answers very well to perform an operation about the time when the patient would be ready for another meal ... It is impossible to prevent vomiting in some cases with best precautions ... the breakfast may be rejected in an unaltered state hours after it has been taken. In other cases the patient does not vomit, even when he inhales chloroform shortly after a full meal."

By 1881 Lyman[5] warned of the danger of inhalation of gastric contents. He recommended an interval of 4 hours between a light meal of liquids and semisolids and administration of ether. Two years later in 1883 Lister[6] recommended that there should be no solids in the stomach when chloroform was used but that clear liquids were beneficial until 2 hours before surgery. In 1920 Buxton[7] recommended a 7 hour fast for solids and 3 hours for clear liquids. Thus, if surgery was scheduled for 2:00 pm, breakfast should be taken at 7:00 am, followed by tea or beef tea at 11:00 am. Fasting recommendations continued to distinguish between liquids and solids at least until 1960 when Leigh[8] recommended 6 hours for solids and 2 hours for clear liquids for children.

NPO after midnight

No documentation has been found that states precisely when, why or by whom 'NPO after midnight' (nothing by mouth after midnight) was introduced, or why no distinction was made between solids and clear liquids. The danger of aspiration of solids was well recognized,[9] but many text books from the 1960s through the 1980s applied the rule to liquids as well as solids, their authors ignoring the physiology of gastric emptying and providing no clinical evidence to support this change.[10-11]

Possible explanations include Mendelson's description of the liquid acid aspiration syndrome in 1946,[12] in which acid liquid without any food particles caused a severe and sometimes fatal form of pulmonary oedema. In 1972 Roberts and Shirley[13] suggested that patients with > 25 ml in the stomach were at high risk of developing the acid aspiration syndrome on the basis of one experiment in one monkey into whose right main bronchus they injected 0.4 ml.kg^{-1}.[14] A generation of anaesthetists failed to recognize that a much larger volume of fluid would need to be in the stomach for 25 ml to reach the lungs.[15] The normal accumulation and emptying of gastric secretions and the rapid emptying of clear liquids were forgotten, and patients in many centres were denied any oral intake on the day of surgery.

False premises

When false premises are accepted, sound logic can lead to invalid conclusions. The first of these premises was that 25 ml in the stomach was equivalent to 25 ml in the lungs. The second was that fasting from midnight produced an empty stomach while any liquid ingested on the day of surgery would produce a 'full stomach'. Finally, the term 'leading cause' was used to imply frequent in relation to deaths from pulmonary aspiration by investigators who advocated the use of H_2 receptor blockers and other pharmacological prophylaxis.

Randomized clinical trials 1983-96

In 1977 Hester and Heath[16] made an incidental finding that fasting for > 4 hours did not influence the volume or pH of gastric contents at induction of anaesthesia. Miller, Wishart and Nimmo[17] conducted the first randomized clinical trial to compare gastric fluid volume and pH in patients who fasted < 4 hours versus those who fasted overnight from 22:00. There were wide ranges of volume and pH in both groups and mean values were not significantly different. Since then, randomized clinical trials with water, tea, coffee and pulp-free fruit juices have consistently shown no significant differences in either gastric volume or pH in patients who drink unlimited clear fluid until 2 hours before induction of anesthesia compared with those who remain 'NPO after midnight' which often means a fast of 12-14 hours.[18]

Evidence based fasting guidelines

The emptying time for solids depends on the type, particle size and total volume of food that is ingested. Solid material must be broken down to semifluid chyme with particle size < 2 mm before it can pass through the pylorus.[19] Clear liquids empty very rapidly with a half-emptying time of 12 minutes.[20] Opinions in editorials[21-22] and Refresher Courses[23] favour a change in fasting guidelines that would allow patients to drink clear liquids until 2-3 hours before surgery. Since 1996, the Canadian Anaesthetists' Society has recommended no solids on the day of surgery but clear liquids until 3 hours before elective surgery in healthy patients. A task force of the American Society of Anesthesiologists is expected to make similar recommendations for publication in 1998. We shall thus have come full circle to fasting guidelines based on Beaumont's description of the physiology of digestion and gastric emptying that he published more than 160 years ago.

References:

[1] Beaumont W: Experiments and Observations on the Gastric Juice and the Physiology of Digestion. Plattsburgh: Allen, 1833

[2] Robinson J: A Treatise on the Inhalation of the Vapour of Ether. Webster, London 1847

[3] Snow J: On the Inhalation of the Vapour of Ether in Surgical Operations. Churchill, London 1847

[4] Snow J: On Chloroform and Other Anaesthetics. Churchill, London 1858

[5] Lyman HM: Artificial Anaesthesia and Anaesthetics. Wood, New York 1881:287

[6] Lister J: On Anaesthetics. In: The Collected Papers of Joseph Baron Lister. Vol 1. Oxford: Clarendon Press, 1909: 135-75. (Originally published in Holmes System of Surgery Vol iii, 3rd ed. London, 1883.)

[7] Buxton DW: Anaesthetics: Their Uses and Administration. 6th ed. Lewis, London 1920: 24

[8] Leigh MD, Belton MK: Pediatric Anaesthesiology. 2nd ed. New York: Macmillan 1960: 145

[9] Guedel AE: Inhalation Anaesthesia. 2nd ed. Macmillan, New York 1951: 89-101

[10] Lee JA, Atkinson RS: A Synopsis of Anaesthesia. 5th ed. Wright, Bristol 1964: 64

[11] Cohen DD, Dillon GB: Anesthesia for Outpatient Surgery. Thomas, Springfield 1970

[12] Mendelson CL: The aspiration of stomach contents into the lungs during obstetric anesthesia. Am J Obstet Gynec 1946; 52: 191-205

[13] Roberts RB, Shirley MA: Reducing the risk of gastric aspiration during cesarean section. Anesthanaly 1974; 53: 859-868

[14] Roberts RB, Shirley MA: Antacid therapy in obstetrics. Anesthesiology 1980; 83: 53

[15] Coté CJ: NPO after midnight in children - a reappraisal. Anesthesiology 1990; 72: 589-92

[16] Hester JB: Heath ML. Pulmonary acid aspiration syndrome: should prophylaxis be routine? Br J Anaesth 1977; 49: 595-599

[17] Miller M: Wishart HY, Nimmo WS. Gastric contents at induction of anaesthesia. Br J Anaesth 1983; 55: 1185-8

[18] Maltby JR: Preoperative fasting. Current Anaesthesia and Critical Care 1996; 7: 276-280

[19] Minani H, McCallum RW: The physiology and pathophysiology of gastric emptying in humans. Gastroenterology 1984; 86: 1592-1610

[20] Hunt JN: Some properties of an elementary osmoreceptor mechansim. Journal of Physiology (London) 1956; 132: 267-88

[21] Goresky GV, Maltby JR: Fasting guidelines for elective surgical patients. Can J Anaesth 1990; 37: 493-5

[22] Strunin L: How long should patients fast before surgery? Time for new guidelines. Br J Anaesth 1993; 70: 1-3

[23] Stoelting RK: NPO and Aspiration Pneumonitis. 46th Annual Refresher Course Lectures and Clinical Update Program. Park Ridge, Illinois: American Society of Anesthesiologists, Inc., 1995: 432

The Contribution of Anesthesiology to the Development of Palliative Care in Germany

T. Krause and B. Wiedemann
Department of Anaesthesiology, St. Georg Hospital Leipzig, Germany

In the twentieth century, curing diseases has increasingly been seen as the overriding objective of medical intervention; such intervention usually followed a highly technicized, functional approach. Especially in the areas of anesthesiology and intensive care this process can easily be observed. During the last few decades development of palliative care has set new standards.[1] In 1990, the WHO stated (retranslated from German): "Palliative care attends to patients with active, progressive diseases and limited prognosis, whose treatment centers on the optimal quality of life."[2,3] The founder of the first modern hospice, the British social worker, nurse and physician Cicely Mary Strode Saunders formulated: "You matter because you are you, and you matter to the last moment of life. We will do all we can not only for you to die peacefully, but also to live until you die."[4] As early as 1953, John Bonica expressed the commitment of anesthetists to the same objective in his textbook "The Management of Pain", which called attention to adequate pain therapy as an essential factor for the control of symptoms.[5,6,7]

German anaesthesiologists played an important role in the development of palliative care, which emerged in the early seventies in this part of the world, although Martin Kirschner and other were active in this area at the beginning of the century.[8]

Speaking about palliative care means to speak about a quite recent phenomenon. Confronted with chronic cancer pain, German anesthetists recognized that effective care for such patients required the development of new concepts.[9] Of course, palliative medicine can only be realized in a multidisciplinary approach. Nevertheless - an anaesthesiologist's knowledge about pain management is essential in this field. 1971 the first in-patient unit for pain therapy was established in Mainz under U.Gerbershagen. Anaesthesiologists were also instrumental in founding the Association for the Study of Pain (Gesellschaft zum Studium des Schmerzes (GSS)) in 1976.

At its annual meeting in 1982, the key topic was Cancer Pain. Five years later in 1987, the association organized the World Congress of Pain on behalf of the International Association for the Study of Pain; it was also held in Hamburg.[10] Nevertheless, palliative care in Germany developed slowly and a widespread resistance to the very idea of hospices which were often misnamed "Sterbeklinik" was evident. Translated into English word by word this term means "hospital for dying". But in the German language the term contains a lot of negative implications. It sounds like "ghetto of the dying". Where does the word "Sterbeklinik" come from? In 1971 the catholic priest Iblacker produced a documentary movie, named: "Noch 16 Tage ... eine Sterbeklinik in London" (16 days left...a hospital for dying in London). The movie discribed the work and the concept of St. Christophers Hospice in London. Being brought to the homes of German public via television, this movie led to a widespread discussion. The German "Ministry of Youth, Family and Health" asked the church, representatives of the medical profession and public corporations whether or not they saw a need for special units in cases of terminal illness or not. The evangelical and catholic churches and the medical representatives stated that their opinion, there was no need for such units. They believed that it was possible to manage the problem with in existing structures in Germany.[11] Both the state and the major churches rejected the concept of hospices. Such resistance and ignorance of the international hospice movement led to a deficit of expertise in the areas of terminal and palliative care.

Additionally, regulations concerning the prescription of strong opioids were highly restrictive, a fact much criticized by anesthetists.[12] In the early eighties, the University of Goettingen university was among the first to establish, in its department of anesthesiology, an out-patient unit for pain therapy. In 1989, Göttingen was the first German university to create a chair of algesiology and appointed J. Hildebrandt to it.[13]

Living in Leipzig, we would like to ad a few words about developments in the east of Germany. In East Germany, the anesthetist M.Tschirner established the first pain unit at the "Charité" hospital in Berlin in 1980, and in 1986, oral morphine therapy was introduced.

In intensive care units, anesthetists were under increasing pressure to take ethically problematic decisions and with growing interest in palliative care,[14,15,16] issues of ethics concerning the end of life became ever more important and called for new solutions.[17,18,19,20]

In Cologne, D. Zech and his colleagues of the university hospital's out-patient pain clinic cooperated with the department of surgery in establishing a palliative care unit in 1983.[21,22,23] Following these precedents and building on the experience of the "Paul Lechler Hospital" of Internal Medicine in Tübingen, two hospitals in Bonn founded palliative care units in 1988 and 1990, respectively.[24,25] The palliative care ward at the "Bonn Malteser Order Hospital" was the first unit of its kind in Germany under the direction of an anesthetist - E. Klaschik. After federal funds became available in 1991, a whole series of palliative care units have been founded. In addition, several hospices have been opened.[26] Anesthetists are involved in most of them, either as consultants or in some cases, as directors. In 1992, the first continuing training course in pain therapy and which was organized by a professional association of anesthetists was held in Bochum.[27] In the following year, a first list of palliative care units and hospices in Germany was prepared by anesthetists from Cologne;[28] In 1993, the first German textbook of pain therapy was published.[29] In order to maximize interdisciplinary cooperation, the "German Society of Palliative Medicine" was founded in 1994, and the following year, the "Interdisciplinary Association of Pain Therapy" was born.[30]

In sum, anesthetists have been most instrumental in the introduction of palliative care into German medicine and in achieving public acceptance.

References:

1. Meuret G: Palliative Krebsbehandlung und terminal care - eine Empfehlung für Ärztinnen und Ärzte, Pflegende und psychosoziale Fachkräfte. Ministerium für Arbeit, Gesundheit und Sozialordnung Baden - Württemberg, Reihe Gesundheitspolitik, Stuttgart 1995; 34:13

2. Palliativmedizin, Neurologie und Psychiatrie: RV Maydell, R Voltz (ed), Deutsche Gesellschaft für Palliativmedizin, 1996; 2

3. Zech D: Entwicklung der Palliativmedizin in Deutschland. In: Palliativmedizin heute, E Klaschik, F Nauck (ed), Springer, Berlin, 1994: 88-89

4. Saunders CM: Hospice and Palliative Care - an Interdisciplinary Approach. E Arnold (ed), UK 1990

5. Hildebrandt J: Die Therapie chronischer Schmerzen - eine Aufgabe des Anaesthesisten? Anaesthesie-Intensivtherapie-Notfallmedizin 1990; 25: 247

6. Bonica J: The Management of Pain. Lea & Febiger, Philadelphia 1953

7. Kiss J: Das Ende einer Ära, Gedanken zum Treffen „The Bonicas Remembered" in Seattle am 7. und 8. März 1996. Der Schmerz 1996; 10:216

8. Goerig M, Schulte am Esch J: Martin Kirschner - Anästhesist, Intensivmediziner, Schmerztherapeut. AINS 1994; 6:343-353

9. Hildebrandt J: Die Therapie chronischer Schmerzen - eine Aufgabe des Anästhesisten? Anaesthesiologie-Intensivtherapie-Notfallmedizin 1990; 25: 247

10. Zimmermann M, Druell-Zimmermann, D: Gesellschaft zum Studium des Schmerzes 1975 - 1995, eine Chronik. Heidelberg 1995: 5-11

11. Godzik P: Die Hospizbewegung in der Bundesrepublik Deutschland, Texte aus der VELKD, Lutherisches Kirchenamt der VELKD, Hannover, 3. Auflage 1992; 47:12-16

12. Zenz M: Status of cancer pain and palliative care. J Pain Symptom Man. 1993; 8:416-418

13. Zimmermann M: Druell-Zimmermann D: Gesellschaft zum Studium des Schmerzes 1975 - 1995, eine Chronik. Heidelberg 1995 : 5-12

14. Schara J: Was darf die Intensivmedizin? In: Prüfsteine med. Ethik. H R Zielinski, Dadder (ed), Saarbrücken-Scheidt 1984

15. Opderbecke HW: Grenzen der Intensivmedizin. Klinikarzt 1984; 13:797-802

16. Weis K-H: Ethik und Grenzen der Intensivmedizin. Anästhesiologie-Intensivmedizin-Notfallmedizin 1984; 33:1-3

17. Salomon F: Beatmung - Ja oder Nein? Ethische Überlegungen zu Grenzfragen der Intensivmedizin. Anaesthesiologie-Intensivmedizin-Notfallmedizin 1985; 20:143-146

18. Zielinski HR: Palliative Therapie und Hospizbewegung in der Bundesrepublik Deutschland. In: Prüfsteine medizinischer Ethik XIII. H R Zielinski, Dadder (ed), Saarbrücken-Scheidt 1993: 29

19. Hermanns K, Salomon F: Sterben und Tod auf einer operativen Intensivstation aus der Sicht der Angehörigen - eine Fragebogenuntersuchung. Anästhesiologie-Intensivmedizin-Notfallmedizin 1993; 28:75-80

20. Prien Th, Lawin P: Therapiereduktion in der Intensivmedizin, "Sterben zulassen" durch bewußte Begrenzung medizinischer Möglichkeiten. Anaesthesist 1996,45:176-182

21. Pichlmaier H, Thielemann-Jonen, J Zech, D: Die palliative Behandlung von terminal Tumorkranken. Der Internist 1988; 26:26-33

22. Lehmann K A: In memoriam Dr. med. Detlev Zech. Anaesthesist 1995; 44: 886

23. Jonen-Thielemann J : Zehn Jahre Palliativstation: Chirurgische Universitätsklinik Köln. In: Palliativmedizin heute. E Klaschik, F Nauck (ed), Springer, Berlin 1994; 103-116

24. Zech D: Entwicklung der Palliativmedizin in Deutschland. In: Palliativmedizin heute. E Klaschik, F Nauck (ed). Springer, Berlin 1994

[25] Klaschik E : Drei Jahre Palliativstation: Malteser Krankenhaus Bonn. In: Palliativmedizin heute. E Klaschik, F Nauck (ed), Springer, Berlin 1994; 117-126

[26] Zech D : Entwicklung der Palliativmedizin in Deutschland. In: Palliativmedizin heute. E. Klaschik, F Nauck (ed). Springer, Berlin 1994; 92

[27] Zimmermann M, Druell-Zimmermann D: Gesellschaft zum Studium des Schmerzes 1975 - 1995, eine Chronik. Heidelberg 1995; 14

[28] Stationäre Hospize und Palliativeinrichtungen in Deutschland. Schmerzambulanz der Klinik und Poliklinik für Anästhesiologie und Operative Intensivmedizin der Universitätsklinik zu Köln (ed), Köln 1993

[29] Zenz M, J Jurna : Lehrbuch der Schmerztherapie. Wissenschaftliche Verlagsgesellschaft, Stuttgart 1993

[30] Zimmermann M, Druell-Zimmermann D: Gesellschaft zum Studium des Schmerzes 1975 - 1995, eine Chronik. Heidelberg 1995; 16

The Impact of the Copenhagen Anaesthesiology Centre on the Practice of Anaesthesiology in the Czech and Slovak Republics

B. Dworacek, M. Buroš, J. Pokorný
Medical School, Prague, Czech Republic

In the years before World War II, the standards of anaesthesiology in the Czech and Slovak Republic (former Czechoslovakia) were determined by the needs of the surgical profession. Surgical practice followed the traditions of the surgical school of Vienna, dating from the time that the region was part of the Austro-Hungarian Empire. There were no independent anaesthesiologists at that time. Anaesthesiology was treated as a part of the surgical profession: It was included in the surgical curriculum and administered by the surgeons who were operating on the patients[1,2].

After World War II, anaesthesiology in the Republic started to differentiate itself from the surgical profession. This was to the merit of physicians who had returned to their native country from the United Kingdom and the United States. L. Spinadel founded the first independent anaesthesiological department in the military hospital in Prague and for some years this remained a unique situation. But soon, the rapid development of surgical techniques (especially in thoracic surgery) led to the evolution of a separate group of physicians who were willing to devote their full effort to anaesthesia. This was most apparent in hospitals with large surgical departments. However, these new specialists remained within their surgical departments and their activities were limited to the more complicated operations. Anaesthesia for common operations was still administered by the surgeons themselves and was often delegated to junior staff and sometimes even to the nurses[2].

An important milestone for the profession was in 1952, when the Chief Surgical Advisor of the Republic decided that anaesthesia should be administered only by physicians. However, he did not specify which specialization these physicians should have because, at that time, there were only a few specialized anaesthesiologists.

At the same time, a new organization for the medical professions was introduced and anaesthesiology was then recognized as a separate specialization. A regional structure was chosen and Regional Medical Officers were appointed from every medical profession, including anaesthesiology. The function of institutional anaesthesiologist was introduced in every hospital, and had the responsibility for the quality of anaesthesia administered by members of the surgical professions. The Institute for Advanced Training of Physicians was founded and included a chair for anaesthesiology. This Chair was founded for the further training and examination of anaesthesiological specialists[2].

Those who were already specialized in this profession founded a new society that formed a section of the Surgical Society. In 1956, this section became a member of the newly founded World Federation of Societies of Anaesthesiologists. Many favourable circumstances combined and guaranteed a high quality of anaesthetic practice. Technical research and development was stimulated by well-developed pharmaceutical, mechanical and rubber industries. Intensive contacts were maintained with anaesthesiologists from abroad. At the Institute for Clinical and Experimental Surgery, the leading anaesthesiologist Hugo Keszler and his colleagues tackled the problems of resuscitation.

In spite of these developments, anaesthesiologists still remained within the framework of the surgical departments. In 1959, B. Dworacek was sent for a year-long anaesthesiology course at the WHO Training Centre in Copenhagen. A year later, M. Buroš was also sent there[3]. They were most impressed with the position and organization of anaesthesiology in this Centre. Anaesthesiology formed a separate discipline there and it was professionally and economically independent from the surgical departments. Because of this independence, anaesthesiologists could apply the experience they had gained in surgical anaesthesia to new areas that were not directly related to surgery.

We would like to mention four of the people who played a significant role in the exploration of these new areas. In 1952, Bjørn Ibsen returned from his training in the United States. Soon afterwards, he took care of the artificial ventilation of patients who had been paralyzed during the outbreak of poliomyelitis in Denmark. At that time, no automatic respirators were available in Copenhagen. As a result, Ibsen mobilized a large group of medical students who applied artificial ventilation manually, using Waters sets that were in abundant supply. In a short time, the mortality rate was decreased by a large percentage[4]. After this experience, Ibsen started admitting into his anaesthesiological department critically ill patients whose vital functions were failing, without regard for the cause of their condition. An anaesthesiologist was always present and could support vital functions without any delay. At the same time, the cause of the illness was treated by a team led by an anaesthesiologist and further consisted of a surgeon, neurologist, internist and, if necessary, other specialists. This team-approach proved to be quite effective. Because of this, Bjørn Ibsen can be seen as the founding father of the intensive care unit in the anaesthesia department[5].

H. Ruben turned his attention to the organization and equipment of rescue teams. Because of his technical expertise, he fostered the development of effective tools for resuscitation that are known under the name of AMBU. W. Dam used his experiences with resuscitation in the toxicological department of his hospital and, in this way, contributed to the optimal treatment of victims of poisoning. J. Kirchhoff used his experience with regional anaesthesia for the policlinical treatment of patients with chronic pain.

After returning to their native country, Dworacek and Buroš were able to easily convince their colleagues of the effectiveness of the Danish organization of anaesthesiology. In 1961, the anaesthesiological section separated from the surgical society and founded its own independent association. Without delay, a new concept for the future development of anaesthesiology was worked out. Anaesthesiology was defined as a separate profession that was independent from surgery and included the responsibility for the organization of intensive care units. These principles were quickly assimilated between 1965 and 1969 and were also adopted by the Public Health Department.

As a result, anaesthesiologists could then begin to apply their experience outside of the operating room. For example, Dworacek successfully promoted the training of basic resuscitation in schools. In 1968, this training was included in the curricula of all schools in the Republic.

This new concept of anaesthesiological organization and practice from the WHO Training Centre in Copenhagen became the starting point for the organization of anaesthesiology and the function of anaesthesiologists in former Czechoslovakia.

This concept improved the position of the anaesthesiologist and made him an equal member of the operating team. The experience that was gained in the operating room could be applied to the treatment of critically ill patients in the intensive care units of the anaesthesia departments, the treatment of chronic pain symptoms and resuscitation in a general sense. Proof of this improved position and organization is demonstrated by the following numbers: Before 1960, there were only a handful of anaesthesiologists in what is now the Czech and Slovak Republics. At this moment, there are more than 1,200 specialists in the Czech Republic alone.

References:

[1] Dworacek B, Keszler H: The Development of Anaesthesiology in Czechoslovakia. Anaesthesia: Essays on its History. Springer-Verlag, Berlin Heidelberg 1985; 258-261

[2] Pokorný J, Bohuš, O et al: Anesthesiologie a resuscitace v České a Slovenské republice na cestě k oborové samostatnosti (Anaesthesiology and Resuscitation in the Czech and Slovak Republics on the Way to Professional Independence). Pražká vydavatelská společnost, Praha 1996; 11-14, 27-30, 46-52.

[3] Secher O: Anaesthesiology Centre Copenhagen. Anaesthesia: Essays on its History. Springer-Verlag, Berlin Heidelberg 1985; 321-334

[4] Ibsen B: The treatment of Shock with Vasodilating Agents. Anaesthesia: Essays on its History. Springer-Verlag, Berlin Heidelberg 1985; 112-15

[5] Mushin WW: Clinician versus Researcher in Anaesthesia. Anaesthesia: Essays on its History. Springer-Verlag, Berlin Heidelberg 1985; 381

History of Blood Gas Analysis

W. Severinghaus[*], P. Astrup[**]

[*] University of California, San Francisco, USA
[**] Rigshospitalet Copenhagen, Denmark

I. Introduction

From the earliest studies of blood by Robert Boyle (1627-1691) and the earlier understanding of similarities between fermentation of wine and respiration of animals, the history of both the physiology and measurement of CO_2 is coupled to studies of acids and bases. The alkalinity of blood was discovered by Hilaire Marin Rouelle (1718-1779) in Paris, using titration and color indicators. Henry Bence Jones (1813-1878), a physician at St. George's Hospital in London, about 1849 recognized the connection between blood alkalinity and stomach acid secretion. Cholera had been shown to reduce the "free alkali" of blood in 1831 by an Irish physician working in India, William B. O'Shaughnessy (1809-1889). The connection between the CO_2 content and alkalinity was established in his 1877 thesis by Friedrich Walter (b.1850) studying in Strasbourg under fellow-Latvian Oswald Schmiedeberg (1838-1921), making it possible to study acidosis by extracting and quantifying the CO_2 from blood.

From Walter's discovery until the introduction of electrochemical analysis in the mid 20th century, measurement of blood O_2 and CO_2 contents thus depended on vacuum extraction, usually in combination with acidification to free CO_2, and chemical (e.g ferricyanide) alteration of oxyhemoglobin to free O_2. The freed gases were measured volumetrically until Donald D. van Slyke (1883-1971) at the Rockefeller Institute in New York introduced a more accurate manometric apparatus in 1924 [1], still the standard but seldom used method.

2. Analysis of pH

Physical chemistry as a discipline began about 1884 when Jacobus Hendricus van't Hoff (1852-1911) in Amsterdam, following the thermodynamic theories of Josiah Willard Gibbs (1839-1903) and Henri Louis Le Chatelier (1850-1936), realized that osmotic pressure of molecules (or, later, ions) in solution was precisely the same as they would exert at the same concentration in a gas, thus linking solution theory to the long established laws describing the behavior of gases. The most dramatic, major change in understanding of electrolyte solutions occurred when Svante Arrhenius (1859-1927) in Uppsala used conductivity to prove the reality of the existence of ions in his 1884 thesis [2]. The Arrhenius thesis stimulated Wilhelm Ostwald (1853-1932), shortly after moving from Riga to Leipzig in 1887, to make the first electrometric measurement of H+ ions, and to identify the relationship between acid strength and H+ ion concentration and activity. Ostwald's student Hermann Walther Nernst (1864-1941) discovered the energetic equivalence of Faraday's constant F, the charge in coulombs per mole, to PV/n of the old gas laws, mathematically linking the gas laws to electrometric ion activity with his equation for the EMF generated by a concentration (C) gradient of a single ion:

$E = (RT/nF)(\log C)$ where R is the gas constant, T temperature and n the valence [3].

After Nernst moved to Göttingen, his assistant Heinrich Ludwig Danneel (1867-1942) discovered the reaction of oxygen with a negatively charged metal (cathode), the basis of oxygen polarography later developed by Jaroslav Heyrovsky (1890-1967) in Prague. Nobel prizes in chemistry were awarded to van't Hoff (1901), Arrhenius (1903), Ostwald (1909), Nernst (1920) and Heyrovsky (1959).

3. The carbonic acid buffer system

The astonishing ability of blood to neutralize large amounts of acid led Lawrence J. Henderson (1878-1942), Professor of physiology at Harvard, to clarify the buffer system composed of bicarbonate and free CO_2 in 1907. Even before H+ could be measured in CO_2 - HCO_3^- mixtures with electrodes, he rewrote the law of mass action for weak acids and their salts. In terms of CO_2 and $NaHCO_3$, this was: $[H+] = K(H_2CO_3/NaHCO_3)$, recognizing that K, the dissociation constant, for practical purposes assumes dissolved CO_2 to be H_2CO_3 (actually only 1 part in 300 is carbonic acid).

Ostwald's platinum hydrogen electrode was useless in blood because the CO_2 was lost during equilibration with H_2. Following Nernst's discovery of ion potentials, in 1906, a biologist and biochemist, Max Cremer (1865-1935) discovered an electrical potential proportional to the $[H^+]$ difference across thin glass membranes, making possible the glass pH electrode. By 1909, Fritz Jacob Haber (1868-1934, Nobel prize 1918) and Zygamunt Klemensiewicz (1886-?) constructed and carefully studied a glass pH electrode in Karlsruhe.

The term pH, the negative log of H^+ ion concentration, was suggested by S. P. L. Sørensen as a simplification to save writing about 8 zeros, in a paper on enzyme activity, written while he directed the Copenhagen Carlsberg laboratory [4]. Although use of pH rather than nanomoles of H+ has often been attacked, it seems to have survived largely because most acid-base and titration chemical reactions show symmetry around their pK when expressed in terms of pH, or of relative changes in H+, but not H+ concentration per se. Following his lead, in 1917 Karl Albert Hasselbalch (1874-1962), director of the Finsen Laboratory in Copenhagen, adapted Henderson's mass law for carbonic acid to the logarithmic form known as the Henderson-Hasselbalch equation: $pH=pK'+\{log[HCO_3^-]/S.Pco_2\}$.

Hasselbalch devised a method of measuring pH of blood or plasma without loss of CO_2 despite equilibration with H_2, by re-equilibrating the same H_2 bubble with repeated aliquots of sample until CO_2 came to equilibrium - a very impractical method for clinical use! The first blood glass pH electrode, designed to keep Pco_2 in solution, was constructed by Phyllis T. Kerridge (1902-1940) in London in 1925. D. A. McInnes and D. Belcher replaced the cup with capillary tubing in 1932, added a clever 3-way glass stop-cock for making a fresh liquid junction with saturated KCl, to make the first truly precise blood pH electrode, although it was designed to operate at room temperature. Thermostatted blood pH apparatus was described in 1931 by W. C. Stadie, H. O'Brien and P. E. Laug, but did not become available commercially until the mid 1950's. Accurate temperature correction factors for blood were not known until T. B. Rosenthal's work published in 1948.

Measurement for clinical patient care of pH and Pco_2 was stimulated by the polio epidemics in 1950-53. In Copenhagen, anesthesiologist Bjorn Ibsen (1915-) and clinical chemist Poul Astrup (1915-) demonstrated to the clinicians that the high blood CO_2 content did not represent metabolic alkalosis, but hypercapnic acidosis, using the established Van Slyke method and the Henderson-Hasselbalch equation to compute Pco_2. The subsequent artificial ventilation of as many as 100 patients at one time led to establishment by Ibsen of the first intensive care unit. Astrup soon devised a simpler method using only a pH electrode before and after equilibrating blood with known Pco_2 gas. A review of Van Slyke's work suggested to him that a blood pH-log Pco_2 plot, generated by equilibrating a sample with differing CO_2 concentrations in oxygen, would be linear over the physiologic range. The unknown Pco_2 could then be read from the originally measured pH on the line connecting two known pH-Pco_2 points. Furthermore, the horizontal displacement of this line (on the pH axis) revealed the non-respiratory acid base abnormality. Siggaard Andersen, Engel, Jørgensen and Astrup [5] first computed a "standard bicarbonate", later defining "base excess" (BE) in mM/L of blood, dependent only on pH, Pco_2 and Hb measurements.

Although BE is now the dominant measure of metabolic acid base balance, its introduction initiated a 20 year trans-atlantic acid-base debate between two groups, one consisting largely of internists using HCO_3- as the metabolic parameter, the other largely anesthesiologists and critical care physicians using BE. The debate arose partly because in-vivo alterations of Pco_2 result in movement of HCO_3- between blood and the body's ECF, which generally has about 3 times the volume of blood. In response, the terms standard base excess (SBE) was later introduced by the simple expedient of assuming an effective ECF hemoglobin concentration of 5 gm/dl.

Some internists prefer to work with the calculated HCO_3- and 6 "simple" remembered equations to estimate patient acid-base states. Stewart has proposed to measure every ion and compute the abnormality equivalent to base excess as strong ion difference [6]. It too is altered by Pco_2 variations driving HCO_3- in or out of ECF. Schlichtig, Grogono and I have converted the 6 bicarbonate-based compensation equations into the expected relationship of SBE and Pco_2 [unpublished].

4. CO_2 electrode

Richard Stow in Columbus, Ohio, faced with the same polio ventilation problem, conceived an electrode for measuring Pco_2 [7]. He knew that CO_2 permeated rubber freely, and that CO_2 acidified water. He constructed his own glass pH and reference electrode, wrapped it with thin rubber membrane over a film of distilled water, and showed it could measure Pco_2. Stow felt it would never be stable enough to be accurate and refused to patent the idea. In order to stabilize Stow's electrode Severinghaus and Bradley added HCO_3- to the electrolyte, and incorporated Po_2 and Pco_2 electrodes in a common thermostat [8].

5. O_2 electrode

In 1922, Jaroslav Heyrovsky [9] accidentally discovered a method to measure dissolved oxygen using a "dropping mercury cathode" with which the continuously renewed surface avoided "poisoning" by protein or other substances. He developed polarography as a method of analyzing many ionizable substances after eliminating O_2, which in his view was a contaminant. Otto Müller (1908-) and Percy Baumberger (1892-1973) at Stanford reported biologic O_2 analysis with dropping mercury in 1935, and Henry K. Beecher (1904-1976) at Massachusetts General Hospital's Anesthesia department was first to accurately measure human plasma Po_2 in this way. Among others who measured tissue O_2 with implanted bare platinum cathodes were Lawrence R. Blinks (1900-1989) at Stanford and Philip W. Davies (1915-), Detlev W. Bronk (1897-1975) and Frank Brink, Jr (1910-) at the University of Pennsylvania.

In 1952, Leland Clark adapted polarography to measure performance of his blood oxygenator by covering a platinum cathode with cellophane to exclude protein. Although this electrode was extremely sensitive to blood flow in his pump oxygenator stream, poisoning was prevented. He also tried a polyethylene membrane successfully, but at first he rejected it, thinking it could not be dependable since the reference electrode was outside the membrane, depending on leak under the membrane edge or through microscopic holes in the polyethylene. On Oct 4, 1954 he suddenly realized he could put a reference anode under the polyethylene with the cathode, and constructed that day the first modern O_2 electrode [10].

Clark and Stow independently discovered the technique of using a differentially permeable membrane to separate an electrochemical cell from a substance to be analyzed. Clark's O_2 electrode required stirring and calibration with tonometered blood. Need for stirring and tonometry was eliminated by miniaturizing the O_2 cathode in 1959. Astrup's equilibration method was gradually supplanted by three electrode systems in the mid 1960's. Blood gas analysis has been judged to be the test most often altering therapy, and has greatly facilitated developments in respiratory physiology.

6. Other blood gas methods

About 1976, transcutaneous measurement of Po_2 especially in neonates was made possible by heating the skin, by Renate Huch, Albert Huch, Dietrich Lübbers and Patrick Eberhardt in Marburg, Germany [11]. Transcutaneous Pco_2 electrodes were developed in 1978. Optical (fluorescence) techniques for measuring pH, Pco_2 and Po_2, developed by Lübbers and associates, are now competing with electrode methods both in bench and in-vivo (cardio-pulmonary by-pass apparatus control and intra-vascular) applications.

7. Oximetry

The concepts underlying oximetry had their beginning in the early 1860's. In 1862, Felix Hoppe Seyler (1825-1895), the founder of physiologic chemistry in Germany at Tübingen crystalized the red coloring material of blood and named it haemoglobin. He later studied its spectrum, and showed that it was oxygen that changed the color by forming a loose combination he termed "oxyhaemoglobin". Georg Gabriel Stokes (1819-1903) reported in London in 1864 that hemoglobin was the carrier of oxygen. By 1874, Karl von Vierordt (1818-1884), a German physiologist, had spectroscopically measured the rate of oxygen consumption of his own hand after applying a tourniquet.

In 1929, a young American physiology graduate student Glen Millikan (1906-1947), working with Francis John Worsley Roughton (1899-1972) in the laboratory of Joseph Barcroft (1872-1947) at Cambridge, optically measured the speed of combination of oxygen with hemoglobin, using purple and yellow filters and photocells to record the change of color in glass tubing downstream from a point where hemoglobin was mixed with oxygenated saline. In the physiology department of Göttingen in 1932, Ludwig Nicolai (1904-) resurrected Karl von Vierordt's work, adding photoelectric light detection. His associate Kurt Kramer (1906-1985) continued that work, introducing the new German barrier layer photocells into physiology to record saturation in-vivo by transilluminating the arteries of animals. In Leipzig about 1936, Karl Matthes (1905-1962), after working with both (Sir) Henry Dale in London and (Sir) Charles Sherrington at Oxford, developed the first two wavelength ear saturation meter with red and green filters, again based on Nicolai's studies. He later switched to red and infra-red filters.

At the outbreak of war in 1939, Millikan returned to the US and began unpaid research at the University of Pennsylvania on in-vivo oxygen measurement at the request of the British Admiralty. Both Millikan and Kramer became deeply involved in developing optical blood oxygen saturation methods for their respective air forces because fighter pilots were blacking out at high altitude. In 1942, Millikan published [12] his light-weight ear "oximeter" (a term he coined) using the two German ideas, Kramer's copper oxide barrier photocells and Matthes' two wavelengths for total light and thickness compensation, with red and green filters. By good luck Millikan's green filter and photocell proved to be responding only to infra-red light, the ear being essentially opaque to green. After the war, Millikan became chairman of physiology at Vanderbilt University but was killed by a falling rock in 1947 while climbing in Tennessee's Smoky Mountains.

Earl Wood (1912-) at the Mayo Clinic added a pressure capsule to squeeze the blood out of the ear to obtain a zero setting, a method discovered in 1940 by J. R. Squire at University College in London. Robert Brinkman (1894-?) and Willem Zilstra (1925-) in Groningen developed a "reflectance" oximeter called "cyclops" for forehead operation in the 1950's.

None of the preceeding devices could be depended upon for accurate analysis without in-vivo calibration while the patient breathed oxygen. In order to take account of COHb, MetHb, and hemoglobin concentration, M. Polanyi at the American Optical Company, in 1961-62 introduced the concept of using multiple wavelengths of light to distinguish between pigments, constructing a fiberoptic catheter oximeter. About 1964, Robert Shaw, a surgeon in San Francisco, assembled a multi-wavelength fiberoptic absolute-reading ear oximeter, accurate without in-vivo calibration down to 70% SaO_2 (marketed by Hewlett-Packard). Perhaps because of cost and weight, its use was largely limited to pulmonary and cardiac function laboratories.

In 1972 in Tokyo, Takuo Aoyagi invented the pulse oximeter while working with an ear piece densitometer, attempting to measure cardiac output by I.V. dye injection. He tried to cancel out the pulsatility of the red signal by subtracting an equally pulsatile infra red signal which was insensitive to the dye. By chance he noted that changes in SaO_2 reintroduced pulsatility in the record. He then studied the literature on oximetry, and developed the now-famous equation for pulse oximetry:

$SpO_2 = f(Rac/Rdc)/(IRac/IRdc)$ where R and IR are red and infrared signals, ac and dc referring to the pulsatile and total components of each. This equation makes it possible to compute arterial saturation without precalibration, independent of ear thickness, skin pigment, hemoglobin concentration or light intensity. Aoyagi has recently extended the method to permit non-invasive analysis of cardiac output, plasma volume and liver blood flow by pulse oximetry after cardio green dye injection [13].

For more complete historic information and references see [14,15].

References:

[1] Van Slyke DD, O'Neill JM: The determination of gases in blood and other solutions by vacuum extraction and manometric measurement. J Biol Chem 1924; 61:523

[2] Arrhenius SA: über die Dissociation der in Wasser gelösten Stoffe. Z Physik Chemie 1887; 1:631-658

[3] Nernst WH: Die elektromotorische Wirksamkeit de Jonen. Z Physik Chemie 1889; 4:129-181

[4] Sørensen SPL: Enzymstudien II. Mitteilung über die Messung und die Bedeutung der Wasserstoffionenkonzentration bein enzymatischen Prozessen. Biochem Z 1909; 21:131-304

[5] Siggaard-Andersen O, Engel K, Jørgensen K, Astrup P: A micro method for determination of pH, carbon dioxide tension, base excess and standard bicarbonate in capillary blood. Scand J Clin Lab Invest 1960; 12:172-176

[6] Stewart PA: Modern quantitative acid-base chemistry. Can J Physiol Pharmacol 61: 1444-61, 1983

[7] Stow RW, Baer RF, Randall B: Rapid measurement of the tension of carbon dioxide in blood. Arch Phys Med Rehabil 1957;38:646-650

[8] Severinghaus JW, Bradley AF: Electrodes for blood PO_2 and PcO_2 determination. J Appl Physiol 1958; 13:515-520

[9] Heyrovsky J: Electrolysis with the dropping mercury electrode. Chemicke Listy 1922; 16:256-304

[10] Clark LC, Jr: Measurement of oxygen tension: a historical perspective. Crit Care Med 1981; 9:960-962

[11] Huch R, Huch A, Lübbers D: Transcutaneous measurement of blood PO_2 ($tcPO_2$). J Perinat Med 1973; 1:183-190

[12] Milliken GA: The oximeter: an instrument for measuring continuously oxygen saturation of arterial blood in man. Rev Sci Instr 1942; 13:434-444

[13] Iijima T, Aoyagi T, Iwao Y, Masuda J, Fuse M, Kobayashi N, Sankawa H. Cardiac output and circulating blood volume analysis by pulse dye-densitometry. J Clin Monit 13:81-89, 1997

[14] Astrup P, Severinghaus JW: The History of Blood Gases and Acid Base Balance. Munksgaard, Copenhagen, 1986, pp1-332

[15] Severinghaus JW, Astrup PB: History of Blood Gas Analysis. Int Anes Clinics 25:(4), 1987, pp1-224

Historical Interactions of Pharmacology and Anesthesia

J. Parascandola
Public Health Service Historian, Fishers Lane, Rockville, Maryland U.S.A.

The histories of pharmacology and anesthesia are closely intertwined. Pharmacology began to emerge as a distinct professional discipline at about the same time that inhalation anesthesia was being developed in the 19th century, although the antecedents of both pharmacology and anesthesia date back many centuries and have certain common threads. Since anesthetic agents (whether general or local) are drugs, it is understandable that the science of pharmacology would contribute to the discovery of anesthetics and to an understanding of their physiological action and appropriate use.

The interaction between the two fields, however, is a two-way street. The study of anesthetics has also influenced the development of pharmacology. Efforts to explain the action of general anesthetics in the late 19th and early 20th centuries, for example, led to an enhanced understanding of the mechanisms by which drugs act, as will be discussed later in this paper.

Chauncey Leake, an eminent pharmacologist and medical historian who also contributed to the field of anesthesia, has referred to the study of drugs before the 19th century as "protopharmacology."[1] Knowledge of drugs in this period was primarily empirical, based largely on the clinical experience of the physician. The great majority of drugs used in the era of protopharmacology were botanical in origin. Few of these substances cured disease, but rather they alleviated the symptoms of illness and injury. One of the chief among these symptoms, of course, was pain.

Humans have sought drugs for the relief of pain probably since before the dawn of recorded history. The narcotic effects of substances such as alcohol and opium was known in antiquity, and these drugs were used for therapeutic as well as what we might call recreational purposes. Alcohol and opium are among our oldest anesthetics.[2] Oswald Schmiedeberg (1838-1921), one of the founders of modern pharmacology, argued that the Greek poet Homer was alluding to opium when he speaks in The Odyssey of the substance that Helen put in wine "to quit any pain and strife, and bring forgetfulness of every ill." Others have disagreed about the nature of the drug involved, and some scholars have even argued that Homer was not referring to a drug at all, but to the charm of Helen's conversation.[3] Be that as it may, we can see that the history of "protoanesthesiology," to use an analogy with Leake's terminology, is bound up with the history of protopharmacology.

Mandragora, or mandrake, is another example of a drug that was used in antiquity to relieve pain and induce sleep. The root of the plant was believed to resemble the human body, and it was often depicted in later herbals rather fancifully, with the root literally displaying a human form, sometimes in both male and female varieties. The legend surrounding this plant claimed that when it was pulled from the ground it would utter such unearthly shrieks that anyone who heard them would be driven mad or die. Elaborate schemes were proposed for avoiding this fate,

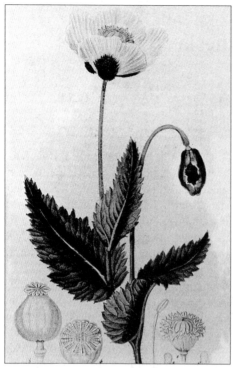

An illustration of the opium poppy, which has been used to ease pain since antiquity, from F. P. Chaumeton's Flore medicale decrite, Paris, 1815-20. (Courtesy of National Library of Medicine)

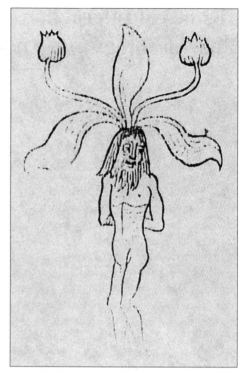

A fanciful illustration of the mandrake plant, whose root was believe to resemble the human body, from Hortus sanitatus, Mainz, 1491. (Courtesy of National Library of Medicine)

such as having a dog tied to the plant by a rope pull it up. One cannot help but wonder whether such legends were propagated by herb-gatherers as a way of limiting competition.[4]

Alcohol, opium, mandragora, and other substances came to be used at times over the centuries for the purposes of anesthesia in surgical operations, though as we know they proved to be less than reliable anesthetics. Dioscorides, in the first century B.C., for example, mentions the use of mandragora by physicians "when they are about to cut, or cauterize."[5]

From early times, medical practitioners and natural philosophers tried to understand how drugs exerted their action on the body, the basis of the science of pharmacology. For much of Western history, the explanation of drug action was couched in terms of humoral theory, with therapy based upon a principal of opposites. Substances with hot and dry properties, for example, would be used to treat diseases characterized as being caused by an excess of phlegm, a cold and wet humor, in the body.[6]

As alternatives to the Galenic humoral theory began to be postulated in the post-Renaissance period, other explanations of drug action were offered. So, for example, the corpuscular theory espoused by Robert Boyle (1627-1691) and others hypothesized that the physiological effects of drugs was based upon the size and shapes of the corpuscles or atoms which composed these substances. The so-called iatrochemists attributed the action of drugs to their acidic and basic properties.[7]

As a result of the attention given to animal experimentation by William Harvey (1578-1657) and his contemporaries in the 17th century, experimentation involving the study of the effects of drugs on animals became more common. Particular attention was focused on the action of potent poisons, perhaps because it was relatively easy to observe and measure severe toxic effects. Death is a convenient end point. In the words of one historian, however, few of these studies "contributed anything to pharmacology, the majority serving only to confirm that poisons were poisonous."[8]

It was not until the 19th century that pharmacology emerged as a modern experimental science, especially beginning with the work of François Magendie (1783-1855) in France. At the same time that he was helping to establish physiology as an experimental science in the early part of the 19th century, Magendie was laying the groundwork for experimental pharmacology as well. Magendie's experiments on strychnine-containing plant poisons, on the alkaloid emetine, and on other substances established the site of action of these drugs in the body. He also developed or refined methods that were invaluable to pharmacological research.[9] His pupil Claude Bernard (1813-1878) further contributed to the development of pharmacological theory and technique in his studies of carbon monoxide and curare. This latter substance came to play an important role in producing muscular relaxation in surgery, but that development had to await the 20th century.[10]

At about the same time that Magendie was carrying out his pioneering work establishing the foundations of pharmacology, experiments with gases in Britain were leading man closer to the discovery of inhalation anesthesia. One may cite in this connection, for example, Humphrey Davy's (1778-1829) studies of nitrous oxide and his suggestion at the turn of the 19th century that this gas might possibly be useful for controlling pain in surgical operations, as well as Henry Hill Hickman's experiments in the 1820s using carbon dioxide to induce a state of insensibility in animals.[11]

Just as these experiments with gases, however, did not immediately result in a practical application of anesthetics and the creation of a field of anesthesiology, Magendie's researches on drugs did not establish pharmacology as a distinct discipline. This latter step, like the discovery of inhalation anesthesia, had to await the 1840s.

The story of the discover of inhalation anesthesia in the United States in the 1840s, and the cast of characters involved, is too well known to repeat it here. It should be noted, however, that the beginnings of the establishment of pharmacology as a separate academic discipline occurred in this same general period. The first institute of pharmacology was established at the University of Dorpat by Rudolf Buchheim (1820-1879). Although located in Russian-controlled Estonia, the University of Dorpat was essentially a German institution in language and faculty, and it was in the German-speaking world that pharmacology was to first receive recognition as an independent discipline.

Buchheim, a German, was appointed to the chair of materia medica at Dorpat in 1846, but soon transformed the teaching of that traditional didactic subject into experimental pharmacology. He called for the creation of a specialist in pharmacology, separate from the chemist and the pharmacist. Buchheim's first laboratory of pharmacology, however, was located in the basement of his home, and the university did not establish a laboratory for him until some years after his appointment.

It took several decades for pharmacology to become firmly established as a medical school subject on a par with the other medical sciences, first in Germany and then spreading to other countries. The man who was most influential in making Buchheim's dream of an independent discipline of pharmacology into a reality was another German, Oswald Schmiedeberg. A pupil of Buchheim, Schmiedeberg succeeded his master at Dorpat in 1869, but it was after he moved to Strassburg in 1872 that he had his greatest impact. His institute at Strassburg became a mecca for the study of the new field. More than 150 students from around the world, many of whom went on to become leaders in pharmacology, received their training in his laboratory. One of these was John Jacob Abel (1857-1938), the father of American pharmacology.[12]

The practitioners of this new science began to subject the whole array of substances in the known pharmacopeia, as well as the many new chemicals that were being isolated or synthesized at the time, to experimental investigation to evaluate (or reevaluate) their therapeutic effectiveness and to understand the mechanism of their pharmacological action. Naturally this work included substances with anesthetic properties.

It was a German pharmacologist, Oscar Liebreich (1839-1908), who in 1869 discovered the sedative properties of choral hydrate, for example, as will be discussed in more detail later in this paper. Another German pharmacologist, Rudolf Kobert, first demonstrated the sedative action of scopolamine in 1887. Yet another German pharmacologist, Walter Straub (1874-1944), developed the first electrically-developed roller pump in 1911 and suggested that it be used for the infusion therapy during anesthesia.[13]

Ludwig Burkhardt (1872-1922) played an important role in the development of intravenous anesthesia in the early years of the 20th century. Although Burkhardt was a surgeon, he first became involved in basic research at the Department of Pharmacology at the University of Würzburg. This period of pharmacological research may well have contributed to his interest and success in the area of intravenous anesthesia.[14]

Anesthetic substances also presented a challenge to pharmacologists to explain their mechanism of action. The general anesthetics created a particular problem which will be the focus of the rest of this paper. It is necessary to begin this discussion by providing some general background about theories of drug action in the late 19th century. Chemistry, which was just emerging as a modern science at the end of the 18th century, had a significant impact on the field of experimental pharmacology as it developed in the 19th century. In the early part of the century, the isolation of alkaloids such as morphine from opium and quinine from cinchona bark enabled pharmacological investigators to begin to study the physiological effects of pure chemicals, as opposed to the mixtures of substances typically present in crude plant drugs or their extracts. Scientists could also begin to investigate the chemical composition and structure of the pure substances from plant drugs. As the century progressed, chemists also began to synthesize new organic compounds, some of which had useful pharmacological effects.[15]

In the midst of this burst of chemical activity, it is not surprising that many investigators began to interpret drug action in terms of chemical reactions. For example, Thomas Lauder Brunton in England postulated in 1871 that certain chemicals enter into a reversible combination with the cell, altering its chemical and functional properties in the process, and Thomas Fraser in Scotland argued in the following year that pharmacological action was often, if not always, the result of the reaction between a drug and certain constituents of the body. The involvement of chemical reactions in drug action had been suggested earlier, but chemistry and pharmacology had by the 1870s advanced to the point where more concrete evidence was accumulating to support such a view.[16]

Studies of the relationship between chemical structure and physiological activity in this period undoubtedly influenced the thinking of pharmacological researchers such as Brunton and Fraser. Indeed, both of them made significant contributions to this area of research.[17]

Perhaps the first person to make a serious beginning in the field of structure-activity relationships was James Blake, an English physician who later emigrated to America. Given the lack of knowledge about the structure of organic compounds in the 1830s and 1840s, when Blake did his work, it is not surprising that he focused on inorganic chemicals. He first was able to show that the different salts of a given metal often produced identical pharmacological effects. Later he reported that elements that were isomorphous (i.e., which have the same crystalline form) generally have very similar pharmacological properties. He concluded that: "...there exists some intimate connection between the chemical properties of substances, and their physiological action."[18]

Blake's work was important in demonstrating that a relationship could be established between the pharmacological action and the chemical nature of a substance. As chemists began to understand more about the structure of organic compounds, and to draw structural formulas for some of these molecules, attention began to be focused on the relationship between structure and function in these chemicals. Most drugs are after all organic compounds.

In the 1860s, while structural organic chemistry was still in its infancy, Benjamin Ward Richardson (1828-1896), an English physician, investigated the relationship between structure and activity in a series of hydrocarbon compounds. Richardson was able to associate certain functional groups with specific physiological properties. For example, the nitrite group was shown to be associated with vasodilation and quickening of the heart, and the hydroxy (alcohol) group with depression of the active functions of the cerebrospinal system. He was thus able to establish at least a crude relationship between structure and activity.[19]

The study which really drew attention to the field of structure-activity relationships, however, was that of Alexander Crum Brown, a chemist, and Thomas Fraser, a pharmacologist, of Edinburgh University. Their first paper on the subject, published in 1869, began with a declaration of faith: "There can be no reasonable doubt that a relation exists between the physiological action of a substance and its chemical constitution, understanding by the latter term the mutual relations of the atoms."[20]

Although the structures of most organic compounds was not known, Brown and Fraser refused to be deterred from their investigation. They reasoned that they could attain some understanding of the subject by producing the same known change in structure in a number of different compounds and observing the effect on their physiological activity. For various reasons, they chose to work with a series of alkaloids. Each of the alkaloids was subjected to methylation (i.e., the addition of a methyl group) because there was some evidence in the literature that this reaction removed or diminished physiological activity.

They found that upon methylation the ability of the alkaloids to produce convulsions disappeared. The narcotic properties of morphine and codeine, two of the alkaloids in their study, were also diminished. At the same time, the methylated compounds exhibited a new and different pharmacological property. They all showed a paralyzing, curare-like effect. A relatively small change in structure had thus produced a dramatic change in the pharmacological properties of the alkaloids.

Brown and Fraser expanded their studies to other substances, and soon found that in general the compounds now known as quaternary ammonium salts (which includes the methylated alkaloids) were associated with a paralyzing action. They had been quite fortunate in their choice of compounds to study, because such clear-cut relationships between structure and activity are not common. Their success encouraged other investigators to undertake research in this area.

At first there was considerable optimism that a general law, or perhaps a few generalizations, describing the relationship between structure and activity would be found. High hopes were also held out for therapeutics. Brunton suggested, for example, that the time might not be far off when scientists would be able to synthesize substances that would act on the body in any desired way and would be able to predict the pharmacological action of a substance from its chemical structure.[21]

Some synthetic drugs were developed in the late 19th century based on structural considerations, such as the analgesic phenacetin, but success in discovering new useful therapeutic agents was often based more on luck that correct reasoning on structural grounds. Oscar Liebreich's discovery of the sedative properties of chloral hydrate was noted earlier. Liebreich was indeed influenced by structural considerations in this work. Since choral hydrate was known to decompose to chloroform in caustic alkaline solutions, Liebreich hypothesized that the same reaction should take place in the alkaline body fluids. In his view, chloroform would thus be slowly released in the body, inducing a state of unconsciousness. Choral hydrate did of course prove to be a successful hypnotic, but it was soon shown that Liebreich's theory concerning its mode of action was incorrect. The alkalinity of the body is not strong enough to decompose the choral hydrate into chloroform.

Supporters of the view that drugs act by forming a chemical combination with the cell pointed to the results of structure-activity studies as evidence in favor of their views. Whatever the limitations of these studies, they had demonstrated relationships between specific structural features of molecules and particular pharmacological effects in some cases. These relationships could be interpreted as involving chemical combinations between a specific chemical grouping on a drug molecule and some constituent of the cell.

Not all drug researchers, however, were enthusiastic about the structural approach or convinced that the action of drugs could best be explained in terms of chemical combination with the cell. Some pharmacologists, such as Arthur Cushny, thought it more likely that most drugs induce their effects by altering such physicochemical characteristics of the cell as surface tension, electrolytic balance, and osmotic pressure, rather than by entering into a chemical combination with the cell. In their view, the structure of a drug molecule was important in so far as it determined the physical properties of the molecule, not because of the presence of some specific chemical group which combined with a cell constituent.[22]

Probably the most difficult class of pharmacological agents for the supporters of the chemical view to explain was the anesthetics, a fact that their opponents did not let them forget. By the late 19th century, it was obvious that a number of substances of widely different chemical composition (such as ether, chloroform, pentane, ethanol, and urethane) all had the ability to produce narcosis in the organism. This situation was difficult to explain from a structural viewpoint, as one could not associate any particular grouping of atoms in these molecules with the narcotic or anesthetic properties. Many anesthetics, in fact, were chemically rather inert. Their action was also of a relatively transitory and readily reversible nature, also arguing against a firm chemical combination with the cell.

How then could one explain the similarity of action of these compounds?

Various unsuccessful attempts had been made before the end of the 19th century to explain the action of narcotics and anesthetics. It was not until 1899, however, that Hans Horst Meyer and Charles Overton (1865-1933) independently provided a useful and influential analysis of the action of anesthetics. Meyer was a pharmacologist who had been one of the successors of Buchheim and Schmiedeberg at Dorpat, but who had moved to Marburg by the mid-1880s. Overton was a botanist by training, and was in Zürich at the time of his work on narcosis. Whereas Meyer and his students had been specifically investigating the phenomenon of narcosis, Overton came to the problem indirectly through a study of the permeability of plant and animal cells to various substances.

Both men recognized that lipid solubility plays a key role in the action of anesthetics, a fact that Ernst von Bibra (1806-1878) and Harless had suggested half a century earlier. But Bibra and Harless believed that narcotics acted by actually dissolving the fat out of brain cells, a view that was difficult to reconcile with the reversible and transitory action of anesthetic agents. Meyer and Overton agreed that anesthetics probably exerted their effects on the cholesterol and lecithin-related constituents of the cells, but postulated, in the words of Overton, that these "compounds probably change the normal state of these cell constituents without causing them to be removed from the cells." Furthermore, they were able to demonstrate quantitatively that anesthetic action was directly proportional to the coefficient of partition between solubility in lipids and water. In other words, anesthetic action somehow depends upon the distribution of the narcotic agent in the body.[23]

Although Meyer and Overton were not able to offer a detailed explanation of the mechanism of action of anesthesia, their

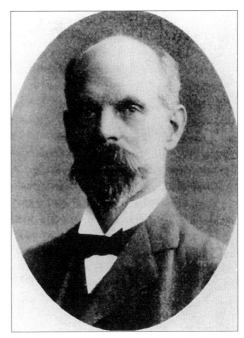

Botanist Charles E. Overton, cofounder of the Meyer-Overton theory of narcosis. (Courtesy of the National Library of Medicine)

results certainly argued for the key role of physical properties such as solubility in the process. As one modern pharmacologist has commented, the Meyer-Overton hypothesis was deeply disturbing to those attempting to relate structure and activity.[24] It should also be noted in passing that the fact that such chemically unrelated substances as cocaine, benzyl alcohol, antipyrine, and certain inorganic salts all exhibit some local anesthetic action was another source of concern for proponents of the structural chemistry viewpoint.[25]

Of course, in retrospect we realize that both sides were in a sense correct, in that both the physical and chemical properties of a drug influence its action. In fact, the borderline between "physical" and "chemical" has become blurred as our understanding of molecular interactions has progressed. We must keep in mind, however, that in the period under consideration little was known of the biochemistry

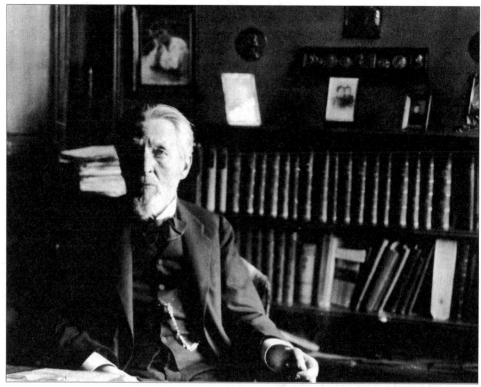

Pharmacologist Hans Horst Meyer, cofounder of the Meyer-Overton theory of narcosis. (Courtesy of National Library of Medicine)

of the cell, and the concept of the electronic nature of chemical bonding was only just emerging. We should therefore not be surprised if distinctions were made between physical and chemical factors which seem to us to be rigid and artificial. To scientists at the beginning of this century, a chemical bond or union implied a covalent bond, as concepts of weaker linkages such as hydrogen bonds and Van der Waals forces had not yet been developed. While some investigators were beginning to recognize that the term "chemical" might be interpreted more broadly, there was still a lack of agreement about the involvement of "true chemical bonding" in drug action.

The questions raised in the struggle to explain the action of anesthetics helped to refine views about the mechanism of drug action. The challenge offered by anesthetics, for example, helped to curb overzealous and oversimplified efforts to related structure and activity. Some pharmacologists and medicinal chemists of the late 19th and early 20th centuries tended to oversimplify the relationship between structure and activity by striving too hard to relate a particular pharmacological activity to the presence of a specific chemical grouping in the molecule. There was perhaps too much emphasis on attempting to assign stimulant, depressant, and other specific pharmacological properties to particular chemical groups. Unfortunately drug action is not that simply explained. The problem in understanding anesthetics helped to remind physicians and scientists of this fact.

The action of anesthetics and certain other compounds also served as a reminder of the need to take physicochemical factors such as solubility and surface tension into account in explaining drug action. It came to be more clearly recognized that a change in the structure of the molecule might modify its pharmacological action in some cases by altering some physicochemical property, such as solubility, rather than be affecting a chemical bond between specific functional groups in the drug molecule and in the cell.

The discussion of these questions helped pave the way for a broader view of drug action, one which essentially absorbed both the physical and chemical positions and thereby made the controversy no longer meaningful. While there is still ample room for controversy, and still much to be learned about the molecular mechanisms of drug action, pharmacologists are generally agreed upon the importance of both physical chemistry and structural organic chemistry in probing this subject. The problem of explaining the action of anesthetics played an important role in shaping this outcome, one of the ways in which anesthesia has contributed to pharmacology.

References:

[1] Leake C: Prolegomenon to current pharmacology. Univ California Pub Pharmacol 1 1938; 1:1-30 and Leake C: An historical account of pharmacology to the twentieth century. Springfield, IL: Charles C. Thomas 1975, p. 17

[2] On the early use of opium, alcohol, and other drugs for anesthetic purposes, see, for example, Robinson V: Victory over pain: a history of anesthesia. New York: Henry Schuman 1946, pp. 3-26

[3] Ibid., p. 4 and Holmstedt B, Liljestrand G: Readings in pharmacology. New York: Pergamon Press 1963, pp. 4-5

[4] Holmstedt B, Liljestrand G: Readings (n.3), pp. 9-16; Robinson V: Victory (n. 2), pp. 8-9

[5] Quoted from the English translation in Holmstedt B, Liljestrand G: Readings (n. 3), p. 16

[6] On Galenical theory, see Temkin O: Galenicals and Galenism in the history of medicine. In: Galdston I (Ed). The impact of the antibiotics on society. New York: International Universities Press 1958, pp. 18-37

[7] For a discussion of early theories of drug action, see Earles MP: Early theories of the mode of action of drugs and poisons. Ann Sci 1961; 17:97-110 and Earles MP: Early scientific studies on drugs and poisons. Pharm J 1962; 188:47-51

[8] Earles MP: Early scientific studies (n. 7), p. 49

[9] On Magendie and the beginnings of experimental physiology and pharmacology, see Lesch J: Science and medicine in France: The emergence of experimental physiology, 1790-1855. Cambridge, MA: Harvard University Press 1984 and Olmsted JMD: Francois Magendie. New York: Schumann's 1944

[10] Olmsted JMD: Claude Bernard, physiologist. New York: Harper and Brothers 1939

[11] Rushman GB:, Davies NJH:, Atkinson RS: A short history of anaesthesia: The first 150 years. Oxford: Butterworth-Heinemann 1996, pp. 4-7

[12] On the emergence of pharmacology as an independent discipline in the German-speaking world, see Kuschinsky G: The influence of Dorpat on the emergence of pharmacology as a distinct discipline," J Hist Med All Sci 1968; 23:258-271; Haberman, ER: Rudolf Buchheim and the beginnings of pharmacology as a science. Ann Rev of

Pharmacol 1974; 14:1-8; Bruppacher-Cellier M: Rudolf Buchheim (1820-1879) und die Entwicklung einer experimentellen Pharmakologie. Zürich: Julius Druck 1971; Koch-Weser P, Schechter PJ: Schmiedeberg in Strassburg, 1872-1918: the making of modern pharmacology," Life Sci 1978; 22: 1361-1372. On Abel and pharmacology in the United States, see Parascandola, J: The development of American pharmacology: John J. Abel and the shaping of a discipline. Baltimore: Johns Hopkins University Press 1992

[13] Holmstedt B, Liljestrand G: Readings (n. 3), pp. 106-110, 122-126 and am Esch JS, Goerig M: Anaesthetic equipment in the history of German anaesthesia. Lübeck: Dräger 1997, pp. 110-111

[14] Goerig M, Schulte am Esch J: Historical remarks regarding intravenous ether anesthesia. Bull Anesth Hist July, 1996; 14[3]: 1, 4-6

[15] For further information, see Lesch J: Conceptual change in an empirical science: the discovery of the first alkaloids," Hist Stud Phys Sci 1981; 11: 305-328 and Rose FL: Origin and rise of the synthetic drugs. In: Poynter FNL (Ed). Chemistry in the service of medicine. Philadelphia: J. B. Lippincott 1963, pp. 179-97

[16] Brunton TL: Lectures on the experimental investigation of the action of medicines. British Med J 1871; 1:413-415 and Fraser TR: Lectures on the connection between the chemical properties and the physiological action of active substances. British Med J 1872; 2:401-403

[17] The discussion of the history of structure-activity relationships that follows is drawn from my earlier publications on the subject. For more detailed information, see Parascandola J: Structure-activity relationships: the early mirage. Pharm Hist 1971; 13:3-10; Parascandola J: The controversy over structure-activity relationships in the early twentieth century. Pharm Hist 1974; 15:54-63; Parascandola J: Form and function: early efforts to relate chemical structure and pharmacological activity. Canadian Bull Med Hist 1988; 5:61-72

[18] Blake J: On the action of certain inorganic compounds when introduced directly into the blood. Edinburgh Med Surg J 1841; 56:124

[19] See, for example, Richardson BW: Report on the physiological action of the methyl compounds. British Assoc Rep 1867; 37:47-57

[20] Crum Brown A, Fraser T: On the connection between chemical constitution and physiological action. Part I. - On the physiological action of the salts of the ammonium bases, derived from strychnia, brucia, thebaia, codeia, morphia, and nicotia. Trans Roy Soc Edinburgh 1869; 25:151

[21] Brunton TL: An introduction to modern therapeutics. London: Macmillan 1892, p. 4

[22] For a fuller discuss over this dispute, see Parascandola J: The controversy (n. 17)

[23] On the work of Meyer and Overton, see Lipnick RL: Hans Horst Meyer and the lipid theory of narcosis. Trends Pharmacol Sci 1989; 10:265-269; Overton CE, Studies of narcosis [English translation, ed. by Lipnick, RL]. London: Chapman and Hall and Parkridge, IL: Wood Library-Museum of Anesthesiology 1991; Faulconer, Jr., A, Keys TE: Foundations of anesthesiology. Parkridge, IL: Wood Library-Museum of Anesthesiology 1993, pp. 1261-1266; Holmstedt B, Liljestrand G: Readings (n. 3), pp. 146-154

[24] Albert A: Relations between molecular structure and biological activity: stages in the evolution of current concepts. Ann Rev Pharmacol 1971; 11:15-16

[25] Parascandola J: "The controversy (n. 17), p. 59

Development of Skeletal Muscle Relaxants

R. Hughes
Formerly: The Wellcome Research Laboratories, Beckenham, UK and
The Royal College of Surgeons of England, London, UK

INTRODUCTION

The development of skeletal muscle relaxants from the curare poisons of the South American Indians has already been reported including the historical background, identification of the plants and their curare alkaloids, and the early pharmacological and clinical studies (1). The present review, therefore, concentrates on recent developments in the search for more specific and shorter neuromuscular blocking agents.

Pancuronium

The introduction of pancuronium into anaesthetic practice was an important advance in its time. The drug was synthesized by Savage and his co-workers in 1967 and its design was based on the steroid nucleus (2). The pharmacology of pancuronium was reported by Buckett and his colleagues in 1968 (3) and the drug was first used clinically by Baird and Reid in 1967 (4). Pancuronium is 5-10 times more potent than tubocurarine but is long acting. However, unlike tubocurarine, it does not cause ganglion blockade, but tachycardia and hypertension are associated with its vagal blocking properties and a parasympathomimetic action. It is now recognised that long acting agents have a limited usefulness because of their slow onset, long duration and variability in clinical use.

Clinical Considerations

Because of the advancements in surgical and anaesthetic techniques, surgery is now being carried out on patients who, formerly, would have been regarded as too ill for such treatment to be attempted. Consequently, it becomes even more important that the drugs used in anaesthetic practice are free from unwanted effects. Furthermore, there is an increasing awareness of the drawbacks of the older neuromuscular blocking agents which cause undesirable cardiovascular side-effects. The breakthrough came with the discovery of the non-depolarizing agents atracurium and vecuronium, with a duration of action intermediate between that of suxamethonium and pancuronium. Both agents offer particular advantages in the development of neuromuscular blockade.

Vecuronium

Vecuronium is an analogue of pancuronium and its chemical properties were described by Buckett and his colleagues in 1973 (5) and by Savage and his collaborators in 1980 (6). Durant and his co-workers (1979) showed, in animal studies, that the drug exhibited pronounced neuromuscular blocking activity with only very weak actions at sympathetic ganglia and on the cardiac vagus (7). The first clinical experience was reported by Crul and Booij in 1980 who found that the potency of vecuronium was similar to that of pancuronium but with no significant cardiovascular effects or histamine release (8). The shorter action of vecuronium was associated with rapid uptake by the liver.

Atracurium

Atracurium represented a new approach in the development of skeletal muscle relaxants. The drug was designed uniquely by Stenlake (1978) to undergo spontaneous degradation at physiological temperature and pH by a self-destruction mechanism called Hofmann elimination which proceeds independently of renal and hepatic function (9); atracurium also undergoes an enzymic ester hydrolysis. Pharmacological studies by Hughes and Chapple in 1981 demonstrated that neuromuscular blocking doses were virtually free of autonomic side effects and cumulation was negligible when successive doses were administered (10). The first quantitative clinical evaluation of atracurium was reported by Payne and Hughes in 1981, who found that its neuromuscular blocking potency was similar to that of tubocurarine but the cardiovascular effects of the drug were minimal (11). Atracurium is a weak histamine liberator with a potency of about one third that of tubocurarine. The drug can also be administered as a continuous infusion which provides a constant and more controllable neuromuscular block for long operations (12). Atracurium has also been used in the intensive care unit to provide neuromuscular relaxation for those patients where an adequate gaseous exchange could not be achieved with the use of analgesic and sedative drugs alone (13).

OBJECTIVES

The development of new non-depolarizing blocking agents concentrates on improvements to minimise cardiovascular effects and histamine release. Also, to speed onset and to shorten duration of action in an effort to find a replacement for the depolarizing agent, suxamethonium. No single drug yet incorporates all these desirable characteristics, yet all of the potential new agents display at least one of them.

AMINO STEROIDS

Pipecuronium

The chemical structure associated with the vagolytic effects of pancuronium has been identified and removed to produce the long-acting agent, pipecuronium. The drug was developed in Hungary and the first clinical experience was reported by Alánt and his co-workers in 1980 (14). Pipecuronium is about 20 per cent more potent than pancuronium and is free of cardiovascular effects and histamine release in the clinical dose range. However, long acting agents have a limited usefulness in anaesthetic practice as already mentioned.

Rocuronium

The steroidal substances are undergoing extensive study with the aim of increasing liver uptake in the new compounds in order to reduce onset time and to shorten duration of action. The skeletal muscle relaxant, rocuronium (Org 9426) has been developed as a product of this research. The drug has a more rapid onset time than other available non-depolarizing neuromuscular blocking agents and which is associated with its low potency and the large number of molecules available to occupy the cholinergic receptors. The pharmacology of rocuronium was reported by Muir and his associates in 1989 (15) and Wierda and his colleagues described their clinical experiences with the drug in 1990 (16). Rocuronium is 6-8 times less potent that vecuronium but its onset of action, within 60 seconds, is twice as rapid (Table 1 and Fig. 1). Intubating conditions at 1 minute compare favourably to those after suxamethonium which may be attributable to the possibility that the laryngeal muscles are affected before the adductor pollicis muscle (17). The duration of action and recovery index of rocuronium is similar to that of vecuronium; cardiovascular

Type of Anaesthesia	Fentanyl (2-3 µg/kg)		Halothane (0.5-0.75%)	
Rocuronium	0.6 mg/kg	0.9 mg/kg	0.6 mg/kg	0.9 mg/kg
Time to maximum block (s)	58 (10.6)	47 (7.0)	59 (15.3)	44 (8.1)
$T_{25\%}$ (min)	34 (7.4)	51 (10.7)	33 (4.4)	58 (7.8)
$T_{90\%}$ (min)	54 (17.4)	77 (21.0)	52 (10.6)	86 (14.7)
Recovery Index (min)	13 (6.7)	17 (5.4)	13 (4.4)	20 (4.0)

$T_{25\%}$ - time to 25% recovery; $T_{90\%}$ - time to 90% recovery; Recovery Index - time from 25% to 75% recovery. Values expressed as mean±SD
From Cooper RA, Mirakhur RK, Maddineni VR Anesthesia 1993; 48:103-105

Table 1: Onset and duration of action of rocuronium bromide during fentanyl or halothane anaesthesia

effects and histamine release are minimal at the clinical dose. The vagolytic activity of the drug falls within the range between vecuronium and pancuronium and higher doses may cause some tachycardia and hypertension. If the neuromuscular blocking dose is increased by 50%, the time to complete block is reduced to about 45 seconds but the clinical duration and recovery index are significantly prolonged (18). Rocuronium is proving useful for facilitating rapid endotracheal intubation.

Rapacuronium

Rapacuronium (Org 9487) is the latest steroidal agent which is undergoing development; its clinical profile was reported by Wierda and his co-workers in 1993 (19). It is

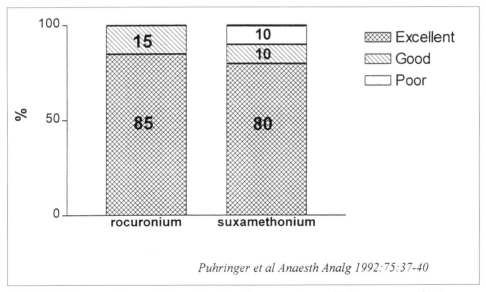

Puhringer et al Anaesth Analg 1992;75:37-40

Fig. 1: Intubating conditions at 60 sec. after 0.6mg/kg rocuronium and 1.0mg/kg suxamethonium

Group	n	Lag Time (s)	Block at Maximal 1 min (%)	block (%)	Onset (s)
A Suxamethonium	15	25 (11)	95 (11)	99 (0.2)	67 (20)
B + C (Rapacuronium + neostigmine and Rapacuronium)	30	18 (7)	93 (10)	99 (1.7)	83 (38)

Intubating conditions 1 min after muscle relaxant

Group	n	Excellent	Intubating conditions[a] Good	Poor	Impossible
A Suxamethonium	15	7	7	-	1
B + C (Rapacuronium + neostigmine and Rapacuronium)	30	16	14	-	-

[a] Scores according to the Goldberg system; results expressed as mean±SD.
Data adapted from Wierda et al Anesth Analg 1993; 77: 579-584

Table 2: Onset variables of the neuromuscular block

characterised by low potency, since it is almost 3 times less potent than rocuronium, and by its rapid rate of onset. The fast onset of action coincides with the development of good to excellent intubating conditions in 1 minute which is similar to suxamethonium (Table 2). The duration of action of rocuronium is at least half that of vecuronium but is somewhat longer than suxamethonium. However, it is claimed that the neuromuscular block can be rapidly reversed if neostigmine is given within 2 minutes of the administration of rapacuronium (Table 3); under these conditions the clinical profile of rapacuronium is comparable to that of suxamethonium. Cardiovascular effects are minimal at clinical dosage but higher doses may cause small increases in heart rate and small decreases in blood pressure which are not associated with histamine release. The short action of rapacuronium has been attributed to rapid redistribution into the liver followed by hepato-biliary excretion. The drug is showing promise for facilitating rapid endotracheal intubation and for providing neuromuscular relaxation for short surgical procedures.

Group	n	Time (in minutes until)			
		$T_1 = 25\%$	TOF = 70%	$T_1 = 90\%$	TOF = 70%
A. Suxamethonium	15	8.0 (2.5)	-	10.6 (3.3)[a]	-
B. Rapacuronium + neo	15	5.7 (0.6)	6.6 (1.2)	10.8 (3.5)	11.6 (1.4)[b]
C. Rapacuronium	15	8.0 (1.9)[b]	12.0 (3.2)	16.4 (5.8)	24.1 (6.2)

Group A = patients receiving suxamethonium; Group B = patients receiving rapacuronium followed by neostigmine: Group C = patients receiving rapacuronium without neostigmine. TOF, train-of-four.
Results expressed as mean±SD; * P<0.05; [a] compared to [b] P = not significant
From Wierda et al., Anesth Analg 1993;77:579-584

Table 3: Recovery Variables of neuromuscular block

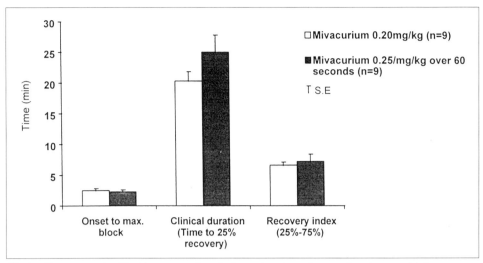

Fig. 2: Neuromuscular blocking properties of mivacurium in patients under nitrous oxide/oxygen fentanyl-thiopentone anaesthesia

BENZOISOQUINOLINES

Doxacurium

The structure of the benzylisoquinolinium esters can be easily modified to produce stable and highly specific neuromuscular blocking agents. Such a drug is doxacurium which was described by Basta and his colleagues in 1988 (20). Like pipecuronium it is more potent than pancuronium but free of cardiovascular effects and histamine release at multiples of the clinical dose. The drug is excreted by the kidneys with the liver as a secondary route. However, like pancuronium and pipecuronium, doxacurium is long acting and therefore is of limited usefulness.

Mivacurium

The benzylisoquinolinium nucleus can also be manipulated chemically to undergo rapid hydrolysis by plasma cholinesterase of which mivacurium is an example; its clinical pharmacology was described by Savarese and his collaborators in 1988 (21). Mivacurium is approximately 3 times more potent than atracurium; the onset of neuromuscular block is similar, but slower than that of suxamethonium. However, its duration of action and time to recovery is about half that of atracurium (Fig. 2) but twice as long as suxamethonium. If the clinical dose is increased to shorten the onset time and improve intubating conditions, hypotension and tachycardia may occur due to histamine release (22) (Fig. 3). These cardiovascular effects may be minimised if the drug is administered in divided doses or by slow injection. Mivacurium does not have significant vagal or ganglionic blocking effects in the recommended dose range. The drug is particularly suitable for providing neuromuscular relaxation for short surgical procedures and it is claimed that induced reversal with neostigmine may not always be necessary. As mivacurium is virtually non-cumulative, it may be administered by continuous infusion for longer operations (23).

Cisatracurium

Atracurium is a mixture of 10 stereoisomers which can now be separated by high pressure liquid chromatography. These

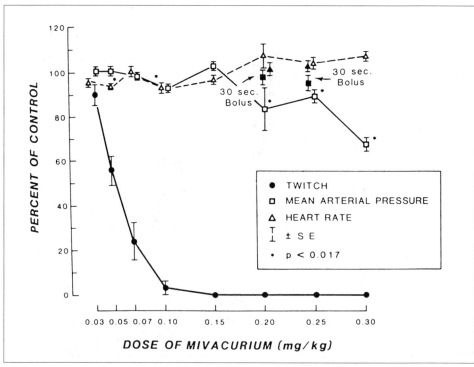

Fig. 3: Neuromuscular and cardiovascular dose-response of mivacurium

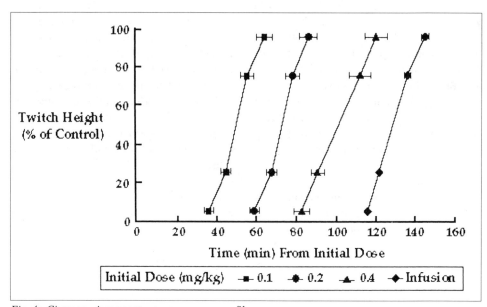

Fig. 4: Cisatracurium spontaneous recovery profile

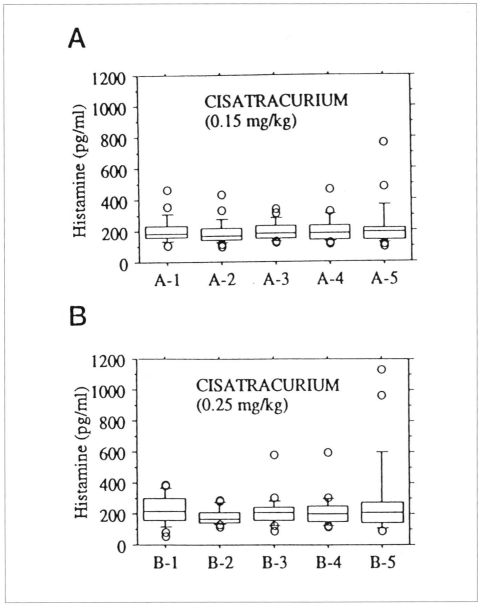

Fig. 5: Box plot of plasma histamine (pg/mL). Samples were taken 5 min. before thiopental (A1, B1), 3 and 5 min after thiopental (A2, B2 and A3, B3), and 3 and 5 min after muscle relaxant (A4, B4 and A5, B5)

isomers have the same molecular structure as the parent compound but a different spacial configuration of the various chemical groups within the molecule. The cisisomer (51W89) is of particular interest and represents approximately 15% of the atracurium mixture. Studies by Wastila and Maehr in 1993 showed that its pharmacological profile was similar to that of atracurium with a wide separation between the neuromuscular blocking doses and those which affect the autonomic nervous system (24). Clinical studies by Lien and his co-workers in 1993 demonstrated that the cisisomer was approximately 3 times more potent than the isometric mixture but the time course of neuromuscular blockade was similar to that of atracurium mixture (25) (Fig. 4). The drug appears to be virtually free of cardiovascular effects and histamine release at doses within the clinical range (26) (Fig. 5). Cisatracurium has been administered as a continuous infusion and provides greater flexibility and controllability in the management of neuromuscular block during long operations with a predictable rate of recovery (27). The drug has also shown promise when given by infusion to patients in the intensive care unit who required neuromuscular relaxation to facilitate mechanical ventilation (28). Metabolic studies have indicated that Hofmann elimination is the predominant pathway for the spontaneous breakdown of cisatracurium and, unlike the atracurium mixture, ester hydrolysis does not appear to play a significant role in this process (29).

CONCLUSION

The search for a non-depolarizing agent to replace suxamethonium is proving difficult to achieve in man but some progress has been made towards fulfilling this objective. Suxamethonium acts by mimicking the action of acetylcholine and rapidly depolarizing the muscle, whereas the non-depolarizing agents act by competing with acetylcholine for occupancy of the cholinergic receptors which is a relatively slow process. Furthermore, the non-depolarizing drugs which have been found to be very short-acting have a low potency. Consequently there is the risk that the large doses required to produce neuromuscular paralysis may cause unacceptable side-effects and histamine release.

However, there is now a greater understanding of the physiology and pharmacology of the neuromuscular junction which may lead to the development of more specific and safer neuromuscular blocking drugs. It is also conceivable that new skeletal muscle relaxants may be designed with a unique mode of action as yet unknown. For example, relatively large doses of neuromuscular blocking agents are used to provide surgical relaxation by paralyzing the responses to motor nerve stimulation whereas, ideally, all that is needed is to abolish muscle tone. The resting tone of a muscle is controlled by the fusimotor system which is a reflex arc involving the spinal cord and the (y - efferent nerves. If drugs could be discovered which would selectively block this pathway, then it may be possible to provide adequate surgical relaxation without some of the drawbacks associated with the use of neuromuscular blocking agents. Meanwhile it is now commonplace to use neuromuscular paralysis to ease the work of the surgeon during operations.

Acknowledgements

I am indebted to Mr A Freeman of Glaxo Wellcome Plc and to Dr A W Muir of Organon Laboratories Ltd for their assistance in the preparation of this review and to Mrs Claire Ryan of Glaxo Wellcome Plc for preparing the manuscript.

References:

1. Hughes R: Development of skeletal muscle relaxants from the curare arrow poisons. In: Atkinson S, Boulton T B, ed. The History of Anaesthesia, International Congress and Symposium Series 134. Royal Society of Medicine Services Ltd. London New York 1989, p 257-267

2. Buckett W R, Hewett C L, Savage D S: Potent steroidal neuromuscular blocking agents. Chemie Therapeutique 1967;2: 186

3. Buckett W R, Marjoribanks C E B, Marwick F A, Morton M B: The pharmacology of pancuronium bromide (Org NA97) a new steroidal neuromuscular blocking agent. Br J Pharmac 1968; 32: 671-682

4. Baird W L M, Reid A M: The neuromuscular blocking properties of a new steroid compound, pancuronium bromide (a pilot study in man). Br J Anaesth 1967; 39: 775-780

5. Buckett W R, Hewett C L, Savage D S: Pancuronium bromide and other steroidal neuromuscular blocking agents containing acetylcholine fragments. J Med Chem 1973; 16: 1116-1124

6. Savage D S, Sleigh T, Carlyle I: The emergence of Org NC45; 1-[(2β, 3α, 5α, 16β, 17β) - 3, 17-bis (acetyloxyl) - 2 - (1 - piperidinyl) - androstan - 16 - yl] - 1- methyl piperidinium bromide from the pancuronium series. By J Anaesth 1980; 52: 3S-9S

7. Durant N N, Marshall I G, Savage D S, Nelson D J, Sleigh T, Carlyle I C: The neuromuscular blocking activities of pancuronium, Org NC45 and other pancuronium analogues in the cat. J Pharm Pharmac 1979; 31: 831-836

8. Crul J F, Booij L H D J: First clinical experience of Org NC45. Br J Anaesth 1980; 52: 49S-52S

9. Stenlake J B: Biodegradable neuromuscular blocking agents. In: Stoclet J C, ed. Advances in Pharmacology and Therapeutics, Vol 3, Ions - Cyclic Nucleotides-Cholinergy. Oxford: Pergamon Press 1978: 303-311

10. Hughes R, Chapple D J: The pharmacology of atracurium; a new competitive neuromuscular blocking agent. Br J Anaesth 1981; 53: 31-44

11. Payne J P, Hughes R: Evaluation of atracurium in anaesthetised man. Br J Anaesth 1981; 53: 45-54

12. Eagar B M, Flynn P J, Hughes R: Infusion of atracurium for long surgical procedures. Br J Anaesth 1984; 56: 447-452

13. Wadon A J, Dogra S, Anand S: Atracurium infusion in the intensive care unit. Br J Anaesth 1986; 58: 64S-67S

14. Alánt O, Darvas K, Pulay I: First clinical experiences with a new neuromuscular blocker pipecuronium bromide. Arzneinittelforsch 1980; 20: 374-379

15. Muir A W, Houston J, Green K L, Marshall R J, Bowman W C, Marshall I G: Effects of a new neuromuscular blocking agent (Org 9426) in anaesthetised cats and pigs and in isolated nerve-muscle preparations. Br J Anaesth 1989; 63: 400-410

16. Wierda J M K H, De Wit A P M, Kuizenga K, Agoston S: Clinical observations on the neuromuscular blocking action of Org 9426, a new steroidal non de-polarising agent. Br J Anaesth 1990; 64; 521-523.

17. Meistelman C, Plaud B, Donat F: Rocuronium (Org 9426) neuromuscular blockade at the adductor muscles of the larynx and adductor pollicis in humans. Can J Anaesth 1992; 39: 665-669

[18] Cooper R A, Mirakhur R K, Maddineni V R: Neuromuscular effects of rocuronium bromide (Org 9426) during fentanyl and halothane anaesthesia. Anaesthesia 1993; 48: 103-105

[19] Wierda J M K H, Van der Broek L, Proost J H, Verbaan B W, Hennis P J: Time course of action and endotracheal intubating conditions of Org 9847, a new short-acting steroidal muscle relaxant; a comparison with succinylcholine. Anesth Analg 1993; 77: 579-584

[20] Basta S J, Savarese J J, Ali H H, Embree P B, Schwartz A F:
Rudd G D. Clinical pharmacology of doxacuriuim chloride, a new long-acting non-depolarising muscle relaxant. Anesthesiology 1988; 69; 478-486

[21] Savarese J J, Ali H H, Basta S J, Embree P B, Scott R P F, Sunder N, Weakly J N, Wastila W B, El-Sayad H A: The clinical neuromuscular pharmacology of mivacurium chloride (BW1090U). A short acting non-depolarising ester neuromuscular blocking drug. Anesthesiology 1988; 68: 723-732

[22] Savarese J J, Ali H H, Basta S J, Scott R P F, Embree P B, Wastila W B, Abou-Donia M M, Gelb C: The cardiovascular effects of mivacurium chloride (BW109OU) in patients receiving nitrous oxide-opiate barbiturate anesthesia. Anesthesiology 1989; 70: 386-394

[23] Ali H H, Savarese J J, Embree P B, Basta S J, Stout R G, Bottros L H, Weakly J N: Clinical pharmacology of mivacurium chloride (BW 109OU) infusion: comparison with vecuronium and atracurium. Br J Anaesth 1988; 61; 541-546

[24] Wastila W B, Maehr R B: The pharmacological profile of 51W89, the R, as - R' cis isomer of atracurium in cats. Anesthesiology 1993; 79: A496

[25] Lien C A, Belmont M R, Abalos R N, Abou-Donia M, Savarese J J: Dose-response relations of 51W9 under nitrous oxide opioid-barbiturate anesthesia. Anesthesiology 1993; 79: A948

[26] Lien C A, Belmont M R, Abalos R N, Quessy S, Savarese J J: Cardiovascular effects of 51W89 under nitrous-oxide-opioid-barbiturate anesthesia. Anesth Analg 1994; 78: S247

[27] Mellinghoff H, Pirpiri P, Buzello W: Comparison of 51W89 and atracurium administered by continuous infusion. Anesth Analg 1994; 78; S283

[28] Stone A J, Polland B J, Harper N J N: Infusion requirements of patients receiving 51W89 in the intensive care unit. Br J Anaesth 1994; 73; 486P-487P

[29] Welch R M, Brown A, Dahl R: The degradation and metabolism of 51W89, the Rcis-R'cis isomer of atracurium in human and rat plasma. Anesthesiology 1994; 81: A1091

More than 100 Years Development of Analgesics and General and Local Anaesthetics at Hoechst: a Historical Review

R. Muschaweck, Frankfurt am Main, Germany

Introduction
Ladies and Gentlemen,

Let me first say how grateful I am for your invitation to this symposium in Hamburg which aims to pay tribute to a hundred and fifty years of development work in analgesia. It is a great honour to be asked to report on the more than a century of pharmaceutical research into pain relief at Hoechst AG. I may add, incidentally, that in my scientific work as a pharmacologist, I myself have been involved in this development for nigh on fifty years, and have had close personal contacts with many of the researchers.

I should like to begin by quoting the great nineteenth century Munich surgeon Johann Nepomuk Nussbaum (1878), words which are undoubtedly still very true today:

Pain is a change in the way we felt The power of pain tames the wildest beast and can send the tamest into the wildest frenzy. Everybody fears pain and would like to be rid of it as quickly as possible

Elimination of pain has been the aim of compassionate fellow men and doctors of every age. The development of medicine, chemistry, and pharmaceutical formulation science provided the impetus and contributed to progress towards alleviation of pain.

Like many chemical and pharmaceutical companies all over the world, the chemical and synthetic dyes factory founded in 1863 in Hoechst am Main (now part of Frankfurt am Main) set about the task of manufacturing pharmaceutical products. Antipyretics and analgesics were brought onto the market. A further objective at the time one based on social concerns was to make good and cheap medicines available to works employees. The workers description of the products as the Höchster Hausapotheke or Höchst medicine chest gained widespread currency.

The above developments were also reflected in a change of name. Farbwerke Hoechst AG, which was previously known as Meister Lucius und Brüning and had lions in its emblem, subsequently adopted the tower and bridge as its symbol and became Hoechst AG. The pharmaceutical group will in future go under the joint name of Hoechst Marion Roussel and will be part of Hoechst Holdings.

Strong and mild analgesics at Hoechst

As regards the strong analgesics, it is very likely that the properties of the poppy *(Papaver somniferum)* were already known in the early days of human history; descriptions of the pain-relieving effects of opium the dried milk of the unripe seed capsule undoubtedly go back as far as the third century BC. Sydenham was perfectly justified when he said "Nolem esse medicus sine opio", or "I do not want to be a doctor without opium", and in many respects this is largely true to this day. However, it was not until 1805 that the pharmacist Friedrich Wilhelm Adam Sertürner (1783-1841) succeeded in isolating the principal alkaloid of opium, which he called morphium.

It was through Gay-Lussac that the alkaloid came to be generally known as morphium. However, nearly one hundred and fifty years were to go by before the chemical constitution of morphine was definitively established and it could be synthesized. Many morphine derivatives were produced, some with stronger and some with weaker action, and with slight differences they have continued to be used to the present day. Hoechst too carried out studies on the structure of the morphine molecule (Vongerichten and Schröder 1881, and also Knorr and Hörlein 1907). Finally, a contribution came from Schaumann, who regarded morphine as a 4-phenylpiperidine derivative, hoping thereby to explain the morphine-like analgesic action of pethidine. However, ...

In the laboratories of Farbwerke Hoechst AG entirely new avenues were being explored as part of investigations aiming to develop new spasmolytics. In 1938 Otto Eisleb synthesized 1-methyl-4-phenylpiperidine-4-carboxylic acid ethyl ester, and a Hoechst pharmacologist by name of Otto Schaumann noticed that in addition to the desired spasmolysis this new substance had an unexpected secondary effect, namely central-analgesic activity like that of morphine. The compound produced a characteristic reaction described by Walter Straub (1874-1944) after administration to mice, the so-called mouse-tail phenomenon. This consists of a peculiar S-shaped posture of the tail, which is held up and often over the back; cats show timidity and fear as well. These phenomena in mice and cats are also observed after administration of morphine. The new compound was not such a powerful analgesic as morphine, but it was better tolerated, and it entered the doctors arsenal under the name of Dolantin® (pethidine, meperidine).

The discovery of Dolantin and its pain-relieving action did indeed point the way towards new methods of controlling pain, but Schaumann was quick to see its dangers as well, and he drew critical attention to the possible side effects: "even though people under physical stress can never be totally prevented from misusing such drugs, which can of course suppress not only genuine pain but other unwanted feelings as well, a way will be found" and this was Schaumanns hope "of reducing this risk to a minimum". Unfortunately, however, this hope has not been fulfilled; dependence and addiction remain the scourge of our century.

Continuing his work on modifications of the pethidine molecule, Otto Eisler synthesized Hoechst compound 10720, ketobemidone (1942, 1944), which was also manufactured under the name Cliradon (1949).

Meanwhile, Ehrhart and Bockmühl, exploring new lines of investigation during the Second World War, succeeded in making a new class of powerful synthetic analgesics. These new analgesics were characterized by a carbon skeleton which had twophenyl groups, a basic residue, and an ester or keto

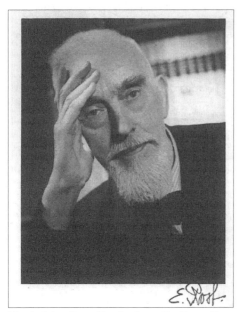

Fig. 1: Privy Councillor Professor Dr. Eugen Rost, pharmacologist, more than thirty years member of the Reichsgesundheitsamt Berlin (1900-1935), was working on the morphinelike and related drugs (Betäubungsmittelverordnung).

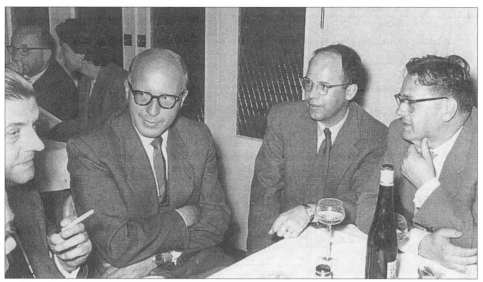

Fig. 2: Dr. Eugen Dörzbach (Hoechst), Prof. Norbert Brocks (Brackwede)

group. The analgesic Hoechst 10820, 2-dimethylamino-4,4-diphenylheptan-5-one hydrochloride, was considerably more powerful than morphine (Schaumann) and under the generic name methadone, or the commercial name Polamidon, was greeted with worldwide interest. A note is in order here, however: because of decisions connected with the war, methadone did not become generally available in Germany until after other countries. Although the general side effects are not as severe under methadone, habituation, addiction, and dependence are observed with the drug. However, since the withdrawal symptoms have a slower onset and are milder than those of morphine and morphine derivatives, for example, methadone is often used as a substitute narcotic in the treatment of severe withdrawal syndromes.

There are marked differences between the effects of the two optical antipodes of methadone, and separation of the racemate was therefore undertaken. It was found that the l-form of Polamidon is some 11-13 times stronger than the racemate as an analgesic, but only 1.3-1.5 times as toxic (1954-1964).

It is well known that there are certain connections between the analgesic and antitussive effects of the opium alkaloids, though with differences in their action. The conclusion drawn from this was that powerful synthetic analgesics might also have antitussive activity. Methadone in particular was a prime candidate here, and its chemical variants with more specific antitussive efficacy were prepared. Bockmühl and Ehrhart developed normethadone (Ticarda), for example; its analgesic activity corresponds to that of codeine, but its antitussive activity is twice as strong (Berger, 1951; Buchheim, Angermann 1951).

In the course of further investigations in the field of central-acting cough remedies, Lindner and Stein (1959) also investigated diphepanol (Tussukal®). While studying the links between central-analgesic and central-antitussive activity in terms of chemical structure and toxicity, the above authors found that the analgesic action component could be practically switched out, which would also reduce the risk of habituation and addiction.

With the strong analgesics pethidine and methadone and its derivatives, Hoechst research laboratories have undoubtedly made an outstanding contribution in the field of pain control. The scientific importance of drug research cannot be overlooked.

Let us now turn to the area of so-called mild analgesics, in which Hoechst researchers were involved at a very early stage. This group includes the antipyretic and antiinflammatory drugs in general. Research here thus began mainly with work aimed at antipyretic activity alone. In 1882 Otto Fischer described (ahydroxyhydromethylquinoline in particular as an outstanding antipyretic, putting its effects on a par with those of quinine. He wanted to bring about a considerable reduction in quinine consumption.

In the very same year the pharmacologist Filehne (1844-1927) indicated that the chemical company of Meister Lucius und Brüning would shortly be bringing out a synthetic alkaloid under the name of Kairin. However, because of the side effects that soon became apparent in man, the use of Kairin as a medicinal drug was abandoned.

Finally, however, Hoechst turned to the synthesis of pyrazolone derivatives. The initial impetus for this came from Ludwig Knorr (1859-1921), who synthesized the first representative of this series of compounds way back in 1883. The errors and confusion concerning the chemistry of the first analgesics and antipyretics from this period were later cleared up. Knorr had discovered the pyrazolone derivative 1-phenyl-2,3-dimethylpyrazolin-5-one. This was marketed by Hoechst under the name suggested by Knorr, i.e. antipyrine.

As is usually the case when new avenues are being opened in the area of therapy and in chemistry and synthesis, Knorr came up against fairly considerable resistance. Emil Fischer (1852-1919), who was Knorrs teacher and who had suggested reacting phenylhydrazine with ethyl acetoacetate, was initially against patenting the antipyrine synthesis method. He believed that if such a patent were taken out the entire area of the reactions between hydrazines and ketones would be blocked, thus being barred to further scientific research. Fischer eventually came round to Knorrs view, but only after the importance of patent protection and economic development to his young company had been clearly demonstrated. There was also a lengthy discussion over names between Knorr and Filehne, who was then at the University of Erlangen. Filehne thought that the new drug could not possibly be brought out under the name of antipyrine. Knorr insisted, however, and brought the discussion to an end with a message telegraphed back from Venice where he was on his honeymoon. The message read simply Antipyrine stays.

In 1897 there was a further development, in the form of the synthesis of aminophenazone, later named Pyramidon. Filehne was just about to suggest that Hoechst incorporate the dimethylamino group in the phenyl residue of antipyrine. In the meantime, however, this compound had been synthesized by Friedrich Stolz (1860-1936) in the form of 1-phenyl-2,3-dimethyl-4-dimethylaminopyrazolin-5-one, also known as aminophenazone and Pyramidon.

Pyramidon in its turn was passed to Filehne for pharmacological investigation. It was characterized by a multifaceted pattern of activity, exerting not only an antipyretic and analgesic action more powerful than that of antipyrine, but also antiinflammatory and spasmolytic properties. Because of its therapeutic effects, it was also added to a whole series of mixed products. After misuse in particular or after many years of use side effects were observed with Pyramidon, such as occur in practice with many other drugs in people who are specially predisposed. These included changes in corpuscular constituents of the blood, such as the dreaded agranulocytosis. These adverse reactions, though rare, eventually led to the use of aminophenazone being limited or discontinued in many countries. On the other hand, a considerable number of pharmaceutical companies have manufactured pyrazolone derivatives.

Thus at Hoechst an attempt was finally made to find a water-soluble product for pain control and spasmolysis. Bockmühl and Windisch succeeded in this when they synthesized 1-phenyl-2,3-dimethyl-5-pyrazolone-4-methylaminomethanesulfonate sodium, which was marketed under the name of Novalgin (metamizol).

The low toxicity of Novalgin, good general tolerability, and extremely good solubility in water mean that it can be administered parenterally, even in high doses. However, because of the high concentration of the product (the solution is highly hypertonic), it must be injected slowly by the intravenous route. With Novalgin, therefore, there is the possibility of treating the patient both ente-rally and parenterally. The analgesic and spasmolytic effects of metamizol mean that it is often the drug of choice for the treatment of colic in human and veterinary medicine, where it can also largely be used in place of opiates to treat severe attacks of pain. Even severe renal colic can thus be controlled in human patients. This kept Novalgin among the drugs in medical use. Other metamizol-containing products made by Hoechst, such as baralgin and arantil, will only be mentioned in passing here.

We can thus say that Hoechst has repeatedly endeavoured to carry out pioneering work with both strong and mild analgesics and to lay milestones in the field of agents for general therapeutic use and for preoperative and postoperative pain control.

Drugs for general anaesthesia (narcosis) and for local pain neutralization (local anaesthesia, local analgesia)

As the company's history shows, Hoechst also produced volatile anaesthetics for clinical and surgical use, e.g. for general anaesthesia. Above all, however, Hoechst developed drugs for local-regional and superficial elimination of adverse reactions or pain, i.e. the surface anaesthetics and the injectable local anaesthetics or local analgesics.

General anaesthesia, volatile anaesthetics, diethyl ether, chloroform, and nitrous oxide or laughing gas (N_2O) were already in use and well-known as general anaesthetics in the nineteenth century. As a chemical company, Hoechst naturally had a very wide range of solvents. For example, in 1913 the company sold chloroform protected from light in dark cobalt-blue bottles to prevent the formation of chlorine under the name of Chloroformium pro narcosi Hoechst. Aether pro narcosi Hoechst was manufactured in a particularly pure form and was protected against the formation of oxidation products (especially peroxides) through the use of an antioxidant (butylhydroxytoluene) and of dark brown bottles to protect it from light. Supplies were delivered to doctors as specified in the German Pharmacopoeia (1920 and 1927). Whereas ether is occasionally still used even if very rarely (chloroform can now be considered completely obsolete on account of its familiar side effects. The Hoechst subsidiary Messer Knappsack - Griesheim produced industrial gases. It was thus inevitable that nitrous oxide, N_2O, or laughing gas (1927), for example, would also eventually be introduced as an inhalable general anaesthetic, particularly in dentistry, under the name of Nitrous oxide pro narcosi.

I do not know to what extent acetylene was supplied as a precursor for a general anaesthetic, but I should like to relate an incident from my personal experience. During my clinical studies under the Würzburg gynaecologist Carl Joseph Gauss (1879-1950), the great-nephew of the renowned mathematician C.F. Gauss, I myself witnessed acetylene-induced general anaesthesia. After a demonstration experiment performed on the students we were able to observe the rapid onset of this type of general anaesthesia in patients, and their equally rapid awakening, which was without any after-effects. The one thing that left an impression was the rosy colour of the skin, a sign of good peripheral blood flow. Gauss wanted to introduce general anaesthesia with acetylene chiefly as a narcose la reine for emergence anaesthesia during childbirth. According to Gauss the method seemed ideal for obstetrics, doing no harm to either the mother or child. However, the extremely high risk of explosion (static electricity or copper acetylide formation) and the Second World War put a rapid end to these studies.

For historical reasons I should also mention isopropyl chloride, which was likewise used for general anaesthesia for a time, again in obstetrics. A very pure form of this compound was produced by the Rheinpreußen Aktiengesellschaft für Bergbau und Chemie from 1951 on the advice of Hans Killian (1892-1982), formerly a surgeon in Freiburg and Wroclaw and was to be used for emergence anaesthesia, for example, in the same way as trichloroethylene. Occasional unwanted side effects and Hoechsts takeover of the Rheinpreußen pharmacological group and research led to this halogenated agent being taken off the market in 1955.

Farbwerke Hoechst AG, previously known as Meister Lucius und Brüning, had been working on non-combustible and non-explosive halogenated hydrocarbons (propellants, refrigerants, and many others) and developing new methods for their synthesis. In addition to this, Suckling and Raventos had pointed out the good general-anaesthetic effects of Fluothane. These properties had led O. Scherer and H. Kühn to introduce their own process for Hoechst halothane and to pass it on to anaesthetists. The first patent was granted forty years ago, in 1957. Hoechst halothane contains an admixture of thymol as an antiseptic.

Siegemund, who was from the same group of Hoechst chemists, sent me a whole series of halogenated ethers for investigation. However, further tests of their suitability as general anaesthetics proved unsuccessful despite their generally good efficacy and tolerability one of the reasons being the instability vis—vis the alkaline CO_2 absorber in the closed anaesthetic systems, i.e. technical difficulties.

Volatile anaesthetics thus accounted for only part of the anaesthetic development work at Hoechst. It was rather local pain control that was the repeated object of pharmaceutical, pharmacological, and clinical research.

The development of usable agents for local and regional anaesthesia was a central concern at Hoechst at an early stage. Good general tolerability and good degradability of the chemical substances in the organism were the stipulated aim. Finally, the desired temporary effect had to be reversible once the medical intervention was over.

Although the discovery of the alkaloid of the coca bush (Erythroxylon coca) provided an agent that had many different applications, the known side effects prevented its general use. The search for the action principle began. A few words, or to be more precise a few general critical comments, are in order here:

There is no specific property that makes a substance a local anaesthetic. However, few compounds meet the requisite criteria. Many antihistamines, phenols, and even calcium ions, etc. could be mentioned, and if I were to do so it would probably become clear that there are in principle no uniform criteria. Nevertheless.

The good surface-anaesthetic efficacy of 4-aminobenzoic acid ethyl ester, also known as Anesthesin or Benzocaine, had been recognized by K. Ritsert way back in 1890, but it was not until 1902 that this compound became one of Hoechst pharmaceutical products. It was subsequently sold as a surface-acting local anaesthetic over a number of decades, and is still available today. However, attempts to formulate it as a usable aqueous solution were unsuccessful on account of its inadequate solubility. Further developments followed in fairly rapid succession.

In 1897 the ortho form and the new ortho form were developed by Alfred Einhorn (1857-1917) and Robert Heinz (1865-1924) in the light of the findings with Benzocaine. However, these compounds too foundered on the rock of poor solubility. The attempt to introduce an anilide derivative synthesized by Einhorn and Oppenheimer (1900) as a local anaesthetic (Nirvanin) was likewise abandoned, on account of poor local tolerability. Further efforts to produce a well-tolerated local anaesthetic came up against the same problems.

A great advance was finally made at Hoechst when Einhorn and Uhlfelder succeeded in developing a Benzocaine product that was soluble in water. On 27th November 1904 a patent application was filed for a basic ester of 4-aminobenzoic acid. To endow Benzocaine with good solubility, the ethyl group of the ester was replaced by the basic diethylaminoethyl residue, allowing the formation of a salt. The hydrochloride was readily soluble in water and, in addition, the solution was practically neutral as a result of the free amino group on the benzene ring. The compound was named Novocain®.

Only a year after it was announced, the new anaesthetic was already in medical use. I do not think that registration of this kind would be possible today. Later, in a summary, Einhorn, Fiedler, Ladisch, and Uhlfelder wrote, the monohydrochloride of p-aminobenzoic acid diethylaminoethyl ester so completely fulfilled expectations in the pharmacological and clinical trials that in 1905 it proved possible to introduce it into medical use under the name Novocain®.

The local anaesthetic Novocain was characterized by a relatively low general toxicity (roughly a quarter of that of cocaine), excellent tissue tolerability, and a high degree of stability even in solution. For many years it held its position as an almost unbelievable standard for other local anaesthetics. It found its way into the pharmacopoeias of many countries, indeed virtually every country in the world. The seizure of the patented process as enemy property during the First World War (1917) may have contributed to this distribution. The generic name procaine, as the US Pharmacopeia calls it, dates from this time. After more than 90 years the product and the drug is still in use even if much reduced use in hospitals and general practices.

Novocain had little surface-anaesthetic efficacy, and so for a long time cocaine was retained for mucosae and conjunctivae, for anaesthesia of the eyes, and for topical use in ENT. A usable topical anaesthetic did not come into being until the synthesis of Pantocaine (tetracaine, Amethocaine, etc.) by Eisleb and the pharmacological investigations of Fuszgänger and Schaumann. Appropriately formulated, Pantocaine or 4-(butylamino)benzoic acid 2-(dimethylamino) ethyl ester could be used for virtually any kind of local anaesthesia. For practical reasons, however, it was reserved for surface anaesthesia and mucosal anaesthesia. It was also intended that Pantocaine would be used for specific anaesthesia of the injection site prior to nerve-block anaesthesia in dentistry, in the form of a metered-dose spray, but because of the rapid evaporation of the solvent and the fairly low solubility of Pantocaine in this solvent, the applicator nozzles often became irreversibly blocked.

Since I had worked on the degradation products of local anaesthetics of the ester

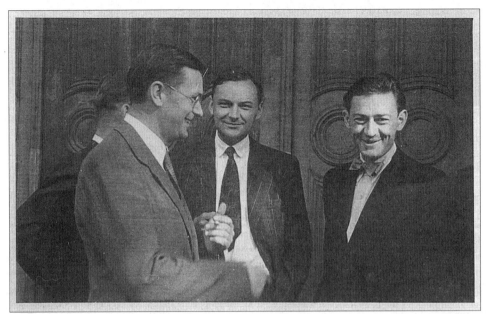

Fig. 3: Professor Dr. Albrecht Fleckenstein (m.) was working about pain and endoanesthesia (1949), Pharmacological Institute Heidelberg.

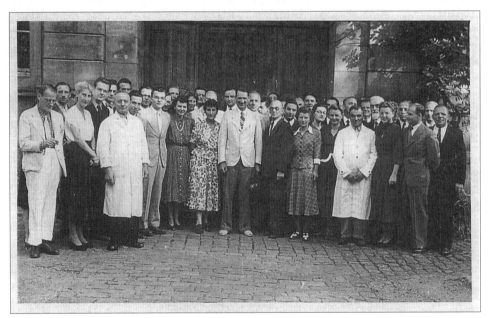

Fig. 4: Professor Dr. Fritz Eichholtz, on his 60th birthday in the middle in front of the Pharmacological Institute Heidelberg (1949).

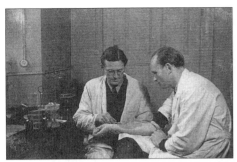

Fig. 5: Intracutaneous testing of local anesthethics.

group years earlier (1950), I was able to kill two birds with one stone. The salts of 4-aminobenzoic acid or 4-(butylamino)benzoic acid and also of a number of other organic acids, e.g. with procaine and tetracaine, and similar local anaesthetics are better dissolved in certain solvents, with their water solubility maintained. The curious discovery of a reduction in toxicity which was greater than one would expect for the increase in molecular weight was a happy bonus. This product, which was made by Hoechst under the name of Gingicain, was brought out as a metered-dose mucosal anaesthetic for use in dentistry..

Finally, mention should be made of a late development at Hoechst: Cornecain(, which was introduced specially for ophthalmology by Ther and Mügge.

When Hoechst took over the pharmaceutical department of Rheinpreussen Aktiengesellschaft für Bergbau und Chemie in 1955 it naturally also inherited the local anaesthetics which had been developed there. These were synthesized in the course of work on aminosalicylic acid manufactured for therapeutic purposes (treatment of tuberculosis) by W. Grimme and H. Schmitz, and were tested pharmacologically, toxicologically, and from the general point of view by Keil and his associates. They included the procaine analogue hydroxyprocaine, whose general tolerability was as good as that of procaine, the homologue of tetracaine, hydroxytetracaine (Salicain®, Rhenocain), bronchiocain (Gynodal), and prusocain. Hydroxytetracaine was somewhat stronger than tetracaine, and as it was also less toxic than the latter it was added to hydroxyprocaine to strengthen its action, particularly for local anaesthesia of the mouth and jaw region. In terms of surface-anaesthetic efficacy, however, bronchiocain and prusocain were superior to tetracaine.

However, for various reasons and competition from the companys other products played a part here the derivatives of 4-aminohydroxybenzoic acid were not developed further and disappeared from the Hoechst range.

Research in the area of local anaesthetics had in the meantime also gone down other pathways, including some forgotten avenues. The local anasthetic efficacy of anilidine was rediscovered.

This was not taken up again until about 40 years later, when Löfgren found the long-acting and strongly active diethylamino-2,6-dimethylacetanilide or lidocaine. At Hoechst too people remembered the work carried out by Einhorn and Oppenheimer at the turn of the century. However, scientists set out to search for a product that would be better degraded, and in 1953 they found one, in the form of 2-butylamino-2-chloro-6-methylacetanilide, butanilicaine (Hostacaine®) (Ehrhart et al., Häussler and Ther). In the body Hostacaine is rapidly broken down by enzymatic degradation at the peptide-like NH-CO bond, mainly in the liver, and the toxic cleavage products (principally o-chlorotoluidine) are excreted in the urine. Hostacaine was detoxified rapidly and well.

Hostacaine has low subcutaneous toxicity, of much the same order as that of Novocain®, whereas its acute intravenous toxicity is about twice that of Novocain. The phosphate salt of Hostacaine® was finally introduced for

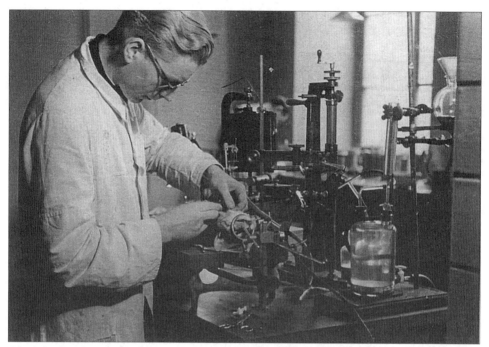

Fig. 6: Studies on endoanesthesia (E.Roesch) with very antique apparatus.

nerve-block and local anaesthesia, especially for jaw surgery. The good deep nerve-block anaesthesia and the rapid onset of action with Hostacaine have for years made it a leading dental drug, especially in Germany.

The most recent advances in the development of a new local anaesthetic at Hoechst have for me been a personal experience of a special kind. Despite decades of research, no-one has yet succeeded in finding an ideal local anaesthetic, and I do not believe one ever will.

Nevertheless, no effort should be spared to at least come closer to this goal. One should, perhaps, make progress in other substance classes. It should be worth the effort. It was a stroke of good fortune that the chemist R. Rippel was working on the synthesis of new heterocyclics from the thiophene series. This group was an obvious candidate for pharmacological investigations, and the local-anaesthetic properties especially looked extremely interesting. On account of its specific properties, the hydrochloride of 4-methyl-3-(2-propylaminopropionylamino)-2-thiophenecarboxylic acid methyl ester in particular seemed to offer a number of new advantages. In 1974 Muschaweck and Rippel presented a new local anaesthetic carticaine (Ultracain®), and reported on its chemical and pharmacological properties. At the same time, investigations were carried out into its tolerability (Baeder et al.), degradation (Uihlein), and kinetics, using the 35 S-labelled product (Hofer et al.), and the first clinical results were obtained (Eberl, Glatzel, Hecksher-Sorensen, Eerola, Reng, Auberger and Hendolin). Numerous publications have appeared since the official introduction of carticaine (Ultracain®). A few months ago (22nd/23rd November 1996), the twentieth anniversary of its general clinical use was celebrated in dentistry (Rheinhartshausen Symposium, Rhg., chaired by G. Frenkel; proceedings not yet published). Its indication, anaesthesia, had after all been discovered in this field. Over 70% of German dentists use

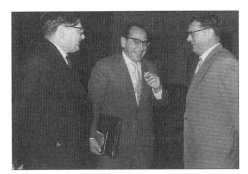

Fig. 7: Professor Klaus Soehring (m.)

Ultracain® for infiltration anaesthesia and nerve-block anaesthesia.

The successful development and use of modern local anaesthetics was helped, finally, by the discovery, isolation, and synthesis of vasoconstrictors. In contrast to cocaine, virtually all synthetic local anaesthetics cause vasoparalysis or vasodilation, making it impossible to ensure the surgeons need for a blood-free site of operation. Here too Hoechst has been able to make another valuable contribution.

Vasoconstrictors

The general development of local anaesthesia was helped, finally, by the development, isolation, and synthesis of the vasoconstrictors. Synthesis of pure adrenomedullary hormones in particular played an important role. By adding these to the local-anaesthetic solutions for injection it was finally possible to dispense with cocaine.

The vasoconstricting and thus haemostatic action of adrenal hormones had been known for a long time. The active principle isolated by Otto von Fürth (1867-1938), John Jacob Abel (1857-1938), Jokichi Takamine (1854-1922), and Aldrich was already known and had been given the names adrenaline and epinephrine. Then, in 1903, Friedrich Stolz (1860-1936) succeeded in synthesizing the D, L form of adrenaline, and a year later Flächer managed to separate the two optical antipodes. Complete identity with natural l-adrenaline was confirmed. This product was launched by Hoechst under the name of Suprarenin®. Epinephrine became the international non-proprietary name.

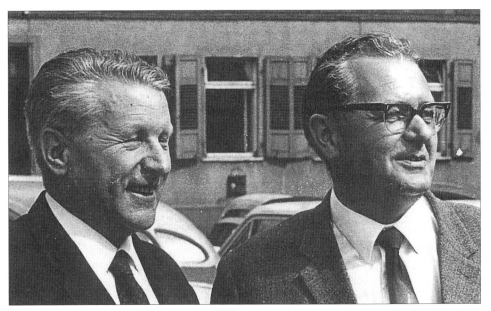

Fig. 8: Professor Dr. Leopold Ther (left) (HOSTACAIN® – Butanillicain), Roman Muschawek (right) (ULTRACAIN® – Anticain) – Pharmacological Institute HOECHST AG.

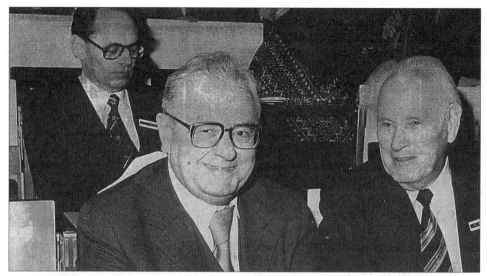

Fig. 9: Professor Hans Killian (r.), the great old man, on of the most important promotor of the graduation and position of the German anesthesists, speaking about the textbook "Lokalanaesthesie und Lokalanaesthetika" with the coauthor Roman Muschaweck.

The physiological significance of l-noradrenaline or norepinephrine, formed during the synthesis, remained unrecognized, and it was not until 1950 that noradrenaline (Arterenol®) gained importance as a vasoconstricting agent. A further sympathomimetic made and sold by Hoechst (and others) was used as a vasoconstrictor; the drug in question was corbadrine (Cobefrin or Lirotil), and had the company name Corbasil®. However, the use of Corbasil® as a vasoconstricting additive to local anaesthetics in dentistry was of only temporary importance. Other sympathomimetics developed by Hoechst need not be mentioned in connection with local anaesthesia.

Only one thing is certain: without the isolation of an endogenous hormone and its synthesis for the very first time, local anaesthesia for surgical interventions would remain of very limited value. Not until the anaesthetics could be combined with a vasoconstrictor, particularly adrenaline (Suprarenin), did the way really become clear for their use in medical, dental, and veterinary surgical practice.

Closing remarks

The data presented in this paper cover more than a century of work by researchers in the field of analgesia and anaesthesia at Hoechst. Tribute should be paid, above all, to the collaborative endeavours of chemists, pharmacologists, anaesthetists, surgeons, and other doctors, as they all contributed to significant progress in treatment and research.

a) Thanks to their efforts, it has been possible to bring out a diverse range of analgesics in smooth succession, starting with Kairin (1882) and antipyrine (1883), then Novalgin, and finally the powerful analgesics Dolantin (1939) and Polamidon (1949).

b) Volatile general anaesthetics such as nitrous oxide, chloroform, and diethyl ether were naturally also made available. The company developed its own methods for the chlorinated and fluorinated hydrocarbons; Hoechst halothane comes into this category.

c) The development of synthetic local anaesthetics must also be considered a

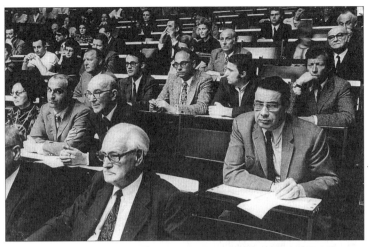

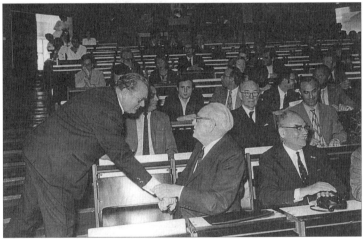

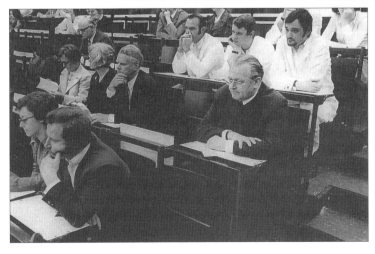

*Fig. 10:
Symposium at the
Pain Clinic at Mainz.*

particular Hoechst achievement, starting with Anesthesin (1893/1902), then Novocain® (1905) and Pantocaine® (tetracaine) (1932), and finally Ultracain® (1974).

d) The first ever synthesis (1903-1905) of an endogenous hormone, l-epinephrine (Suprarenin) and l-norepinephrine (Arterenol), was of epoch-making significance, not least for local anaesthesia. Without this achievement relatively bloodless surgical interventions would not have become possible.

Thank you for giving me the opportunity to report on over a century of successful development work in analgesia and anaesthesia at Hoechst. General medical practice, surgery, anaesthesia, and emergency medicine have all benefited. Thanks must finally go to those who paved the way of this development up to the present day.

Postspinal Headache – its Prevention over the Decades

St. Wilhelm, M. Goerig, Th. Standl
Department of Anaesthesiology, University Hospital Hamburg, Hamburg, Germany

The problem of spinal headache

The successful introduction of spinal anaesthesia in Germany by the surgeon August Bier at Kiel in 1898 was associated with the occurrence of headache in almost all patients. It is known that even Bier and his assistant Hildebrandt themselves suffered from severe headache the day after they had injected cocaine one another into the subarachnoid space. Leakage of cerebrospinal fluid through the dural rent was assumed to contribute to this complication by several early investigators and Bier was widely criticized on the grounds that the large diameter of his 15- or 17-gauge instrument was responsible for unnecessary pain and tissue trauma to the patient.

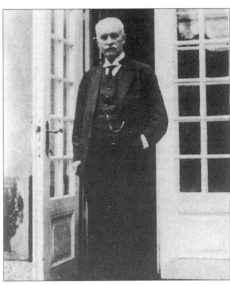

Portrait of the German surgeon August Bier (1861-1949) who introduced spinal anaesthesia in clinical practice at Kiel in 1898

Rationale for the use of small bore needles

In 1904, Babcock of Philadelphia realized the advantages of the spinal needle that was designed by the American neurologist Corning of New York in 1900 and proposed the use of a spinal needle with a 20-gauge diameter "with a well-fitted stylette so that the needle cannot become clogged in the introduction". Later in 1922, Corning's two-needle device for lumbar dural puncture was recommended again by Hoyt of New York. He was convinced that on the one hand rigidity was required to penetrate the dense tissue but on the other hand the "infamous spinal headache" could possibly be reduced by the use of a smaller inner needle for piercing the dura. In 1923, Greene had begun to investigate various spinal needles on cadavers at the University of Oregon. His work led him to two important conclusions. At first, "postdural puncture headache (PDPH) is due to the trauma of the spinal dura severe enough to produce excessive leakage of cerebrospinal fluid" and secondly, "a small needle having a smooth round point would separate rather than sever the fibers of the dura". The marked decrease in the frequency of PDPH using smaller bore atraumatic spinal needles resulted in the reintroduction of introducers in the late 1920's.

Coverpage of Bier`s article on spinal anaesthesia

XVI.
Aus der Königlichen chirurgischen Klinik zu Kiel.
Versuche über Cocainisirung des Rückenmarkes.
Von
Prof. Dr. August Bier.

Die Schleich'sche Infiltrations- und die Oberst'sche regionäre Cocainanästhesie haben die gefährliche allgemeine Narkose in sehr wesentlicher und erfreulicher Weise beschränkt. Aber für „grosse" Operationen sind beide Verfahren doch nur im geringen Grade verwendbar. Ich habe den Versuch gemacht, durch Cocainisirung des Rückenmarkes grosse Strecken des Körpers unempfindlich gegen Schmerz zu machen. Dies wurde in folgender Weise ausgeführt:

Bei dem in Seitenlage befindlichen Kranken wird die Quincke-sche Lumbalpunktion in bekannter Weise vorgenommen. Die Hohlnadel wählt man sehr dünn. Nachdem sie in den Sack der Rückenmarkshäute eingedrungen ist, entfernt man den Stöpsel, welcher die Lichtung der Nadel verschliesst, und setzt sofort den Finger auf die Mündung, damit möglichst wenig Liquor cerebrospinalis ausfliesst. Mit einer Pravaz'schen Spritze, welche genau auf die Punktionsnadel passt, wird die gewünschte Menge Cocain eingespritzt. Dabei muss man natürlich bei der Länge der Nadel so viel Cocainlösung mehr nehmen, als die Lichtung derselben fasst. (Bei unserer Nadel 1½ Theilstriche der Pravaz'schen Spritze.) Damit das Cocain nicht aus dem Stichkanale der Rückenmarkshäute in die Gewebe sickert, lässt man die Nadel mit der daraufsitzenden Spritze 2 Minuten stecken und entfernt sie dann. Die Stichöffnung in der Haut wird mit Collodium verklebt.

Die Lumbalpunktion wird unter Schleich's Infiltrationsanästhesie schmerzlos ausgeführt. Zuerst wird die Haut, dann werden mit einer langen Nadel die übrigen Weichtheile bis auf die Wirbelsäule infiltrirt.

Greene's cadaver experiments at the University of Oregon focusing tissue trauma after dural puncture were published in JAMA 1926

LUMBAR PUNCTURE AND THE PREVENTION OF POSTPUNCTURE HEADACHE *

H. M. GREENE, M.D.
Member of the teaching staff, University of Oregon Medical School
PORTLAND, ORE.

As the result of experiments made during 1923 and my experience since that time with the use of a small needle [1] having a round, sharp, tapering point, I am convinced that postpuncture headache is caused by trauma to the spinal dura sufficient to result in excessive leakage of cerebrospinal fluid to the point at which the brain is left without a water cushion.

These experiments demonstrated that a greater trauma was produced by the use of a needle with a blunt cutting point than by a needle of the same caliber with a point rounded, tapering and sharp. It was also shown that leakage followed puncture of the spinal dura in every instance in which the membrane was suspended and filled with water, and that the amount of leakage was in direct relation to the size of the needle used (Fig. 1).

The problem is, then, to do the puncture by ways and means that produce the least possible trauma to the spinal dural sac.

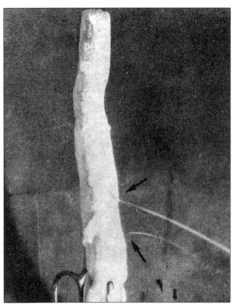

Greene's experiment: Spinal dural sac suspended and filled with water. The large stream (upper arrow) results from a puncture with a 19-gauge needle with a cutting point; a small stream (lower arrow) from a 22-gauge needle with a round point.

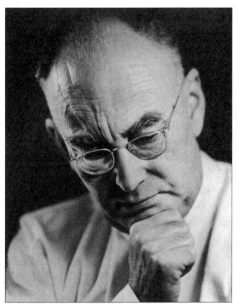

Portrait of the Hamburg surgeon Helmut Schmidt (1895-1979) whose contributions to regional anaesthesia have fallen into oblivition during the past decades.

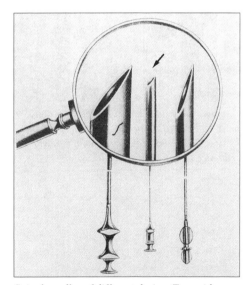

Spinal needles of different design. To avoid unnecessary trauma to the dura, Schmidt recommended the use of the short-bevel needle (arrow)

Modifications and improvements

In 1932 the German Helmut Schmidt could demonstrate that the use of a 20-22-gauge short-bevel needle, developed by George Pitkin of New Jersey in 1924, resulted in the comparable low incidence of PDPH of less than 5%. This needle made of rustless steel was less likely to break, retained its sharp point longer and it withstood considerable manipulation without bending. However, Schmidt was also convinced that severe headache could only be avoided if patients were strictly placed in a down-head position for at least 12-24 hours following lumbar puncture and the question of PDPH, alleviated but not entirely answered, continued to capture the interest of several investigators.

Newer spinal needles

In the United States the concept of the two needle-device that already Hoyt had espoused in 1922 led to the routine use of a fine 26-gauge spinal cannula that was inserted through a 21-gauge introducer needle, at first described by Greene in 1950. Shortly thereafter in 1951, Hart and Whitacre of Cleveland were responsible for the introduction of a 20-gauge solid-end needle that was drawn to a sharp pencil-like point with the orifice on the side of the needle, just proximal to the tip. This new concept of a non-cutting spinal needle was improved by the use of a 22-gauge Whitacre needle by Cappe in 1960 and the development of blunt needles of different sizes by Sprotte in Germany since 1987. Disposable spinal needles of different design and size made of stainless steel are now available. Like their predecessors, several requirements must be met. The cutting edges of the needle may be dulled somewhat during the manufacturing process as an aid in both spreading rather than cutting tissues. Today, there is agreement that PDPH is dependent on needle design and size. As a consequence, non-cutting needles should be preferred over cutting needles and the smallest gauge needle available should be used.

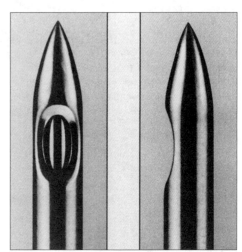

Scanning electron micrograph of a 25-gauge, 90 mm Sprotte needle. Special attention has to be focused on the outlet of the cannula both with reference of its form and surface.

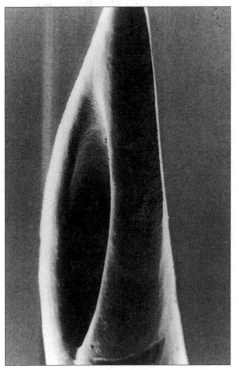

Scanning electron micrograph of the fang tip of an elapid snake which produces only minimal tissue damage.

Had the Beginning of Modern Anaesthesia been possible in the 16th Century ?

H. Petermann
Department of Anaesthesiology, University Erlangen-Nuremberg, Germany

Summary

Speaking of modern anaesthesia means considering the time between 1846 and today. What has been before 1800 ? Right now there are only few information about anaesthesia in former times existing. There are hints that even the medicine man in Egypt (10.-1.Jh.v.Chr.) had knowledge about agents inducing sleep. Pedanios Dioskurides (1.Jh.n.Chr.) described plants that include narcotic active substances in his Materia medica. This knowledge was traded up to the 16. century. It is possible that the beginning for modern anaesthesia has been set in this century?

Looking for early notes on narcosis you will find: V. Cordus gives a description how to distill and to use ether, Paracelsus noted the inducing sleep effect of it to chicken and at least A. Vesal did an endotracheal intubation on a pig during an anatomical examination. All these understandings are still the basic components of modern anaesthesia:
• the drug and how to produce it
• the knowledge about the narcotic effect
• the technique of avoiding lack of air.

Situation in the 16th Century

In the middle ages public health was in the hand of priests or monk doctors. The ecclesiastics were well educated and the first ones, whom people consulted having problems with their health. Layman doctors called "medici" or "magistri" were described in the literature since the 12th century. Having studied medicine at Universities in the 15th century "gelehrte Doktores" (scientific doctors) could be distinguished from "Wundaerzte or Chirurgen" (doctors for wound or surgeons) who underwent an education like a craftsman. Besides this we also had midwives and pharmacists as well as a lot of travelling healing men, mainly called "Kurpfuscher."

The studied doctors at that time only made urinoscopy and pulse diagnosis. They treated the internal diseases with medicines from the chemist's shop. For special cases they had to be consulted by the Wundaerzte. The

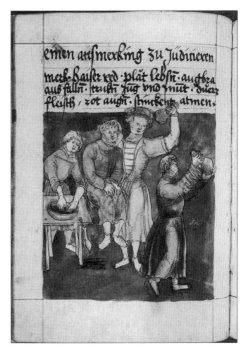

Doctor, Barber-surgeon and Assistant.
In: Liber quod libetarius. Nürnberg 1547. fol. 72v.

Wundaerzte, the early surgeons, did the real treatment of the patient. They made trepanations, amputations, resections of ulcers, cured inflammations of the skin and epidemic diseases like cholera, plague and dysentery, and took care of fractures and luxations. For treatment they used pilulae, klistiery, infusions and decoctions, unguents, bandages and plaster, as well as special instruments for surgical therapy. As an instruction the Wundaerzte could use the different Wundarzneien (vulnerary medicine) like those of Hans von Gersdorff (1517).

Valerius Cordus (1515-1544):
Preparation of Oil of Vitriol

The various chapters are entitled:
I. Preparation of Oil of Vitriol.
II. Selection of the Vitriol
III. Preparation of the Vitriol.
IV. Calcination of the Vitriol.
V. Construction of the Furnace.
VI. Distillation of the Vitriol
VII. Separation of the Water Which Had Been Added.
VIII. Rectification of the Oil of Vitriol.
IX. Its Properties.
X. How the Sweet Is Made From the Sour.
XI. Method of Separation.
Properties of the Substance Which Has Been Separated.

Valerius Cordus studied medicine at the University of Wittenberg and was the author of the first German pharmacopoeia (1547). In his "… Annotationes in P. Dioscoridis Anarzeibei Medica materia …" (remarks to Dioscurides Materia medica) he described the preparation of oil of vitriol in 12 chapters. But he also gave three prescriptions of its application: *Against Stones, For a Debile Stomach* and also *For the Heat and Thirst of Fevers.* There is not any notice, that sulfuric ether might be inducing sleep.

Paracelsus (1492-1541):
Effects of Sulfuric Ether

However, the following should be noted here with regard to this sulphur, that of all things extracted from vitriol it is most remarkable because it is stable. And besides, it has associated with it such a sweetness that it is taken even by chickens, and they fall asleep from it for a while but awaken later without harm. On this sulphur no other judgment should be passed that in diseases which need to be treated with anodynes it quiets all suffering without any harm, and relieves all pain, and quenches all fevers, and prevents complications in all illnesses.[2]

Aurelius Philipp Theophrast Bombast von Hohenheim, called "Paracelsus", studied medicine in Ferrara and then practiced in Strasbourg and Basle. Afterwards he wandered around, restless and impatient, and published a lot of books. In "Operum Medico-Chimicorum sive Paradoxorum", book seven, chapter seven, he described the "suesses Vitriol" (sulfuric ether).

He recognized the anaesthetic effect of sulfuric ether and that it had no negative side effects (for chicken). Before he came to this description he wrote about the "Spongia somnifera" (sporific sponge), that was used for inducing sleep or causing insensibility against pain. He probably had recognized, in which way "suesses Vitriol" (sulfuric ether) might be applied.

Andreas Vesalius (1514-1564):
Artificial Respiration on a Sow

Next you will begin the section which I promised a little while ago, I would describe, that on a pregnant bitch or sow, although from the point of view of the voice it is better to take a pig, since when a dog is bound for some time, no matter what you do, he neither barks nor howls after a while and so you cannot judge the weakening or cessation of the voice … .

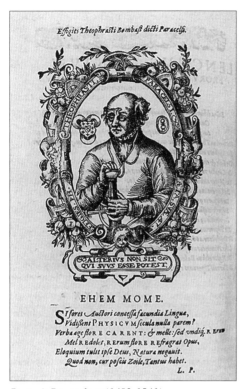

Portrait Paracelsus (1492-1541).
In: Paracelsus: Opera medico-chemica sive paradoxa. T.7. Frankfurt 1605.

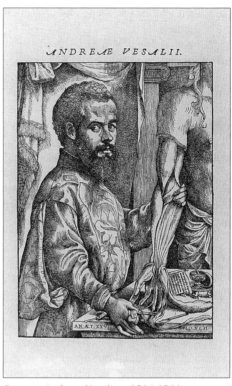

Portrait Andreas Vesalius (1514-1564).
In: A. Vesal: De humani corporis fabrica libri septem. Basel 1543.

And then I make a long cutting in the throat with a rather sharp knife which can lay back the skin and the muscles beneath it right down to the trachea, taking care that the cutting does not slip off to the side and injure some important vein. ...

But that life may in a manner of speaking be restored to the animal, an opening must be attempted in the trunk of the trachea, into which a tube of reed or cane should be put; you will then blow into this, so that the lung may rise again and the animal take in air. Indeed, with a slight breath in the case of this living animal the lung will swell to the full extent of the thoracic cavity, and the heart become strong and exhibit a wondrous variety of motions. So, with the lung inflated once and a second time, you examine the motion of the heart by sight and touch as much as you wish ....

With this observed, the lung should again be inflated, and with this device, which I have learned nothing more pleasing to me in Anatomy, great knowledge of the differences in the beats should be acquired. For when the lung, long falcid, has collapsed, the beat of heart and arteries appears wavy, creepy, twisting, but when the lung is inflated, it becomes strong again and swifst and displays wondrous variations ....

And as I do this, and take care that the lung is inflated at intervals, the motion of heart and arteries does not stop ....[3]

Andreas Vesal studied medicine in Paris, but then gave his attention mainly to anatomy.

He gained a lot of knowledge by dissecting entire animals.

The above description of Vesal is part of his anatomical studies. He did not look for ways of artificial respiration of animals, but wrote down his observations. If his experimental animals lived longer, he was able to study their anatomy for a longer time. This was the reason why he did not publish this fact in a special work, it was part of his anatomical book Fabrica of 1543. He might have realized the importance of his observation, since this experimental scene illustrated the first letter of the seventh book, the "Q".

Why did the Knowledge of V. Cordus, Paracelsus and A. Vesal not lead to the Beginning of Modern Anaesthesia ?

Valerius Cordus described a drug - namely oil of vitriol - and how to produce it, Paracelsus recognized the effect of inducing sleep and Vesal found out a technique of a voiding lack of air. Circumstances in those times were not quite favourable for introducing new inventions. Surgical interventions were part of the work of the 'Wundaerzte' (surgeons). Most of them had not studied at an university or got to read any book. All there knowledge had been brought to them by word of mouth. To be able to realize the importance of the understandings of V. Cordus, Paracelsus and A. Vesal, the Wundaerzte should have read books and studied at universities. But most of them did not have the time nor the money to do so.

The 'gelehrte Doctor' (scientific doctor) did not take care of the knowledge of those surgeons. The felt they were superior to them, that is why they had no interest in helping them. There was no way that the important discoveries of V. Cordus, Paracelsus and A. Vesal could have been seen as an entierety. According to their lives since V. Cordus died early, Paracelsus fell into disgrace and A. Vesal was only respected for his anatomical wok this cirkumstance is understandable.

Conclusions

1. In the 16. century nobody used anaesthetic agents to cause unconsciousness, i.e. anaesthesia.
2. The major basic findings for modern anaesthesia were already known at that time.
3. It did not come to anybody`s mind to combine all of the above mentioned results.
4. Because of these reaons people still had to wait another three hundred years for operations without pain.

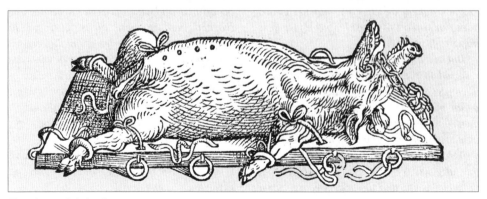

Experimental Animal.
In: A. Vesal: De humani corporis fabrica libri septem. Basel 1543.

References:

1. Cordus V: Annotationes in Pedacii Dioscoridis Anazarbei de medica materia libros V... . Straßburg 1561. English Translation from: Foundations of Anesthesiology. A Faulconer and Th Keys (ed), Springfield 1965. Vol.1, P 267-275

2. Paracelsus: Opera medico-chemica sive paradoxa... T.7. Frankfurt 1605. English Translation from: Foundations of Anesthesiology. A Faulconer and Th Keys (ed), Springfield 1965. Vol.1, P 266

3. Vesal A: De humani corporis fabrica libri septem. Basel 1543. English Translation from: Foundations of Anesthesiology. A Faulconer and Th Keys (ed), Springfield 1965. Vol.1, P 10-11

4. Keys Th E : Die Geschichte der chirurgischen Anaesthesie. Springer, Berlin 1968

5. Petermann H: Die Wundaerzte in der freien Reichsstadt Nuernberg im 16. Jahrhundert. Erlangen 1995. (Magisterarbeit, unpublished)

A Quantitative Analysis of Newspaper Reports on the Introduction of Anaesthesia

H. Connor
County Hospital Hereford, UK

Introduction

Reading the reports about anaesthesia in the newspapers gives a qualitative impression of the public and professional reaction to the introduction of anaesthesia, but can numerical analysis of the reports be used to quantitate the magnitude of the reaction and to compare it with that to other events? An objective measure of public reaction to an event is difficult to define, but certainly the number of reports about cholera in the London Times newspaper correlated closely with the number of deaths (Figure 1), and it seems reasonable to assume that the number of deaths would be a reflection of the extent of public interest.

Methodology

The Hereford Times and the Hereford Journal were scanned from January 1847 to December 1849, and counts made of the numbers of articles about anaesthesia, Chartism and the reform movement, cholera and railway accidents. In some instances a

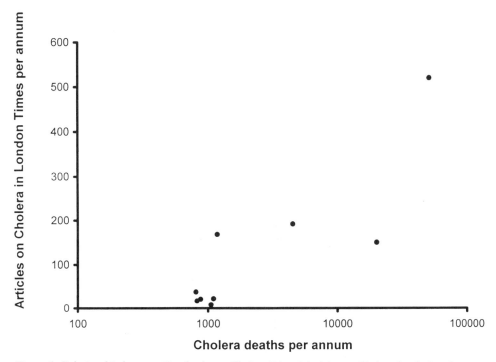

Figure 1. Relationship between Deaths due to Cholera(1) and Articles on Cholera in the London Times 1847 - 1855(2). Spearman rank correlation test r=0.65, p < 0.05.

Topic	Dates	Reports Indices and (Reports Ratios)									
		London Newspapers				Provincial Newspapers					
		London Times	Morning Chronicle	Evening Chronicle	The Globe	Hereford Times	Hereford Journal	Shropshire Journal	Shropshire Chronicle	Cheltenham Examiner	Manchester Guardian
Anaesthesia	Jan - Mar 1847	0.8 *(1.0)*	0.8 *(1.0)*	2.8 *(1.0)*	3.5 *(1.0)*	3.7 *(1.0)*	3.8 *(1.0)*	3.5 *(1.0)*	1.8 *(1.0)*	5.0 *(1.0)*	2.1 *(1.0)*
Cholera	Oct - Dec 1848	10.5 *(12.7)*	18.3 *(24.3)*	- *(-)*	46.3 *(13.2)*	3.8 *(1.0)*	3.5 *(0.9)*	9.8 *(2.8)*	6.0 *(3.4)*	7.0 *(1.4)*	5.4 *(2.6)*
Chartism	Apr - Jun 1848	10.8 *(12.9)*	15.9 *(19.9)*	- *(-)*	44.8 *(12.8)*	6.5 *(1.8)*	4.3 *(1.1)*	12.2 *(3.5)*	- *(-)*	10.3 *(2.1)*	20.4 *(9.7)*
Railway Accidents	July - Dec 1848	2.2 *(2.7)*	4.0 *(6.7)*	- *(-)*	9.4 *(2.7)*	1.3 *(0.3)*	0.8 *(0.2)*	4.3 *(2.4)*	2.6 *(1.5)*	4.3 *(0.9)*	3.9 *(1.9)*
Crimean War	Jan - Mar 1855	51.3 *(61.6)*	- *(-)*	- *(-)*	- *(-)*	67.8 *(18.3)*	61.3 *(16.1)*	30.8 *(17.6)*	- *(-)*	53.6 *(10.7)*	- *(-)*

Table 1. Reports Indices and Ratios for Anaesthesia and other topics in London and provincial newspapers. (–) = data not collected)

single article contained information which related to more than one event. For example, an article under a single headline might contain information about separate uses of anaesthesia in Hereford, London and Bristol. The following definitions have therefore been used: a report is defined as the information given under a single headline or sub-headline, and items are defined as the information given about separate events within a report. A report may therefore contain one or more items.

The periods of peak reporting for each topic were identified for the Hereford newspapers. To ensure a reasonably representative time interval, the reports were counted over three month periods for anaesthesia, Chartism and cholera, but over six months for railway accidents because of the smaller number of reports; the number of reports on railway accidents was then halved to obtain a three month average. Having identified the peak reporting periods for each topic in the Hereford newspapers, these same periods were then used to count the numbers of reports in newspapers from London, Manchester, Shrewsbury and Cheltenham. In the case of the London Times, reports were initially identified by using Palmer's Index of the Times(2). Complete concordance was found between the reports identified using Palmer's Index and visual scanning of the newspaper for the first month of each topic period. Scanning of the London Times newspaper was therefore limited to the first month of each topic, and only those reports identified in Palmer's Index for subsequent months were read. To compare reporting of anaesthesia, Chartism, cholera and railway accidents with reporting of an event of

Topic	Dates	Reports Indices					
		London Newspapers			Provincial Newspapers		
		mean ± SEM	n	comparison with anaesthesia	mean ± SEM	n	comparison with anaesthesia
Anaesthesia	Jan - Mar 1847	2.0 ± 1.2	4		3.3 ± 1.1	6	
Cholera	Oct - Dec 1848	25.0 ± 4.4	3	p = 0.028	5.9 ± 1.5	6	p = 0.021
Chartism	Apr - Jun 1848	23.8 ± 4.3	3	p = 0.028	10.7 ± 2.5	5	p = 0.004
Railway Accidents	July - Dec 1848	5.2 ± 1.9	3	p = 0.028	2.9 ± 1.2	6	p = ns
Crimean War	Jan - Mar 1855	51.3	1		53.4 ± 4.0	4	p = 0.005

Table 2. Reports Indices for Anaesthesia and other topics in London compared with provincial newspapers.

unequivocally major public interest the same methodology was applied to the reporting of a three month period of the Crimean war in five of the ten newspapers.

The different newspapers varied considerably in their size. For example, during 1848 the average number of pages published each week (excluding occasional supplements) was 72 in the London Times (six issues, each of 12 pages) and six in the Hereford Times (one issue of six pages). To allow for this difference results have been expressed as a reports index, in which the number of reports in each newspaper have been divided by the average number of pages in each issue of that paper. Editorial policy on the use of sub-headlines also varied between the different newspapers. To allow for this the findings have also been expressed as a reports ratio, which is calculated by dividing the number of reports on each non-anaesthetic topic by the number of reports on anaesthesia. News items in the Herefordshire newspapers were also categorised, according to their content, as being either purely factual, purely opinion, or a mixture of fact and opinion.

Results are expressed as the mean ± SEM, and statistical differences and relationships have been assessed using the Mann-Whitney U test, Fisher's exact test and the Spearman rank correlation test.

Results

The Reports Index results (Tables 1 and 2) show that, with the exception of railway accidents in the provincial newspapers, coverage of anaesthesia was less than that of all the other topics. In comparison with the provincial papers the London newspapers carried fewer reports on anaesthesia ($p = 0.045$), and more reports on cholera ($p = 0.012$); there were no statistically significant differences between London and the provinces in coverage of other topics. Similar results were found using the Reports Ratio (Table 1), except that coverage of cholera in the provincial papers was now similar to that of anaesthesia.

Examination of news items showed marked differences between the two Hereford newspapers (Figure 2). The Hereford Times carried more items which were overtly favourable to the introduction of anaesthesia (11/52) than did the Hereford Journal (1/35), $p = 0.012$. In comparison with items which were favourable to anaesthesia, the Journal published more items which were adverse or described anaesthesia deaths (1 v 7), whereas the opposite was true of the Times (11 v 4), $p = 0.002$. Reports of deaths attributed to anaesthesia were commoner in the second 13 months than in the first 12 months ($p = 0.002$).

Discussion

The introduction of anaesthesia appears to have generated relatively little newspaper coverage compared with that on the other topics. In the Hereford newspapers only railway accidents generated fewer reports, possibly because the editors thought readers would have little interest in this subject as the railway had not yet reached Hereford, and did not do so until 1853(3). In the six months to the end of June 1848 there were 90 deaths as the result of railway accidents(4); that coverage in all the newspapers was not higher than it was must be an indication of public tolerance and acceptance of such a high fatality rate as a necessary by-product of the benefits of rail travel. The cholera epidemic of 1848 was the subject of intensive coverage in London, but less so in the provinces and least of all in Hereford which was fortunate in that it escaped the epidemic of 1848 completely(5). The Chartist and other reform associations were relatively inactive in Herefordshire, moderately active in Cheltenham and Shrewsbury and most active of all in the big cities(6), and this is reflected in the different emphasis given to reports of the movement in the different areas. Analysis of the Reports Indices for Chartism in London (capital city) and in Manchester (a large industrial city) compared with those for the non-industrial towns of Cheltenham, Shrewsbury and Hereford shows a statistically significant difference (23.0 ± 3.8 versus 8.3 ± 0.9, p = 0.029). Coverage of the Crimean war was vastly more intensive than that of any other topic in all five of the newspapers in which it was studied.

Coverage of anaesthesia in the London papers was, relative to the number of pages published each week, less than in the provincial newspapers. This may be an indication of the disillusionment with anaesthesia which occurred among many London surgeons after the initial euphoria of January 1847, and which was a consequence of the high anaesthetic failure rate in the capital at that time (7).

More detailed analysis of the reporting in the Hereford newspapers is shown in Figure 2. During the first two years after the introduction of anaesthesia the Hereford Times carried 58 items and the Hereford Journal 36 items on the subject. When allowance is made for the different number of pages in the two papers, this represents a similar level of coverage. In both papers about 70 percent of items were purely factual. However, where an opinion was expressed the two papers differed markedly. The Hereford Times was enthusiastically in favour of anaesthesia taking every opportunity to extol its benefits, whereas the Hereford Journal, in line with its stated editorial policy(8), published a greater percentage of more neutral items. Although the Hereford Times was politically Liberal and the Hereford Journal Conservative, difference in the reporting of anaesthesia is unlikely to reflect any difference in opinion associated with political ideology because no such distinction is apparent between the two Shrewsbury newspapers, the Shropshire Chronicle (Liberal) and Eddowe's Shropshire Journal (Conservative).

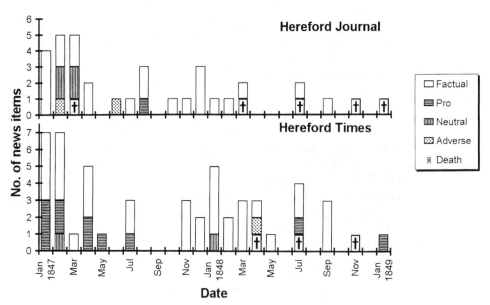

Figure 2. Categorisation of news items on anaesthesia in the Hereford Journal and Hereford Times, January 1847 - January 1849.

As time went by the coverage of anaesthesia decreased, although both papers were now more likely to publish items about death (either medical or accidental) resulting from anaesthetic agents. It seems probable that, as anaesthesia became more widely accepted, the only news deemed worthy of reporting was when something went wrong. In the mid-nineteenth century, as in the late twentieth, good news was not newsworthy. Serious diseases (cholera), the threat of outright rebellion (Chartism at a time when rebellion was rife in mainland Europe), accidents and, above all, war, are what have gripped the public imagination and interest throughout the ages.

Acknowledgements

I am grateful to David Griffin, Andrew Connor and Tom Connor for their help in scanning some of the newspapers, to librarians in the reference libraries in Hereford, Shrewsbury, Cheltenham and Colindale (London) for their assistance, to Dr. S. Jones for help in producing the figures, and to Miss V. Bailey for typing the manuscript.

References:

[1] Annual Reports of the Registrar General. 1847-1855. HMSO, London

[2] Palmer's Index of the London Times Newspaper. 1847-1855. Kraus Reprint Int. Ltd., Vaduz 1965

[3] Howse WH: A History of the City of Hereford. In: Herefordshire: Its Natural History, Archaeology and History. (Ed) Woolhope Naturalists Field Club, SR Publishers Ltd., Gloucester 1954, p 202

[4] Morning Chronicle 25 August 1848, p7 col.2

[5] Ross J : Hereford and the cholera - why did we escape it? J Roy Coll Phys (Lond), 1990; 24: 238-241

[6] Thompson D: The Chartists. Temple Smith Ltd., London 1984 pp341-368

[7] Ellis RH: James Robinson, England's true pioneer of anaesthesia. In: The History of Anaesthesia Third International Symposium, Eds BR Fink, LE Morris and CR Stephen. Wood Library, Museum of Anaesthesiology, Atlanta 1992 pp158-164

[8] Hereford Journal 10 February 1847, p1 col.4

Notes of the History of Anaesthesia for Cardiac Surgery in Southern Moravia

I. Čundrle, J. Pokorný, D. Řehořková
University Hospital Brno - Bohunice, Czech Republic

The beginnings of modern anaesthesiology in Brno, south of Moravia, were greatly influenced by Prof. B. Hejduk, the head of the Brno Second Department of Surgery. During World War II Hejduk took a complete course for anaesthesiology specialists organized by the Academy of Medicine in London. At the beginning of 1947 he persuaded M. Hrdlica (1910 – 1983), an assistant at the Orthopedic Department, to devote his full efforts to anaesthesiology and promised him his support. Hrdlica accepted the proposal and Prof. Hejduk kept his promise. He helped him to deal with modern procedures in general and regional anaesthesia. Hrdlica gradually educated more doctors of his own department and also of other departments and hospitals. Finally he became an adviser for anaesthesiology to the Regional Surgeon (1953) and the head doctor for anaesthesiology at the Regional Institute for National Health in Brno (1957). He was a Regional Anaesthesiologist up to 1967. In 1956 he received a specialists diploma for anaesthesiology. He cooperated over the long - term with the Brno Second Department of Surgery which was later taken over by a prominent cardiac surgeon Prof. J. Navrátil after Prof. Hejduk had left for abroad. M. Hrdlica worked on a number of research

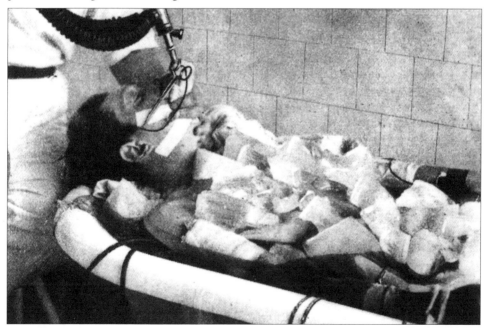

Fig. 1: Artificial hypothermia

projects, such as artificial hypothermia or hibernation (Fig.1). Together with surgeons he worked on both experimental cardiac and vascular surgery including open heart surgery and revascularization (Fig.2). Great credit is owed to Hrdlica as an anaesthesiologist in the advancement of Brno cardiosurgery which is now renowned world - wide. He published 21 scientific works. He is a co-author of the monography Anaesthesiology from 1965. At the end of 1966 he was sent by the Ministry of Health to Greifswald in the former GDR as an expert to found an anaesthesiology department. His successor was doctor Frantisek Zeman.

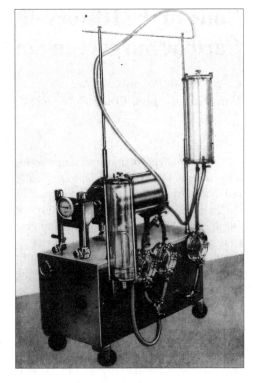

Fig.2: Aparatus for ECCO Premacard II (Czech made).

From Boston Massachusetts, to Timişoara, 5 February 1847 - the First Surgical Use of Anaesthetic Ether in Romania

Sorin Ghişoiu
Timişoara, România

On 16 October 1846 William Thomas Green Morton (1819-1868) of Boston Massachusetts introduced ether as an anaesthetic agent for an operation performed by John Collins Warren (1778-1856) - the excision of a vascular malformation of the mouth and tongue of the patient, Gilbert Abbot (1825-1855). In the same institution, Massachusetts General Hospital, and on the following day, an excision of an arm tumour was performed by George Hayward under ether anaesthesia, also by Morton. Robert Hinkley`s (1853-1941) painting of an operation for the amputation of a leg under ether anaesthesia being performed by Frederick Heywood, is thought to show a procedure which took place on 17 November of the same year; on 21 November, the term "anaesthesia" was coined by Oliver Wendell Holmes (1809-1894). On 26 November 1846, the first partnership of anaesthetists was created between Nathan C. Keep (1800-1875) and William T. G. Morton, the former founding, and later becoming Dean, of the first Harvard Dental School.

The news crossed the Atlantic amazingly quickly due to the excellent postal system and mail-boats of those days. On 14 December 1846 Jobert de Lamballe (1799-1867) gave the first administration of ether in Paris to a patient, Pierre Dihet, with an apparatus constructed at the suggestion of Dr. Willis Fisher. This "first" was a failure but some days later, experiments with ether proved successful according to publications dated 23 January 1847.

Meanwhile, on 19 December 1846 the extraction of an impacted molar tooth under ether was carried out in London by J. Robinson (1813-1861) and Dr. Francis Boott, the patient being a Miss Lonsdale; ether was being used at about the same time in the Dumfries and Galloway Hospital in Scotland by Dr. William Scott and Wiilliam Fraser. On 21 December the surgeon, Robert Liston (1794-1847), declared after carrying out his first amputation with ether anaesthesia given by Wm Squire, "This Yankee dodge beats mesmerism hollow". On 22-23 December ether was given to his son by Dr. Buchanan and on 30 December Francis Plomley described the physical signs of ether anaesthesia. On 31 December 1846, William Herpath (1796-1868) of Bristol administered ether through a large tube with an ivory mouthpiece.

The beginning of 1847 produced a great deal of data on ether anaesthesia in England and in Continental Europe. This may be summarised:

4 January	Glasgow; dental extraction by J. H. H. Lewelin (1818-1886)
9	Edinburgh Royal Infirmary, Dr. James Mathew Duncan (1826-1890)
12	Paris; Hopital Saint Louis, Joseph-François Malgaigne (1806-1865); P. F. Blandin (1789-1849); Ph. Ricord (1800-1889).
17	Edinburgh; James Miller, using an inhaler sent by Robert Liston (1800-1889)

17	Paris; Academy of Science names Charles Thoma Jackson (1805-1880) discoverer of ether	
19	Edinburgh; Sir James Young Simpson (1811-1870) gives ether during labour	
21	Paris; Joseph F. E. Charrière (1803-1876) made an inhaler for surgeon Guersant, of the Hôpital des Enfants	
23	Berne; Hermann Asken Demme (1802-1867) ether during an operation	
24	Erlangen; Johann Ferdinad Heyfelder (1798-1869) ether unsuccessfully for an operation Leipzig; H. E. Weichert & C. F. E. Obenhaus - successful administration at the „Jakobsspital"	
25	London; J. Tomes - Middlesex Hospital, ether for an operation	
27	Vienna; Franz Schuh (1804-1865), ether for operation described by Joseph Skoda (1805-1881)	
29	Vienna; von Watman & Joseph Weigert, ether for operation, also 1st use in veterinary practice	
1st February	Paris; further operations under ether anaesthesia; Jaques G. T. Maissoneuve (1809-1865), Pierre J. Roux (1780-1854), Alfred-Armand-Louis Marie Velpeau (1795-1867), François Magendie (1783-1855). Speeches vehemently against "inebriation by ether"	

And then on 5 February 1847 at Timişoara, ether anaesthesia by Mathias Musil and J. K. Seiss

This story began for the author in 1985 with an article by Thomas Breier published in the Timişoara Medical,, magazine, in which he reported the administration of sulphuric ether at the Military Hospital of Timişoara: "The narcosis method, discovered by the north-American doctor Gh. (sic) Jackson in 1841 (sic) but applied only in 1846 in USA is being used in Timişoara for the first time in February 1847 in a surgical procedure by a chief doctor Giess (sic) and Dr. Musil in the Military Hospital, on the soldier patient named Nikola Muntyan.[1]

This detailed passage obviously contained interesting and verifiable historical details causing the author to search in the archives of "Temesvarer Wochenblatt" from 1842 to 1847. From the issue of 13 February 1847 the exact date of the ether anaesthetic was shown to be 5 February 1847, 112 days after Morton's first successful demonstration (Fig.1). A continental information network, involving Vienna, has been established as the route by which the news of the discovery came to Timişoara. The correct names of the military doctors - from the Gothic text - are Musil and Siehs, the patient was indeed Nikola Muntyan and the device for the ether inhalation had been made just before the procedure by the army doctors, following drawings in the Illustrated London Gazette. [?News?]

This information was shown in a poster presentation, at the Bavaria-România Anaesthesia and Intensive Therapy Symposium held in Bucharest in May 1987 and was later published,[2] establishing an undeniable medical priority for my country. The reference to the London journal was given incorrectly, but in February 1991 the author discovered data in the Budapest Semmelweis

Temesvárer Wochenblatt
für
nützliche Unterhaltung und heimatliche Interessen.

Nro 7. Sonnabend den 13. Februar. **1847.**

Redacteur: **Dr. David Wachtel.** (Achter Jahrgang.) Herausgeber: **Joseph Beichel.**

Lokales.

Ueber die Einathmung des Schwefeläthers bei chirurgischen Operationen, um den Kranken jedem Schmerzgefühle unzugänglich zu machen, eine Erfindung des nordamerikanischen Arztes Jackson, hat man, angeregt durch die günstigen Erfolge, welche diesfalls vorzüglich von Wien aus gemeldet worden, auch bei uns, und zwar im hiesigen Militärspitale einen Versuch angestellt. Es geschah dies in der zweiten Abtheilung vom dritten Bataillonsspital des 61. Lin. Inf. Regimentes Baron Rukavina, unter der Aufsicht der HH. Regimentsarzt Dr. Russl und Oberarzt Dr. Sieß. Wir geben hiemit den sämtlichen Bericht, welcher uns hierüber vorliegt: „Gemeiner Nikola Muntyan, der 1. Compagnie des 3. Rukavina Regimentes ist, am 16. Nov. v. J. mit Entzündung der Beinhaut des Mittelfingers der rechten Hand zugewachsen, in deren Folge Brandfraß des Nägelgliedes eintrat, welcher die Absetzung des Gliedes nothwendig machte. Die Operation wurde den 5. Februar Nachmittag vollzogen und hiebei ein Versuch zur Erprobung der neuen amerikanischen Entdeckung mit dem Einathmen der Schwefelätherdämpfe behufs der hiedurch zu erzeugenden Schmerzlosigkeit gemacht. Der Kranke athmete aus dem nach der „London illustrat. Gazette" verfertigten, etwas unvollkommenen Apparate die Dämpfe über eine halbe Minute, worauf sich sein Gesicht röthete, und die Augen ich schlossen. In diesem Momente wurde der Hautschnitt gemacht und sodann der Knochen abgesägt. Als dieses beinahe gänzlich geschehen war, erwachte der Kranke, ohne jedoch Schmerz zu verrathen, und erst bei Anlegung der blutigen Hefte zur Vereinigung der Wunde zuckte er schmerzhaft zusammen. Die ganze Operation hatte eine Minute gedauert. Drei Minuten nach der Operation, nachdem sich der Kranke vollkommen erholt hatte, versicherte er, während des Schnittes gar keinen Schmerz, sondern nur das Anwehen eines kalten Luftstromes an seinem Finger gefühlt zu haben; nur die Nadelstiche bei Anlegung der Hefte seien schmerzhaft gewesen. Fünf Minuten nach der Operation zeigte der Puls bei sonstigem Wohlbefinden 58 Schläge, später jedoch wurde er ganz normal und in dem Wohlbefinden trat keine Veränderung ein. Es ist hiemit der Beweis geliefert, daß durch Einathmung der Schwefelätherdämpfe wirklich eine Empfindungslosigkeit bei Operationen ohne Nachtheil des Kranken herbeigeführt werden könne. Ob jedoch bei größern, längere Zeit erfordernden und ein wiederholtes Einathmen bedingenden Operationen derselbe Erfolg würde erzielt werden, müssen fernere Versuche erweisen."

Fig. 1

Museum on K. J. Siehs. It appears that Joseph Siehs (1813-1850) was the secretary of the first medical organisation in Banat and Timişoara between 1838 and 1841, the "Verein für praktische Heilkunde".[4,5] Meanwhile, on 5 February 1994, the Medical Stamps Group of the Red Cross had designed an anniversary postmark (designer Dr. M. Mârginean) for Timişoara commemorating the first anaesthetic performed there. The mark was also presented in the German magazine Philatelia Medica, with an appeal for information about the two doctors who gave the anaesthetic. Another article appeared in the Românian magazine Medifila in 1994. Due to these philatelic representations, information was soon at hand on Mathius Musil (1806-1889) and Joseph Siehs (1813-1850). It was provided by Dr. Walter Nissel of Vienna and came from the Kriegsarchiv Wien, and we thank him for his contribution. In June 1994, Philatelia Medica published biographies of the two doctors with a leading article Locales reprinted from the Temesvara Wochenblatt newspaper.

In April 1995, Dr. Hannelore Müller discovered in the Robert Musil book collection of the Austrian Library of Timişoara University, a portrait in oils (1849) by Zoma, of Mathias Musil, Robert Musil`s grandfather. (Fig. 2)

We were then able to present the biographies of the first anaesthetists of Timişoara (the operation was for the amputation of a finger of the right hand) with a picture of Musil and this was published: S. Ghişoiu, M. Mârginean. New information about the first ether anaesthesia in Timişoara, February the 5th 1847. Jurnalul Societatii Romane de Anestezie Terapie Intensiva, 2, number 1, Martie 1995, pp 69-71.

The two men had very different lives but shared some things in common, beginning with their philosophical studies and followed by the medical course at the "Josephinum" in Vienna and, of course, by the anaesthetic at Timişoara.

It is of interest that the progressive training centre, the "Josephinum" was opened in 1785 in Vienna for training army doctors. Established by the enlightened Emperor Joseph II (1741-1790), it was built between 1783 and 1785 by the architect Isadore Canevale (1730-1785). A commemorative plaque, made by Wilhelm Voertel, still exists in he Lorraine room at Franzesburg, south of Vienna and shows the plan presented by the architect to the Emperor and to his personal physician, Giovanni Alessandre von Brambilla (1728-1800), known for his beautiful ornaments on medical instruments.

In the "Joseph-Akademie" is the History of Medicine Museum of the University of Vienna[6] which contains many unique collections. Musil and Siehs, while training at the Josephinum must have faced difficulties and

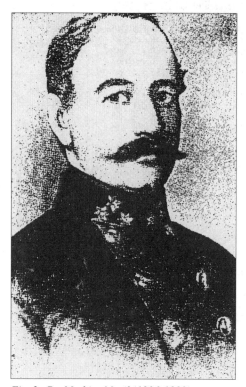

Fig. 2: Dr. Mathias Musil (1806-1889)

tensions inherent in the conservative University of Medicine of Vienna, founded in 1365.

In 1833 the Director of the Josephinum was a doctor originating from Banat, Ferdinand Zimmermann (1775-1854), Professor and Academician who had practised as a surgeon in Vienna, Budapest, Zemum and Belgrade. In 1798 he had been in the "Rheinarmee".[5]

The Military Hospital at Timişoara, where the first ether anaesthetic was given, still exists. Built in 1766, it was enlarged with further floors during and after the Napoleonic wars in 1817-1818, having then 350 beds. It is possible that at that time the operating rooms were put on the first floor. In 1855 a warm air heating system was installed which was designed by a doctor born in Medias, Paul Traugot Meissner (1778-1865).

This splendid building has now been in continuous use for more than 230 years and is older than Massachusetts General Hospital (of 1821) with which it is often compared. It is a square structure with three interior courtyards and was once close to a Vauban-style fort which no longer exists; the ground floors have massive bomb-resistant walls. The Army hospital served as the medical faculty of the university temporarily to 1914, and later was concerned with the rise in importance of the University of Medicine of Timişoara. This recently celebrated its half century as the fourth University Medical School in România and the only one to have been founded during the 20th century. Many well-known Romanian people have been treated there - Ana Aslan, I. Făgărăşanu, H. Aubert etc. CT scanning became available in 1992. Few cities in Europe had three hospitals permanently active during the 19th century like Timişoara.

M. Musil's grandson, Robert von Musil, (1880-1942) became an important Austrian writer. Born in Klagenfurt and undergoing military training in Eisenstadt, he studied at Mährisch-Weisskirchen (today`s Hranice, Cehia) and like his father, became an engineer and mathematician and then an author whose works were translated into Romanian. His first book Peregrinations of pupil Törless was inspired by the atmosphere of the military school but his main work "Der Mann ohne Eigenschaften" was about Berlin in 1930-1933, the last part appearing during his voluntary exile in Vienna which continued until his death in Geneva. The book describes the fall of the Danube Empire (Karl Dinklage, Robert Musil, Leben Werk, Wirkung, Amathea Verlag 1960)[7]

The grandson must have known something of his grandfather`s activities in Timişoara because in his book we find a passage: „... while the artistic spirit should be admired as Goethe, Michelangelo and Luther are today, we barely know the name of one who gave society the blessing of anaesthesia; no-one does research into the lives of Gauss, Euler or Maxwell (after a certain Mrs. Stein) and too few are interested in where Lavoisier and Cardanus died ...".

What Timişoara would like is a portrait of Siehs and a drawing of the apparatus described in the Locales article, but this is going to be difficult when a century and a half has elapsed since the event.

The anaesthesiologists of Timişoara have organised a symposium on the history of Romanian anaesthesia for 1 March 1997 as a celebration of the first administration of ether by the Army doctors, Mathias Musil and Joseph Siehs. On this sesquicentenary, a commemorative plaque will be unveiled in honour of our great predecessors..

As a footnote, it is interesting to see how ether came to the Danube principalities:

– Iaşi (Iassi) - no date, ether administration by Dr. Ludovic Laurentiu Russ (1816-1889). See "Albina Românescâ" nr. 12

of 9 February 1847 pp 54-6; also G. Barbu 1967, C. Arseni, H. Aldea 1988
- Bucaresti - 21 February 1847 by Demetrius P. Wartiadis (1807-1862) and Johan Franz Traugot Rissdörfer (1809-1849) for a leg amputation published in "Vestitorul Românesc" nr. 19, 8 March 1848 p 76. See also Bercuş Cl. 1981 Barbu G. 1967.
- Târgu-Mureş - Army Hospital, ether administerd by Johann Rummel, Militärarzt 22 February 1847
- Cluj/Klausenburg/Kolosvar - ether administered by Dr. Bogdán Abraham Pattantyús (1817-1865) and Simon Vélics at Carolina Hospital, published in "Termeszetbarát" nr. 33, 11 March 1847, p587 ("Aethereli kisérlet és jeszánalku kérelem")(see also Bologa V. 1955)
- Brasov/Kronstadt - also an ether anaesthetic by Kraft but no date; see also Bologa V. 1955

References:

[1] Breier T: Din istoricul starii de sanatate a populatiei timisorene (secolul al XIX-lea) Timişoara Medicala nr. 4, Tomul XXX, 1985, p. 55-58

[2] Ghişoiu S: Prima aestezie cu eter la Timişoara (5 februarie 1847). Timişoara Medicală nr. 4, Tomul XXXII, 1987, p.95-99

[3] Snow J: On Narcotism by Inhalation of Vapours. A Facsilime Edition with an Introductory Essay by Richard H. Ellis. Royal Society of Medicine Services Limited, 1991

[4] Szinnyey J (ed): Magyar Irok Elete es Munkai Budapest 1903-1914, I-XXVI vol. (Vol. XII, p. 980)

[5] Petri AP: Heilwasser im Banat. Th. Brelt, 1988

[6] Reuter HH, Reuter MA : Philipp Bozzini and Endoscopy in the 19 the Century. Max Nitze Museum, Stuttgart 1988

[7] Berghahn W: "Robert Musil". Rowohlt Taschenbuch-Verlag GmbH, Reinbeck-Hamburg, 1988

Introduction of Ether Anesthesia into Japan

A. Matsuki
Department of Anesthesiology
University of Hiosaki School of Medicine, Hirosaki, Japan

Introduction

During the Edo period (1603-1867) Dejima of Nagasaki was the only door to Japan available to western counties. This artificial island of Nagasaki was used almost exclusively by Dutch traders and so it is not surprising that through this portal there was a rapid influx of information, including medical science. Among conveyed information, there was a news concerning the publication of Dutch text book on ether anesthesia published in 1847. The Tokugawa shogunate asked Dutch traders to import it to Japan. On request of the shogunate they brought six copies of the text book written in Dutch, but the exact date when they came to Japan unclear but possibly by the summer of 1849.

Investigation of the copies imported

A most distinguisthel Japanese physician in this period was Seikei Sugita. He mastered not only Dutch but German and Latin. His linguistic ability inherited from his grand

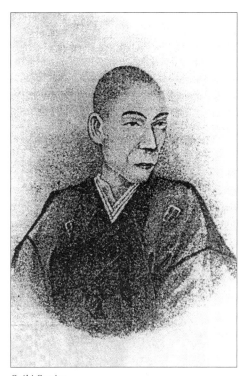

Seiki Sugita

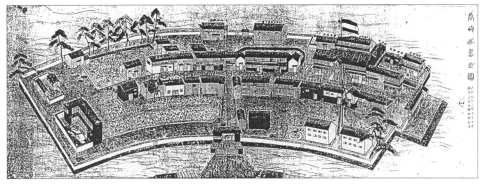

Dejima of Nagasaki

father Genpaku Sugita (1733-1817) who had translated into Japanese J. Adam Kulmus' Dutch text book of anatomy. S. Sugita was asked by the shogunate to translate the Dutch text book on ether anesthesia, which reached Japan at least by the summer of 1849. He finished his translation to publish it in 1850 as entitled "A ether Kyuho shisetsu" (A treatise of ether inhalation). It included in the second volume of his "Saisei bikou (Notes on medical Science)". This was the Japanese translation of Sarluis' book on ether anesthesia and the first monograph on anesthesia in Japan. Sarluis' book was Dutch translation of Schlesinger's text book in German. All six copies has been preserved in the National Diet Library in Tokyo.

In 1855, five years after S. Sugita published his Japanese translation, he succeeded in giving ether anesthesia to a patient with breast cancer and a burn patient, However, detailed records about these patients remain unclear. He must have used imported ether from Holland by the Dutch traders for these patients, because ether was not yet produced in Japan at that time.

Conclusion

Dutch edition of Schlesinger's German text book published in 1847 was brought to Japan in about 1849 and this is the earliest information on ether anesthesia in Japan. The book was translated by Seikei Sugita into Japanese in 1850 to be published. Thereafter ether anesthesia prevailed widely in Japan, but it was gradually replaced by chloroform anesthesia in the next twenty years.

Acknowledgement

Erdmann W: Professor and Chairman, Department of Anaesthesiology, Erasmus University

Goerig M: Department of Anaesthesiology, University of Hamburg, School of Medicine

McIntyre JWR: Emeritus professor, Department of Anaesthesiology, University of Albert Faculty of Medicine

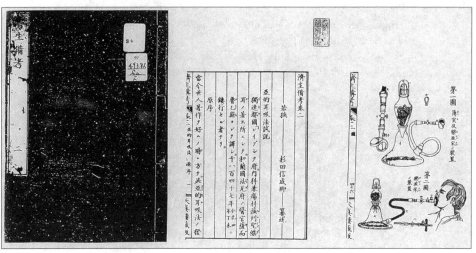

Sugita's Japanese translation included in "Saiseibiko" vol. 2 published in 1850. The cover, first page and Figure 1 and 2.

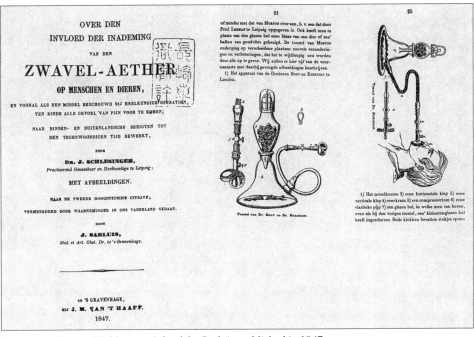

Dutch translation of Schlesinger's book by Sarluis, published in 1847.

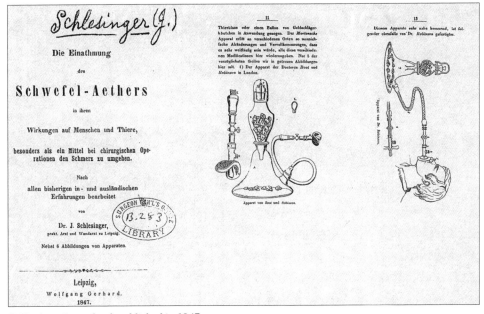

Schlesinger's text book published in 1847.

Priority to Whom?
Who was the First to Apply Ether by Inhalation?

H. Petermann
Department of Anaesthesiology, University Erlangen-Nuremberg, Germany

Summary

According to the discussion in 1847 a lot of people claim to have been the first one in using sulphuric ether for 'operations without pain'. Relating to their arguments there can not be a sole discoverer or inventor of the great benefit insensibility during surgical operations.

It all began around 1800 involving a lot of people and resulted in the first public demonstration on October 16th, 1846, in Boston, Massachusetts, which we owe to Dr. Jackson and Dr. Morton. In this article I would like to introduce known and unknown persons who have applied sulphuric ether.

Beginnings in the 16th Century

The first person to describe the distillation and application of ether was Valerius Cordus (1515-1544). His book "Remarks to the Materia medica of P. Diskurides", was published after his death in 1561. The effects of „suesses Vitriol", how sulphuric ether was named because of its smell, were reported by his contemporary Paracelsus (1493-1541). *Sulphuric ether is associated which such a sweetness that it is taken by chickens and they fall asleep from it for a while but awaken later without harm*[1, p.266]. The pharmacist Buchner wrote in 1847 that ether had been known for its properties reducing sensitivity, relieving pain and inducing sleep for more than 100 years. Because of its characteristic Anodynia (pain reliever) it was recommended by Friedrich Hoffmann (1660-1742). Like most of the other drugs it was given orally. In the 18th century it was known that the inhalation of ether induces sleep, relieves pain and lowers heart rate. This knowledge was not common in the 17th and 18th century, so around 1800 sulphuric ether was introduced to clinical practice again.

Pneumatic Researches

In 1772/74 Joseph Priestley (1733-1804) and Carl Wilhelm Scheele (1742-1786) discovered oxygen and soon started investigations on therapeutic use of gases. Humphry Davy (1778-1829) worked at the pneumatic institute of Thomas Beddoes (1760-1808) and stated: *An immense mass of pneumatological, chemical, and medical information must be collected, before we shall be able to operate with certainty on the human constitution. Pneumatic chemistry, in its application to medicine, is an art in infancy, weak, almost useless, but apparently possessed of capabilities of improvement. To be rendered strong and mature, she must be nourished by facts, strengthened by exercise, and cautiously directed in the application of her powers, by external skepticism*[2, p.447]. He described the effects of nitrous oxide, that was the subject of his research, as follows: *As nitrous oxide in its extensive operation appears capable of destroying physical pain, it may probably be used with advantage during surgical operations in which no great effusion of blood takes place*[3, p.556]. This book was already translated into German in 1812/14. Henry Hickman (1800-1830) conducted further experiments on nitrous oxide with similar results.

Around 1800 – "Nitrous Oxide and Ether Frolics"

Thos. Lee titled his short article "The Sedative Effects of Vaporous Ether Recognized Forty Years Since" describing that he had observed the inhaling of ether by Dr. Graham in Bristol in a drug shop[2, p.164]. Michael Faraday (1791-1867), co-worker of H. Davy described the sedative effect of sulfuric ether in 1818: *When the vapor of ether mixed with common air is inhaled, it produces effects very similar to those occasioned by nitrous oxide. ... By the imprudent inspiration of ether, a gentleman was thrown into a very lethargic state, which continued with occasional periods of intermission for more than thirty hours ...*[4, p.476]. A thesis was written "On ether inhalation", in Philadelphia in 1824 by Matthew B. Caleb. This essay was cited by B. Schuchardt (?) 1898[5]. Unfortunately we do not have any details except the title (Fig. 1).

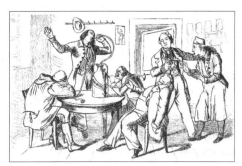

Fig. 1 Illustration of German students geltring high during an ether frolic, around 1847

On March 30th, 1842, William Crawford Long (1815-1878) performed an operation on two small tumors on the nape of the neck of James Venable. He did not publish his results until 1849 and therefore did not have any influence on the invention of ether for surgical operations. He wrote: *I was anxious, before making my publication, to try etherization in a sufficient number of cases to fully satisfy my mind that anesthesia was produced by ether, and that it was not the effect of imagination or owed to any peculiar insusceptibility to pain in the person experimented on*[8].

Horace Wells (1815-1848) claimed to have been the first person who applied ether, because he had performed tests with sulfuric ether in Boston in December 1845 and reported this to Dr. Morton and Dr. Jackson. He mentioned this fact in a letter to the Académie de Médecine de Paris.

First Publication on October 16th, 1846

On November 9th, 1846, Dr. Henry J. Bigelow (1818-1890) gave a lecture to the Boston Society of Medical Improvement, that was published in the Boston Medical and Surgical Journal 35 (1846), (p. 309-317): *It has long been an important problem in medical science to devise some method of mitigating the pain of surgical operations. An efficient agent for this purpose has at length been discovered. ... On the 16th of October, 1846, an operation was performed at the hospital upon a patient who had inhaled a preparation administered by Dr. Morton, a dentist of this city, with the alleged intention of producing insensibility to pain. Dr. Morton was understood to have extracted teeth under similar circumstances, without knowledge of the patient. The present operation was performed by Dr. Warren ...*[1, p.286].

U.S. Patent No. 4848

In order to make money with their invention Dr. Morton and Dr. Jackson applied for a patent on "Letheon" as they called the substance.

IMPROVEMENT IN SURGICAL OPERATIONS

Specification forming part of Letter Patent No. 4848, dated November 12, 1846. Be it known that we, Charles T. Jackson and William T.G. Morton, of Boston ... have invented or discovered a new and useful improvement in Surgical Operations on Animals, whereby we are enabled to accomplish many, if not all operations, such as are usually attended with more or less pain and suffering, without any or with very little pain to or muscular action of person who undergo the same; and we do hereby declare that the following is a full and exact description of our said invention or discovery[8, p.552].

At the end of the text of the patent it is said: *What we claim as our invention is - The herinbefore described means by which we are enabled to effect the above highly important improvement in surgical operations - viz., by combining therewith the application of ether or the vapor thereof - substantially as above specified*[8, p.554]. Morton and Jackson did not mention the drug they used, ether is named as a drug that may also be used.

Discussion about Priority in The Lancet

Note in the Lancet on December 26th, 1846: *The means used is believed to be the inhalation of the vapour of sulphuric ether for two or three minutes, which, it is stated, produces insensibility for about an equal length of time.* "This information was given on a paper by Dr. Bigelow, read before one of the medical societies.

Dr. Morton's and Dr. Jackson's patent for "The Letheon" was point of discussion in The Lancet. R.H. Collyer gave the following answer to the editor in January 1847: *Years since, I gave the process of inhalation to produce unconsciousness to the world ... The process of inhalation to produce unconsciousness, so that all kinds of surgical operations might be performed without pain to the patient, I have publicly advocated since 1842, and published in 1843.* In a note to the editor the author of this note was regarded as a jump-up-behinder, because he has given no further information on his statement[2, p.163].

Future issues of the Lancet still dealt with the question, who had been real inventor of the application of ether on surgical operations. In March Dr. Henry Bennet published the information that Dr. Horace Wells from Connecticut was the first one using ether for medical applications for the first time. *I would draw the attention of your readers to the important fact, (testified by Dr. Marcy from New York), that Mr. Wells had resorted to the use of nitrous oxide and sulphuric ether to produce insensibility during operations, as far back as October 1844, and, that is was only several months subsequently that he himself communicated the results which he had obtained to Drs. Jackson and Morton, results which Dr. Jackson then treated with incredulity"*[2, p.265]. Even articles from the "Boston Medical and Surgical Journal" and "Galignani's Messenger, Paris" were cited, that name Dr. Horace Wells of Hartford, Connecticut, to be the one discovering the effects of sulphuric ether.

In the further discussion both parties, Dr. Wells and Dr. Jackson and Dr. Morton, had witnesses gaving the benefit of the discovery of ether to one party or the other. *The discovery of this method has been boldly claimed by Dr. Jackson and Morton: and to them must certainly be accorded the chief merit of bringing it into use. No sooner was the discovery announced, that Dr. Collyer claimed priority of invention, without, however, adducing those proofs which could alone substantiate his pretensions. Still another aspirant Mr. Horace Wells appears in the field, with apparently better-founded claims. History will, in due course, assign to each his just award citing*[2, p.447], so the words of Robert Barnes. In order to strenghten his position Dr. Horace Wells gave a pamphlet to the editor of The Lancet, in which nearly thirty people testified him having performed extraction of teeth without any pain on several patients[2, p.471-474]. This was followed by a public letter, that admissions were conclusive and fatal to the pretensions of Mr. Horace Wells[2, p.547]. With a letter of W.T.G. Morton the discussion in the Lancet came to an end.

Besides all discussion about 'who can claim priority' no one can avoid his destiny.

Horace Wells committed suicide in drunkenness from ether, William T.G. Morton died pretty poor having become a drunkard, Charles T. Jackson was hopelessly bereft of reason. Only William C. Long lived a long and easy life. As. A.B. Gould puts it: *It appears that if Jackson and Morton had not patented the discovery and had accepted the decision of the French Academy of Arts and Sciences, both would have become wealthy and famous as the men who gave pain-free surgery to mankind.*[6, p.387].

Priority in German speaking Countries

The news about operations without pain was first published in the "Deutsche Allgemeine Zeitung" on January 1st, 1847, and on January 10th, 1847, in the "Allgemeine Zeitung, Augsburg". Very soon physicians started utilizing ether, e.g. in Erlangen according to an order by the Ministry for Internal Affairs of January 19th, 1847. The first operations were performed in Berne on the 23rd, in Erlangen and Leipzig on the 24th, in Munich and Tübingen on the 25th, in Vienna on the 28th of January and in Würzburg on the 3rd of February. So the merit of being the first German doctor using sulfuric ether can not be given to one person only because of the fact there are a few days in between the various tests. Aloys Martin (1818-1891) did a lot for spreading the knowledge.

In a review of the monograph of J. Bergson, Dr. Phil. H. Wolff wrote in 1847:

Also when I have proofed herewith that I have used the vapours of ether for inhalation and published this earlier than Jackson, I will not claim the priority instead of Jackson because I only used few ether ... so I did not recognize the effects, that make the importance of this invention, the unraising of sensibility and consciousness[7, p.307f].

Conclusions

- It has to be made a difference between the discovery of the drug and the invention of the first medical application.
- There has been knowledge about sulphuric ether ("Suesses Vitriol") in the 16. century. The effect of producing unconsciousness was only observed in experiments with animals.
- At the beginning of the 19. century sulphuric ether was used for so called "Ether Frolics".
- Horace Wells was probably the first person using ether for painless extractions of teeth. But he did not publish any data or demonstrate this in public.
- Dr. Morton and Dr. Warren performed the first public demonstration on the effects of ether for medical applications. Without any pain a patient was operated on October 16th, 1846.
- Priority for discovering the effects of sulphuric ether and using it for clinical applications can not be given to one person alone. A lot of people have merits discovering this great benefit.
- The discussion about priority will still continue and might bring some new aspects in future.

References:

[1] Foundations of Anaesthesiology, Vol 1
[2] The Lancet. London. 1847; Vol 2
[3] Davy H: Researches, Chemical and Philosophical; Chiefly Concerning Nitrous Oxide or Dephlogisticated Nitrous Air and its Respiration. London 1800
[4] Pharmaceutical Journals and Transactions. 1847; Vol 6-7
[5] Janus: 1898; Vol.3 : p 55
[6] Anaesthesia. Essays on its History. Springer, Berlin 1985
[7] Allgemeine Medicinische Central-Zeitung. 1847; Vol 16 : p.307f
[8] Duncum B: The Development of Inhalation Anaesthesia. Oxford University Press. London 1947

The first Day of Chloroform Anesthesia in Spain

J.C. Diz, A. Franco, J. Alvarez, J. Cortés
Servicio de Anestesiología y Reanimación Hospital General de Galicia-Clínico Universitario, Spain

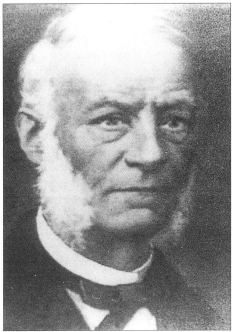

Figure 1: Prof. Antonio Casares Rodrigo (1812-1888), chairman of organic chemistry of the University of Santiago. He was the first in obtaining chloroform in Spain, and also the first in clinical experiments and self-experimentation.

Introduction

Chloroform was discovered, independently, in 1831, by Samuel Guthrie in New York, Eugène Souberain in Paris and Justus von Liebig in Germany, but until 1847 the anesthetic properties it were unknown. On March 1847, the French physiologist Flourens found that it had an anesthetic effect on animals similar to that of ether. David Waldie, a chemist from Liverpool, advised Prof. Simpson the use of chloroform in October 1847.

The discovery of chloroform anesthesia

The night of November 4th, 1847, is considered as the starting date of chloroform anesthesia. James Y. Simpson (1811-1870) and his collaborators Drs. Duncan and Keith inhaled chloroform after dinner, in his house of 32 Queen St. in Edinburgh. They reached a certain state of drunkenness and insensibility, during which they even missed the elemental rules of etiquette. In the following days, Simpson administered chloroform to his patients, and on November 10th he read a paper to the Medico-Chirurgical Society of Edinburgh. On November 20th, chloroform was used as anesthetic in several operations in St. Bartholomew's Hospital of London. From that experiences, the news of chloroform anesthesia spread quickly throughout the world, and the daily press played a very important role in the propagation of the news (1-3).

The introduction of chloroform anesthesia in Spain

At the end of November 1847, several medical journals of Barcelona (4) and Cadiz (5), and some daily and political newspapers of Barcelona published the first news of the discovery. In Madrid the news were published a few days later (6). In the meantime, more news about the discovery arrived to Santiago, probably at the

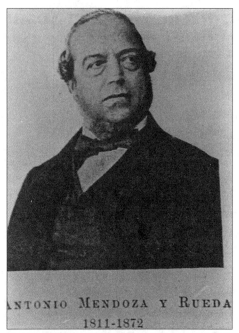

Figure 2: Prof. Antonio Mendoza Rueda (1811-1872), professor of surgery in Barcelona. He was one of the pioneers in Spain of ether and chloroform anesthesia.

end of November or in the first days of December. We know certainly that on December 4th, a surgeon of the School of Medicine of Santiago, Prof. Vicente Guarnerio, had read in the Journal des Debats from Paris news about the experiments made in London on November 20 th (7).

First experiments in laboratory

In Santiago de Compostela, Prof. Antonio Casares Rodrigo (Fig.1), chairman of chemistry of this University, prepared a little amount of chloroform on December 5th. In the following days he continued his experiments, trying to get a sufficient amount of chloroform for using it as an anesthetic. He used a procedure similar to that reported by M. Soubiran to the Academy of Sciences on November 28th, although Prof. Casares did not know that report (8). There were another experiments in Barcelona, by the pharmacist Francisco Domenech, and in Madrid the pharmacist Dr. Merino could get a little quantity of chloroform on December 15th.

First experiments in animals

It the last years several authors demonstrated that the first experiments with chloroform as an anesthetic in Spain were in animals, on December 19th, 1847, in Barcelona and in Santiago (4, 9). Prof. Antonio Mendoza (Fig.2) anesthetized a dog in Barcelona (10), and also did Prof. Casares in Santiago (8), and in both experiments they could achieve quickly a state of complete insensibility in animals, making painful interventions on them (section and pulling of nerves, arterial sutures, skin pricking and so). The animals did not show any sign of pain and there were no significative alterations of vital constants. The dogs recovered completely in a few minutes in both experiments.

Self-experiments

After the experiments with a dog in Santiago, on sunday December 19th, and with several surgeons of the school of medicine as witnesses (Profs. Vicente Guarnerio, José González Olivares and Andrés Laorden), Prof. Casares inhaled chloroform during a few minutes. He got a state of drowsiness and insensibility, in which he did not feel any pain after skin pinching and puncture. He had optic and acoustic sensations, without any alteration in pulse rate or breathing, and he recovered completely in half an hour (7-8).

First clinical trials

After the laboratory studies and self-experiments of Prof. Casares in Santiago and the experiments of Francisco Domenech and the surgeon Antonio Mendoza in Barcelona (10), all of them on December 19th, on Monday 20th there were the first clinical trials with chloroform in Spain.

On Monday 20th, Dr. Antonio Mendoza in Barcelona, amputated a leg in a state of complete insensibility to Joaquina Stivill, a 38 years old patient, who had a giant sarcoma in the knee (10). The same day, in Santiago de Compostela, Drs. Vicente Guarnerio (Fig.3) and José González Olivares also tested the new anesthetic. Dr. Guarnerio made an amputation of the penis to Domingo Barreiro, a 60 years old patient, and Dr. González Olivares a mastectomy with axillary lymph node dissection to Georgina Camaño, 38 years, and a partial amputation of the penis to the soldier José Salvador (11). All these operations were made in a state of complete insensibility, something that did not happen during the first experiments with ether in Spain at the beginning of January 1847, and the surgeons were completely pleased with this new anesthetic. In Madrid and in other places of Spain there was a delay of several days to obtain and test the chloroform, using it in Madrid on December 30 (9).

First publications about chloroform

The journal Gaceta Médica (Madrid) published, on December 30th, the news about the experiments of Dr. Guarnerio in Santiago, in a paper entitled "Ensayos sobre el cloroformo" (7). This paper was reprinted in several medical journals and newspapers of Madrid, in the first days of January 1848 (6). A more detailed report of the operations of Santiago was published in Madrid in the journal Boletín de Medicina, Cirugía y Farmacia, on January 2nd, 1848. The operation made in Barcelona by Dr. Mendoza had little echo in the Spanish scientific press, and the first and sole paper that we know was published in the journal La Abeja Médica, on January 1848 (10).

More experiments with chloroform in Santiago

During the first days of January 1848, Profs. Antonio Casares and Andrés Laorden made more experiments with dogs and rabbits. They studied the endurance of the animals to increasing doses of chloroform and the possibility of resuscitation of the animals with electrical stimulation. They concluded that this was the only method available for resuscitation in certain situations of chloroform intoxication (12-13).

First reports about the potential dangers of chloroform

With the knowledge they had with the experiments in animals and the clinical application of chloroform in Santiago, the surgeons of the School of Medicine of Santiago advised about the potential dangers of chlo-

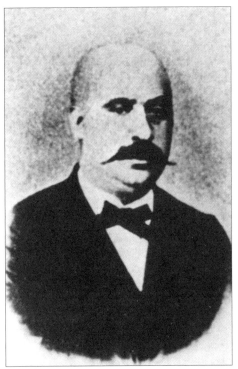

Figure 3: Prof. Vicente Guarnerio Gómez (1818-1880), professor of surgery in Santiago. He was, with Prof. González Olivares in Santiago and Prof. Mendoza in Barcelona, the first in using chloroform in patients in Spain on December 20 1847.

665

roform and anesthesia, in several papers published in Spain in the first months of 1848 (14-16).

Conclusions

We consider that the first day of chloroform anesthesia in Spain is December 20th, 1847, when in Santiago and Barcelona occurred the first clinical administrations of chloroform as an anesthetic. These clinical trials were preceded, also in Santiago and Barcelona, by experiments in animals and self-experiments. Later, and from the surgeons of Santiago, aroused the first warnings in Spain about the potential dangers of chloroform.

References:

[1] Keys TE: "Die Geschichte der chirurgischen Anaesthesie." Springer-Verlag, Berlin-New York, 1968.

[2] Armstrong-Davidson MH: "The Evolution of Anaesthesia." John Sherratt and son, Altrincham, 1965.

[3] Duncum BM: "The Development of inhalation anaesthesia." Oxford University Press, London, New York, Toronto, 1947.

[4] Hervás J: "La anestesia en Cataluña. Historia y evolución." Tesis Doctoral, Barcelona, 1986.

[5] Márquez C: "La introducción de la anestesiología en España a través de la prensa médica gaditana de la segunda mitad del siglo XIX." Tesis Doctoral, Cádiz, 1987.

[6] Franco A, Alvarez J, Cortés J: et al "Importancia de la prensa diaria y política de Madrid en el proceso de introducción y popularización de la anestesia." Rev. Esp. Anestesiol. Reanim., 1994, 41: 100-108.

[7] Guarnerio V: "Ensayos sobre el cloroformo". Gaceta Medica, 1847, 3: 282.

[8] Casares A: "Preparación del cloroformo." Bol. Med. Cir. Farm. 1848, 3: 7.

[9] Cortés J. "Contribuciones al conocimiento de la historia de la introducción de la anestesia en Madrid y Santiago de Compostela." Tesis Doctoral, Santiago, 1992.

[10] Mendoza A: "Sarcoma: amputación del muslo, inspiración del cloroformo." La Abeja Medica, 1848, 2: 11-12.

[11] González Olivares J: "Inhalaciones del cloroformo." Bol. Med. Cir. Farm. 1848, 3: 6.

[12] Casares A, Laorden A: "Experimentos con el cloroformo." Bol. Med. Cir. Farm., 1848, 3: 27-28.

[13] Laorden A: "Reflexiones sobre los efectos del cloroformo, y conveniencia de su uso, aplicaciones que de él pueden hacerse a la Medicina, y medios de contraruar sus efectos." Rev. Med. (Santiago), 1848, 1: 10-13; 2: 17-24.

[14] Baeza J: "Revista Clínica de Guarnerio." Rev. Med. (Santiago), 1848, 1: 88; 5: 142.

[15] Magaz J: "Inconvenientes graves del uso de las inhalaciones clorofórmicas: medio de evitarlas." Rev. Med. (Santiago), 1848, 1: 236-240.

[16] Pintado M: "Reseña de las contraindicaciones del cloroformo." Rev. Med. (Santiago), 1848, 1/7: 129-135.

The Search for the Holy Grail
John Harrison and the Bimetallic Strip

C. A. B. McLaren, *Ridgeway Hospital, Swindon, UK*

The search for the Holy Grail continues unabated in all walks of life. In anaesthesia one hundred and fifty years after the introduction of ether, we are still searching for the ideal inhalation anaesthetic agent.

The long evaluation of the substituted hydrocarbons resulted in the production of halothane, which at first seemed to be the answer to the requirements of the ideal agent.

The potency of the new agent required the design and construction of vaporizers which would ensure an accurate concentration and delivery of the anaesthetic vapour, throughout the range of the ambient working temperatures. In nearly all modern temperature compensated vaporizers a bimetallic strip is used to regulate the gas flow into the vaporising chamber.

When two strips of dissimilar metals are joined tightly together side by side and subjected to a change in temperature, one will expand more than the other, this produces a deflection of the strip. This movement can be used to vary the size of the entry port in the vaporising chamber, which in turn alters the volume of the carrier gas passing into the chamber. It is this change which is fundamental to the accurate working of most of the vaporizers in use today.

At this time the bimetallic strips are made of invar and brass. Invar is an iron nickel alloy which has a negligible coefficient of expansion, whilst brass has a good coefficient.

We must now go back in time more than four hundred years, to the city of Pisa, where on 15 February 1564, Galileo Galilei was born. What is the connection between him and modern anaesthesia? His claim to fame is that one of his first discoveries and investigations resulted in the development of the pendulum. His later works got him into terrible trouble with the Catholic Church and the Pope of that period (URBAN VIII), especially his paper declaring that all the previous tenets were wrong, and that the earth was not the centre of the universe, so it is of interest that his discovery was made whilst attending Sunday mass, listening to a very boring sermon.

He noted the regular periodicity of a swinging lamp. Many further experiments with the pendulum led him to suggest that the pendulum could be used to construct an accurate clock and prove the answer to one of the holy grails of the day ... an accurate method of keeping time. He did not follow up this suggestion, but fifteen years after his death, Christmas 1656, the first pendulum clock was invented.

The invention is credited to Christian Huygens (1629-1695), a Dutch scholar, who seems to have been more interested in the scientific development rather than the inherent difficulties at this time on perfecting a working machine.

As we shall see, the Holy Grail at this time was the problem of establishing longitude at sea, a follow-up of Galilei's project proposed to the Dutch States General in 1636.

From the time man first went to sea, there had been great problems in the determination of longitude, latitude gave no such problems, sun and star shots giving the answer.

However, the determination of longitude was much more difficult, many ingenious but cumbersome instruments were devised, but without much success.

The solution of this problem of maritime navigation had assumed great importance with the development of England as a maritime power, with the resulting increase in wealth and prestige.

One of the main reasons for the foundation of the Royal Observatory in 1675 was an attempt to find a solution, but 40 years later the answer was as elusive as ever.

There were so many shipwrecks with the resulting loss of life, and valuable cargo, that the Lords of the Admiralty were driven to petitioning Parliament to do something about it.

The disaster which finally broke the camel's back took place on the night of 22/23 October 1707. The War of the Spanish Succession had by this time been in progress for seven years.

Admiral Sir Cloudesley Shovell's fleet of five ships was returning from Gibraltar, which had been captured in 1704. In a thick fog, loaded with the spoils of war, four of the five ships, including the flagship HMS Association, a 90 gun, three decker, launched in 1697 were wrecked on the Gilstone rocks in the South West Approaches to the English Channel - in all more than 2000 lives were lost. The Admiral survived the wreck, only to be murdered on reaching one of the inhabited Scilly Islands.

This disaster led to the Lords of the Admiralty petitioning Parliament to do something about the problems of the accurate determination of longitude, whilst at sea, out of sight of land.

On the eighth of July 1714, Act 12, Queen Anne Chapter 15, was passed. Large financial rewards were offered for anyone devising a system for the accurate determination of longitude.

The rewards were up to £20000 (in today's currency almost a million pounds), dependent upon the accuracy of the method. The full amount for error within 30 miles, £15000 for 40 miles, and £10000 for not exceeding 60 miles, to be tested on a voyage from England to the West Indies.

During the deliberations on the Bill, Sir Isaac Newton enumerated various methods for determining longitude which had already been suggested, „true in theory but difficult to execute ...one of which is by a watch ... but by reason of the motion of the ship ... variation of heat and cold such a watch hath not yet been made" - prophetic words indeed.

The offers of such large sums of money by Parliament stimulated many ideas to win the prize, many publishing their own books on exactly why their ideas were correct.

At this time, 1714, the hero of our story, John Harrison, the eldest son of a carpenter, was 21. He was born in the West Riding of Yorkshire in March 1693, and baptised in the village church of Wragby, before the family moved to Barrow on Humber in Lincolnshire.

Even as a small boy he had been fascinated by machinery, and without any formal education or apprenticeship was already making clocks, the movements and dials of his first three clocks are still in working order.

To keep a clock accurate it is necessary to produce a pulse of accurate and constant duration, ie Galileo's pendulum theory. At this time the principal problems in respect of the accuracy of all the pendulum clocks in use were the effects of changes in temperature and the effects of friction.

Harrison, who had now been joined by his younger brother, set about trying to solve the problems. The difficulties with friction arose from the poor quality of any available lubricating oils at this time. As a result the early Harrison clock movements were in the main of wooden construction, metals likely to rust were avoided, if necessary brass was used.

The parts requiring lubrication were made from lignum vitae, a tropical hardwood which exudes its own grease.

He noted that in all pendulum clocks there were large swings in accuracy depending upon the ambient temperature. In 1730 he comments „but there is no wire of any metal whatever, whereof to make a pendulum, but what it is continually altering its length according to ye degrees of heat or cold; this I discovered two years ago". Clocks running to time in the winter will lose a little in summer and vice versa. „And to correct this altering of ye Length of ye Pendulum, I compose it of nine wires, viz 5 of steel and 4 of brass", and so in 1730 first bimetallic strip was described. Astonishingly, the new pendulum was accurate to within one second in a hundred days.

Harrison and his brother had by this time heard of the prize to be awarded for the discovery of a method to determine accurately longitude at sea.

They produced a series of clocks H1 H2 H3 which were transported in turn to London and their accuracy demonstrated.

In 1736, the first sea trial was made, but as the clock was four feet square, and weighed 30kg, even though it proved accurate, Harrison elected to make a smaller clock with other improvements - this took a further 22 years to construct, H4 being unveiled in 1760.

Eventually H4 was produced and performed excellently when taken by Harrison's son, William, to the West Indies. By a quirk of fate the beer, the staple fluid for the sailors of the time, had been contaminated. It was therefore necessary to put into Madeira for provisions. Using the H4, William was able to predict that really they were 100 miles nearer to land than judged by the navigations officer - much joy all round. The voyage to Jamaica was equally successful.

The Board of Longitude, however, were not so enthusiastic, and once again moved the goal posts, although they did award Harrison £7500, instead of the full amount. The wrangling went on despite further successful trials. Harrison, by this time 79 years old, petitioned George III on 31 January 1772.

The King is alleged to have remarked "these people have been cruelly wronged", and then exclaimed, "By God Harrison, I will see you righted". It took another eighteen months, 21 June 1773, before Act 13 George III Chapter 77 duly received the Royal Assent and Harrison was awarded the sum of £8750.

In addition to all the other sums previously received from the Board of Longitude, the final sum came to more than £20000. At last John Harrison had won the great longitude prize despite considerable opposition.

Within three years, 24 March 1776, Harrison died on his 83rd birthday. Thus, just over three hundred years ago, one Holy Grail was finalised. However, even with the use of the bimetallic strip, now made of Invar (36% nickel and 64% iron) and brass (63% copper and 37% zinc), we are still looking for our Holy Grail.

Where have all the Bellows Gone?
Ten manual Respiratory Devices reviewed

K. P. Kötter[1], W. H. Maleck[2], G. A. Petroianu[3]

[1] Department of Neurological Intensive Care Unit, Leopoldina-Hospital, Schweinfurt, Germany
[2] Department of Anesthesiology, Klinikum Ludwigshafen, Germany
[3] Department of Pharmacology, University of Heidelberg at Mannheim, Mannheim, Germany

Introduction:

Baker cited Galen having used bellows to inflate lungs of a dead animal in the second century, and that Paracelsus possibly tried bellows on a "dead subject" without success.[1] Bellows must have been invented before 1667, i.e. the first description of ventilation of dogs with bellows by Hooke[2]. In 1744 Fothergill gave a lecture on artificial ventilation. He discussed the use of bellows, but considered mouth-to-mouth ventilation to be superior[3]. In 1776 the experiments on artificial ventilation of dogs with bellows were repeated by Hunter.[4,5] In 1827 Leroy described a pair of "safety" bellows (soufflet calibré) with adjustable tidal volumes (according to age)[5-7] (Fig. 1).

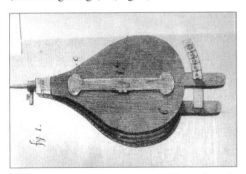

Fig.1: The bellows of Leroy in 1827, graduated for age (4, 6, 10, 16, and 20 years).[5] Reproduced according the 170 year old original.

The resuscitation set of the Royal Humane Society in 1829 included a pair of bellows, too[7]. The Fell-O'Dwyer bellows of the late 19th century allowed successful long-time-ventilation for over 24 hours in patients with opioid intoxications and head trauma[5,8,9,10]. A modification by Matas favors an adjustable tidal volume between 0 and 700 cm^3 and airway pressure monitoring[11]. In 1943 Kreiselman invented a ventilator with 1,6 l bellows and a non-rebreathing valve, a 27 mbar pressure relief valve and oxygen inlet[12]. The "Oxford inflating bellows" were described by Macintosh and Mushin in 1953[13,14]. Dönhardt described the Dräger Resutator in 1955, which was included in our experiment (Fig. 2)[15].

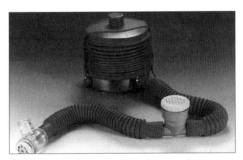

Fig.2: Dräger Resutator 63 (historical) Photo property of the authors.

Lucas et al. described a 3 l bellows with a non-rebreathing valve and a 30 mbar audible pressure relief valve in 1958.[16,17] The first self-expanding bag ventilator with a volume of 1,3 l and a non-rebreathing valve (precursor of the Ambu bag) was described by Ruben 1957[18,19]. As early as June 1957 this Ruben-bag was part of a resuscitation set commercially available in Germany[20]. Simple balls without any valve for ventilation of newborns were described as early as in the 19th century[10]. In the sixties the bags/balls superseded the bellows. The rationale remains unclear, but one reason might be an inferior quality of many bellows at that time[21]. The Dräger Company, Germany, stopped the production of bellows for manual ventilation in 1972[22,23]. In 1988 Frimberger reinvented graduated bellows with a 50 mbar pressure relief valve, oxygen inlet, and adjustable tidal volumes[24,25]. This device was introduced (Kendall Cardiovent) in 1994 and has been sold in Germany since 1996 (Fig. 3).

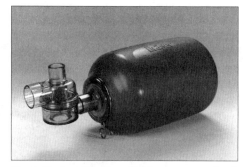

Fig.4: *Dräger Resutator 2000 as an example of a ball ventilator.*
Photo property of the authors.

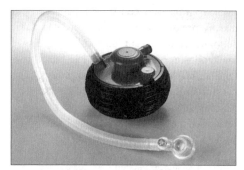

Fig.3: *Kendall Cardiovent (1994 prototype, slightly different from 1997 model)*
Photo property of the authors.

Methods

We compared the Kendall Cardiovent to two other bellows (historical Dräger Resutator 63; Tagg Breathsaver) and seven bags/balls (Ambu Mark 3; Ambu Silicon; Laerdal Resu; Dräger Resutator 2000 (Fig. 4); Aerodyne Hope 4; Mercury; Weinmann Combibag). Twelve paramedics carried out mask ventilation for two minutes with each device on a Laerdal Recording Anne lying on the floor (using the FATS-technique[26,27] and in a bed, trying to achieve a tidal volume of 800-1200 ml as recommended by the AHA [28,29]. The participants scored handling of the devices on a 6-point-scale (1 = very good, 6 = insufficient).

Discussion

The Kendall Cardiovent allowed an exact ventilation comparable to the best bag or ball devices. Its handling was also comparable to the best bag or ball devices. Even the historical Dräger Resutator 63, manufactured until 1972, compared on floor favourably with the most bag/ball ventilators. It should be noted that this device had been stored for many years and was used for the study without special preparation.

Conclusion

The principle of the graduated bellows as realized in the Kendall Cardiovent is promising. It is not clear why the bellows ventilators disappeared in the 1960's and 1970's.

Results	TV on floor (l)			TV in bed (l)			Score
	<.8	.8-1.2	>1.2	<.8	.8-1.2	>1.2	Mean
Ambu Mark 3	2%	94%	4%	50%	50%	0%	1.7
Ambu Silicon	2%	58%	40%	16%	84%	0%	2.8
Laerdal Resu	4%	63%	33%	28%	71%	1%	2.5
Dräger Resutator 2000	3%	70%	27%	35%	65%	0%	3.4
Aerodyne Hope 4	5%	77%	18%	39%	60%	1%	4.6
Mercury	10%	52%	38%	32%	68%	0%	3.4
Weinmann Combibag	34%	66%	0%	92%	8%	0%	4.6
Kendall Cardiovent	3%	95%	2%	22%	78%	0%	1.8
Dräger Resutator 63	9%	91%	0%	38%	62%	0%	3.4
Tagg Breathsaver	25%	75%	0%	52%	48%	0%	4.9

References:

[1] Baker AB: Artificial respiration, the history of an idea. Medical History 1971; 15:336-351

[2] Hooke R: An Account of an experiment made by M. Hook[e], of preserving animals Alive by blowing through their lungs with bellows. In: Falconer A, Keys TE, Foundations of Anesthesiology, Vol.1, Wood Library-Museum of Anesthesiology, Parkridge 1993, p. 13-14

[3] Fothergill J: Observation on a case published in the last volume of the medical essays, of recovering a man dead in appearance, by distending the lungs with air. Philosophical Transactions of the Royal Society of London 1744/45; 43:275-281

[4] Hunter J: Proposals for the recovery of people apparently drowned. Philosophical Transactions of the Royal Society of London 1776; 66:412-425

[5] Klippe HJ, Löhr J, Kroeger C: Historische Aspekte zur Entwicklung der endotrachealen Intubation. Praxis der Pneumologie 1981; 35:413-420

[6] Leroy J: Recherches sur l'asphyxie. Journal de la Physiologie expérimentale et pathologique 1827; 7:45-65

[7] McLellan I: Nineteenth century resuscitation apparatus. Anaesthesia 1981;36:307-311

[8] Dobell ARC: The origins of endotracheal ventilation. Annals of Thoracic Surgery 1994; 58:578-584

[9] Matas R: On the management of acute traumatic pneumothorax. Annals of Surgery 1899; 29:409-434

[10] Matas R: Intralaryngeal insufflation for the relief of acute surgical pneumothorax. JAMA 1900; 34:1371-1375 and 1468-1473

[11] Matas R: Artificial respiration by direct intralaryngeal intubation with a modified O'Dwyer tube and a new graduated air-pump, in its applications to medical and surgical practice. American Medicine 1902; 3:97-103

[12] Kreiselman J: A new resuscitation apparatus. Anesthesiology 1943; 4:608-611

[13] Macintosh RR: Oxford inflating bellows. Br Med J 1953;ii:202

[14] Mushin WW: Cardiff Inflating Valve. British Medical Journal 1953; ii:202

[15] Dönhardt A: Zur Indikation der künstlichen Beatmung: Tracheotomiebeatmung oder Eiserne Lunge. Anaesthesist 1957; 6:31-33

[16] Lucas BGB, Whitcher TD: Artificial respiration: Comparison between manual and intermittent positive-pressure methods. Br Med J 1958; ii:887-889

[17] Lucas BGB, Trotman CG, Whitcher TD: A hand-operated resuscitator. Br Med J 1959; i:1165-1166

[18] Ruben H, Ruben A: Apparatus for resuscitation and suction. Lancet 1957; ii:373-374

[19] Ruben H: Self-Contained Resuscitation Equipment. Canadian Medical Association Journal 1959; 80:44-45

[20] Loennecken SJ: Ein Notfallsbesteck zur Atmungs- und Kreislauf-Wiederbelebung für dringliche ärztliche Hilfe an Ort und Stelle. Anaesthesist 1958; 7:275-278

[21] Anonymous (ECRI): Evaluation: Manually operated resuscitators. Health Devices 1971; 1:13-17

[22] Anonymous (Drägerwerk, Medizintechnik): Balg-Resutator 63. Gerät zur manuellen künstlichen Beatmung. Gebrauchsanweisung. 5th Edition, July 1972.

[23] Busch (Drägerwerk, Geräte-Archiv): Personal communication, November 1994.

[24] Frimberger E, Claasen M: Gerät zur Einmann-Reanimation. Dtsch Med Wochenschr 1988; 113:1761-1763

[25] Frimberger E: A new device for ventilation and cardio-pulmonary resuscitation (CPR). Second PECEMS, Abano Terme 1994, Book of Abstracts p. 9

[26] Cummins RO, Austin D, Graves JR, Litwin PE, Pierce J: Ventilation skills of emergency medical technicians: A teaching challenge for emergency medicine. Annals of Emergency Medicine 1986; 15:1187-1192

[27] Barnes TA: Emergency ventilation techniques and related equipment. Respiratory Care 1992; 37:673-694

[28] American Heart Association: Guidelines for cardiopulmonary resuscitation and emergency cardiac care. Part II: Adult basic life support. JAMA 1992; 268:2187

[29] American Heart Association: Guidelines for cardiopulmonary resuscitation and emergency cardiac care. Part III: Adult advanced cardiac life support. JAMA 1992; 268:2200

The Oesophageal Detector Device (ODD)

W. H. Maleck[2], G. A. Petroianu[3], K. P. Kötter[1],

[1] Department of Neurological Intensive Care Unit, Leopoldina-Hospital, Schweinfurt, Germany
[2] Department of Anesthesiology, Klinikum Ludwigshafen, Germany
[3] Department of Pharmacology, University of Heidelberg at Mannheim, Mannheim, Germany

As early as 1956 oesophageal intubation was recognized to be a possible cause of mortality resulting from anaesthesia[1]. This report, studying 1000 deaths associated with anaesthesia occurring in the United Kingdom between 1950 and 1955, revealed at least one, but less than 16 deaths by oesophageal intubation (exact number not given) out of 589 deaths attributed to anaesthesia. In contrast, there were 110 deaths from regurgitation. No recommendations for detection of oesophageal intubation were given.

In 1979 a review on anaesthetic accidents forwarded between 1970 and 1977 to the Medical Defence Union of the United Kingdom found unrecognized oesophageal intubation as the cause of 37 out of 277 cases of death and 13 out of 71 cases of brain damage, making it the most common cause[2]. Opposed to this, acid aspiration was responsible for 22 deaths only. The authors recommended not to rely on movements of the reservoir bag and the chest and suggested "When in doubt, take it out".

Clearly, the general acceptance of tracheal intubation and paralytic agents lead to a decline in the percentage of deaths caused by aspiration and a definite increase in the percentage of deaths because of oesophageal intubation in the 1970's when compared to the 1950's.

Until the 1970's most anaesthesiologists assumed clinical signs prove the correct position of the tracheal tube. A 1973 report on a death caused by oesophageal intubation stated that death could have been avoided by adherence to a 5-point checklist (preoxygenation - cord visualization - epigastric auscultation - thoracic auscultation - auscultation of expiratory breathing tube)[3].

Another report on a death from unrecognized esophageal intubation published in 1978 stated that abnormal sounds accompanying respiration had been heard by the assisting nurse. This was not taken seriously by the physician in charge until death ensued. Subsequently he was sentenced to 5 years in prison in absentia[4].

In 1980, however, two groups from the UK and Australia described five cases of

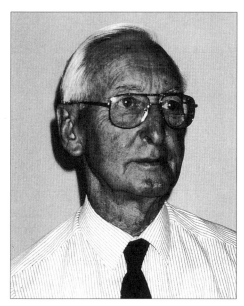

B. J. Pollard, proposed aspiration of air for control of tube position in 1980. With kind permission of B. J. Pollard.

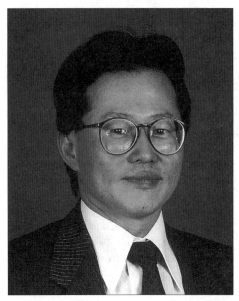

M. Y. K. Wee, reinvented and named the ODD in 1988. With kind permission of M. Y. K. Wee.

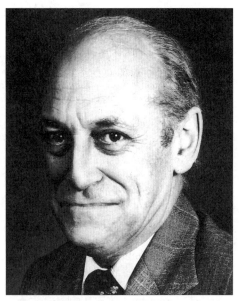

J. F. Nunn, proposed the bulb type ODD in 1988. With kind permission of J. F. Nunn.

oesophageal intubation with normal clinical signs leading to delayed recognition and two cases of brain damage[5,6]. The message that clinical signs were unreliable was not accepted easily: "There was difficulty having this article published ... because its conclusions, directly opposing the conventional understanding, were suspicious."[7].

Pollard and Junius, the authors of one of these reports, developed a "Test to verify accurate placement of an endotracheal tube". This was presented as a poster at the 7th World Congress of Anaesthesiologists in 1980 in Hamburg. They proposed aspiration of air from the tube immediately after intubation with a 20 ml syringe and stated that "Air is easily aspirated when the tube is located in the trachea but none when it is in the oesophagus".[8] Beside the presentation in Hamburg, the lecture was also given at 3 major hospitals in the United States of America, Canada, and the United Kingdom. The audience was sceptic in spite of a recent death from oesophageal intubation at one of these hospitals[7].

In 1985 Wee carried out experiments on devices to detect oesophageal intubation by means of pH differences between the oesophagus and the lungs. He noticed that when suction was applied to the oesophagus there was a large negative pressure, as compared to the trachea. Sometime in 1986 he rediscovered the idea of aspirating air with a 60 ml syringe from the tube[9]. He named it the Oesophageal Detector Device (ODD) and performed a study on 100 patients[10]. Later that year Pollard's group published a study using a 60 ml syringe, too[11].

In 1988, in the correspondence section of Anaesthesia, the question of priority was cleared as the first description being Pollard's and Wee being an independent reinventor[12,13]. Later modifications included the use of a bulb or a concertina instead of the syringe and the integration of an acoustic control or electronics into the ODD[14-17]. In the mid 1990's the

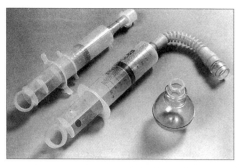

From left to right: Ambu TubeCheck-Syringe, a Self-made syringe type ODD, and Ambu Tube-Check-Bulb. Property of the authors.

ODD was believed to be the most reliable method of detection of tracheal intubation when capnometry is not available or unreliable (i.e. in CPR)[18-24]. Since 1995 ODD's are commercially available from Ambu as TubeCheck-Syringe and TubeCheck-Bulb.

From a clinical point of view the ODD is a device that fulfills its task. From a scientific point of view there are several questions that still have to be solved:

– except for two small investigations of our group, the syringe technique has never been compared to the bulb technique directly[25,26]

– with both syringe and bulb the optimum volume(s) have rarely been investigated[26,27]

– the optimum aspiration rate is unclear, since it is defined by material and design in the case of the bulb and depending on the user with the syringe,

– the question of inflation of the lungs before aspiration vs. aspiration only is not solved.

Footnote:

After finishing this paper we discovered a further case report on undetected oesophageal intubation published in the 1970's (British Medical Journal 1973;i:365-366).

Here the case of a 28-year-old nurse is reported who suffered severe brain damage with spastic quadriplegia following cardiac arrest during operation on wisdom teeth.

The anaesthetist in charge was found at court to be guilty of not having performed the necessary tests, especially not detecting the malposition of the nasally introduced tube by direct laryngoscopy (the anaesthetist claimed to have seen the tube in the correct place).

The patient was awarded 55.000 British Pounds, the highest sum up to this date ever awarded in the United Kingdom for medical malpractice.

References:

1. Edwards G, Morton HJV, Pask EA, Wylie WD: Deaths associated with anaesthesia. A report of 1000 cases. Anaesthesia 1956; 11:194-220
2. Utting JE, Gray TC, Shelley FC: Human misadventure in anaesthesia. Can Anaesth Soc J 1979; 26:472-478
3. Peterson AW, Jacker LM: Death following inadvertent esophageal intubation. Anesthesia and Analgesia 1973; 52:398-401
4. Gordh T, Mostert JW: Improper Endotracheal Intubation. International Anesthesiology Clinics 1978; 16/3:27-33
5. Pollard BJ, Junius F: Accidental Intubation of the Oesophagus. Anaesth Intens Care 1980; 8:183-186
6. Howells TH, Riethmuller RJ: Signs of endotracheal intubation. Anaesthesia 1980; 35:984-986
7. Pollard BJ: Personal communication, December 1995 and January 1996
8. Pollard BJ: A test to verify accurate placement of an endotracheal tube. In: Abstracts of the 7th World Congress of Anaesthesiologists Hamburg 1980 Excerpta Medica, International Congress Series 533, Amsterdam 1980, p. 494, Abstract 1112
9. Wee M: Personal communication, October 1995
10. Wee MYK: The oesophageal detector device. Anaesthesia 1988; 43:27-29
11. O'Leary JJ, Pollard BJ, Ryan MJ: A method of detecting oesophageal intubation or confirming tracheal intubation. Anaesth and Intens Care 1988; 16:299-301
12. Pollard B: Oesophageal detector device. Anaesthesia 1988; 43:713-714
13. Wee M: A reply. Anaesthesia 1988;43:714
14. Nunn JF: The oesophageal detector device. Anaesthesia 1988;43:804
15. Welsh BE: Yet another aid to detect oesophageal intubation. Anaesthesia 1996;51:606
16. Schafer PG, Johnson SE, Lu JK, Pace NL: Use of the esophageal intubation detector whistle for detecting esophageal or tracheal intubation. Anesthesiology 1995; 83:A222
17. Schafer PG, Matsumura KS, Lind GH, LU JK, Pace NL: The electronic esophageal detector device for detection of tracheal and esophageal intubation: does it work? Anesthesiology 1996; 85:A987
18. Clyburn P, Rosen M: Accidental oesophageal intubation. Br J Anaesth 1994;73:55-63
19. Petroianu G, Maleck W, Bergler WF, Ellinger K, Osswald PM, Rüfer R: Präklinische Kontrolle von Tubuslage und Beatmung. Anaesthesist 1995; 44:613-623
20. Benumof JL: The ASA difficult airway algorithm: New thoughts/considerations In: Annual Refresher Course Lectures, ASA, Atlanta 1995, Lecture 253
21. Salem MR, Baraka A: Confirmation of tracheal intubation. In: Benumof JL, Airway Management. Mosby, St.Louis 1996, pp. 531-560
22. Ardagh M: A review of detection techniques for oesophageal intubation. Emergency Medicine (Carlton, Victoria) 1996; 8:147-151
23. White SJ, Slovis CM: Inadvertent esophageal intubation in the field: Reliance on a fool's "Gold Standard". Academic Emergency Medicine 1997; 4:89-91
24. Clyburn PA: The detection of accidental oesophageal intubation. In: Latto IP, Vaughan RS Difficulties in Tracheal Intubation. 2nd Edition, Saunders, London 1997, pp. 231-240
25. Petroianu G, Bergler WF, Widjaja B: The "Oesophageal Detector Device" (ODD): Which one is the best? South African Society of Anaesthesiologists Annual Congress, Johannesburg 1992
26. Maleck WH, Koetter KP, Herchet J, Petroianu GA: Syringe or bulb? Three Esophageal Detector Devices in test. Journal of Emergency Medical Services 1996; 21/3:S10
27. Wafai Y, Salem MR, Czinn EA, Barbella J, Baraka A: The self-inflating bulb in detecting esophageal intubation: effect of bulb size and technique used. Anesthesiology 1993; 79:A496

Some Notes on the History of Capnometry, its Use for Detection of Oesophageal Intubation and Hand-Held Capnometers

W. Maleck[1], G. Petroianu[2], K. Kötter[3]

[1] Department of Neurological Intensive Care Unit, Leopoldina-Hospital, Schweinfurt, Germany
[2] Department of Anesthesiology, Klinikum Ludwigshafen, Germany
[3] Department of Pharmacology, University of Heidelberg at Mannheim, Mannheim, Germany

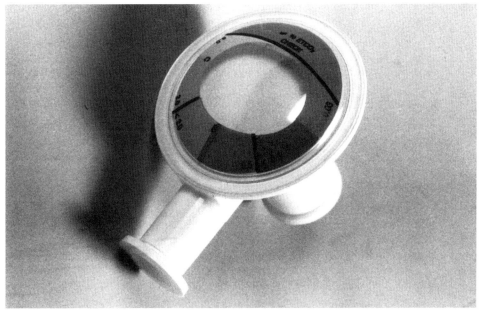

Fig. 1: FENEM FEF-detector, introduced in 1988 and now sold as Nellcor EASYCAP.

It might be assumed that capnometry is a very recent technique. When the main author of this article started to work at the Klinikum Ludwigshafen (a 1,000 bed teaching hospital) in 1992, only a few of the operating theatres and none of the induction rooms had the capnometry monitor devices available. It was not before 1997 that all places where anaesthesia was being performed were equipped with capnometry.

However, the capnogram has been described in text and picture as early as 1949. Both infrared [1,2] and mass spectrography devices [3] were already used at this time.

In 1950 a "portable" mass spectrometer of the size of a cupboard was used in operating theatre [4]. In 1952 the influence of hyperventilation, breath holding, forced expiration, ergometry and lung disease on the capnogram was recognized [5,6]. In 1955 the capnometer was used for controlled ventilation in Polio [7] and to monitor the respirator and the CO_2 absorber [8-11]. It was described that end-tidal CO_2 approximates alveolar CO_2 only if a plateau is seen [8-11]. In 1957 the influence of cardiac output on alveolar carbon dioxide was described and the capnometer was used as a guide to effective cardiac massage during cardiac arrest [12]. An analysis of the difference between arterial and end-tidal CO_2 tension was published in 1960 [13]. In 1961 an article on the use of capnometry for detection of an obstructed airway was published [14].

In 1967 a monography on capnography was published in Dutch language (with an English summary) [15]. Some years later, a monography in English followed [16].

The application of capnometry for the detection of oesophageal tube malposition was first proposed in 1981 and formally studied in 1983 [17-22]. The idea had been proposed at about the same time by different groups from the Netherlands [17,18] Finland [19,20], USA [21] and South Africa [22].

Interestingly, it was not easy for the Finnish group to publish their message: *"We had in one hospital in Helsinki ... a fatal critical incident due to inability to detect an oesophageal intubation. ... this sad complication stimulated me to wonder whether capnometry ... might be of some value in avoiding this kind of complications. ... We then performed the study and Dr. Linko reported the results at our national meeting in 1981 ... I can vividly remember the cheerful laughter from the audience and the difficulties to get the results published ..."* [23]. In 1986 a review on oesophageal intubation established capnometry as the "gold standard" in checking the position of the tube [24]. A colorimetric CO_2 detector, introduced in 1988 [25,26] and a paperback size infrared device, introduced in 1990 [27] made hand-held (i.e. < 1 kg) qualitative capnometry in out-of-hospital settings available. Since 1995 hand-held quantitative capnometry is available [28].

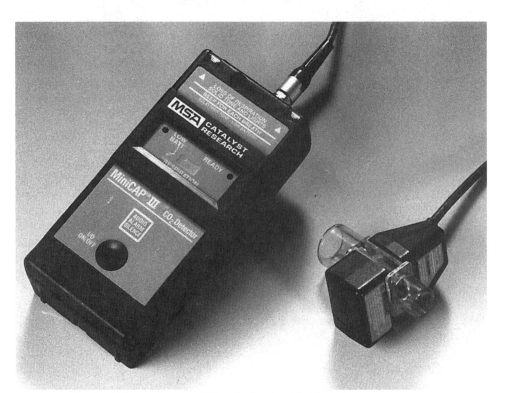

Fig. 2.:   MSA MiniCAP, introduced in 1990,   the first hand-held infrared capnometer

References:

1. Luft KF: Über eine neue Methode der registrierenden Gasanalyse mit Hilfe der Absorption ultraroter Strahlen ohne spektrale Zerlegung. Zeitschrift für technische Physik 1943; 24: 97-104
2. Fowler RC: A rapid infra-red gas analyzer. Review of Scientific Instruments 1949; 20: 175-178
3. Kydd GH, Hitchcock FA: Mass spectrographic studies on expired and alveolar air. Federation Proceedings 1949;8:89-90
4. Miller FA, Hemingway A, Nier AO, Knight RT, Brown EB, Varco RL: The development of, and certain clinical applications for a portable mass spectrometer. J Thorac Surg 1950; 20: 714-728
5. DuBois AB, Fowler RC, Soffer A, Fenn WO: Alveolar CO_2 measured by expiration into the rapid infrared gas analyzer. J Appl Physiol 1952; 4: 526-534
6. DuBois AB, Britt AG, Fenn WO: Alveolar CO_2 during the respiratory cycle. J Appl Physiol 1952; 4: 535-548
7. Collier CR, Affeldt JE, Farr AF: Continuous rapid infrared CO_2 analysis. J Lab Clin Med 1955; 45: 526-539
8. Elam JO, Brown ES, Ten Pas RH: Carbon dioxide homeostasis during anesthesia. I. Instrumentation. Anesthesiology 1955; 16: 876-885
9. Elam JO, Brown ES: Carbon dioxide homeostasis during anesthesia. II. Total sampling for determination of dead space, alveolar ventilation, and carbon dioxide output. Anesthesiology 1955; 16: 886-902
10. Elam JO, Brown ES: Carbon dioxide homeostasis during anesthesia. III. Ventilation and carbon dioxide elimination. Anesthesiology 1956; 17: 116-127
11. Elam JO, Brown ES: Carbon dioxide homeostasis during anesthesia. IV. An evaluation of the partial rebreathing system. Anesthesiology 1956; 17: 128-134
12. Leigh MD, Jenkins LC, Belton MK, Lewis GB: Continuous alveolar carbon dioxide analysis as a monitor of pulmonary blood flow. Anesthesiology 1957; 18: 878-882
13. Nunn JF, Hill DW: Respiratory dead space and arterial to end-tidal CO_2 tension difference in anesthetized man. J Appl Physiol 1960; 15: 383-389
14. Leigh MD, Jones JC, Motley HL: The exspired carbon dioxide as a continuous guide of the pulmonary and circulatory systems during anesthesia and surgery. J Thorac Cardiovasc Surg 1961;41:597-610
15. Smalhout B: Capnografie bij de Diagnostiek, Operatie en Nabehandeling van Neurochirurgische Aandoeningen. Oosthoek, Utrecht 1967
16. Smalhout B, Kalenda Z: An Atlas of Capnography. Volume 1. 2nd Edition, Kerckebosch-Zeist, Utrecht 1981
17. Ionescu T: Signs of endotracheal intubation. Anaesthesia 1981; 36: 422-423
18. Kalenda Z, van der Vliest O: Tracheal intubation guided by the capnogram. 6th European Congress of Anaesthesiology, 8-15 Sep 1982, Volume of Summaries, p. 478-479
19. Linko K, Paloheimo M, Tammisto T: Capnography for detection of accidental intubation. Acta Anaesthesiol Scand 1983; 27: 199-202
20. Linko K, Paloheimo M: Capnography facilitates blind nasotracheal intubation. Acta Anaesthesiol Belg 1983; 34: 117-122
21. Murray IP, Modell JH: Early detection of endotracheal tube accidents by monitoring carbon dioxide concentration in respiratory gas. Anesthesiology 1983; 59: 344-346
22. Klein MTD, Moyes DG: Accidental oesophageal intubation - a practical solution. South African Medical Journal 1984; 66: 4-5
23. Tammisto T: Personal communication, January 1996.
24. Birmingham PK, Cheney FW, Ward RJ: Esophageal intubation: A review of detection techniques. Anesthesia and Analgesia 1986; 65: 886-891
25. Fehder CG: Carbon Dioxide Indicator Device. US patent 4,728,499. Filed August 13, 1986; patented March 1, 1988
26. O'Callaghan JP, Williams RT: Confirmation of tracheal intubation using a chemical device. Can J Anaesth 1988; 35: S59
27. Vukmir RB, Heller MB, Stein KL: Confirmation of endotracheal tube position: a miniaturized infrared qualitative CO2 detector. Ann Emerg Med 1990;19:465
28. Petroianu GA, Junker HM, Maleck WH, Rüfer R: A portable quantitative capnometer in test. Am J Emerg Med 1996;14:586-587

Using Things Right out of Home – Apparatus for Inhaling Ether and Chloroform in 1847

H. Petermann
Department of Anaesthesiology, University Erlangen-Nuremberg, Germany

Summary

Shortly after the news about painless surgery due to the application of ether had spread, people already started employing this promising method. This is why we conclude that doctors must already have been familiar with the devices that were used for the inhalation of ether, namely equipment of fine mechanical kind or glass of the laboratory or of daily use. Anyhow, constructing devices for physiological experiments and tests must have been common in the 19th century.

Introduction

"Mikroskope und Fernroehre verwirren eigentlich den reinen Menschensinn." – Johann Wolfgang Goethe (1749 -1832)[1]
More than 15 years passed, and regarding this statement, nobody thought of disturbances that apparatus for biological phenomena could bring. The development of medical devices can only be carried out, if the following considerations are taken into account:
1. similar biological processes occur under definite conditions in a similar way.
2. there is a fundamental conformity in the dead and the living nature
3. one has to be convinced that physical or chemical measurements describe vital processes.

Already in 1844 Carl Vierodt measured the carbon dioxide concentration at certain respiratory levels. In the years 1840/50 Theodor Schwann (1809-1885), Hermann Helmholtz (1821-1894), Emil du Bois-Reymond (1818-1896), Ludwig Bruecke (1819-1892) und Carl Ludwig (1816-1895), five young German physiologist, were engaged in developing useful principles, that were received by experiments. A lot of their work was carried out by using physical apparatus and devices. In 1847 G.G. Valentin described 159 apparatus for physiological measurements.

The apparatus for ether and chloroform inhalation emerged as part of the development of apparatus for biological processes.

In the first experiments a piece of cloth or sponge was saturated with sulfuric ether and placed to the nostrils or mouth of the patient, in order to make inhale the vapors of ether. This is how William Crawford Long (1815-1878) used ether in his first experiments in 1842. During the following years a lot of people tested the use of ether as an anaesthetic agent. This lead to the well-known date: the 16th of October 1846 – the beginning of modern anesthesia.

The First Apparatus for Ether Inhalation

The first public application of ether in Boston, Mass. was already carried out with a special constructed device made of glass. This device had been constructed by N.B. Chamberlain, Boston.

In the U.S. Patent No.4848, dated November 12, 1846, the Drs. W.T.G. Morton (1819-1868) and C.T. Jackson (1805-1880) described it as follows:

Various modes may be adopted for conveying the ethereal vapor into the lungs. ... A more effective one is to take a glass or other proper vessel, like a common bottle or flask and place in it a sponge saturated with sulphuric ether. Let there be a hole made through the side of the vessel for the admission of atmospheric air, which hole may or may not be provided with a valve opening downward, or so as to allow air to pass into the vessel, a valve on the outside of the neck opening upward, and another valve in the neck and between that last mentioned and the body of the vessel or flask, which latter valve in the neck should open toward the mouth of the neck or bottle. The extremity of the neck is to be placed in the mouth of the patient, and his nostrils stopped or closed in such manner as to cause him to inhale air through the bottle, and to exhale it through the neck and out of the valve on the outside of the neck. The air thus breathed, by passing in contact with the sponge, will be charged with the ethereal vapors, which will be conveyed by it into the lungs of the patient. This will soon produce the state of insensibility or nervous quiet required. (4, S.553)*

Exactly a year after the first one Dr. Morton, this time together with August A. Gould, took out a patent on a new inhaler (U.S. Patent No.5365).

This time the construction included a modification. If necessary the bottle with ether could be put into a warm or hot water bath to vaporize the ether.

Apparatus for Ether Inhalation in Europe

Centers for making of apparatus in 1847 were Paris, Berlin and Leipzig. Different kinds of apparatus could be found in 1847:
– Apparatus of fine mechanical kind or made of glass
– Flask- (Morton) or bladder apparatus (Herapath)
– Devices without sponge or water (Charrière, Heyfelder, Herapath), apparatus with a sponge, and vessel with water topped with ether.

John Snow wrote the following note about the devices mentioned above:

Many of the apparatuses at first invented did not allow of easy respiration, but offered obstruction to it - by sponges, by the ether itself, by valves of insufficient size, but more particularly by tubes of too narrow caliber: and there is reason to believe that, in many instances, this was the cause of failure, and that in others the insensibility, when produced, was partly due to asphyxia - a circumstance especially to be avoided. (7, p.21)

Considering these objections some general principles for constructing inhalers were put up:
– the diameters of the tubes for inspiration and expiration have to be wide enough
– the air passing through the ether or sponges full with ether have to be the same, that will be inspired
– the inspiratory air has to be fresh, i.e. there should be no circulation of already exspired air
– the exspiration should not be stenous to the patient
– the mouthpiece has to be tight fit at the mouth in order to avoid inspiration of atmospheric air
– there should be a device to regulate the air stream
– the nose has to be closed by a fitting device

We would like to introduce you to different types of apparatus, representative of those common in 1847 or being very special

For the first application in London Mr. Hooper constructed his first ether inhaler, build up according to the specifications of Drs. Boot and Robinson. (4, p.131)

This apparatus consisted of the following parts:
1. Pad for mouth, to be held by the operator.
2. Horizontal valve for the escape of expired air
3. Vertical flap valve
4. Stop-cock

5. Nasal spring
6. Elastic tube
7. Glass vessel, with a smaller one having pieces of sponge saturated with ether, and having a small perforated stopper, to be opened when the apparatus is in use.
8. Sectional view of the pad, showing the mouthpiece.

The device invented by Charrière in Paris is quite similar. It was covered with a wire netting to avoid the firing of the vapor of ether. Both apparatus were widely spread over Europe.

Other modifications are those of Luer in Paris and Bouchacourt, Bonnet und Ferrand, Pomis and Diday in Lyon. One can compare those apparatus a little bit to a wine bottle.

Another glass inhaler is the one by J.F. Heyfelder (1798-1869). It resembles a bottle for spirits used at that time. Other types are compared e.g. with beer bottles.

Alfred Smees was convinced, that a faster vaporization of ether would lead to more satisfying results. His apparatus is cylindrical made of tin and about 8 inches long and 3 inches wide.

The bottom third was partitioned off and could be filled with hot water. A diaphragm

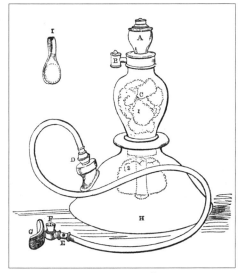

Paris: Apparatus of Charrière[15]

placed diagonally across the interior of the vaporizer forced the air drawn in by the patient to pass over the surface of the ether before reaching the mouthpiece. Immediately behind the mouthpiece was an expiratory valve.[4, p.140]

John Snow (1813-1858), probably the first anesthetists, constructed an inhaler made of tin. It had a spiral inside in order to elongate the way of inspired air through the ether. It

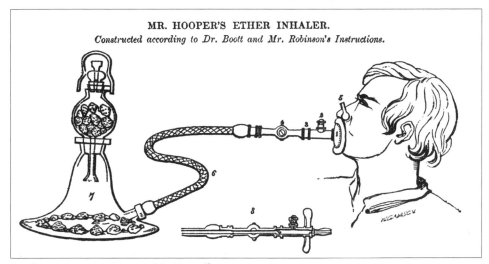

London: Apparatus of Boot and Robinson[15]

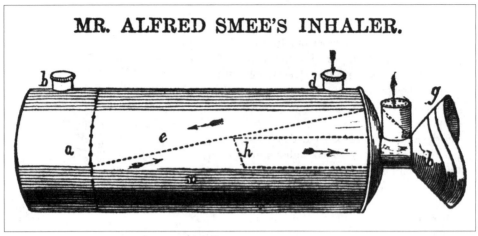

London: Smeeth`s Sulfuric Ether Instrument[15]

also came in variation with a water bath to assure that the ether had a constant temperature.

In his booklet "Die Einathmung der Aether-Dämpfe in ihrer verschiedenen Wirkungsweise ..., Würzburg 1847", Robert von Welz (1814-1879) described the apparatus he used for inhalation of the vapor of ether, which had been constructed by the metalworker-master Gerster in Würzburg.

Dr. Textor, Dr. von Marcus and Dr. Rinecker testified in July 1847 that the apparatus of Welz was safe, fast and pleasant.

On July 22, 1847, Welz sent his monograph as well as an apparatus to King Ludwig I. of Bavaria:

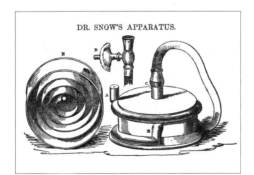

London: Snow`s Ether Inhaler[15]

The enclosed certificates of Mr. Hofrath Textor und Marcus and the recommendations of my booklet including a description of the ether apparatus of Your Royal Majesty governments of Unterfranken and Aschaffenburg, dated June 22, and of Oberfranken, dated July 8 this year, to all Court and practical doctors, I will name as proof for my words ...[12]

On October 29, 1847, a note was published in the "Intelligenzblatt für Mittelfranken", according to a expert opinion by Dr. F.Ch. Rothmund (1801-1891). The apparatus of Welz is characterized as following[13]:

1. Recommendable is its simplicity, solidity and cheapness
2. the apparatus is easy to take along and especially suitable for private surgery
3. the handling is easy and allows ether vapors to be inhaled by mouth or nose
4. it does no use more ether to induce narcosis for comparable apparatus
5. the narcosis can be induced slow or fast, each time in a pleasant way for the patient.

This information should be given to the medical staff.

Other apparatus were similar to sprinkling cans or special constructions like portable, pneumatic, hydrostatic or experimental inhalers. Mr. Hooper even constructed one to be used for horses.

Prices for the Apparatus

In an article Dr. Hammerschmidt[9] described the various types of apparatus and gives their prices.

1. bladder apparatus by Dr. F. Heller according to those of Dr. Ragsky
   price: 40 kr. C.M. to 2 fl. C.M.
2. apparatus by Reisser, flask made of wood with valve
   price: 2 fl. C.M. to 12 fl. C.M.
3. flask apparatus by Prof. Pleischl, made of glass
   price: 6 to 10 fl. C.M.
4. bladder apparatus by Dr. S. Eckstein for surgical operations in the face
   price: 2 fl. bis 8 fl. C.M.

The following advertisement could be found in "Nürnberger Kurier" in February 1847; Mechanikus J.J. Heller offers his *Apparate zum Athmen von Aether-Daempfen, vollständig, alles Noethiges enthaltend zu 3 fl. 30 kr. und hoeher* (apparatus for inhalation of vapor of ether, complete, including everything necessary for 3 fl. 30 kr. and more) for Aerzte und Wundaerzte (doctors and surgeons).

R. v. Welz named a price of 2 Kronenthalern for his apparatus.

To compare these prices:
The yearly budget for an household was[12, p.111]

People to live in	Budget for the year (in fl.)
the poor	65 *(5.5 per month)*
worker	155 *(12.9 per month)*
petit bourgeoisie	400 *(33.3 per month)*
bourgeois	over 800 *(66.6 per month)*

The price for Aether sulphuric was 24 kr. for about 29 ml and 4 kr. for about 3.6 ml.

Conclusions

1. Most of the used apparatus in 1847 have two parts: one for taking up ether and vaporizing the agent, the other part as a supply line for the vapors.
2. At that time any available and convenient material was used for these devices
3. Various modifications according to different theories were available.
4. Constructing devices for medical use was common in the 19. century.

References:

1. Goethe W: Werke. Hamburger Ausgabe. ND München 1982. Bd.12. S.430
2. Rothschuh K E: Die Bedeutung apparativer Hilfsmittel für die Entwicklung der biologischen Wissenschaften im 19. Jahrhundert. In: Naturwissenschaft, Technik und Wirtschaft im 19. Jahrhundert. Goettingen 1976. S.161-185
3. Illustrierte Zeitung, Leipzig. Bd.8 (1847)
4. Duncum B: The Development of Inhalation Anaesthesia. Oxford University, London 1947
5. Bauer A: Ueber Schwefelther und seine neueste Anwendung ... Prag 1847
6. Rosenfeld: Die Schwefelther-Daempfe und ihre Wirksamkeit, vorzueglich in Bezug auf operative Chirurgie. Pest 1847
7. Snow I: On The Inhalation of the Vapour of Ether in Surgical Operations. London 1847
8. Bergson I: Die medicinische Anwendung der Aether-Daempfe ... Berlin 1847
9. Schlesinger I: Die Einathmung des Schwefel-Aethers ... Leipzig 1847
10. Hammerschmidt: Über die verschiedenen Apparate zur Aethernarkotisirung. In: Notizen aus dem Gebiete der Natur- und Heilkunde. 1847, Bd.3. Sp.104-110, 119-127
11. Nürnberger Kurier. Jg. 173 (1847), No.44 (13.Feb.)
12. Lutz, H: Zwischen Habsburg und Preußen, Deutschland 1815-1866. Berlin 1985
13. Kgl. Bayer. Intelligenz-Blatt fuer Mittelfranken. Ansbach. 1847, No.86
14. Deneke I: Volkskunst. Katalog GNM. Nuernberg 1985
15. Pharmaceutical Journal and Transactions. Vol.6 (1846/47)

(All figures of No. 15)

Administration of Ether Anesthesia per Rectum in Spain

J.C. Diz, A. Franco, J. Alvarez, J. Cortés
Servicio de Anestesiología y Reanimación, Hospital General de Galicia-Clínico Universitario, Spain

Introduction

In the history of rectal ether anesthesia we can differentiate three basic periods: the first period, in 1847, in which several European authors made experiments administering liquid ether or its vapors per rectum, trying to avoid the inconvenients of the inhalation of ether. The second period was in the eighties of XIXth century, after a paper of Oscar Wanscher in the International Congress of Medicine in Copenhagen. And the third period occurred at the beginning of XXth century, when we can outline the work of the American James Taylor Gwathmey, with his method of oil-ether-anesthesia.

First period (1847)

On February 20th 1847, the surgeon of the Hospital General of Madrid Antonio Saez operated a patient of a giant breast tumor that weighed 7 kg. after the administration of one drachm of sulfuric ether and one ounce of distilled water per rectum, making the mixture at the moment of the injection (1). He repeated twice the procedure and extirpated the tumor, although he had to use also the inhalation of ether. The patient died a few hours after the operation. In the spring of 1847, the Spanish Juan Vicente Hedo made several experiments with pure ether per rectum in animals, and he reported his experiences to the Gazette Médicale de Paris (2). In this communication he points out that his experiments were later than those of Marc Dupuy (3), but claims the priority of the method for the surgeon Antonio Saez (1-4), since he used the ether per rectum one month before Dupuy, and three before Pirogoff (5-6).

Second period

After the paper of Oscar Wanscher, in 1882, there was a revival of rectal ether anesthesia, that had been almost completely forgotten since 1847. In 1884 the Danish Axel Yversen visited Daniel Mollière, in Lyon (France), and advised him the technique of rectal etherization (7). Mollière used this technique, initially with a skin bladder, and later warming ether in a waterbath at 48 °C. He did not have very good results, and sometimes he observed serious mucous injuries, with pain, diarrhoea, rectal bleeding and one death.

In 1884, the Spanish surgeon Federico Rubio y Galí used the technique of Mollière, in the Hospital de la Princesa in Madrid in several patients, and he previously warmed up the ether in a waterbath to 25-30 centigrades (8). The opinion of this surgeon was that rectal etherization is fast, but its action is too soft, although he could associate inhalation of chloroform in low doses. This surgeon believed that the complications of the technique (abdominal pain, diarrhoea, and so), are caused by excessive intestinal distension, and the way of avoiding this is administering ether progressively in low doses, and discontinuing its administration if the patient has tenesmus. Sojo y Battle used a similar technique in Barcelona in 1885 (9). Also in 1884, Dr. José Godoy used ether per rectum in a cholera epidemic that affected the city of Granada causing 4.000 dead in little more than a month (10). The experiments of Dr. Godoy were based on the experiences of another physician of Granada, Dr. Maestre, who in 1859 used chloroform against the malaria. These experiments of ether per rectum had little success in surgery, since the patients scarcely reached a state of drowsiness, although the analgesia was sufficient for doing the operation in some instances. Regarding the ether per rectum in the treatment of the cholera, several authors state that it offered positive results in 94% of the cases (11).

Third period

The American John Henry Cunningham, in 1903, and Frank Howard Lahey, in 1905, began a new period in the history of rectal anesthesia, as they administered a mixture of vapors of ether with air (12). Walter S. Sutton used in 1910 a modification of this technique, since he used oxygen instead of air (13).

In 1913 James Taylor Gwathmey proposed, after animal and clinical experimentation, his method of oil-ether-anesthesia (14), which had a certain acceptance among surgeons. In Spain, Dr. José Soler Juliá was probably the first surgeon who used the method of oil-ether-anesthesia after 1917, in Barcelona. He made a mixture of one part of ether and half of oil, with a prior injection of one centigram of morphine 15 minutes before the operation 15). In the IX Congress of the International Society of Surgery in Madrid in 1932, he reported 50 cases of rectal etherization with good results, although he recognized that sometimes he had problems with the estimation of the doses.

Dr. José Sancho Castellano, from Zaragoza, used the method of Gwathmey in obstetric analgesia, in 1926. Although he reported good results with this technique, after 1927 he used the method of Kahn, this is, the use of Luminal instead of magnesium sulfate, paraffin wax instead of olive oil and cocoa butter instead of alcohol (16).

Conclusions

In summary, rectal ether as a surgical anesthetic was probably used for the first time in Spain, in February of 1847, this is, a month before Dupuy. It was used later in 1884, as in several other European countries, although this route of administration did not reach popularity.

References:

[1] Roel F G: "Tumor escirroso enquistado de la mama derecha que pesó trece libras (de á 16 onzas) y un cuarterón. La facultad, 1847; 10: 155-157

[2] Vicente Hedo J: "Note sur l'injection de l'ether dans le rectum." Gazette medicale de Paris, 317, 1847

[3] Dupuy M: "Note sur les effects de l'injection de l'ether dans le rectum." Comptes rendus de l'académie des sciences, 1847, 24 (april): 605-607

[4] Vicente Hedo J: "Análisis de cuanto se ha dicho sobre el éter como medio de acallar el dolor en las operaciones quirúrgicas y obstétricas, con algunas reflexiones acerca de los experimentos hechos: 1º En los animales. 2º En el hombre sano. 3º En los enfermos ú operandos. 64 pp. Imprenta del Presidio, Valencia, 1847

[5] Pirogoff NI: "Noveau procédé paur producire, au mayur de la vapeur d'ether, l'insensibilité chez les individus soumis à des operations chirurgicals. Comptes rendus de l'académie des sciences, 1847, 24 (may): 789

[6] Pirogoff NI: "Effets des vapeurs d'ether administreés par la rectum." Comptes rendus de l'académie des sciences, 1847, 24 (june): 1110

[7] Mollière D: "Note sur l'etherisation por la voie rectale." Lyon medidale, 1884, 44: 419-422

[8] Rubio y Galí F: "Eterización por el recto." Reseña del cuarto ejercicio del Instituto de Terapéutica operatoria del Hospital de la Princesa, Madrid, 1884, 4: 122-131

[9] Sojo y Battle F: "De la eterización por vía rectal." Revista de ciencias medicas, 1885, 11: 151-155

[10] Granizo F: "El eter y la eterización intestinal en el tratamiento del cólera morbo asiático." pp.29, Granada, 1884.

[11] Rodríguez Méndez, J: "Eterización rectal." Gaceta medica catalana, 1885, 196: 507-509

[12] Cunningham JH, Lahey FH: "A method of producing ether narcosis by rectum, with the report of forty-one cases." Bost. Med. Surg. J. 1905, 152: 450-457

[13] Sutton WS: "Anaesthesia by colonic absorption of ether." Ann. Surg. 1910, 5: 457-459

[14] Gwathmey JT: "Oil-ether anesthesia." Lancet, 1913, 2: 1756-1758

[15] Soler Juliá J: "Anestesia rectal." Rev. Esp. Obst. Gin., 1918, 3: 20-204

[16] Sancho Castellano J: "La anestesia en el parto normal, con referencia especial al método de Gwathmey y a su modificación de Kahn." Rev. Esp. Obst. Gin. 1928, 13: 444-466

James Young Simpson and American Women in Medicine

S. H. Calmes,
Olive View-UCLA Medical Center
Sylmar, California, USA

In 1854, there were no women medical practitioners in the United Kingdom, on the Continent or in Scandinavia or Russia[1]. Only in the United States (U.S.) could women enter medicine, and this entry began only five years earlier when Elizabeth Blackwell (1821-1910) received the first M.D. degree awarded to a woman[2]. Enormous hostility to women's entry into medicine was present, and opportunities for women to study medicine were extremely limited. Also, American medical practice and education were less advanced than European medicine. Many graduates of U.S. medical schools traveled to Europe seeking further study, to augment their limited medical education[3]. Study consisted of attending lectures at several European medical schools and following established practitioners on their hospital, office and home visits. Typically, letters of introduction to noted European physicians were sent with the student by their American professors with European ties. This entry to the superior European medicine was difficult for the few American women medical graduates because of the lack of women physicians in Europe and because American professors were reluctant to write the needed letters of introduction, fearful of putting their friends in Europe in the difficult situation of advocating for women in medicine.

In this setting, it is quite surprising that James Young Simpson (1811-1870[4]) allowed a recent female American medical graduate Emily Blackwell (1826-1910; sister of Elizabeth Blackwell) to study with him for four months[5]. Although Elizabeth Blackwell had gone to Europe for study after her own graduation, family contacts there paved the way for her study (the Blackwell family was originally from England), and she did not spend long periods of time with prominent practitioners who became identified with her. The situation with Emily Blackwell was different. Simpson was very well-known by then for his work in obstetrics, his discovery of chloroform's anesthetic properties and his advocacy for anesthesia in obstetrics. She showed up unintroduced, Simpson became identified as actively helping her, and his subsequent letters introduced her to other leading European practitioners. Also, Elizabeth Blackwell returned to England in 1859, practicing only ten years in the U.S. Emily Blackwell ran the women's medical institutions which the two founded for another forty years. Overall, this accomplishment probably had more long-term effect on American women in medicine.

This paper examines why Simpson might have broken with tradition and accepted Blackwell, what Blackwell learned during her study with Simpson and what the results of her study were. Sources used were standard biographic sources on both Simpson and Elizabeth and Emily Blackwell, Elizabeth Blackwell's letters to Emily and Emily Blackwell's letters to her family during her time in Europe. ("Blackwell" refers to only Emily Blackwell. Elizabeth Blackwell will be referred to by her full name.)

Emily Blackwell graduated with honors

from the medical college of Western Reserve University in Cleveland, Ohio, in March 1854. She then sailed for London for advanced study. Apparently contact with Simpson was not arranged beforehand, and no personal go-between was available. Her plans were to discuss her needs with *"Dr.s Oldham and Simpson"* first. This letter also mentions the possible need for a disguise while studying in Europe[6]. She arrived in Edinburgh in mid-May 1854 and found Simpson ill and unable to receive visitors. She then wrote,

"At last I have the satisfaction of seeing Dr. Simpson, hearing yesterday that he was well enough to receive patients. I called and sent my card. I was immediately ushered in, (Simpson) enjoying most heartily the amazed looks of some of them (patients) when he addressed me as Dr. Blackwell."[7]

The letters do not document how Dr. Simpson came to first accept her as a student or his initial feelings about this situation. Letters later in the summer document long discussions with him on walks and rides about how she could best educate herself, given the difficult situation for women in medicine.

Dr. Blackwell's quarters were at Minto House, not in the Simpson home at 52 Queen Street[8], as is frequently stated. She spent most of her time in his office, which was in his home[9]. Simpson's practice was extremely busy; patients were seen every two minutes. *"I see a great deal at Dr. S's that I could not see elsewhere."* She was stationed in the *"green room,"* and Simpson would send in patients, ordering her to make a diagnosis or to apply a treatment. Patients were also sent in to her as a "case of such-and- such." She used his medical library and examined his instruments. Another assistant, a Dr. Priestly, was also working.

Simpson's diagnosis was nearly always by touch. She described his treatments: cupping, leeching, giving injections and, in one case, acupuncture. *"He gives as little medicine as anyone I ever saw."* Consumption (tuberculosis) was treated by rubbing the patient all over with olive oil. She observed him giving chloroform and observed operations, which nearly always were done as soon as the need was determined. She was given a few poor patients to care for herself. In July, she was left with his "list" (of patients to care for) when he went out of town for the weekend.

Simpson's attitude towards her appeared to be one of tolerance and not active help.

"Dr. S has given a little more. I do not count on any positive aid from him. However he rather liked the novelty of a woman. Dr. S has no objection to my being as far as possible indoctrinated into his views, and as I am sometimes useful, does not dislike my being about his house and picking up what I can ... he will not in the least put himself out to trouble to aid me."[10]

Later, Blackwell did not expect to get the official assistantship with him she desired.

"However considering how illiberal the general feeling in Edinburgh is, it is a good deal for the Dr. to have given me what he has. My residence with Dr S has however fully proved to me how superficial the opposition that women make to the idea is, it is violent at first but soon fades away when you are brought in contact with them"[11]

Blackwell finally acknowledged what she did learn, *"and Dr. S did me altogether good in that way for he used to throw troublesome cases on me and abandon me to my own resources in a way that made a Dr. of me.."*[12]

She left Edinburgh in August, as she unable to study much there. Simpson was not on good terms with the trustees of the Maternity Hospital, and he was unable to get her in there. Apparently access to the University Hospital was also limited. And, perhaps it was time to move on: *"Dr. S has more than once most decidedly expressed his conviction that*

London is quite ready for us."[13] Apparently she left for London without any letters from Simpson. She then had to care for a sick sister-in-law in London for several months. Although never documented in the letters, she apparently received some introductions from Simpson and then went on to Paris, Berlin, and Dresden. She returned to the U.S. in 1856 as one of the best trained physicians in European medicine.

Why did Simpson help, even in a passive way, this early medical woman? He often took unusual stands, as demonstrated by his early use and then advocacy of anesthesia for obstetrics. He was well known to have an argumentative personality and boldness, which were helpful in the fight for acceptance of anesthesia in obstetrics. Agreeing to have a woman doctor work in his office – an outrageous situation in 1854 – attracted further attention to him, attention which he no doubt desired. Finally, it is known that Simpson had sympathy towards women, especially sick women, the result of his close relation with his mother, whose final years were marked by illness.

Simpson's support of Emily Blackwell's graduate medical study had a significant effect for American women in medicine. On Blackwell's return, she helped her sister develop a dispensary into a hospital, the New York Infirmary for Women and Children, which opened in 1857. A woman's medical school was added in 1868. This was the first U.S. medical school to have a three year, graded curriculum, educational requirements for entry and examinations for graduation.[14] Both the hospital and medical school provided vital and superior opportunities for women to enter medicine. Both were run by Emily Blackwell after her sister's return to England in 1859. Simpson's personality, which often generated considerable hostility against him, ultimately led to great improvement of women's health by relieving pain in obstetrics and by improving American women's medical training.

References:

1. Bonner T N: To the Ends of the Earth: Women's Search for Education in Medicine. (Harvard University Press, Cambridge) 1992; pp 6-30

2. Elizabeth Blackwell. In Notable American Women. (The Belknap Press of Harvard University, Cambridge) 1971. vol I, pp 161-165

3. Bonner T N: American Doctors and German Universities: A Chapter in International Intellectual Relations. University of Nebraska Press, Lincoln 1988

4. Sir James Young Simpson. In Dictionary of National Biography. Oxford Press, Oxford 1963; vol XVIII, pp 272-273

5. Emily Blackwell. In Notable American Women. The Belknap Press of Harvard University, Cambridge 1971; vol I, pp 165-167

6. Elizabeth Blackwell to Emily Blackwell, April 20, 1854. Blackwell Family Papers, The Schlesinger Library, Radcliffe College, Cambridge (hereafter BFP, SL)

7. Emily Blackwell to "Dear People." May 20, 1854. BFP, SL. (All are written from Edinburgh unless otherwise specified)

8. Emily Blackwell to "Dear People." May 6-10, 1854, p 1. BFP, SL. Minto House is described in Wright D. Sights and sites in Edinburgh. In Barr AM, Boutlon TB and DJ Wilkinson, eds. Essays on the History of Anaesthesia. Royal Society of Medicine Press, London 1996, pp 135-136. This was a hospital run by surgeon James Syme from 1829-1833. During the time Blackwell was in Edinburgh, it was the Maternity Hospital. She mentions both in her letters, as if they were different institutions. Perhaps Minto House was for lodging, and the Maternity Hospital was a connected building

9. The following sections are taken from letters during the summer of 1854. Clinical subjects often appeared in several letters, making citation difficult. Dr. Simpson's office practice is also documented in a report by Dr. Walter Channing, quoted in Duns J. Memoir of Sir James Young Simpson Edmonston and Douglas, Edinburgh 1873, pp 333-337

10. Emily Blackwell to "Dear People." September 4, 1854. BFP, SL

11. Emily Blackwell to "Dear People." November 7, 1854. BFP, SL

12. Emily Blackwell (from London) to "Dear People." January 29, 1855. BFP, SL

13. Emily Blackwell to "Dear People." November 29, 1854. BFP, SL

14. Emily and Elizabeth Blackwell, Notable American Women, op. cit.

Pioneers and Innovators in Anesthesia

L. Rendell-Baker, J. A. Mayer, G. Bause,
Anesthesia History Association (U.S.A.), Loma Linda University, California, American Society of Anesthesiologists', Wood Library-Museum of Anesthesiology, USA

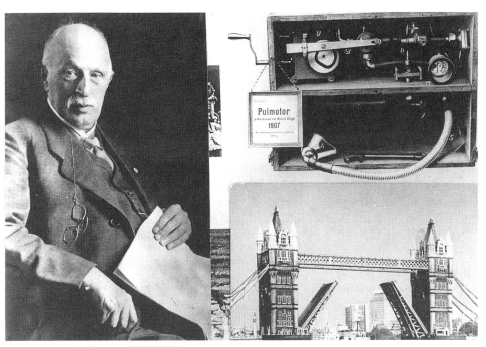

Fig. 1: Heinrich Dräger (1847-1917)

INNOVATORS of EQUIPMENT

Heinrich Dräger (Fig. 1)

Founded Drägerwerk in Lübeck, Germany in the 1880's to make pressure-flow controls for CO_2 to pressurize beer barrels – the „Bierdruck Automat". Pioneered in design of mine rescue, diving and fire rescue breathing apparatus.

Produced:

1902 Roth-Dräger chloroform/oxygen anesthesia apparatus.
1904 Closed circle CO_2 absorption mine rescue apparatus.
1906 Witnessed a failed manual resuscitation from drowning at London's Tower Bridge. This stimulated his design of the Pulmotor.
1907 Pulmotor – the first O_2 powered ventilator.
1907 Roth-Dräger positive pressure anesthesia apparatus for open chest surgery.
1925 First circle CO_2 absorption anesthesia apparatus.

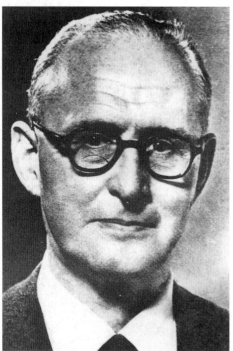

Fig. 2: Sir Ivan W. Magill, KCVO, MB, BCh, DSc (HC), FRCS, FFA.RCS (Hon), (1888-1986)

Sir Ivan W. Magill (Fig. 2)

Born in Larne, Northern Ireland, July 23, 1888.

At the University, he played as a forward in the Rugby football team and represented his university as a heavyweight boxer.

Graduated MB.BCh, BAO in 1913, Belfast University.

During WWI he served in France in the British Army as a regimental medical officer and after the Armistice in 1919 he accepted a posting to the Queen's Hospital, Sidcup, Kent, the Army's maxillo-facial hospital with over 600 patients, even though he had no anesthetic training and little experience. Self-trained with his colleague, Stanley Row-botham, he developed the anesthetic technique and instruments for maxillo-facial surgery – from endotracheal insufflation of ether and air with two separate gum elastic catheters to the method of blind nasal intubation with a wide bore rubber tube with N_2O and O_2 anesthesia. This was a significant breakthrough as it permitted intubation with light anesthesia. He developed a laryngoscope, forceps, connectors and what we now call the Mapleson A breathing system to remove the reservoir bag from the surgical field, and designed a machine to deliver the N_2O/O_2 mixture.

Magill developed the endotracheal technique for harelip and cleft palate operation in infants and later for thoracic surgery he developed endobronchial tubes and bronchus blockers.

Received Henry Hill Hickman Medal in 1938, Robert Campbell Memorial Orator Belfast, 1939 and was knighted by the Queen in 1960. Late Senior Anaesthetist Westminster and Brompton Hospitals, London.

Sponsored foundation of Association of Anaesthetists of Great Britain and Ireland in 1932 and the establishment of the Diploma in Anaesthetic examination in 1935.

David S. Sheridan (Fig. 3)

Born Brooklyn, New York, July 10, 1908.

1940– Founded U.S. Catheter and Instrument Corp. with Norman Jeckel.
1945

1942 Produced the cardiac catheters that Cournand used to develop the method of cardiac catheterization.

1953 Converted the red barn on his property in Argyle, New York, to a plastics research laboratory.

1955 Sheridan developed PVC tubing with "bubbles" to form connectors and PVC tubing with an X-ray opaque line.

1956 Starting with a technician and three women working in a barn, he started production of extruded PVC catheters and tubing as the Sheridan Catheter and Instrument Corporation. Later he

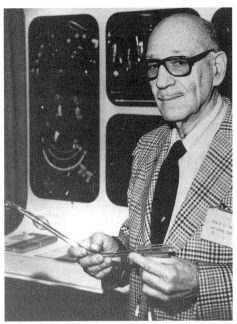

Fig. 3: David S. Sheridan, DSc(Hc) (1908–)

developed suction catheters with a non-stick finish.
1957 Sheridan sold his company to the Brunswick Corporation to become their Sherwood Division.
1959 In cooperation with Dr. Ralph D. Alley, of Albany Medical Center, produced one piece disposable Yankauer suction handles, one piece intravenous cannulas, intra-thoracic drainage catheters and Salem Stomach Sump drains, the Saratoga Sump drains and catheters for open heart operations.
1967 Parted company with the Brunswick Corporation and returned to his red barn to do research.
1970 Built his 2nd plant-The National Catheter Corporation.
1974 Sold this to Mallinckrodt Inc.
1977 Parted from Mallinckrodt and formed the Sheridan Catheter Corporation to make tracheal tubes.

Starting in 1956 with a staff of four in a barn, Sheridan has founded four corporations which now employ 1,150 people and produce 150 million catheters, etc. per year. He pioneered extruded PVC tracheal tubes with the smooth punched Murphy eye, blow molded low pressure cuffs, the electrically formed angled tip suction catheter, the inflation lumen within the wall without increased wall thickness, the X-ray opaque line, the printing on the tube and the incorporated 15 mm. connector, the non-stick surface on suction catheters, the one piece plastic Yankauer suction handles, the Salem Sump drain and the Saratoga Sump drain and open heart catheters.

He endowed a chair of anesthesiology in Harvard University and an MRI Center at Albany University Medical Center.

Henning Ruben (Fig. 4)

In 1948, unable to obtain a Stephen-Slater non-rebreathing valve, he made a copy of it from the diagram in Anesthesiology which became the first Ambu valve.

In 1952 he modified this into a valve which provided for single-handed inflation of the lungs. In 1960 his E valve used silicone membranes instead of valve discs and springs.

1956 Ruben introduced a portable foot operated suction apparatus.
1957 He introduced the first self-filling Ambubag manual resuscitator.
1957 Introduced a mannequin-like „Resusci-Annie" – for teaching artificial respiration and external cardiac compression.
1969–1981 Evolved a new anesthesia breathing system with a „pop off" 1981 valve which never requires adjustment and automatically closes during inflation of the lungs.

(Photograph courtesy of Dr. Henning Ruben)

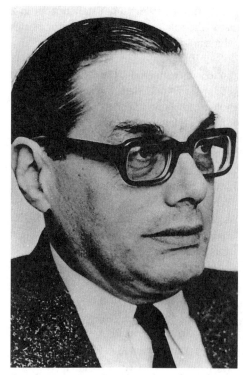

Fig. 4: *Henning Ruben, M.D. Anesthesiologist – Copenhagen, Denmark*

John W. Severinghaus (Fig. 5)

Born in 1922 in Madison, Wisconsin.

Professor of Anesthesia and Director, Anesthesia Research, University of California School of Medicine in San Francisco. During World War II worked on radar at Massachusetts Institute of Technology. Later studied medicine in order to do research in biophysics.

1953 While experimenting with hypothermia at NIH Clinical Center 1958 in Washington he became involved in developing Stow's CO_2 electrode (1954), Clark's O_2 electrode (1956), and the pH electrodes.

1958 Since 1958 has continued to study blood gas and transcutaneous PO_2 and pCO_2 equipment in San Francisco and on sabbaticals in Denmark with Poul Astrup and colleagues, and with Radiometer.

1979 Awarded Doctor of Medicine Honoris Causa by Copenhagen University.

(From Astrup, P. and Severinghaus, J.W. The History of Blood Gases, Acids and Bases. Copenhagen Munsgaard 1986.)

John H. Emerson (Fig. 6)

President, J. H. Emerson Company

Born February 5, 1906, in New York City where his physician father was interested in chest diseases and polio. He was later Commissioner of Health in New York (1914–1916) during the worst NYC polio epidemic in history.

Mr. Emerson recounts that he made little progress at school but found he had a natural aptitude for making things in the workshop.

Mr. Emerson's brothers were applied physiologists who trained with Barcroft and Warburg, but since he was no good at school or exams, he went to work in the Harvard Physics Department Machine Shop. Later he worked in electrophysiology on a light quartz string galvanometer.

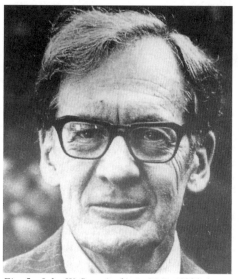

Fig. 5: *John W. Severinghaus, M.D. (1922–)*

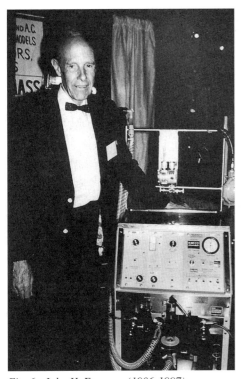

Fig. 6: John H. Emerson (1906-1997)

1928 Emerson set up his own workshop in Harvard Square where he made items of equipment for his brothers and other research workers.

1931 As the polio epidemic increased he was asked by Dr. Jim Wilson, resident physician at the Boston Children's Hospital to make a simple "iron lung". Encouraged by his father he made it in two weeks without an order or drawings. To test it, Jack slept one night in it.

His "iron lung" was first tried on a terminally ill polio patient who was not expected to last the night. Emerson's ventilator worked well right away and the patient survived.

Orders for the Emerson simple, inexpensive, and quiet iron lung, followed, ending sales of Drinker's expensive and noisy iron lung. Emerson still makes and services „iron lungs", particularly the pediatric model.

1952 Emerson added a deep breath or "sigh" attachment to his tank ventilator at the suggestion in 1947 of Dr. Visscher. The value of the "sigh" was rediscovered by Bendixen in 1963.

1952 Anesthesia „Assistor" made for Derrick et al at MGH.

1955 Emerson patented his high frequency "people panter" breathing attachment for an IPPV ventilator. There was little interest. (See Figs. 10 and 23)

1958 Assistor-Controller anesthesia ventilator.

1964 3PV 1st U.S. volume ventilator with a variable I:E ratio introduced to compete with the Swedish Engstrom, designed at request of Don Benson at Johns Hopkins to provide good humidification.

1965 Built 1st U.S. single position hyperbaric chamber for radiotherapy for Columbia Presbyterian Hospital, New York City.

1972 3MV model 1st adult ventilator providing IMV, spontaneous or controlled respiration.

When interest developed in high frequency ventilation Emerson produced prototypes of all three types - oscillators, jets, and HFPPV. These have been used experimentally to many physicians' satisfaction but Emerson has not committed a model to production.

M. Jack Frumin (Fig. 7)

Born September 5, 1919, New Jersey.

1946 M.D., Temple University, Philadelphia, Pennsylvania.

Residency Columbia Presbyterian Medical Center, New York City.

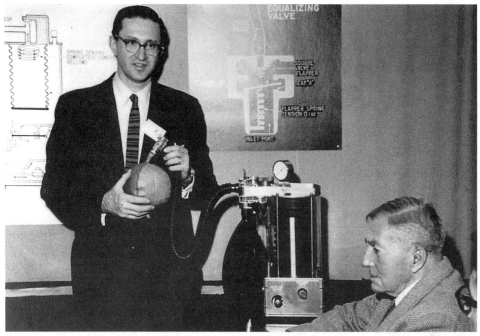

Fig. 7: M. Jack Frumin, M.D. (1919–) and Richard von Foregger

1957 Designed the AutoAnestheton with Arnold Lee. This was a physiologica ventilator which servo-controlled the minute volume ventilation it provided maintain a pre-set end tidal CO_2. This apparatus also incorporated PEEP for the first time.

1959 Introduced the Frumin inflating valve.

1960 Introduced the Frumin positive pressure ventilator.

Research papers published on epidural and spinal blockade, apneic oxygenation, elimination of N_2O and diffusion hypoxia, amnesic action of diazepam and scopolamine.

William W. Mapleson (Fig. 8)

Born in London, United Kingdom, August 2, 1926.

Graduated from Durham University, United Kingdom, BSc 1947, PhD 1953, and DSc 1973.

From 1947 to 1949, he was a radar instructor in the Royal Air Force. In 1952, he was appointed physicist to the Department of Anaesthetics in Cardiff.

As Professor of Physics in Anaesthesia at the University of Wales in Cardiff until 1992, he applied physics and mathematics to the solution of many problems in anesthesia, such as gas exchange within breathing systems and within the body.

He is widely known for his studies, published in 1954, in which he applied mathematical modeling in the functional analysis to predict the fresh gas flow needed for the elimination of expired CO_2 from the single tube breathing systems widely used in the United Kingdom. He labeled these systems A, B, C, D, and E, and later, F, but he did not invent them.

He also evolved a computer-assisted control of the depth of anesthesia.

He was awarded the Pask Certificate and

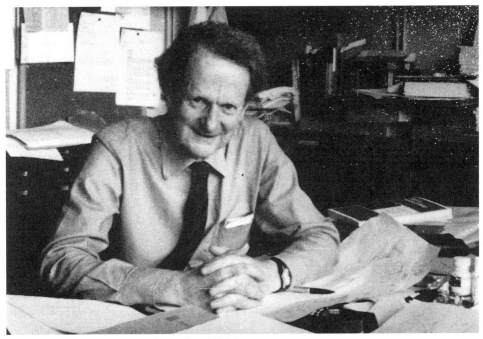

Fig. 8: William W. Mapleson, PhD., DSc. (1926–)

the Clover, Eliasberg, Faculty and Dudley Buxton Medals. He is an honorary member of the Brazilian Society of Anesthesiologists and of the Association of Anaesthetists of Great Britain and Ireland.

Lucien E. Morris (Fig. 9)

Born November 30, 1914, in Mattoon, Illinois

- 1943 M.D., Western Reserve University, Ohio
- 1948 Residency, University of Wisconsin, Madison
- 1954 Professor, University of Washington
- 1968 Professor, University of Toronto
- 1970 Professor and Chair, Medical College of Ohio, Toledo, Ohio
- 1994 President, A.H.A.

Honored world-wide for his contributions.

Introduced:

Equipment - Copper Kettle universal vaporizer with separate metered gas flow. By-pass flowmeter scales for combined fine and coarse flows. Overhead boom to carry gas supply hoses. Vertical double absorber system. Advocate of Revell circulator and totally closed system method.

Publications - 60 scientific, 10 historic, 18 reviews, and chapters in book.

Dr. Lucien Morris is a Swordmaster, and was a university coach for 12 years.

Forrest M. Bird (Fig 10)

Born in Stoughton, Massachusetts in 1921, the son of a WWI pilot who continued to fly and encouraged his son who soloed at 14. He learned to use lathes and other machine tools in his father's workshop. Studied science and engineering at Northeastern University.

On outbreak of WWII, Bird was commissioned as a Transport Command pilot. He became dissatisfied with the BLB O_2 mask control valve then used for high altitude flying.

From a German bomber he flew from

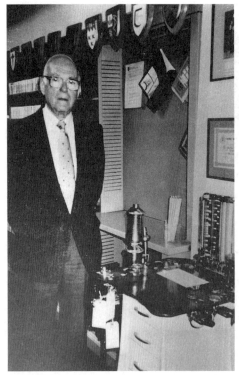

Fig. 9: Lucien E. Morris, M.D., (1914–)
DABA, FACA, FRCP(C), FRCA,
FANZCA, FRSM, D.Sc.

England to Wright-Patterson Air Force Base, he obtained a German O_2 demand valve which he modified to trigger at an inspiratory effort of 1-2 cm. H_2O. Six prototypes were made and tested on flights at over 30,000 feet with excellent results. Bird described the functioning of his demand regulator to the School of Aviation Medicine. Within 3 months it was manufactured and placed in all high flying U.S. aircraft.

Back in civilian life, Bird purchased Army surplus regulators and modified them to provide N_2O mixture during dental procedures. To another regulator he fitted a manual inspiratory control and attached it to a nebulizer so that an emphysematous friend could give himself manually controlled IPPB. Drs. Barach and Cournand suggested an expiratory retard and a flow control be added.

The precursor of the original Bird Mark 7 ventilator magnetic valve design was mounted vertically in the aircraft and used to inflate a pilot's G suit and prevent blackout when he pulled out of a dive.

1957   Bird Mark 7 ventilator was introduced for controlled or assisted respiration.
1958   Mark 4 used with Mark 7 as a ventilator for anesthesia was introduced. The Marks 8,9,10,14, and 17 followed.
1971   Baby Bird ventilator for the first time provided CPAP and IMV.

Since selling the Bird Corporation, Dr. Bird has produced a new line of Percussionaire ventilators for export markets which combine high frequency oscillation with IPPB.

Peter J. Schreiber (Fig. 11)

President North American Drager Company (1968–1996).

Born July 23, 1929 in Dresden, Germany.

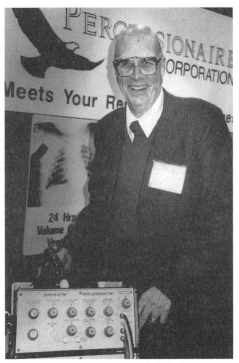

Fig. 10: Forrest M. Bird, Ph.D. (1921–)

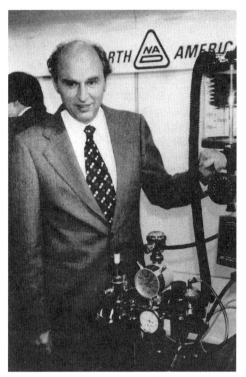

Fig. 11: Peter J. Schreiber (1929–)
President, North American Dräger
Company (1968–1996)

1956 Graduate Engineer from Oskar Von Miller, Polytechnikum, Akademie für angewandte Technik, Munich, Germany.

Contributions:
Design of first commercially available structured anesthesia alarm system.
Design of anesthesia work station.
Keyed filling system for vaporizers.
Device eliminating pumping effect on vaporizers.
Vaporizer interlock systems.
Fluidically controlled anesthesia ventilator.
Electronically controlled anesthesia ventilator.
Narkovet animal anesthesia apparatus.
Drager Vapor vaporizer, Cato drawover vaporizer for NATO forces.
Octavian & Tiberius anesthesia apparatus.
Magnetic controlled Pulmotor.

1970- Clinical Assistant Professor of Anesthesiology,
1978 University of Alabama, Birmingham Director, Anesthesia Patient Safety Foundation, Executive Board Member ASTM, F29 Committee

Author
Anesthesia, Equipment, Performance, Classification and Safety, 1972.
Safety Guidelines for Anesthesia Systems, 1985.
Safety Guidelines for Anesthesia Systems: Risk Analysis and Risk Reduction, 1987.

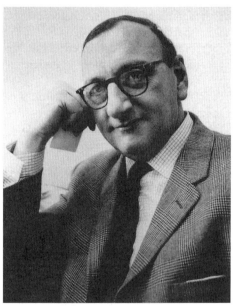

Fig. 12: Gordon Jackson Rees, MB.ChB, FFA.RCS (1918–)

Gordon Jackson Rees (Fig. 12)

A clinical virtuoso who made the practice of neonatal anesthesia look easy.

Born December 8, 1918 in Oswestry, Shropshire.

1942 Graduated MBChB, Liverpool University.
1946 DA England.
1951 FFARCS.
1963 Hon. FFA.RCS.
1946-1948 Residency at Oxford and Liverpool.
1948-1982 Consultant (attending) at Royal Liverpool Children's Hospital and Alder Hey Hospital; Director of Pediatric Anaesthetic Studies, Liverpool University.

Introduced:
1950 The Jackson Rees (Mapleson D) breathing system for controlled respiration in neonates without relaxants.
1960 Amplified use of his method to incorporate apneic doses of relaxants.
1966 Popularized long term nasal intubation for infants on ventilators using a special tube of his design.
1968 First emphasized the need for PEEP in neonatal respiratory deficiency syndrome.
Wrote chapters on Paediatric Anaesthesia, 1950; Neonatal Anaesthesia, 1960; and with T. C. Gray edited Paediatric Anaesthesia, 1981.

Donald H. Soucek, D.D.S., and Leslie Rendell-Baker, M.D. (Fig. 13)

The originators of the RBS pediatric face masks and pediatric anesthesia equipment with standard 15 mm. and 22 mm. fittings.

Donald Soucek, D.D.S., a dental resident in anesthesia at Western Reserve University's Lakeside Hospital in Cleveland, Ohio, in 1960, made face castings from the pediatric patients and modeled the face masks in hard wax from which prototype latex masks were made to fit them by the lost wax process.

Leslie Rendell-Baker, MB.BS, FRCA 1917–

Born March 27, 1917, St. Helen's Lancashire, England

1941 MB.BS Guy's Hospital Medical School, London University
1945-1947 Anesthesia training British Military Hospitals Germany and Guy's Hospital, London
1948-1957 First Assistant to Dr. William W. Mushin, Department of Anaesthesia, Cardiff, Wales
1955-1956 Fulbright Visiting Professor University of Pittsburgh
1957-1962 Assistant-Associate Professor Western Reserve University
1962-1979 Professor and Chairman Emeritus, Department of Anesthesia, Mt. Sinai School of Medicine, New York City
1979- Professor of Anesthesiology, Loma Linda University Present

Introduced:
1950 Narcotic-relaxant-N_2O/O_2 anesthesia in Britain (with Mushin)

Straight and baby connectors, computerized anesthesia record system, RBS pediatric facemasks and pediatric equipment, gas machine with Mapleson A system and jet

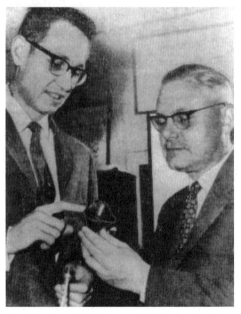

Fig. 13: Donald H. Soucek, D.D.S., and Leslie Rendell-Baker, M.D

ventilator, human engineered gas machine.

1958 to present: Member U.S. Anesthesia Standard Committee.

Produced standards on: 22 mm/15mm fittings, gas machine safety, implantation safety testing for tubes, safe hospital use of ethylene oxide. Legible labels for ampoules, syringe labels, prefilled syringe labels, black caps for vials of concentrated solutions, adopted by USP in 1993.

Author (jointly) - Automatic Ventilation of the Lungs 3 ed. The Origin of Thoracic Anaesthesia, Chapters: Hazards of Gas Machines, Hyperbaric Oxygen, Care of Anesth. Equipment, Development of Pediatric Anesthesia Equipment, Future Anesthesia Workstations, Impact of Standards.

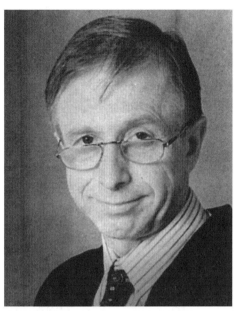

Fig. 14: Archie I. J. Brain, M.A., LMSSA, FFARCS(I) (1942–)

Archie I. J. Brain (Fig. 14)

Born in 1942 in Kobe, Japan.
1970 Graduated from Oxford and London University
Residency - the Royal London Hospital
Honorary Consultant Anaesthetist, Northwick Park Hospital, Harrow, England
Honorary Research Fellow, Institute of Laryngology
1983 Introduced the laryngeal mask airway, a new means of ensuring an airway without intubation.

Dr. Brain divides his time between lecturing worldwide (in five languages on use of the laryngeal mask airway) and research into new forms of airway control.

Robert Bryan Roberts (Fig. 15)

Born January 31, 1933, Holyhead, Wales.
1957 MB.BS., Kings College Hospital Medical School, London University.
1960 DA, England.
1961 FFARCS, England.
1958-1962 Residency at St. Mary Hospital, London and Welsh National School of Medicine, Cardiff.
1962-1968 Senior Resident, Kings College Hospital, London.
1964-1968 Research Fellow and Assistant Attending Anesthesiologist, Mt. Sinai Hospital, New York.
1968 Professor of Anesthesiology and Associate Professor of OB and Gynecology and Director, Obstetrical Anesthesia, Mt. Sinai Hospital, New York.
1968 Designed and produced first plastic disposable anesthesia breathing system (with Thomas J. Mahon).
1970- Chairman of ANSI.Z79 Ethylene Oxide Subcommittee.
1974 First introduction of pre-anesthetic oral antacids in USA to prevent aspiration pneumonitis in parturients with Dr. M. A. Shirley).
1976- Professor and Chairman Department

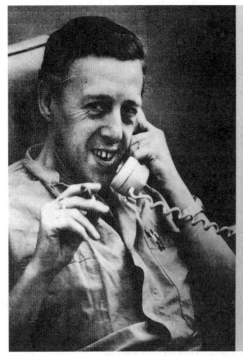
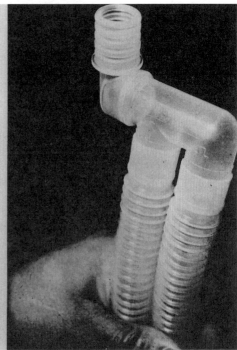

Fig. 15: Robert Bryan Roberts, MB.BS, FFARCS (1933-1983)

of Anesthesiology, Wright State University, Dayton, Ohio.

Publications:

Editor, Infections and Sterilization Problems Int. Anesthesiology Clinic, Vol. 10, #2. 1972. 2nd Edition, January 1976.

Practical Points in Anesthesiology with David C.C. Stark 1973. Medical Examination Publishing Co., New York

Papers on Obstetrical Anesthesiology and Prevention of Aspiration Pneumonitis; Ethylene Oxide versus Stearn Sterilization.

INTRODUCERS of new AGENTS

Dr. James Raventos (Fig. 16 on left)

Pharmacologist at the Imperial Chemical Company's laboratories at Alderley Edge near Macclesfield, England, performed the first animal studies with halothane 1956. These were followed by successful clinical trials in 1957.

An honorary Fellowship in the Faculty of Anaesthetists, Royal College of Surgeons of England was conferred on Dr. Raventos by Dr. John F. Nunn as the Dean of the Faculty on July 14, 1981, in a ceremony held at the ICI Laboratories due to Dr. Raventos' health.

Dr. Charles Suckling (Fig. 16 on right)

The graduate research chemist at Imperial Chemical Industries who with research chemist J. Ferguson worked from 1946-51 to produce a non-flammable volatile anesthetic agent. By 1951 they had synthesized hundreds of fluorocarbon compounds. Of the 10 chosen for biological screening by Raventos, halothane was the most promising. The first patient was anesthetized with halothane by Dr. Michael Johnstone at the Manchester Royal Infirmary on January 20,

1956. Dr.Suckling was awarded the Royal College of Anaesthetists Medal in 1992.

(Photograph courtesy Dr. John F. Nunn, Dean, Faculty of Anaesthetists, Royal College of Surgeons, London)

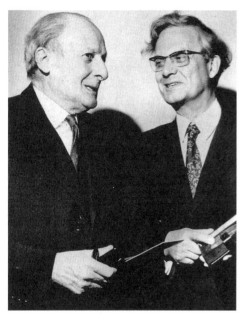

Fig. 16: (on left) Dr. James Raventos
(on right) Dr. Charles Suckling

Paul A. Janssen (Fig. 17)

Born 1926, Tournhout, Belgium.
1951   M.D., Ghent University.
1956   Ph.D., Pharmacology.

A Belgian experimental pharmacologist under whose leadership his staff have since 1954 synthesized over 83000 compounds resulting in 60 new therapeutic drugs being placed on the market. These drugs range from:
Antispasmodics: Lomotil, 1956; Imodium, 1970.
Narcotics: Dextromoramide, 1956; Phenoperidine, 1957; Fentanyl, 1960; Sufentanil, 1974; Alfentanil, 1976; Carfentanil (for animals).
Neuroleptics: Haloperidol; Droperidol.
Short-Acting Hypnotic: Etomidate, 1963.

Anti-fungal agents: Ketoconazole, Miconazole.
Anti-helmitic: Levamisole, originally intended for animals, now also used for colon cancer.
Accelerators of Digestive Tract: Domperidone; Metoclopramide.

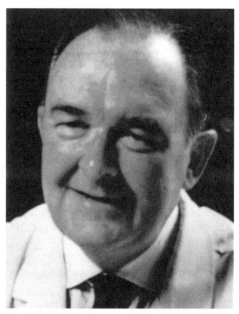

Fig. 17:   Paul A. Janssen, M.D., Ph.D. (1926–)

(Photograph from Schwartz H. Breakthrough; The Discovery of Modern Medicines at Janssen. New Jersey. Skyline Publishing 1989)

Francis F. Foldes (Fig. 18)

Born June 13, 1910, in Budapest, Hungary.
1934   Graduated M.D. from University of Budapest School of Medicine.
1938   Certified in internal medicine.
1941-1947   Specialized anesthesia training and member of staff, Massachusetts General Hospital.
1962-1975   Chairman Department of Anesthesiology, Montefiore Hospital, the Bronx, NY.
1964-   Professor of Anesthesiology, Albert

1975 Einstein College of Medicine, the Bronx, NY. Chairman of the Medical Advisory Board of the Myasthenia Gravis Foundation.

Introduced:
New Agents - Succinylcholine to U.S.A. in 1951, 2-chloroprocaine for epidurals in U.S.A. in 1952, levallorphan and naloxone with narcotics in anesthesia in 1954.
Equipment - Myoscan for assessment of degree of neuromuscular block.
Methods - Intravenous regional neuromuscular block for safe diagnosis of myasthenia gravis; neurolept analgesia for endoscopy.

Publications:
Books - Muscle Relaxants in Anesthesiology, 1957.
Narcotic and Narcotic Antagonists, (with Swerdlow & Siker), 1964. The Clinical Use of Muscle Relaxants, 1966. Enzymes in Anesthesiology, (editor) 1978. Over 500 papers and abstracts.

Honors:
Doctorates from University of Szeged, Berlin, Rostock, and Vienna.
Honorary Fellowships, Faculty of Anaesthetists of Royal College of Surgeons of England, and Royal College of Surgeons of Ireland.
Distinguished Service Award and Award for Excellence in Research, American Society of Anesthesiologists.
Past President, World Federation of Societies of Anesthesiologists.

DEVELOPERS of new METHODS

Virginia Apgar (Fig. 19)
Born Westfield, New Jersey in 1909.
1929 B.S., Mt. Holyoke College.
1933 Graduated M.D. from the College of Physicians and Surgeons, Columbia University, New York.

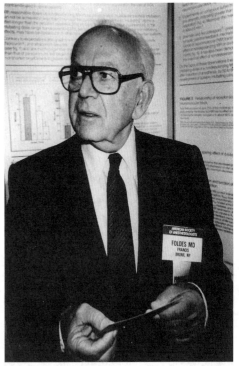

Fig. 18   Francis F. Foldes, M.D. 1910-1997

She intended to take up surgery but was persuaded by Chairman of the Department of Surgery to take up anesthesia as he was well aware of the need for physicians to take up the specialty.

There were then 13 anesthesia training programs in the U.S.A. and only 2 of them paid a salary. Her initial year's anesthesia training was by the head nurse anesthetist at Columbia, followed by 6 months in Madison with Ralph Waters, and then 6 months with Emery Rovenstine at Bellevue Hospital in New York.

In 1938 she was appointed Director, Division of Anesthesia and the sole Attending Physician Anesthetist at Columbia University Hospital. Though enthusiastic, she faced severe problems in recruiting medical staff and handling the clinical work load. However, by 1945, more anesthetics were

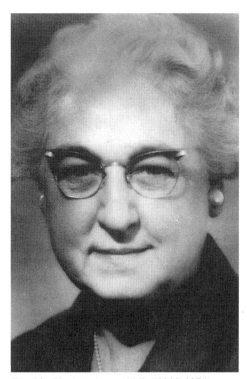

Fig. 19: Virginia Apgar, M.D. (1909-1974)

given by physicians at Columbia than by nurses. The end of WWII ended recruitment problems as demobilized physicians took up anesthesiology whose benefits to the patient and the surgeon they had experienced in the Army. But there was a demand for a strong research oriented department.

In 1949, when E.M. Papper was appointed Chairman of the independent Department of Anesthesiology, Apgar as Professor took over Obstetrical Anesthesia and formed a research group with Duncan Holaday, M.D., an anesthesiologist from 1950 in the blood gas lab, and Stanley James, M.D., a pediatric cardiologist from 1955.

1949-1951 Apgar Score evolved to identify the depressant effect of general anesthetics such as cyclopropane on the fetus. This put OB anesthesia on a scientific basis.

1959 Apgar took a sabbatical at Johns Hopkins to get a Masters degree in Public Health degree with training in statistics and genetics. In April 1959 she was recruited as Vice President for Scientific Research and Director of the National Foundation's (March of Dimes) new Division of Congenital Defects. In this new field she was enormously successful.

Her hobby was making violins!

(Photograph courtesy The Wood Library-Museum)

The Founders of the ICU

Bjorn Ibsen (Fig. 20, Center)
Born August 30, 1915.
1940 M.D. Copenhagen University
1949- Anesthesia residency - Massachusetts
1950 General Hospital

In 1952 Dr. Ibsen was an anesthesiologist at the Rigshospitalet (University Hospital) in Copenhagen. The city possessed only one tank ventilator and six cuirass ventilators when the epidemic of spino-bulbar poliomyelitis struck.

After 27 of 31 patients treated in them died, with more patients requiring artificial respiration being admitted, the Chief of the Blegdam Infectious Diseases Hospital called for Dr. Ibsen's help. On a desperately ill 12-year-old girl Dr. Ibsen demonstrated how tracheostomy with a cuffed tube permitted clearing of airway secretions by suction. This followed by adequate manual artificial respiration with a Waters to and fro CO_2 absorber system produced a prompt improvement in the patient's condition.

By using the same form of controlled ventilation then universally used in Copenhagen for thoracic anesthesia, Ibsen reduced the mortality from 80% to 25%. However, 450 students working in 8-hour shifts were needed to provide manual artificial respiration, thus making mechanical ventilators an

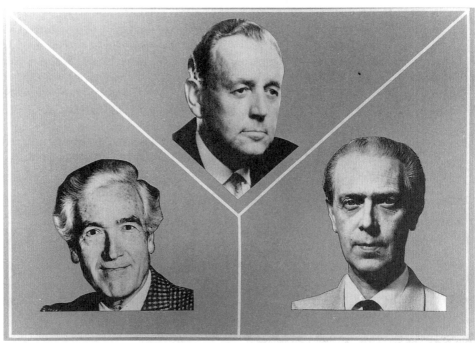

Fig. 20: (Center) Bjorn Ibsen, M.D. (1915–); (Left) Poul Astrup, M.D., Ph.D. (1915–); (Right) Carl-Gunnar Engstrom, M.D. (1913–1987)

urgent necessity. The Engstrom volume ventilator introduced in 1951 filled this need.

Ibsen revolutionized polio respiratory care in units which were copied world wide. In 1953, Ibsen became the chief anesthetist to the Municipal Hospital in Copenhagen where he established the first Intensive Care Unit in a general hospital. Later, Danish anesthetist disciples left for the U.S. and other countries to spread the ICU gospel world wide.

Poul Astrup (Fig. 20, Left)

Born August 14, 1915, Thy, Jutland, Denmark.

1939   M.D. Copenhagen University
1944   Ph.D. Copenhagen University

Astrup was chief of the clinical chemistry laboratory at the Blegdam infectious disease hospital in Copenhagen when the polio epidemic struck in 1952. He became convinced of the need for a faster method of determining the patient's arterial pH and pCO_2. In cooperation with Radiometer he introduced the bedside Astrup apparatus in 1954 which rapidly determined the pH and pCO_2 by the equilibration method, which revolutionized respiratory care.

Author (with John Severinghaus) - The History of Blood Gases, Acids and Bases. Munksgaard Copenhagen 1986, and The History of Blood Gas Analysis, Int. Anesth. Clinics. 1987. 25:4. (Source of this illustration.)

Carl-Gunnar Engstrom (Fig. 20, Right)

Born in Oskarshamn, Sweden in 1913.

1941   M.D. Stockholm University
1949-1950   Treated polio patients at the Stockholm Hospital for Contagious Diseases. Became convinced the positive-negative pressure ventilation in

tank ventilators resulted in hypoventilation which was masked by O_2 administration. So in 1950 he built a ventilator designed to provide predetermined volumes instead of certain pressures.

In 1951, the Engstrom Ventilator and his volume-controlled ventilation method became available in time to help in the Copenhagen polio epidemic

In 1955 the pioneer Swedish cardiac surgeon Viking Bjork and Engstrom introduced postoperative ventilator support for poor risk patients. Bjork's strong advocacy of this therapy after open heart surgery led to the widespread foundation of cardiac ICU's.

(Photograph courtesy Engstrom Medical AB, Bromma, Sweden)

Major R.R. Kirby (Fig. 21, Left) and A. Edward Weninger, (Right)

Bird Corporation in Los Angeles, 1971

With the Baby Bird ventilator they designed for the introduction of IMV and CPAP to treat neonatal respiratory distress syndrome, though these terms were introduced later

This original pneumatically controlled Baby Bird was later superseded by an electronically controlled model and Ed. Weninger went on to design pediatric ventilators for the Sechrist Company.

The Founders of High Frequency Ventilation (Fig. 22)

(Center) Ulf H. Sjostrand, M.D., Ph.D. and colleagues at Uppsala University, Sweden, in 1967 introduced high frequency positive pressure ventilation in an attempt to eliminate the effects fluctuations of intrathoracic pressure had on vascular pressure while investigating the carotid sinus reflexes. Their ventilator delivers high gas flows (175-250 L/min) into a circuit with minimal

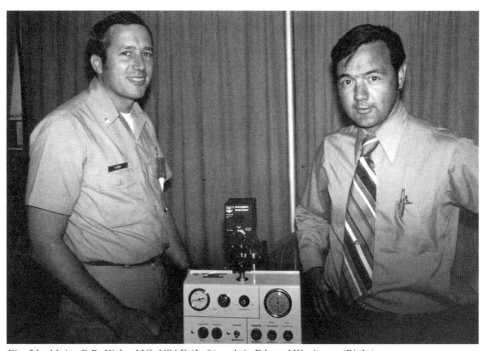

Fig. 21: Major R.R. Kirby, MC, USAF, (Left) and A. Edward Weninger, (Right)

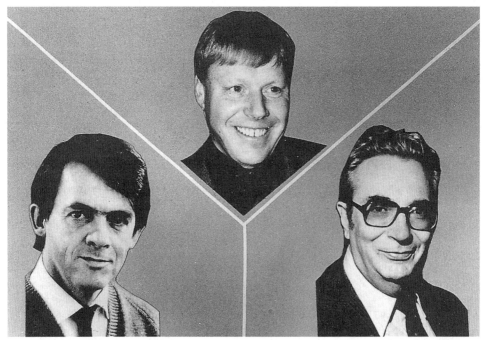

Fig. 22: The Founders of High Frequency Ventilation : (Center) Ulf H. Sjostrand, M.D., Ph.D. and Colleagues, (Left) Peter-Paul Lunkenheimer, M.D. and Colleagues, (Right) Mirislav Klain, M.D. and R.B. Smith, M.D

compressible volume producing 3-4 ml/kg tidal volumes 60-100 breaths/min. It is mainly used for laryngoscopy and bronchoscopy.

(Left) Peter-Paul Lunkenheimer, M.D. and colleagues in the Department of Experimental Surgery, University of Westphalia, Munster, Germany, 1972 wished to measure cardiac performances by myocardial reaction to pericardial pressure oscillations. The method required complete muscular relaxation and no respiratory pressure changes. They produced apneic oxygenation by pressure oscillations in the airway between 1,400 and 2,400 breaths per minute. The CO_2 was removed by a bypass fresh gas flow.

(Right) Mirislav Klain, M.D. and R.B. Smith, M.D. of Pittsburgh, Pennsylvania, successfully converted their fluidic jet ventilator designed for trans-tracheal emergency ventilation to high frequency operation (20 to 400 breaths/minute) after reading Sjostrand's reports.

John H. Emerson (Fig. 23)

patented this high frequency "people panter" breathing attachment for an IPPV ventilator in 1955 but there was little interest in this idea which was developed by Forrest Bird in his Percussionator in 1993 (see Fig. 10).

PIONEER PROFESSORS OF ANESTHESIA

Fig. 24 (Right) Ralph M. Waters, M.D. 1883-1979

Born on a farm in N. Bloomfield, Ohio, on October 9, 1883. Self-taught, he became the

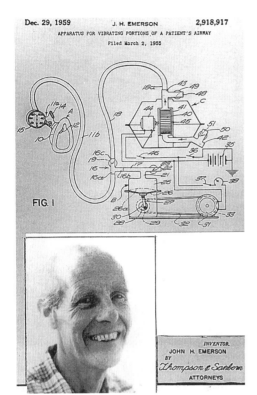

Fig. 23: John H. Emerson

leading professor of anesthesia in the USA in 1933.

- 1907 B.S., Adelbert College WRU Cleveland
- 1912-1913 M.D., Western Reserve University, Cleveland, Ohio. As a student he gave anesthesia and observed Charles K. Teter, D.D.S., pioneer of N_2O/O_2 anesthesia.
- 1912 In general practice, Sioux City, Iowa Began to concentrate his attention on anesthesia. By 1916 his practice was limited to anesthesia.
- 1919 Established first ambulatory surgery center Sioux City's Downtown Anesthesia Clinic, which had the first recovery room.
- 1920 Introduced closed circuit anesthesia with a to and fro soda-lime CO_2 absorber.
- 1926 Moved to Kansas City to take over the practice of an anesthetist there.
- 1927 Appointed head of Department of Anesthesia at University of Wisconsin at Madison where he introduced the anesthesia record system.
- 1928 Established first university residency program in anesthesia.
- 1928 Introduced cuffed tracheal tubes.
- 1930 Introduced cyclopropane into anesthesia.
- 1932 Introduced cuffed endobronchial tubes for chest surgery.
- 1933 Created Professor of Anesthesia at University of Wisconsin where he became the outstanding leader in anesthesia in the USA until he retired in 1949.
- 1936 Popularized "controlled respiration" with cyclopropane.
- 1936 Introduced sodium pentothal into anesthesia.

Dr. Waters trained a whole generation of heads of university departments of anesthesia including Virginia Apgar, Robert Dripps, Torsten Gordh, Merel Harmel, Austin Lamont, Digby Leigh, Lucien Morris, William Neff, Emory Rovenstine, Harvey Slocum, Perry Volpitto, et al.

William B. Neff (Fig. 24, Left)

Born July 1, 1908, in Philadelphia, PA.

- 1930 M.D., Hahnemann University, Philadelphia
- 1930- Residency with Harold Griffith, M.D., Queen Elizabeth Hospital, Montreal and with Ralph Waters, M.D., University of Wisconsin
- 1938- Chairman, Department of Anesthesiology, Stanford University, California
- 1930- As a resident with Dr. Waters and colleagues, he introduced cyclopro-

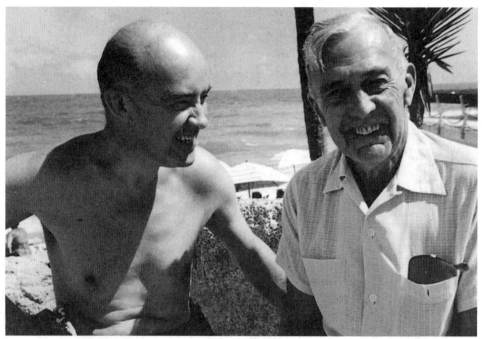

Fig. 24: (Left) William B. Neff, M.D., FFARCS (1908–1997); (right) Ralph M. Waters, M.D. (1883–1979)

1947 Introduced narcotic (Demerol) supplemented nitrous oxide - oxygen, curare anesthesia.
1950
1968 Introduced fresh gas driven venturi circulator for circle anesthesia systems.
1934
1979 Introduced magnetic drive circulator for completely closed CO_2 absorption system.

Neff was influential in establishing the Guedel Memorial Anesthesia Center in San Francisco.

Professor Sir Robert Macintosh (Fig. 25, Left)

Born 17th October 1897 in Timaru, New Zealand. Fighter pilot in WWI. First professor of anesthesia in Europe 1937.
1924 Graduated MB.BS Guy's Hospital Medical School, London University.
1926 FRCSE - took his Surgical Boards intending to become a surgeon. To earn money he gave anesthetics for London dentists and became so successful he gave up idea of surgery.

He gave such an excellent dental anesthetic to the philanthropist Lord Nuffield of Oxford that Nuffield decided to endow an additional University chair for Anaesthetics in Oxford to the four chairs he had proposed. He nominated Macintosh for the post and he was appointed in 1937.

He established the first British Department of Anaesthetics with a research and training program which greatly helped Ralph Tovell train anesthetists for the U.S. European Theatre forces during WWII.

Development of Equipment Vaporizers

1937- Went to Spain to help a maxillofacial surgeon friend operate on civil war casualties. Found there was neither O_2 or N_2O available so had to use a "Flagg
1938

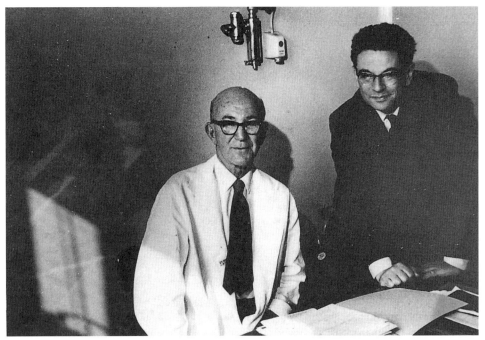

*Fig. 25: (Left) Professor Sir Robert Macintosh, M.A., M.D., FRCSE, FFARCS, (1897-1989),
(Right) Hans G. Epstein, Ph.D. (1913–)*

can" - a drawover air/ether vaporizer. This stimulated him to design, with H.G. Epstein, Ph.D., a range of accurate drawover vaporizers.

1940-1941 Oxford ether/air vaporizer with attached manual resuscitation bellows. These were built in Lord Nuffield's automobile plant and were presented by him to the British Army.

1941 Macintosh curved bladed laryngoscope developed from Davis ENT gag by Macintosh with his technician, Richard Salt.

1942 ESO (Epstein - Suffolk - Oxford) chloroform/air vaporizer built for and used by the British Parachute Medical Units.

1949 Emotril temperature compensated trichloreltrylene/air OB analgesia apparatus.

1950 EMO (Epstein-Macintosh-Oxford) ether/air temperature compensated drawover vaporizer used with Oxford Inflating Bellows in developing countries.

1950 Oxford large bore tracheal tube.

1955 Macintosh-Leatherdale endobronchial tube.

1966 Oxford miniature vaporizer for halothane - used as part of the Tri-Services Apparatus by the British Army in the Falkland Islands campaign 1987.

Books

1940 Macintosh & Bannister, Essentials of General Anesthesia

1944 Macintosh & Mushin, Local Anaesthesia-Brachial Plexus

1947 Macintosh & Mushin, Physics for the Anaesthetist

1955 Macintosh & Ostlene, Local Analgesia - Head and Neck

1957 Macintosh, Lumbar Puncture & Spinal Anaesthesia

1962 Macintosh & Bryce Smith, Local Analgesia - Abdominal Surgery

Hans G. Epstein (Fig. 25 Right)

Physicist to the Nuffield Department of Anaesthetics, 1940-1976.

Operated the research laboratories and designed the Oxford precision drawover vaporizers.

1940-1941 Oxford ether/air vaporizer for British Army.
1942 ESO chloroform/air vaporizer for British parachute medical units.
1949 Emotil trichlorethylene/air OB vaporizer.
1953 EMO ether/air vaporizer for developing countries.
1966 Oxford miniature halothane/air vaporizer - used in British Tri-Services military anesthesia apparatus.

Tested these vaporizers for accuracy.

Author with Macintosh and Mushin of Physics for the Anaesthetist, 1958.

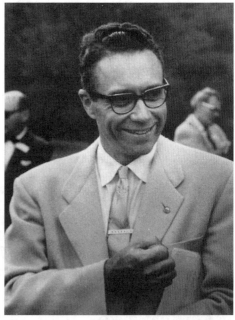

Fig. 26: Robert A. Hingson, M.D. (1913-1996)

Robert A. Hingson (Fig. 26)

Pioneered continuous caudal analgesia for obstetrics, 1942, and jet injection for mass immunizations, 1957.

Born in Anniston, Alabama, April 13, 1913.
A.B.   University of Alabama, 1935.
M.D.   Emory University, 1938.
D.Sc. Thomas Jefferson University, 1964.

Served in U.S. Coastguard in North Atlantic - helped to rescue 300 survivors of torpedoed British liner, SS Athenia.

Fellow in Anesthesia, Mayo Clinic, 1940-1942.

1942 First described continuous caudal analgesia for OB in Lull and Hingson, Control of Pain in Childbirth, 1942, using plastic catheters and malleable steel needles which he introduced. Hingson and Hellman, Anesthesia for Obstetrics.

1943-1945 Established OB caudal analgesia service at Philadelphia Lying-in Hospital, Jefferson Medical College.

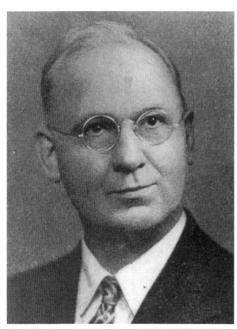

Fig. 27: Dennis E. Jackson, M.D. (1878-1980)

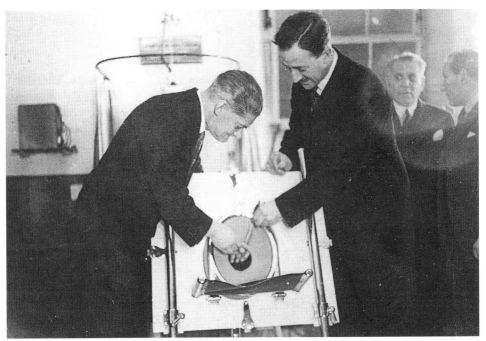

Fig. 28: William Morris, Lord Nuffield of Oxford

1945-1948	Professor of Anesthesia, University of Tennessee.
1948-1951	Associate Professor of Anesthesia, Department of Obstetrics, Johns Hopkins University.
1949	Introduced Xylocaine in United States and United Kingdom.
1951-1951	Chairman, Department of Anesthesiology, Western Reserve University, Cleveland
1954	Edited Pitkin's Conduction Anesthesia, 1954. Introduced portable anesthesia apparatus and resuscitator. Introduced jet injection for mass
1969	immunization against 8 epidemic diseases. Initiated a smallpox eradication campaign in Liberia which preceded the WHO campaign.
1958	Founded Brothers Brothers charitable foundation which continues to provide medical, educational and food resources for populations in need.

Dennis E. Jackson (Fig. 27)

Born September 3, 1878, in Ridgeport, Indiana.

1905	A.B., Indiana University.
1908	Ph.D., Indiana University.
1913	M.D., Rush Medical School, Chicago University.
1910-1918	Taught pharmacology and biochemistry as associate instructor to associate professor at Washington University, St. Louis.
1915	Built first circle CO_2 absorption anesthesia apparatus for use in the dog lab. In spite of his demonstrations of this apparatus, clinical anesthetists were not interested in this method until 1930.
1917	Published Experimental Pharmacology, 2nd edition in 1939; both editions illustrated his anesthesia apparatus and ventilators for use with animals.
1918	Built a portable circle absorption anesthesia apparatus which he offered

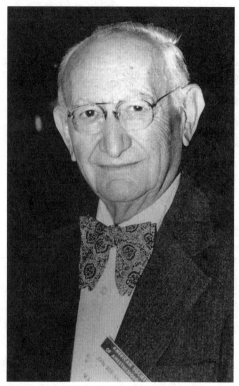

Fig. 29: John Adriani, M.D. (1907-1988)

(Photograph from Thomas E. Keys The History of Surgical Anesthesia. New York. Schuman's. Fig. 36 1945)

William Morris, Lord Nuffield of Oxford (Fig. 28)

This pioneer British automobile manufacturer presenting one of his Both body ventilators to Guy's Hospital, London in 1938.

- 1937 He endowed the first chair in anesthesia in Europe in Oxford and nominated Robert Macintosh as professor.
- 1938 He built and presented "iron lungs" to any British hospital requesting one. Macintosh provided the instruction in their use, producing three films for this purpose.
- 1940 His firm built 1,000 Oxford ether/air drawover vaporizers designed by Macintosh and Epstein and presented them to the British Army.
- 1942 An ESO chloroform/air drawover vaporizer was produced by the Nuffield Department for British Parachute Medical Units.

Nuffield's philanthropies amounted to $120 million.

John Adriani (Fig. 29)

Born December 2, 1907, Bridgeport, Connecticut.

- 1926- A.B., Columbia University, New York.
- 1934 M.D., College of Physicians & Surgeons, Columbia.
- 1934- Intern, Surgery, French Hospital, New York City.
- 1936- Trained in anesthesia under Rovenstine at Bellevue, then became instructor 1939-41.
- 1930
- 1941 He was appointed without an interview as Chief of Anesthesia Services at Charity Hospital, never having been to New Orleans, to oversee 40 OR's,
- 1936

to the U.S. Army. The Army consultant surgeons felt it was too complicated for their anesthetists.

- 1920- Professor and Head of Department of Pharmacology & Materia Medica, Cincinnati College of Medicine.
- 1924 Advised Ralph Waters on the design of his to and fro CO_2 absorption apparatus.
- 1927 Built a combined circle absorption anesthesia apparatus and ventilator. He successfully demonstrated it on one apneic patient but clinicians rejected it in favor of manual chest compression methods of artificial respiration. So it was used in the dog lab. He was 30 years ahead of U.S. anesthetists.
- 1934- Describes the value of trichlorethylene as an anesthetic.
- 1935

Editor: American Lecture Series on Anesthesia, Charles C. Thomas

He was uniquely appointed Professor of Anesthesia at all three universities: Louisiana State University, Tulane, and Loyola School of Dentistry. He was also director of Charity Hospital's Blood Bank and Respiratory Therapy Department. He had a major impact on the teaching of anesthesia in the Southern states.

T. Cecil Gray (Fig. 30)

Born March 11, 1913, in Liverpool.
1937 Graduated MB.ChB, from Liverpool University.
1941 DA, England (Anesthesia Boards).
1946 M.D., Liverpool.
1948 FFA.RCS. Anesthesia training under Dr. R. J. Minuitt at the David Lewis Northern Hospital, Liverpool.
1943-1946 With Halton, performed the first experiments in Britain using tubocurarine during anesthesia. "A milestone in anaesthesia." Proc. Roy Soc Med 1946. 39:400. He also evolved the "Liverpool technique" of using apneic doses of relaxants with N_2O/O_2 anesthesia and controlled respiration.
1947 Appointed Reader in Anaesthetics (Assistant Professor), Liverpool University.
1947-1963 Joint Editor of British Journal of Anaesthesia.
1957-1959 President of Association of Anaesthetists of Great Britain.
1959-1976 Professor of Anaesthetics, Liverpool University.
1964-1967 Dean, Faculty of Anaesthetists, Royal College of Surgeons.
1970-1976 Dean of Faculty of Medicine, Liverpool University.

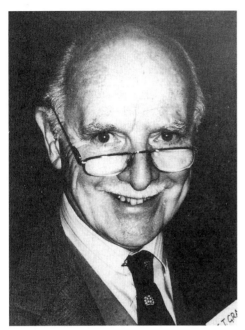

Fig. 30: T. Cecil Gray, CBE, KCSG, MD, FRCP, FRCS, FFA.RCS, (1913–)

1939 10 delivery rooms, and 40 nurse anesthetists, with only 2 laryngoscopes; he succeeded.

His research included:

Evaluation of the function of CO_2 absorbers, soda lime and pH indicators, efficiency of barium and calcium hydroxides as absorbents; effects of humidity on CO_2 absorption; improved pediatric tracheal tube, tracheal tube cuffs, rebreathing in pediatric anesthesia and an improved apparatus; fate of anesthetic drugs in the body, stability of di vinyl ether; effects of anesthetics on bronchi and bronchioles; silent regurgitation and aspiration; Seconal as a basal hypnotic; effect of vasopressors on duration of spinals.

He wrote:

Techniques and Procedures of Anesthesia.
Pharmacology of Anesthetic Drugs, 1941.
The Chemistry and Physics of Anesthesia, 1946.
The Selection of Anesthesia, 1955.

Publications and books:

1959 Operating Theaters and Ancillary Rooms (with Nunn).

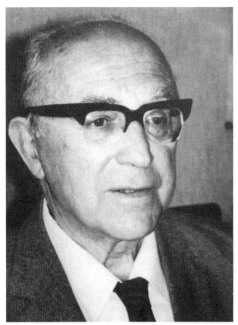

Fig. 31: William W. Mushin, CBE, MB.BS, MA, FRCS, DSC, FC Anaes, (1910-1993)

1964 Modern Trends in Anesthesia (4 editions)
1967 General Anesthesia (4 editions)
1981 Paediatric Anaesthesia (with G. Jackson Rees).

William W. Mushin (Fig. 31)

Born 1910, London, England
1933 MB.BS, London Hospital Medical School, London University, Resident Anaesthetist, London Hospital.
1940 DA, Royal College of Surgeons, London.
1940 Introduced Coxeter-Mushin Absorber & Vaporizer.
1943 Appointed First Assistant to Professor Macintosh in Nuffield Department of Anaesthetics, Oxford.
1946 Published Physics for the Anesthetist with Macintosh with many later editions.
1947 Local Anaesthesia - Brachial Plexus with Macintosh.
1947 Director, and later, Professor of Anaesthetics, Welsh National School of Medicine, Cardiff.
1948 Anaesthesia for the Poor Risk and other essays.
1953 Principles and Practice of Thoracic Anaesthesia with Rendell-Baker.
1963 Editor of Thoracic Anaesthesia.
1965 Automatic Ventilation of the Lungs with Rendell-Baker & Thompson.
1949 Introduced narcotic supplemented N_2O/O_2 relaxant anesthesia in Britain with Rendell-Baker.

Former Dean of Faculty of Anaesthetists of the Royal College of Surgeons.

Former Chairman, Safety of Drugs Committee.

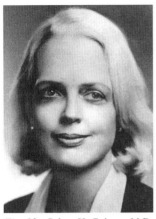 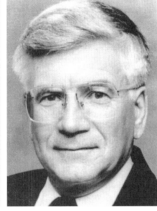 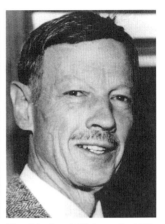

Fig. 32: Selma H. Calmes, M.D. *Fig. 33: Rod K. Calverley, M.D.* *Fig. 34: Jacob Mainzer, Jr., M.D.*

Wood Library-Museum · American Society of Anesthesiologists:

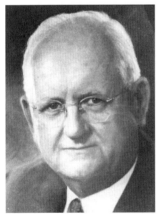 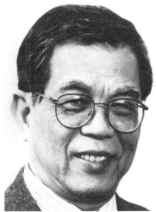 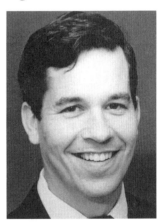

Fig. 35: Founder: Paul M. Wood, MD, FICA, FACA, DABA (1894–1963) *Fig. 36: Librarian: Patrick P.K. Sim, MLS* *Fig. 37: Honorary Curator: George S.L. Bause, M.D.*

Arthur Läwen - his Work in the Field of Anaesthesiology

Ziegler, U., Kohlweyer B., Wiedemann, B.
Clinic of Anaesthesiology, Städtisches Klinikum St. Georg
Leipzig, Germany

Georg Arthur Läwen (Fig. 1) was born on the 6th of February, 1876 as the son of an officer in Waldheim (Saxony) and baptized on the 29th of March in the church of a castle in Waldheim. He initially studied medicine in Rostock but moved to Freiburg and eventually to Munich only to become registered at "Alma Mater Lipsiens" in 1898. During the course of his education he attended lectures in surgery held by Friedrich Trendelenburg (1844-1924) as well as classes in pharmacology under the supervision of Rudolf Böhm (1844-1926). He passed his National Board Examination in medicine in 1900, the year he started his surgical training at the Diakonissen-Hospital in Leipzig under Heinrich Braun (1862-1934) who suggested for him to become an assistant doctor at the Department of Surgery at the University of Leipzig with Friedrich von Trendelenburg being the head. He submitted his "Habilitation" in 1908 and became chairman of the Department of Surgery at the new municipal hospital St. Georg in Leipzig in 1913 being appointed associate professor. Being asked to go to Marburg as a "full" professor he left in 1920 and moved on to Königsberg in 1927. During World War I as well as World War II he became occupied in surgical and anaesthesiological problems relating to injuries acquired during war. After World War II he lived in the area of the Lüneburger Heide with his daughter until he died on the 30th of January, 1958.

His work concerning surgery was honored with a membership in the German Society of Surgery – acknowledgment for his contribu-

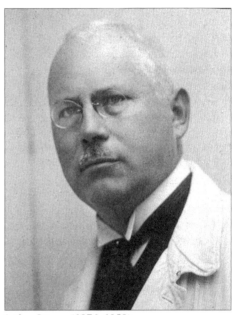

Arthur Läwen (1876–1958)

tion to the development in the field of anaesthesiology was not shed until in the last decade of this century.

Arthur Läwen used nerves of frogs for detailed in vitro investigations on the effect of novocain, cocaine, alypin and stovain. He recognized the danger of the latter substance and thus advised his colleagues not to utilize it. He also introduced sodium bicarbonate in order to enhance the analgesic effect and recommended to prepare a "fresh" solution right before its application and to boil it for a few seconds as to achieve the best possible effect.

By means of a paravertebral injection of 10 ml novocain 0.5% or tutocain per segment, Arthur Läwen was able to achieve analgesia for the first time which made him suggest to apply this method while operating on inguinal hernias, the kidney or the ureter in cases of high risk for general anaesthesia, as well as to secure the diagnosis of a painful gallbladder, kidney or ureter and last but not least to treat postoperative pain. Thus this technique reduced to incidence of intra- and postoperative complications.

Läwen and Roderich Sievers (1878-1943) successfully maintained the action of the heart in a patient suffering from serious brain injury for more than nine hours by artificial respiration herewith sustaining the option of long-term artificial respiration via tracheostomy and proving the effect of adrenaline on the heart. This would not have been possible without Lwens discovery of curarin that had to be applied simultaneously. Visions of thoracic surgery as well as of the treatment of tetanus or poisoning by strychnine came up.

If we look back to the invention of local anaesthetics, Fernand Cathelin (1873-1945) injected cocaine into the hiatus sacralis in the beginning of the 20th century and Walter Stoeckel (1871-1961) applied novocain in order to reduce the pain in obstetrics. Arthur Lwen however was the first person to achieve complete analgesia by the application of a special solution containing novocain injected through the hiatus sacralis to the extradural space. His standard method (sodium bicarbonate ad 20 ml novocain 1,5%) brought about sufficient analgesia of the perineal region - the effect lasting for about two hours.

References:

1. Goerig M, Schulte am Esch J: Arthur Läwen. Ein Wegbereiter moderner Ansthesieverfahren. Anaesthesiol Intensivmed Notfallmed Schmerzther 1993; 29: 315-325
2. Läwen A: Weitere Erfahrungen ber paravertebrale Schmerzaufhebung zur Differentialdiagnose von Erkrankungen der Gallenblase, des Magens, der Niere und des Wurmfortsatzes sowie zur Behandlung postoperativer Lungenkomplikationen. Zbl f Chir 1923 ; 50, 12: 460-465
3. Läwen A: Erinnerungen an Trendelenburg. Der Chirurg 1932; 1: 25-34
4. Läwen A: Über Paravertebralansthesie zur Operation von Leisten- und Schenkelhernien. Der Schmerz 1928; 4: 289-293
5. Läwen A: Die Extraduralansthesie. Ergebnisse der Chirurgie und Orthopädie 1913; 5: 38-84
6. Braun H, Läwen A: Die örtliche Betäubung, ihre wissenschaftlichen Grundlagen und praktische Anwendung . Verlag von Johann Ambrosius Barth, Leipzig 1933
7. Läwen A: Weitere Beitrge zur Sakralanästhesie und zur Paravertebralanästhesie für diagnostische und operative Zwecke. Münch Med Wochenschr 1925; 35: 1449-1452
8. Läwen A: Über segmentäre Schmerzaufhebung durch paravertebrale Novokaininjektionen zur Differentialdiagnose intraabdomineller Erkrankungen. Münch Med Wochenschr 1922; 40: 1423-1426
9. Läwen A: Lokalanästhesie für Nierenoperationen. Münch Med Wochenschr 1911; 26: 1390-1392
10. Läwen A: Alte und neue örtliche Betäubungsmittel. Fortschritte der Therapie 1930; 6: 20-23
11. Läwen A 1906: Vergleichende experimentelle Untersuchungen über die örtliche Wirkung einiger neuer Lokalanästhetika (Stovain, Novokain und Alypin) auf motorische Nervenstämme. Bruns Beiträge zur klin Chir 1906; 50: 623-665
12. Läwen A, Gaza W von 1911: Experimentelle Untersuchungen über Extraduralanästhesie. Deutsch Zeitschr f Chir 1911; 11:289-307
13. Läwen A Jahr: Über die Verwendung des Novokains in Natriumbikarbonat. Kochsalz-lösungen zur lokalen Anästhesie . Münch Med Wochenschr 1911; 39: 2044-2046
14. Läwen A, Sievers R: Zur praktischen Anwendung der instrumentellen künstlichen Respiration am Menschen . Münch Med Wochenschr 1910; 49: 2221-2225

Ernst Jeger - a Nearly Forgotten Pioneer in Cardio-Vascular Surgery and Thoracic Anaesthesia

H. J. Klippe,
Department of Anaesthesiology, Krankenhaus Großhansdorf, Germany

Ernst Jeger (1884-1915), born to Jewish parents in Vienna, performed his medical studies with remarkable results at the University of Vienna (Fig.1). His medical education covered schooling in London, Berlin, New York and Vienna with an emphasis on experimental and clinical surgical work. In 1912 he visited the surgeon Charles Elsberg (1871-1948) at the Mount Sinai Hospital in New York and Alexis Carrel (1873-1944), a vascular surgeon and Noble prize winner in 1912. He also met the physiologists Samuel James Meltzer (1851-1922) and John Auer (1875-1948) at the Rockefeller Institute for Medical Research, investigating apnoeic oxygenation and the solution to the problem of pneumothoraces by their "intratracheal insufflation technique" (Fig.2). This led Jeger to modify their original technique of endotracheal insufflation by a double-lumen endotracheal tube with an inflatable rubber balloon (Fig. 3a, 3b, 3c).

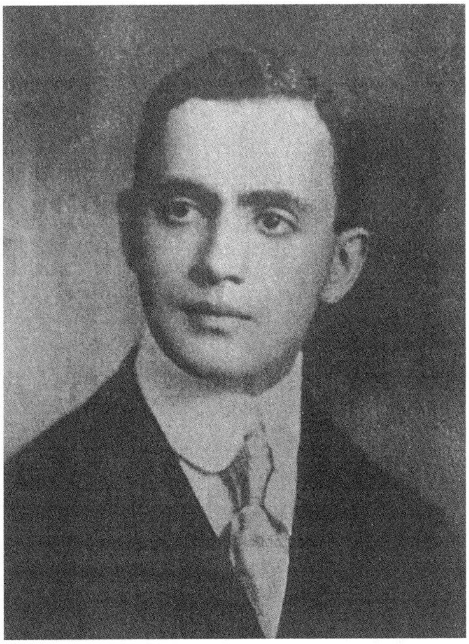

After having returned to Germany he continued his experimental surgical work in Berlin and Breslau, again being involved in vascular surgery mainly. His book "Die Chirurgie der Blutgefaesse und des Herzens" in 1913 can be considered to be a highlight of vascular and experimental heart surgery in the beginning of the 20th century and has to be looked at as one of the "classics" in this field today. His techniques concerning major intrathoracic vessels were important contributions far ahead of that time. At the International Medical Congress in London in 1913, Jeger gave a lecture of a number of vascular operations, that was highly acknowledged by international authorities.

At the beginning of World War I he had to join the German army as a surgeon (Fig. 4). In Przemysl/Poland he worked with Robert Barany (1876-1936), a well-known Austrian surgeon and Noble prize winner in 1915. Again he performed vascular surgery, saving the nearly amputated right arm of a soldier by vascular and nerval reconstruction after stabilization of the humerus (Fig.5).

For the treatment of thoracic injuries he constructed a simplified pressure anaesthesia apparatus with excellent results (Fig.6).

Fig. 1: Portrait of Ernst Jeger, thoracic and vascular surgeon

Taken captive by Russian troops Jeger contracted severe abdominal typhus and died in a Russian hospital on August 30th, 1915, halting a very promising scientific and surgical career far too early (Fig.7,8).

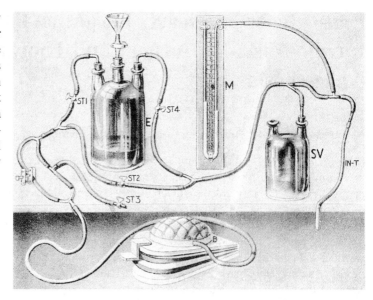

Fig. 2: Meltzer-Auer's device for artificial respiration

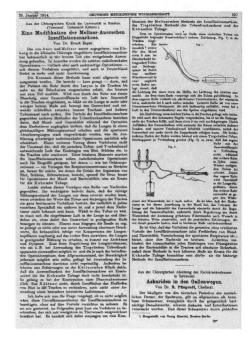

Fig. 3a: Cover page of Jeger's publication in which he decribed the advantageous use of an inflatable tracheal tube for apnoeic insufflation technique

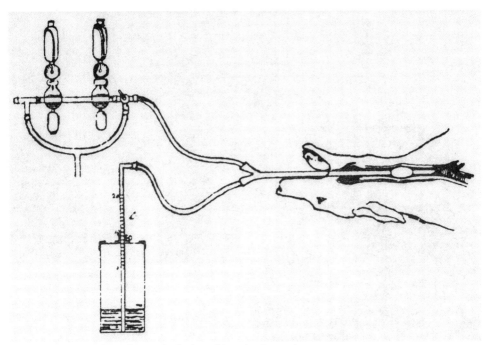

Fig. 3b: Scheme of the technique he had used in animal experiments

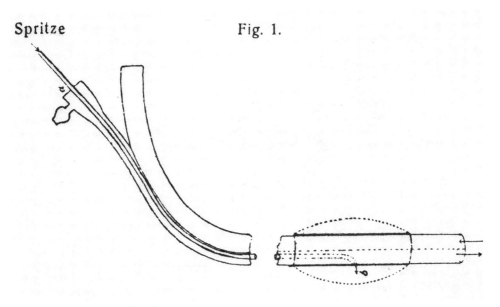

Fig. 3c: The tube he used for his experiments

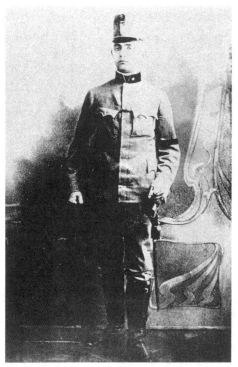

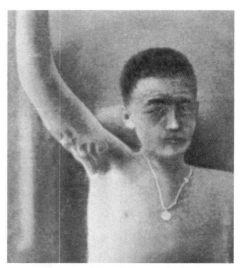

Fig. 5: Portrait of the soldier who had been operated by Jeger and in whom he had performed vascular surgery, saving the nearly amputated right arm of a soldier by vascular and nerval reconstruction after stabilization of the humerus

Fig. 4: Jeger as surgeon of the army during World War I

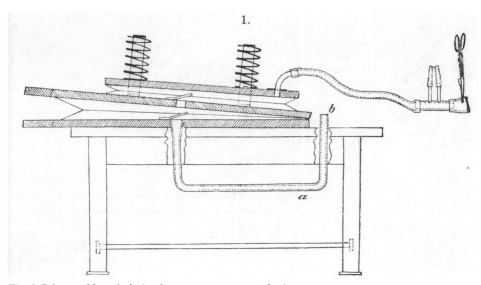

Fig. 6: Scheme of Jeger's device for overpressure anaesthesia

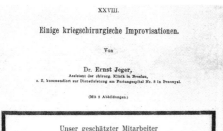

Fig. 7: Cover page of the surgical journal in which his death was announced in 1915

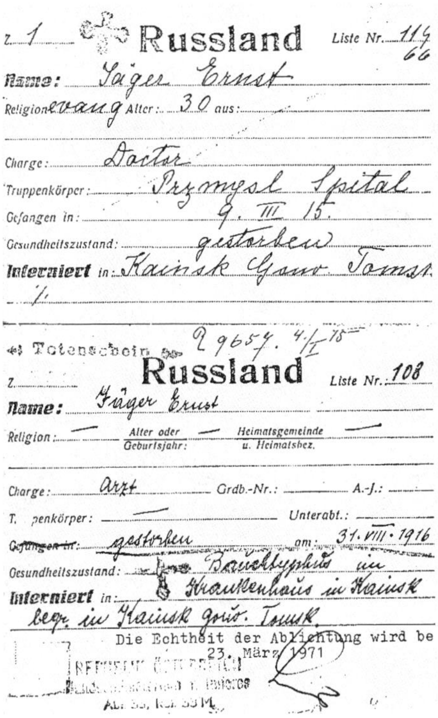

Fig. 8: Ernst Jeger's death certificate

Paul Frenckner - a Swedish Pioneer in Bronchology and Thoracic Anaesthesia

H. J. Klippe
Department of Anaesthesiology, Krankenhaus Großhansdorf, Germany

Paul Frenckner (1896-1967) (Fig. 1) received his medical education at the Karolinska Hospital, Stockholm, being a student of Gunnar Holmgren (1875-1954), the „father of Swedish otorhinolaryngology". Since his visit at Gustav Killian (1860-1921) in 1907, Holmgren had a life-long interest in bronchology. Thus in 1928/29 Holmgren sent Frenckner to Chevalier Jackson senior and junior who were living in Philadelphia - USA and who both were the outstanding specialists world-wide. Hereby and by additional impulse by H. Chr. Jacobaeus (1879-1937) - the Swedish pioneer in thoracoscopy - bronchology became Frenckner`s main field of interest. Back to Stockholm, Holmgren and Frenckner spent a lot of time building up the field of bronchology in Sweden.

In 1934 Frenckner presented his remarkable thesis on „Tracheal and Bronchial Catheterization", including a double lumen bronchoscope in a rigid and a semiflexible version for tracheobronchial intubation and bronchospirometry (Fig.2a,2b,2c). It is a remarkable fact that he presented both in a rigid and a semirigid version, the latter 20 years before comparable other developments were available. This double lumen bronchoscope, still in the 1940`s presented as „Dubbelbronchoskop av Frenckner" in the catalogue of the Swedish Still-Werner AB, Stockholm, is due to be of design quality for the famous double lumen tube which was presented by Carlens the first time in 1949. The thoracic surgeon Clarence Crafoord (1899-1984) asked Frenckner for help since

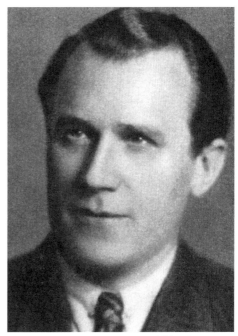

Fig. 1: Paul Frenckner (1896-1967) - the most important Swedish pioneer in bronchology and thoracic anaesthesia.

he was in need of a technique to be able to ventilate patients during thoracic surgery. He also presented his Spiropulsator - manufactured in his company AGA - in the same year (Fig.3). This was a respirator to facilitate IPPB, the frequency being controlled with the so-called „flasher", a bimetal timer invented for marine lighthouses by Gustav Dahlén.

In the forties Frenckner developed cannulae and catheters for surgical and spirometric procedures with Eric Carlens (1908-

1990) and thus had a great impact on Swedish scientific and technical medical development (Fig. 4). In 1957 Frenckner was appointed Professor for ENT. E. Carlens owes a lot of credit to him in the invention of his double lumen endobronchial tube.

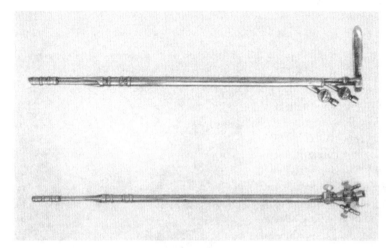

Fig. 2a: Frenckner`s double lumen bronchoscope in a rigid version for tracheo-bronchial intubation and bronchospirometry

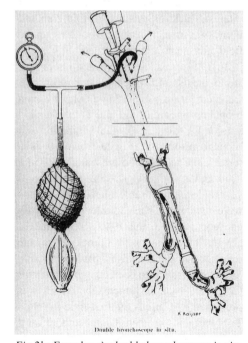

Fig.2b: Frenckner`s double bronchoscope in situ

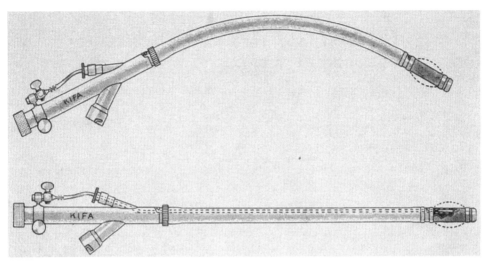

Fig.2c: Frenckner`s double lumen bronchoscope in semiflexible version for tracheobronchial intubation and bronchospirometry

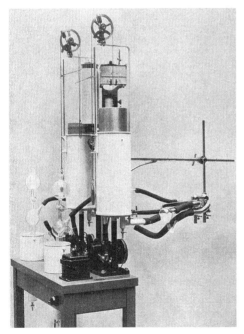

Fig. 3: Double lumen spirometer according to Bjoerkman, developed for the application of Frenckneŕs double lumen bronchoscope.

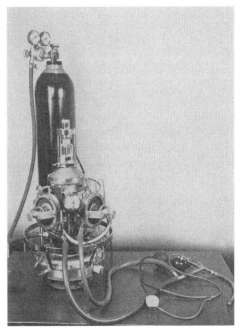

Fig.4: Frenckner's Spiropulsator. This respirator was constructed in 1934 facilitating IPPB. Later – based on the same principle – the Engstroem-Respirator was developed.

Eric Carlens - a Skilful Swedish Pioneer in Bronchology and Thoracic Medicine

H. J. Klippe,
Department of Anesthesiology, Krankenhaus Großhansdorf, Germany

In Sweden diagnosis and therapy of airway and lungs have always been of special interest and a lot of famous people origin from this region, e.g. Gunnar Holmgren (1875-1954), the „father of Swedish otolaryngology", H.C. Jacobaeus (1879-1937), who invented thoracoscopy in 1910 and has always been very interested in pulmonary problems, K.H. Giertz (1876-1950), a disciple of Sauerbruch and founder of Swedish thoracic surgery, as well as Clarence Crafoord (1899-1984), who was an outstanding cardiothoracic surgeon (Fig.1). Eric Carlens had a very remarkable position, too. From 1934 on, he had been trained in ENT together with Paul Frenckner (1896-1967). In 1944 Crafoord asked him to join his cardiothoracic team and Carlens stayed with him until 1975. Carlens' (1908-1990) importance in the field of bronchology and thoracic medicine can not be overestimated (Fig.2). He continued Frenckner's outstanding work in this field and in airway management.

In 1949 he presented his famous double lumen tube for endobronchial intubation, which was originally developed for spirometry (Fig.3). It was Björk, the cardiothoracic surgeon, who recognized its importance for surgery on the lungs. In 1950

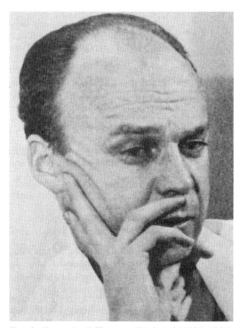

Fig. 1: *Portrait of Clarence Crafoord (1899-1984)*

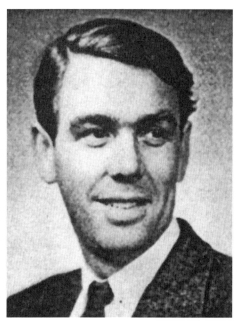

Fig. 2: *Portrait of Eric Carlens (1908-1990)*

Carlens and Björk published results on 15 successfully intubated patients who had undergone pulmonary resections. Due to the invention of this tube the total number of pulmonary operation in Sweden and elsewhere rose rather quickly, and according to this the number of patients in whom intrathoracic lymph node metastases could be detected grew, too. All endobronchial tubes (Norris, Gebauer 1939, Zavod 1940, Frenckner's devices) showed disadvantages of some kind according to Carlens. Thus, in 1949 he introduced his double lumen tube to bronchospirometry. Björk immediately recognized its value for lung surgery and anaesthesia in these patients.Carlens stayed at Stockholm's Sabbatsberg and Karolinska Hospitals with his staff for thoracic surgery

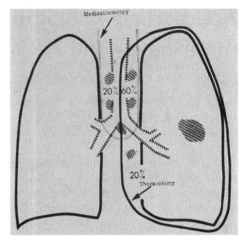

Fig. 4: Mediastinoscopy, as suggested by Clarence Crafoord

from 1944 until 1975 being involved in bronchology, which he had a great skill for.

Clarence Crafoord was an outstanding Swedish cardiothoracic surgeon who invented the endobronchial blocking tube in 1938. Paul Frenckner and Eric Carlens worked with him over decades. His credo was: „Teamwork is the basis for each form of scientific progress." In 1958 Carlens invented mediastinoscopy in order to reach lymphnodes of the mediastinum to be able to carry out preoperative staging of patients with malignant chest tumors (Fig. 4). The main intention was to reduce the number of unnecessary thoracotomies in patients suffering from extensive lymph node infiltration in bronchopulmonary carcinomas. Very soon, though, he and other physicians recognized the far spread diagnostic value of this technique for a variety of bronchopulmonary diseases.

In the early 1960's Carlens was the first to use mediastinoscopy to place cardiac pacemaker electrodes on the atrium directly. In this early stage of cardiac pacing this technique facilitated the procedure, thus avoiding thoracotomy, especially in high risk individuals (Fig.5). In 1968 Carlens was appointed

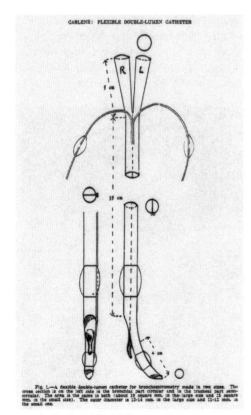

Fig. 3: Carlens' double lumen tube

professor and dedicated a lot of his time to fight tobacco smoking, since it was considered to be one of the main factors causing bronchopulmonary carcinomas.

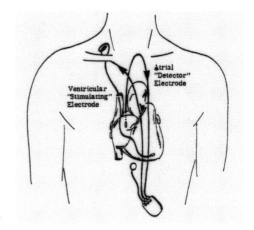

Fig. 5:
The technique of positioning pacemaker-electrodes via mediastinoscopy

Heliodor Święcicki, the Inventor of modern Analgesia for Delivery

W. Jurczyk, J. Kroll and P. Kroll
Department of Anaesthesiology and Intensive Therapy of the Karl Marcinkowski University of Medical Sciences in Poznan, Poland

Heliodor Święcicki was one of the brightest physicians of Polish medicine (Fig. 1). He lived between 1854 and 1923. In the years 1873-1877 he studied at the University of Breslau. While a student he published two dissertations. One of them "The Care of Children in Ancient Greece" became his doctoral dissertation (1877). Between 1882 and 1884 he was gaining his experience and specialisation in the field of gynaecology and obstetrics under such famous personalities as Franz Wilhelm von Winckel (1837 – 1911, Dresden), Paul Zweifel (1848 – 1922, Erlangen). Bernhard S. Schultze (1827 – 1919, Jena), Karl Schröder (1838 – 1887) and A. Gusserow (Berlin) and C. S. Credé (1819 – 1892, Leipzig). At the beginning of the 1885 he settled down in Poznan. He was the first Polish doctor in Poznan working exclusively as a gynaecologist and obstetrician, being at the same time the first modern specialist in this field.

He founded and since 1885 he run his own gynaecological clinic where the recent advances of medical knowledge were used in practice. He designed and introduced to the practice a portable apparatus for inhalation analgesia for delivery using the mixture of compressed nitrous oxide and oxygen. The apparatus he used since 1888 was manufactured by Ash & Sons in London. The company distributed it through its branches in some European cities eg. Berlin. A description of this apparatus states: /cit./ "In the cylinder made up of wrought iron there is a mixture of 4/5 nitrous oxide and 1/5 oxygen".

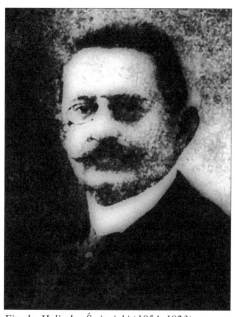

Fig. 1: Heliodor Święcicki (1854–1923)

This cylinder placed in the wooden box contains 220 l of the gas mixture. As shown at the figure, whole apparatus with containing box can be easily transported. The cylinder is supported with cock valve G which can be opened or locked. Soft hose connects the valve with the rubber balloon and also with the face piece. The face piece is a metal face mask with the rubber hose filled with air on its edge to provide a seal between mask and patients face. The gas mixture is delivered to the mask through the adjustable valve H which allows for regulation of its flow. Venting from the mask is done via the expiratory valve situated on the mask. To enable procedures on the mouth or pharynx it is possible to connect straight or bent glass pipe to the valve H instead of the face piece (Fig. 2).

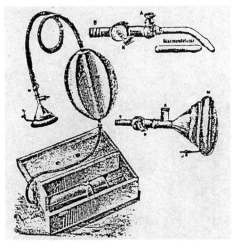

Fig. 2: Swięcicki's apparatus for nitrous oxide-oxygen anaesthesia, around 1883

To use the apparatus the mask must be tightly attached to the parturient's face and she is asked to take deep breaths while valves G and H are being opened so the desired amount of gases delivered.

The apparatus is small and easy to use. Unfortunately, due to low accuracy of the delivery system its use is restricted to short procedures. However the short cases could be satisfactory anaesthetised, so the apparatus gained a wide approval of gynaecologists and obstetricians all over the Europe.

Święcicki published over 100 scientific papers in Polish, German, French and English. In spite of his publication the passage of time concerning the role of the anaesthetic in medicine and set of rectors speeches from the years 1919-1923 remain timeless.

His knowledge and professional skills were highly appreciated in scientific and academic society. This was demonstrated because the was offered the position of the Head of Department of Gynaecology & Obstetrics University in Lvov/1898/ and twice in Cracow/1894 and 1907/.

In 1913 he received his professor's title from the Prussians.

On November 11th, 1918 the last day of World War I, Święcicki organised the first meeting of "Organising Commission of Polish University in Poznan". At that time Poznan belonged to Germany, more precisely to Prussia, and future of this Polish region was not yet certain. Finely, after 6 months of extremely devoted and determined activity at the age of 65 Prof. Święcicki, chef of University Commission, on 7 th May 1919 a solemn Inauguration of University in Poznan took place. Święcicki became the professor of gynaecology at the Faculty of Medicine University in Poznan. Six times he was elected for the rector of University of Poznan (1919, 1919-1920, 1920-1921, 1921-1922, 1922-1923 and 1923-1924). During these years, being the professor of gynaecology & obstetrics he conducted lectures on this subject and in the last part of this period, on theoretical gynaecology and theoretical obstetrics. Święcicki was also extremely active as a member of Association of the Friends of Sciences in Poznan. Since 1889 he held there a position of Vice President. From 1907 till 1915 he was the chief of the Board of Directors, and till his death - a President of Board of Directors. He was the founder of "Nowiny Lekarskie"-the first medical journal in Poznan, founded in 1896. In the years 1896-1897 and 1899-1906 he was the chief editor of this magazine. In 1899 he organised the Vill Congress of Polish Doctors and Natural Historians. Unfortunately, due to political reasons a few days before its opening the Congress was forbidden by Prussian government.

In 1920 in Poznan he initiated deep reforms within the Association of the Friends of Sciences which changed its name to the

Association of the Friends of Sciences in Poznan (PTPN) and changed its character from organisation of people interested in sciences to an association of scientists. Between the First and Second World War PTPN became one of the most famous scientific institutions.

Święcicki also played the leading role in the Society for Scientific Aid of K. Marcinkowski of which he became the member in 1885. The region of Wielkopolska owe this welfare organisation to him giving educational opportunities to more than 7000 holders of scholarships who later played a crucial role in rising in all walks of life after regaining independence by Poland in 1918.

A few months before he died, Święcicki established a Foundation colled "Science and Work" assigning all his personal possessions to financially support professors, assistants and students of Polish universities as well as the families of deceased Polish scientists.

During his life he created three splendid institutions. Two of them, University of Poznan and Association of the Friends of Sciences in Poznan are still working and growing, spreading their influence beyond the country borders. All these facts entile Święcicki to be considered as a creator of Polish science.

Fritz Lotsch - a Forgotten Pioneer in German Anaesthesia

Röse, W.
Department of Anaesthesiology and Critical Care Medicine
Otto-von-Guericke University, Magdeburg, Germany

Professor Fritz Lotsch (1879-1958) (Fig.1) was a surgeon like many other contributors to the early development of anaesthesia in Germany. His well known

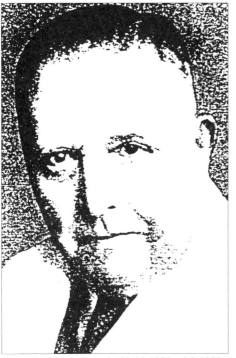

Fig. 1 Prof. Fritz Lotsch (10.10.1879 - 6.8.1958)

clinical teachers were Rudolf Habs for surgery in Magdeburg (1904-1907) and Carl Benda for pathology in Berlin (1909-1911). In Berlin Lotsch worked for Otto Hildebrand (1908-1909 and 1911-1924) and became for a year the temporary director of this department after Hildebrand's death, before Ferdinand Sauerbruch (1875-1951) was the definite successor of the department of surgery at the famous Charité. In 1925 Lotsch was appointed chief surgeon at the district hospital in Burg, where he worked until 1946. From 1946 to 1952 he held the chair at the surgical department of a large hospital in Magdeburg. Lotsch died in 1958.

Lotsch made contributions to the development of a speciality, which nowadays is well known as anaesthesia or anaesthesiology. In 1903, even before finishing his medical studies in Berlin, he published a paper on experiences with the new sleeping drug Veronal (Fig. 2). The results of its application in 30 patients let him conclude: We summarize our experience with Veronal as follows : in cases of simple insomnia, i.e. sleeplessness, that is not related to pain, Veronal can be given over a longer period without hesitation. If and at what point in time addiction occurs, cannot be answered after the short period of observation. Anyhow, disturbances of the general condition or unwanted side-effects on the vital organs are not to be expected. As compared to many other sleeping drugs, Veronal shows clear advantages concerning relative toxicity, solubility and absorption, and nearly complete tastelessness [1].

In his early clinical years Lotsch's interest focussed on problems related to general anaesthesia and to pathophysiological consequences of the iatrogenic open chest. As compared to Sauerbruch he preferred the

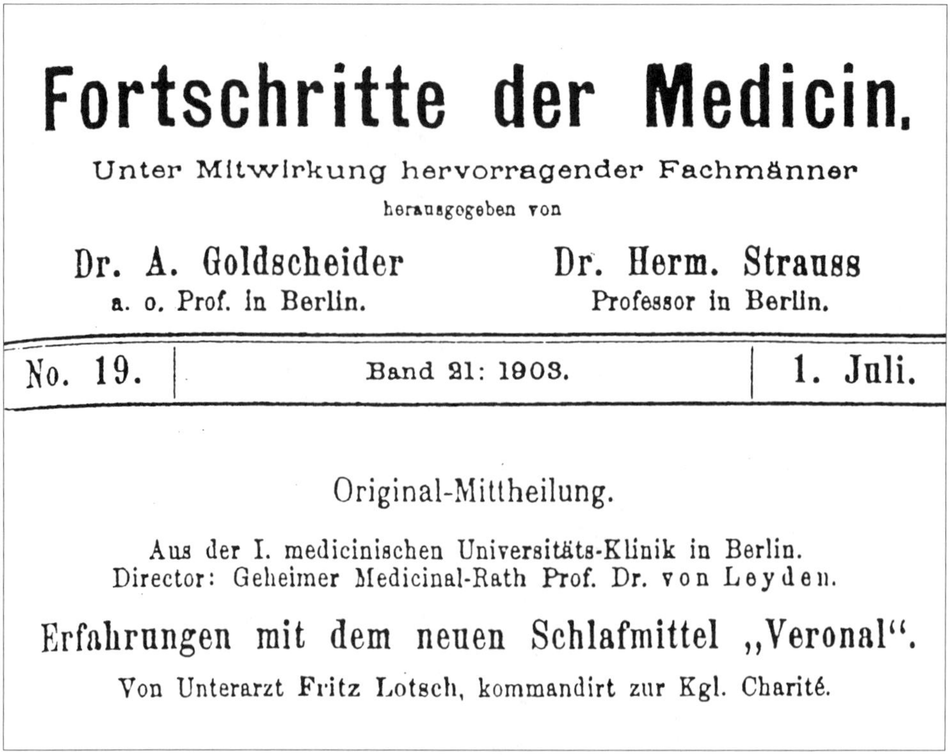

> # Fortschritte der Medicin.
> Unter Mitwirkung hervorragender Fachmänner
> herausgegeben von
>
> **Dr. A. Goldscheider** **Dr. Herm. Strauss**
> a. o. Prof. in Berlin.   Professor in Berlin.
>
> No. 19. | Band 21: 1903. | 1. Juli.
>
> Original-Mittheilung.
>
> Aus der I. medicinischen Universitäts-Klinik in Berlin.
> Director: Geheimer Medicinal-Rath Prof. Dr. von Leyden.
>
> Erfahrungen mit dem neuen Schlafmittel „Veronal".
> Von Unterarzt Fritz Lotsch, kommandirt zur Kgl. Charité.

Fig. 2 Lotsch's first anaestesia-related publication, 1903

concept of Ludolph Brauer (1865-1951) and Franz Kuhn (1869-1929) applying positive pressure to the airways in addition to endotracheal intubation. In 1909 Lotsch published a with consideration of positive pressure ventilation, as suggested by Kuhn[2]. In 1911 another publication followed titled "About procedures in order to eliminate the danger of pneumothorax"[3].

From 1909 until 1914 Lotsch developed different devices for the administration of inhalation anaesthesia in close cooperation with the Georg Haertel company applying the principle of positive airway pressure as well as that of endotracheal intubation [4,5].

Essentials of these apparatusses were:
- an electric motor to fill a 30 - 40 l bag with filtered and moistened air as a reservoir for gas with positive pressure (Fig. 3, 4)
- an oxygen cylinder as an alternate positive pressure generator (Fig. 3, 4)
- different possibilities for the admixture of ether or chloroform (Fig. 3, 4)
- feasibilities for the connection of the apparatus to the patients airway via mask (Fig. 4) or endotracheal tube (Fig. 3)
- the option for exspiration against a variable water resistance (Fig. 4)

Last but not least a very useful recommendation of Lotsch should be mentioned:

A cannula for puncture, injection and infusion, published in 1913. [6] (Fig. 5)

The device consisting of a sharp and pointed inner cannula allowing to insert a blunt outer cannula which is to remain inside the vein for a longer period was followed by improved devices only a few decades later.

Prof. Fritz Lotsch really was a pioneer in German anaesthesia. Some of his ideas, proposals and visions could be realised, some other need further investigations and improvement. In 1931 Lotsch announced: It may be possible to find a new inhalational anaesthetic without the dangers and deficits of ether or chloroform. But it has to be free of the listed possible complications [7]. Sixty six years later we can only agree with Lotsch`s statement. The perfect inhalational anaesthetic as well as the immaculate equipment for the administration of anaesthetic agents still have to be invented.

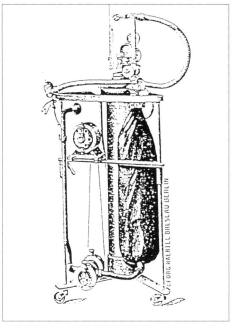

Fig. 3 Lotschs anaesthesia apparatus from 1910

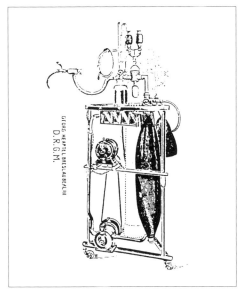

Fig. 4 Improved apparatus for the administration of anaesthetics using positive pressure, 1911

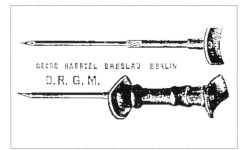

Fig. 5 Lotschs simple cannula for puncture, injection and infusion, 1913

References:

[1] Lotsch F : Erfahrungen mit dem neuen Schlafmittel Veronal. Fortschr Med 1903; 21 : 625-628

[2] Lotsch F : Die Kuhnsche Tubage mit Berücksichtigung des Ueberdruckverfahrens. Dtsch Med Wschr 1909; 35 : 300-302

[3] Lotsch F: Ueber die Methoden zur Beseitigung der Pneumothoraxgefahr. Bln klin Wschr 1911; 48 : 1726-1729

[4] Lotsch F : Ein Apparat zur Ueberdrucknarkose. Arch klin Chir 1910; 93 :285-288

[5] Lotsch F : Verbesserter Ueberdrucknarkoseapparat nach Lotsch. Bln klin Wschr 1911; 48 : 1940-1941

[6] Lotsch F : Eine einfache Kanüle zur Punktion, Injektion und Infusion. Zbl f Chir 1913; 40 : 908-910

Narcosis and Nightshade

A. J. Carter,
North Staffordshire Hospital, Stoke on Trent, UK

Although this year marks the 150th anniversary of the discovery of modern surgical anaesthesia, surgery itself has a much longer history. It is well known that extracts from the opium poppy, Papaver somniferum, were used to dull the pain of surgery during ancient times but less well known that extracts from plants with sedative powers often accompanied them, producing primitive anaesthesia. Most of these sedative plants were members of a large botanical family, the Solanaceae. This paper describes some of them and discusses the ways in which they were administered. It also explains why, during the middle ages, these primitive techniques went out of use but how none the less they provided Shakespeare with the inspiration for some of his greatest plays. When the active principal of the Solanaceae was identified as scopolamine, it came to play a part in 20th century anaesthesia. The combination of omnopon and scopolamine lives on as a premedication, and the presence of poppy heads and mandrake roots on the arms of today's Association of Anaesthetists serves to remind us of the speciality's links with its past.

Seven months after the performance of the first operation under ether anaesthesia the Lancet published a short extract from a paper in a provincial French journal.[1] The extract was entitled "A substitute for the Vapour of Ether to annul Sensation during Operations", and this is what it said:

> At midsummer, when vegetation is at its height, Solanum nigrum, Hyoscyamus niger, Cicuta minor, Datura stramonium, and Lactuca virosa are gathered, and a sponge is plunged into their juice freshly expressed. The sponge is then dried in the sun, the process of dipping and drying is repeated two or three times, and the sponge is then laid up in a dry place.
> When the sponge is required for use, it is soaked for a short time in hot water; afterwards it is placed under the nose of the person to be operated upon, who is quickly plunged into sleep. The operation may then be proceeded with without any fear that the patient has any sensation of pain. He is readily aroused from the stupor by a rag dipped in vinegar, and placed to his nose.
> M Dauriol records five cases in which he has successfully employed this means of bringing about insensibility during operations.[2]

Although described as a "new procedure", Dauriol's method was in fact based on primitive anaesthetic techniques that had been in use from before the time of Christ until well into the middle ages. Those techniques and their legacy today form the subject of this paper.

Materia botanica

Before studying Dauriol's method, however, we must first look at his materials. Of the five plants in Dauriol's list, three, Solanum nigrum, Datura stramonium, and Hyoscyamus niger are members of a large botanical family, the Solanaceae. All three have sedative properties, and Hyoscyamus niger, popularly known as henbane, was cultivated for this property throughout Europe.

Like other medicinal herbs, henbane was grown in herbal, or physic, gardens, and indeed, in one such garden - London's Chelsea Physic Garden, founded in 1673 by the Worshipful Society of Apothecaries - it can still be found growing today. Apothecaries, whose roots lay firmly in the monastery, also studied and catalogued the plants they grew, and in Gerard's Herbal (1597) we find henbane's sedative powers described as follows:

> The leaves seed and juice taken inwardly causeth an unquiet sleepe, like unto the sleepe of drunkennesse, which continueth long and is deadly to the party.[3]

It was this ability of henbane to induce prolonged unconsciousness that particularly impressed the 18th century physician (and benefactor of the Chelsea Physic Garden) Sir Hans Sloane, who recorded the case of four children who accidentally ate henbane seeds. They slept for two days and two nights.[3]

Although not used by Dauriol, one other solanaceous plant must be mentioned, for it is associated with the very earliest attempts at anaesthesia. Mandragora officinarium, popularly known as the mandrake, grows naturally around the Mediterranean, and the plant's anaesthetic power first came to attention during the time of the Roman Empire, when a method for using wine to extract its active constituent was described by the Greek physician, Pediacus Dioscorides:

> The wine of the bark of the root is to be given to such as shall be cut or cauterised. They do not apprehend the pain because they are overborne with dead sleep.[4-5]

However, according to the writer Celsius, the Romans also knew that the anaesthetic power of solanaceous plants was increased when they were combined with extracts from the opium poppy, Papaver somniferum:

> There is another, more efficacious way for producing sleep. It is made from mandrake with opium seed and seed of henbane bruised up with wine.[6]

The spongia somnifera

The roman Empire finally collapsed around the fifth century, and much of our knowledge of it today is due to the custodial work of monks in the early Christian monasteries. In one of these, the Benedictine monastery at Monte Cassino, was found early this century a ninth century method for inducing anaesthesia in the manner described by Dauriol - that is, with the aid of a sponge. According to this description, the sponge was:

> Steeped in a mixture of plant juices, including those of the opium poppy, henbane and mandragora, and dried. When the sponge was moistened, the vapour it produced was ready to be inhaled by the patient.[7]

Although sponges were widely used during the early days of both ether and chloroform anaesthesia, the Roman spongia somnifera is most strongly remembered today for the association it had with the punishment of crucifixion. Traditionally, these sponges contained mandrake wine, which, when used for this purpose, was known as morion, or death wine, because of its ability to make victims appear dead when actually still alive. Although its mode of action is inclear, it was so effective that centurions had orders to spear the bodies of victims before releasing them.

While we do not know whether the Romans used similar methods to induce surgical anaesthesia, the instructions found at Monte Cassino, and more detailed one from the first organised medical school in Europe which opened two centuries later at nearby Salerno,[8] must at least raise the distinct possibility that they might have done.

Decline and fall

The sponge was, however, far from being the only method used to administer ana-

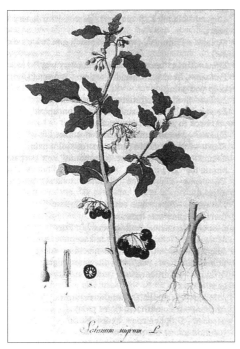

Solanum nigrum (black nightshade)
(Royal Horticultural Society, Lindley Library)

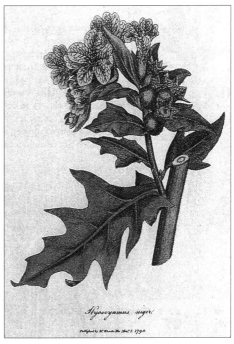

Hyoscycamus niger (henbane)
(Royal Horticultural Society, Lindley Library)

esthesia, as can be seen from an English account dated 1328. Once again we find opium and henbane mentioned, with the following instructions:

> Medle al hem to geder, and boyle ham a lytal, and do hit in a glasen vessel, well stopped, and do ther of III spoonful to apotel of good wine.... and let hym that shall be coruen, sytte agens a good fyre, make hym drynke therof til he falle aslepe, and thou moyst savely corye hym.[9]

A similar, but fictional, account appears in a short story by the popular renaissance writer Giovanni Boccaccio (1313-75):

> Now the doctor, supposing that the patient would never be able to endure the pain without an opiate, deferred the operation till the evening; and in the meantime ordered a water to be distilled from a certain composition, which, being drunk, would throw a person asleep as long as he judged it necessary.[10]

It was around this time that the use of these primitive techniques seems to have reached a peak, but the problems that would eventually lead to their abandonment were now becoming apparent. In his surgical textbook *Chirurgia Magna*, for example, the French surgeon Guy de Chauliac (1300-67) describes the soporific sponge, but then gives asphyxia, congestion, and death as complications of its use.[7]

It is not hard to find reasons why such problems should have arisen. Although the potency of these extracts varied enormously - depending, for example, on the climatic conditions under which the plant had been grown and the method used to concentrate its juices - there was no method of measuring the dose actually administered. Not surprisingly, the results were highly unpredictable for, as the

Italian surgeon Gabriel Fallopius (1523-1562) pointed out:

> If soporifics are weak, they do not help; if they are strong they are exceedingly dangerous.[11]

The use of these techniques now began to decline, but at precisely the time that they were being abandoned by one profession another one was adopting them.

Perchance to dream

The plays of William Shakespeare contain many references to herbal medicines, particularly those with sedative powers. In Othello act III, scene iii, for example, the moor is told that nothing can return to him his once peaceful state of mind:

> Not poppy, nor mandragora
> Nor all the drowsy syrups of the world
> Shall ever medicine thee to that sweet sleep
> Which thou owd'st yesterday.

Like countless other writers since, Shakespeare realised the dramatic potential of substances that could produce temporary unconsciousness, and when, in act IV, scene i of Romeo and Juliet, Juliet asks Friar Lawrence for help in finding a way to avoid the marriage arranged for her the following day to Paris, her fellow Capulet,

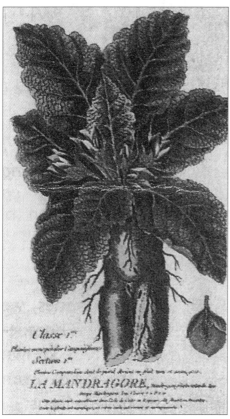

Mandragora officinarium mandrake)
(Royal Porticultural Society, Lindley Library)

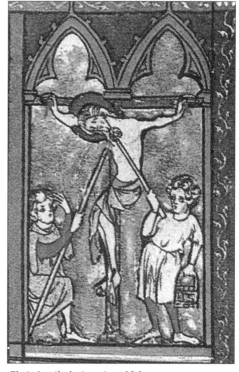

Christ's tribulations in a 13th century
manuscript from Salerno.
Traditonally his sponge contained vinegar
(Sloane manuscript 1977,
by permission of the British Library)

Shakespeare describes a state not unlike that of anaesthesia itself. The friar tells Juliet:

> Take thou this vial, being then in bed,
> and this distilled liquor drink thou off:
> When, presently through all thy veins shall run
> A cold and drowsy humour; for no pulse
> Shall keep his native progress, but surcease:
> No warmth, no breath, shall testify thou liv'st;
> The roses in thy lips and cheeks shall fade
> To paly ashes; thy eyes' windows fall,
> Like death, when he shuts up the day of life;
> Each part, depriv'd of supple government,
> Shall, stiff and stark and cold, appear like death:
> And in this borrow'd likeness of shrunk death
> Thou shalt continue two-and-forty hours,
> And then awake as from a pleasant sleep.

Although much of Shakespeare's remarkable knowledge is said to have come from herbals, it is surely impossible not to find in these words a suggestion of experience more personal in nature.

Twillight sleep

Dauriol's attempt in 1847 to reintroduce, as an alternative to ether, a technique that had been by then long abandoned, was rightly greeted with a dignified silence. It did not, however, take long after the discovery of ether and chloroform for it to become apparent that the use of these agents was also not without risk. The search for a safe anaesthetic went on, and in 1888 the physician Benjamin Ward Richardson decided to investigate the anaesthetic power of the mandrake. Richardson obtained a mandrake root and prepared from it a tincture in exactly the manner described by Dioscorides, which he tested both on animals and on himself. He concluded:

> The wine of mandragora is a general anaesthetic of the most potent quality. The action no doubt depends on the presence of an alkaloid which is like, if

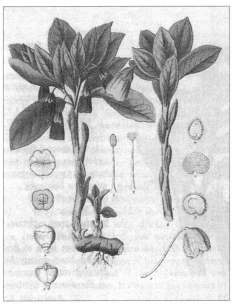

Scopolia camiolica - the source of scopolamine (Royal Horticultural Society, Lindley Library)

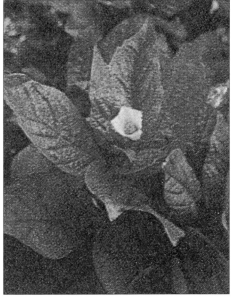

A form of Scopolia carniolica (Blooms of Bressingham)

not identical with, atropine and which would, I have no doubt, be one of the most active anaesthetics we have yet discovered.[12]

Unknown to Richardson, however, the alkaloid had already been isolated from another solanaceous plant, Scopolia carniolica, which grows naturally in the Slovenian province of Carniola. In the same way that atropine, its near relative, had previously been named after Atropa belladonna, the deadly nightshade, so this new alkaloid was now given the name scopolamine.[13]

In 1900, stimulated by continuing concerns about the safety of chloroform, doctors in Germany began to experiment with the use of morphine and scopolamine as an alternative to mask anaesthesia.[11] The technique, which involved giving one or two hourly injections until anaesthesia was considered adequate, never gained popularity in British operating theatres, but in 1910 the anaesthetist DW Buxton wrote:

> A terrified patient after a sleepless night is in the worst condition for an anaesthetic and an operation. In such patients I am convinced that the use of scopolamine and morphine injections before a general anaesthetic is valuable.[11]

Many examples are known of medical techniques that have been abandoned, only to be rediscovered by a new generation. There is, however, surely no finer one than that of this ancient partnership, known to the Romans and perhaps to Shakespeare, and now reborn as the 20th century anaesthetic technique of premedication.

In somno securitas

Although less frequently prescribed today, morphine (or omnopon) and scopolamine still remain in certain situations a pharmacological partnership without equal. Furthermore, like the mandrake roots and poppy heads on the arms of the Association of Anaesthetists, the combination serves as a reminder, in this the quintacentenary year of ether anaesthesia, that the desire to alleviate the fear and pain of surgery, if not always the ability to do so in safety, has been with us since time immemorial.

Today, when we think of plant based medicines, we tend to think of substances that are weak or homoeopathic, but in Shakespeare's day they would have known better. When Friar Lawrence chooses the plant from which he will make Juliet's sleeping potion, he tells us:

> Within the infant rind of this small flower, Poison hath residence, and medicine power.

I thank Dr. Arthur Hollman, medical adviser to the Chelsea Physic Garden, for his invaluable advice and encouragement in the writing of this paper.

The physic garden is open to the public on Wednesday and Sunday afternoons from April to October.

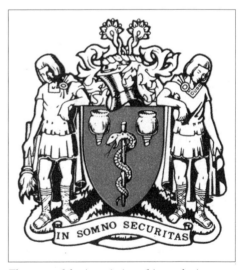

The arms of the Association of Anaesthetists, showing mandrake plants (at top) and opium poppy heads on shield (reproduced by permission of the Association of Anaesthetists of Great Britain and Ireland).

References:

[1] Dauriol M: Nouveau procédé pour plonger dans la strupeur les malades qui doivent subir une opération. Journal de Médecine et Chirurgie de Toulouse 1847; 10:178

[2] Dauriol M: A substitute for ether to annul sensation during operations. Lancet 1847; i:540.

[3] Grieve M: A modern herbal. London: Jonathan Cape, 1931: 397-404

[4] Guthrie D: A history of medicine. London: Thomas Nelson, 1945:116

[5] Bowes JB: In: Atkinson RS, Boulton TB, eds. The history of anaesthesia. London: Royal Society of Medicine, 1989:43

[6] Thompson CJS: The mystic mandrake. London: Rider, 1934:100-101

[7] Keys TE: The History of Surgical Anaesthesia. New York: Schuman, 1945:104

[8] Ellis ES: Ancient Anodynes. London: Heinemann, 1946:137

[9] Husemann T: Weitere Beiträge zur chirurgischen Anästhesie im Mittelalter. Deutsch Zeit F Chir 1900; 57:516

[10] Boccaccio G: Quoted in: Gordon R. The literary companion to medicine. London: Sinclair Stevenson, 1993:295-301

[11] Duncum B: The Development of Inhalation anaesthesia. London: Geoffrey Cumberlege, 1947:375

[12] Richardson BW: Asclepiad 1888; 5:174-83

[13] Atkinson RS, Rushman GB, Davies NJH: Lee's Synopsis of Anaesthesia. London: Butterworth, 1993:92

Anaesthesia in German Military Practice during World War I and World War II - a Comparison

M. Wollbrueck, C.Giese*, G. Hempelmann,
Department of Anaesthesiology, University Gießen, Gießen, Germany

In Europe anaesthesia in field surgery was first established 1847 by N.I. Pirogoff (1810-1881) who used ether for anaesthesia during a military expedition to fight rebels in the Caucasus. At the beginning of World War I application of general anaesthesia had advanced only little beyond the open administration of narcotics using a drop-bottle and a mask inaugurated by Schimmelbusch in 1890. In the first months chloroform was the only substance at hand to induce anaesthesia whereas later on ether and chlorethyl were available. By the end of the war anaesthetic methods were supplemented by the so called Daemmerschlaf with scopolamine and morphine. In a way this procedure was a precursor of the scopolamine – eucodal – ephetonine (S.E.E.) narcosis during World War II. Techniques like regional and local anaesthesia utilizing procaine, which had been introduced in medicine in 1904, were introduced at a later point in time. The

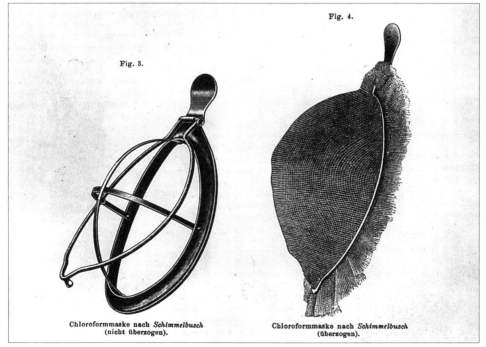

Fig 1: The Schimmelbusch mask inaugurated in 1890 (Curt Schimmelbusch 1860-1895) was used by military surgeons during World War I as well as during World War II. Due to availability mainly chloroform was employed to induce anaesthesia.

anaesthetic procedure for surgery was chosen according to the surgeon's preference (most of them had been educated as civilian physicians) and tactical or logistic aspects. Anaesthesiological approach was adapted to the current military operations - offensive with a great amount of casualties and fast moving troops or frozen lines and fighting in trenches.

During World War II anaesthesia matured a little only as compared to World War I introducing intravenous hexobarbital (Evipan) and a fix combination of Scopolamine - Eucodal - Ephetonine (S.E.E.). Open anaesthesia with the drop-bottle and a preference of ether remained to be the common technique. Unfortunately advantages of hexobarbital in general anaesthesia were ignored by some general surgeons and therefore it was not available in all medical units. Endotracheal intubation - as compared to english surgeons - was employed rarely. Military medicine during World War II showed little acception of technical innovations other than stirring personal constructions. Tactics and warfare dominated medical care in World War II due to the long distances especially at the Eastern front and in North Africa. Therefore first line treatment frequently was analgesia applying morphine rather than anaesthesia. Anaesthesia itself remained a domain of field and military hospitals.

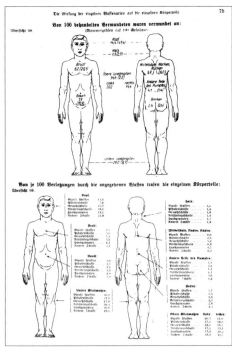

Fig 2: One report on the medical service during World War 1* depicts number and character of wounds. Injuries of the extremities predominanted. Most of them were caused by grenades and shrapnels of the artillery. These casualties could be treated very well with local or regional anaesthesia if procaine was available.

* Sanitätsbericht über das Deutsche Heer im Weltkrieg 1914/18, Heeres-Sanitätsinspection des Reichskriegsministeriums, Bd. 3, Berlin 1934 (Publ.)

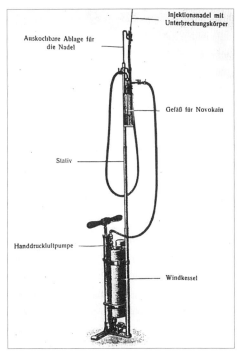
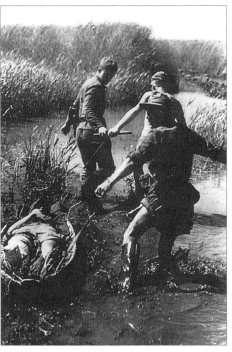

Fig 3: Since surgical treatment of many injuries could be performed applying local anaesthesia, Franz Kuhn (1866-1929) introduced an apparatus for the application of local anaesthesia in mass casualty in 1914. Although it became available commercially soon (Carl Dankert, Berlin-Schoeneberg) the device was not very common.

A reservoir containing 0.5 to 1% procaine was set manually under hyperatmospheric pressure (3-4 atm). With the help of a mechanical interrupter individual application of local anaesthetic was rendered possible.

Fig 4: Medical care in World War II was dominated by problems concerning transport of the wounded soldiers resulting from the long distances and environmental peculiarities. The photograph shows transportation through mud in the Kuban marsh (Caucasus, autumn 1943). First line treatment comprised analgesia utilizing morphine rather than anaesthesia.

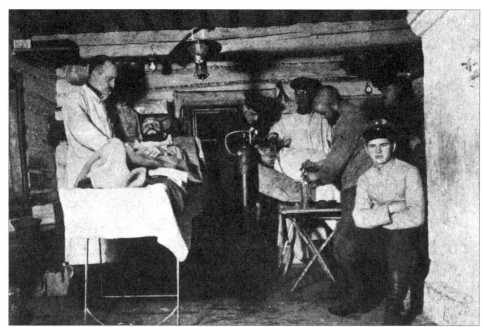

Fig 5 and 6: Anaesthesia during wartime was determined by tactics and warfare. The logistic situation played an important role. The anaesthetic was chosen according to its availability. Many of the general surgeons in World War II had gained experience in World War I making them stick to the substance and the technique they knew. If it was not the uniforms it would have been hard to recognize that Fig 5 (above) shows surgeons during World War I and Fig 6 a field hospital in France in 1944.

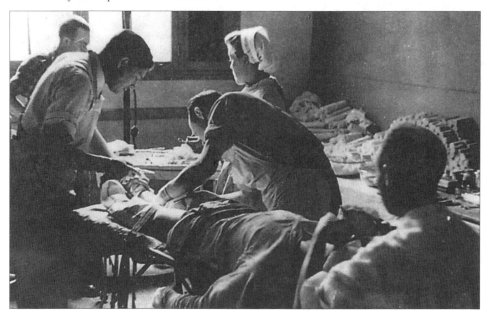

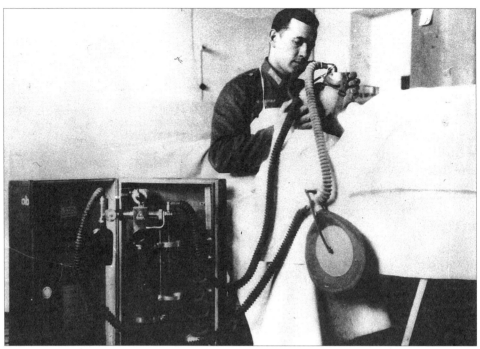

Fig 7: Anaesthesia utilizing the drop-bottle remaind the most common technique during World War II. As compared to World War I, ether was more often employed than chloroform. General anaesthesia using endotracheal intubation was only performed rarely, since this method was not yet accepted in common german surgical practice. Also apparatus for anaesthesia were rather unknown. The photograph depicts a self construction based on the oxygen supply apparatus (SBG 38) with an ether bottle interpositioned in the airway and an excess pressure device.

References:

Albrecht H: Kriegschirurgische Erfahrungen aus dem Feldlazarett. Münch Med Wschr 1915; 63:420-422

Borchard A, Schmieden V: Die deutsche Chirurgie im Weltkrieg 1914 bis 1918. Leipzig 1920

Brandenburg K: Ueber die Versorgung der Verwundeten und Erkrankten im Kriege; die Einrichtung der Militärlazarette im Operationsgebiet. Med Klin 1914; 10: 1377-1379

Danielsen W: Kriegschirurgische Erfahrungen in der Front. Münch Med Wschr 1914; 61: 2294-2296

Drost F: Kriegschirurgische Erfahrungen aus den Jahren 1939-1945. Wehrmed Mit 1963; 7:106-109

Floercken H: Unsere operative Tätigkeit im Feldlazarett. Münch Med Wschr 1915; 62: 241-243

Franz C: Neues in der Kriegschirurgie. Münch Med Wschr 1943; 90: 521-526

Guth E: Sanitätswesen im Zweiten Weltkrieg (Vorträge zur Militärgeschichte, Militärgeschichtliches Forschungsamt (Hrsg.), Bd. 11), Herford und Bonn 1990

Kuhn F: Feld und Lazarettapparat für Lokalanästhesie in Massenanwendung, Dtsch Med Wschr 1914; 43: 1887

Roith N: Zur kombinierten Skopolamin-Morphium-Chloroform-Narkose. Münch Med Wschr 1905; 52: 2213-2218

Sanitätsbericht über das Deutsche Heer im Weltkrieg 1914/18. Heeres-Sanitätsinspektion des Reichskriegsministeriums (Hrsg.), Bd. 3, Berlin 1934

Wollbrueck M: Anästhesie im Krieg: Ein Beitrag zur Geschichte der deutschen Militärmedizin. Med. Diss., Gießen 1995

Zimmer A (Hrsg.): Wehrmedizin. Kriegserfahrungen 1939-43. 1.Bd. Kriegschirurgie I, 2. Bd. Kriegschirurgie II, Wien 1944

S.E.E. (SKOPHEDAL): Wehrmacht's Miracle Drug ?

R. J. Defalque
Department of Anesthesiology
University of Alabama at Birmingham School of Medicine
Birmingham, Alabama, USA

Discovery

The scopolamine-morphine mixtures used to produce twilight sleep in the 1920's occasionally caused severe respiratory or circulatory depression. In 1926, H. Kreitmair[1], a MERCK researcher, found that ephetonin (synthetic, racemic ephedrine) protected his laboratory animals against the depression caused by lethal doses of those scopolamine-morphine mixtures[1]. He also found eukodal (oxycodone), a recently discovered synthetic narcotic to be superior to morphine in safety, efficacy, potency, and freedom of side-effects. In 1928/1929, MERCK released two preparations S.E.E. I (weak), containing 0,5 mg scopolamine, 10 mg eukodal, 25 mg ephetonin/ml solution) and the twice as potent S.E.E. II (forte). In 1942 the preparation was renamed "skophedal". In the late 1930's Martin Kirschner[2], the forceful Heidelberg surgeon, helped popularize S.E.E. and especially its intravenous use, in surgery and in 1938 got it adopted by the Wehrmacht's medical service.

Use in the Wehrmacht

From 1939 through 1943, S.E.E. enjoyed an immense popularity in the German frontline surgical stations[3]. Each of the 30 articles published on anesthesia by German military surgeons in World War II unanimously praised S.E.E.'s speed of action and smoothness, its safety, efficacy, potency and lack of side-effects or depression. It was especially appreciated by the hurried, inexperienced young surgeons facing huge numbers of casulties.

S.E.E. was given intravenously, subcutaneously, or intramuscularly for analgesia in unruly wounded soldiers with intensive pain or to induce rapid quiet, and dry ether anaesthesia and prolonged quiet and safe postanaesthetic sleep. Given alone or as an adjunct to local anaesthetics or evipan (the German equivalent to thiopental), it allowed short surgical procedures, especially around the airway, lung or brain where inhalation anesthesia was impossible or thought to be dangerous. S.E.E., however, was less popular in the rear hospitals, staffed, with older, more conservative surgeons who remained loyal to morphine.

Some "consulting surgeons" (university surgeons attached to an army as medical advisers) were less enthusiastic and felt that S.E.E. had caused some catastrophes in deeply

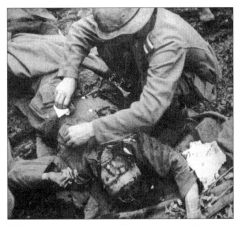

S.E.E. was administered by surgeons facing huge numbers of casulties for analgesia in unruly wounded with intensive pain.

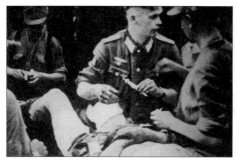

S.E.E. was often used in combination with local anaesthesia.

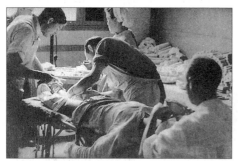

S.E.E. was given intravenously to speed up induction of ether anaesthesia.

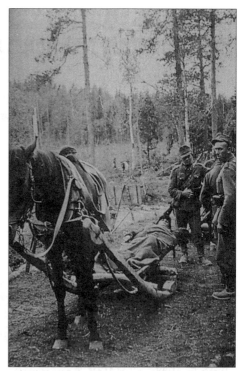

S.E.E. was given during long, painful evacuation.

shocked patients or in patients with lung or brain damage. They also felt that it had caused frostbites in over-sedated patients during their long evacuation in the Russian winter. From mid 1942 on, these consultants surgeons suggested that a morphine-pervitine mixture (pervitine or desoxyephedrine is similar to an amphetamine) be used in such compromised patients, but their advise never became popular. The use of S.E.E. decreased from 1944 to the end of the war for unclear reasons, possibly because of the chaotic supply conditions then existing in the Wehrmacht.

MERCK discontinued S.E.E. in the mid-1980's, apparently because of the civilian surgeos lack of interest. Was S.E.E. a mere pharmacological fad, or was it a superb drug which deserves re-evalution ?

Table I: Discovery

1. In 1920s, Firma Merck's search for antagonists vs twilight depression (Morphine + Scopolamine)

2. In 1926, H. Kreitmair (Merck) tests mixture:
   - **Scopolamine**
   - **Ephetonin** (1926, Synthetic L-Ephedrine): Antagonizes CV, respiratrory, CNS depression
   - **Eukodal** (oxycodone, 1917): Safer, more potent & efficient, less side-effects than morphine

   profound sedation/analgesia without depression

3. SEE (I & II) released in 1928; adopted by Wehrmacht in 1938

Table II: Use in Wehrmacht*

Extensive use by
  - Young surgeons in mass casualties
  - Medical officers in fieled

1. Twilight analgesia for wounded:
   - on battlefield
   - perioperative pain
   - long, painful evacuation

2. Adjunct to I.V. evipan or local anaesthesia in special surgery: brain, chest, jaw, neck

3. To speed up ether induction

4. Sedation for tetanus

5. Euthanasia (?)

* over 30 Publications communications by ex-Wehrmacht Surgeons

Table III: Rare Accidents

1. CNS, CV Depression in shocked wounded
2. Airway obstruction in jaw or neck injuries
3. Respiratory & CV depression in chest or brain injuries
4. Postoperative delirium: wound disruption
5. Frostbites in winter's long evacuations

References:

[1] Kreitmair H: Entgiftung von Skopolamin. Münch Med Wschr 1926; 51:2158

[2] Kirschner M: Die Schmerzbekämpfung im Felde. Chirurg 1936; 8:269

[3] Holle F: Praktische Erfahrungen bei der Schmerzbekämpfung. Dtsch Militärarzt 1942; 7:85

Thanks

Herr W. Schutte, Firma Merck, Darmstadt
Ex-Wehrmacht Surgeons

CODIC – an Universal Therapeutic System Applicable to Automatic Infusion-Controlled General Anaesthesia

J. Stoffregen,
Husterstraße, Hagen, Germany

CODIC is a programmed medication system based on pharmacokinetic principles. These have had a revolutionary impact on traditional drug therapy. With intermittent intravenous medication - for example three times a day routines - the concentration at the receptor site of action is initially too high but is followed by a longer phase during which the agent is below the effective therapeutic level (Fig.1). Clearly, this lessens the desired effect even if not proving totally ineffective, the final result being related to the intensity of the drug's action and to its therapeutic span and half-life.

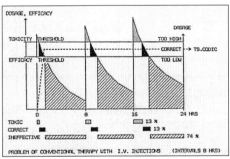

Fig. 1: The concentration of the drug at the side of receptor linking by intravenous application

The situation is not much better if the drug, instead of being given by fractionated i.v. injections, is given by continuous intravenous infusion (Fig.2). With a constant delivery rate and at a given concentration – both have to be estimated by the physician – the time for stopping the infusion to prevent overdosage, has to be decided. Even a two-step infusion (Fig.3) will not solve this

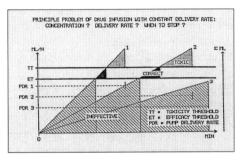

Fig. 2: The pharmacological model when the drug is applied continuously

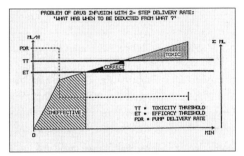

Fig. 3: "Two step infusion" model

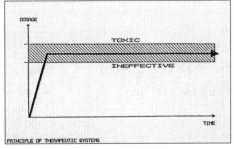

Fig. 4: Therapeutic system

problem because the physician cannot be sure of the initial delivery rate nor "what has to be deducted from what and when".

Therapeutic systems are the answer. Therapeutic levels will be reached quickly and maintained constantly over a pro-grammed period of time, avoiding ineffective or toxic levels (Fig. 4). Louis Lasagne of Rochester University summarised several years ago the potential significance of therapeutic systems as follows: "The future appears as unlimited as our imagination. Therapeutic systems represent a new scientific space whose doors have just been opened for use". This is true for all tasks in intra-venous therapy.

My personal clinical answer to the challenge of pharmacokinetics is CODIC – from COmputeriseD Infusion Control – representing the first programmable therapeutic system of universal application. I began its development in 1978 by using two TTL-prototypes, first for patient-controlled analgesia and then with a computerised exponential profile universally applicable to intensive therapy – balanced anaesthesia being a first-rate example of intensive therapy.

CODIC is an "open" therapeutic system which is pre-programmed but also capable of being programmed by the user. Inputs are made by via a numeric keyboard and function keys. It is empirically programmed for tasks which are either "no demand" or "on demand" based on pharmacokinetic data. In the "on demand" mode for patient controlled analgesia (PCA) CODIC runs via a push-button system. "No demand" is CODIC specifically programmed for anaesthesia by intravenous infusion. For this it contains a "standard infusion profile" - a matrix based on the individual patient's data: - body weight (5kg+), height (50cm+), and the resultant "R" factor as a variable for the harmonic or disharmonic ratio of both factors ("fat reduction factor".

CODIC's "no demand" standard profile is a mathematical function with a fractionated exponential quotient. Its algorithm is:

$$DEF\ FNA(X) = E*Q**((1/(1-T)*(T-(X/T1)))$$

A = initial pump rate Q = E/A
E = final pump rate   T = T2/T1
T1 = start of decreasing X = minutes
T2 = duration of decreasing

The initially high output-rate of the infusion pump is exponentially reduced versus time down to the constant final pump rate necessary for the maintenance of the efficacy level of a given drug to balance elimination pharmacokinetics. CODIC has been succesfully used since 1980 in our hospitals for automated controlled anaesthesia in about 7,000 cases; it has never failed. We have mainly used either Tramadol 1,000mg, or Droperidol 10 mg with Fentanyl 1 mg, or Midazolam 10 mg with Ketamine 200 mg in each 500 ml solution.

The CODIC program has been the same for all three medications:

in adults of 70kg	Initial (A)	kg*10	ml/h	700ml
	for (T1)		5 min	
	final (E)	A/50ml/h	14ml	
	after(T2)		40 min	
in a child of 30kg	Initial (A)	kg*15	ml/h	450ml
	for (T1)		5 min	
	final (E)	A/50ml/h	9ml	
	after (T2)		40 min	
in a 1 year old child of 10kg	Initial (A)	kg*20	ml/h	200ml
	for (T1)		5 min	
	final (E)	A/50ml/h	4ml	
	after (T2)		40 min	

Our experience shows that the same profile can be used for all the above medication combinations in spite of their pharmacokinetic differences ~ as expressed as half-life times. This surprised us, but is probably explicable by our choice of equipotent concentrations.

When using the agonist/antagonist opioid Tramadol, the addition of 10mg/500ml of the potent alpha receptor blocker Droperidol is recommended as Tramadol has an inbuilt tendency to inhibit the receptor de-linking of catecholamines if these have been released, for example by premature intubation during induction, which is typically followed by hypertension for 20-30 minutes.

The capability of varying CODIC's infusion rate by pressing the "change" key has enabled me to adapt this step-wise until the optimum setting has been found. Nine cases were needed to create the setting and dosage for the combination Midazolam 10 mg + Ketamine 200 mg in 500 ml, regardless of age, risk and duration of operation. As an example, figure 5 shows the result in a 57 year old patient under going a Bricker-plasty at the Akademisch Ziekenhuis of the Erasmus University of Rotterdam. My friend Wilhelm Erdmann and I anaesthetised him by a CODIC-controlled method with Midazolam/Ketamine on 13 June 1995. For a procedure lasting almost 9 hours, the 77kg patient needed only 98mg ketamine (!) with 4.9mg midazolam. In standard anaesthetic practice, an adult patient would need at least

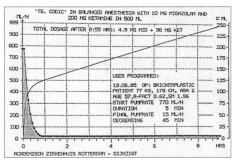

Fig. 5: CODIC - controlled infusion profile when a combination of Ketamine-Midazolame is administered during a surgical procedure lasting nine hours

the same amount of ketamine for induction. This shows CODIC`s outstanding ability to achieve a desired therapeutic result while minimising the dose of a given drug and optimising the desired effect, yet avoiding side-effects. (Fig. 5)

Last but not least, CODIC`s "no demand" program for intravenous anaesthesia can be reproduced simply by using this 5-step decreasing schedule. For example, for a 70kg patient:

Minutes	5	10	20	40	then
ml/hr	700	175	58	29	15
	(1/1)	(1/4)	(1/3)	(1/2)	(1/2)

This means that after 45 minutes the final pump-rate is reached, amounting to only 1/50th (!) of the initial rate, and explaining the remarkably small amounts of ketamine/midazolam needed for the Rotterdam case described above.

A Commentary on:

Johann Sigismund Elsholzt: Clysmatica Nova. Sive Ratio, Qua In Venam Sectam Medicamenta Immitti Possint, Ut Eodem Modo, Ac Si Per Os Assumta Fuissent, Operentur: In Animantibus Per Drastica, In Homine Per Leniora Hactenus Probata, Et Adserta, Beroline: D. Resichelius, 1665

J. W. R. McIntyre †, MD
Department of Anesthesiology, University of Alberta Hospital, Edmonton, Alberta, Canada

Johann Sigismund Elsholtz was born on August 26, 1623, probably in Frankfurt on Oder where his father was imperial notary, but perhaps in Cölln on Spree. This, the hometown of his mother, is presently the district of Neukölln in Berlin. Details of his childhood are scanty but after completing university studies in Frankfurt, Königsberg, and Wittenberg he travelled to various medical centres throughout England and Europe where he met many eminent persons. Finally his doctorate was completed in Padua in 1663. Settling in Berlin he became court physician to the Elector Friedrich Wilhelm of Brandenburg.[1,2]

Diverse interests in natural philosophy continued to develop. Prominent among his numerous publications are a six volume account of dietetics, and a plant catalogue of the Brandenburg March and the electoral gardens in Berlin. His large publication devoted to horticulture in general was highly respected, and a fourth edition was published in 1715 long after his death. His chemical interests are represented by a treatise on certain physical qualities of fluorspar (fluorite, $CaF2$). These scholarly activities led to membership of the German Academy of Natural Scientists[1,2].

A medical interest pursued vigorously in the 50's and 60's of 17th century England was the injection of substances into blood vessels, and this was so in Europe. Elsholtz' major medical publications comprised, in 1665 the CLYSMATICA NOVA, ODER NEWE CLYSTIER, published in German[3] and Latin[4] followed by a second edition in 1667, also published in Berlin. Translations of the 1665 Latin and German versions do not differ substantially in content. The 1665 edition had been expanded in 1667 from nineteen to sixty eight pages, mainly due to his interest in blood transfusion. The particular interest for modern anaesthesiologists is the intravenous injection of opiates described in the 1665 edition.

At the time of Elsholtz' experiments, which must have been conducted during years prior to 1665, the idea of intravenous therapy was extremely controversial. So it remained until by the beginning of the 20th century it had become a generally accepted medical technique. In Elsholtz' time objections were varied; a technique that was too new, too difficult, ill-defined, and stressful for patients. It was sinful to oppose God by attempting to prolong life and it would be too late to save a patient anyway[5]. Interesting examples of medical thinking those may be but more pertinent to this commentary on Elsholtz' 1665 publication are other contemporary events and responses to his work. The man whose activities present us with a most valuable source of such information merits a brief digression.

King Charles II of England granted the first charter to what became the Royal Society on July 15, 1662. John Wilkins and Henry (Henricus) Oldenburg[6,7] became the first secretaries. Wilkins held office for only six years and his successors served only briefly. In contrast Oldenburg served until his death in 1677 and was dominant throughout his period of service. German by birth he was multilingual and in 1653 had been the envoy to England for the Senate of Bremen. Widely read in the classics, theology, and natural philosophy he became deeply involved with Oxford scientific life. His secretarial duties included the minutes of the council and Royal society as well as the registration of its papers, discoveries, and observations. However his intent became not only to facilitate the objectives of Society members within England but to acquire information regarding scientific developments in Europe. To this end he conducted a most extensive correspondence with foreign scientists that on one occasion was misunderstood, resulting in a brief imprisonment in the Tower of London. Nevertheless, these secretarial efforts were rewarded by the Philosophical Transactions of the Royal Society becoming the most prestigious forum for publication in Europe.[8] Some of this massive correspondence is not extant, but the remainder have been collated and annotated[9]. That work and the Philosophical Transactions themselves are an invaluable help to understand the indignation in England regarding Elsholtz' claim for originality expressed in his 1667 publication.

It is likely a copy of Elsholtz' 1665 book reached England[10,11,12]. In his introduction he states his experiments were not unusual or historical but his own special experiments. He pays particular tribute to William Harvey's revolutionary concept of the circulation of the blood[13,14]. That was first published in 1628 at Frankfurt on Oder, and an edition in English appeared in 1653. Though supported by overwhelming experimental evidence, the idea was not universally accepted in Europe for many years.[15] Elsholtz' 1665 text concludes: "I do not seem to be in error or injurious to anyone if I should believe that I was the first to do the experiments with simple infusions upon which the whole discovery rests". This provoked a reviewer for Philosophical Transactions 1670[16] to refute a statement that "there had been nothing printed for ought he (Elsholtz) knew either by English French or Italian of this argument". Evidence cited were previous publications[12,17,18,19]. It could be supposed that both Elsholtz and reviewer referred to the blood transfusion content, but the most prominent of the citations[19] stated, "...Even if I had sweated diligently through more than the last ten years on the mixing of various liquids with the blood of living animals, not only would I have taken care to pour and mix various drinkables, up to two pounds, into the blood mass, but also I would have applied emetics, cathartics, diuretics, cardiacs, and opiates, besides also I would have more often attempted the transfusion of blood itself". This author, Timothy Clarke a physician in ordinary to His Majesty, goes on to mention he had communicated various experiments to the Royal Society about five years previously, had been urged to publish them, but had not done so. It seems extremely unlikely that the reviewer or Elsholtz were referring by inference only to blood transfusion. In this same letter to Oldenburg it is stated "about the end of 1656 or thereabouts the famous mathematician Dr. Christopher Wren first devised and explained at Oxford the infusion of various liquids into the blood mass of living animals. In the following year he communicated to me (Clarke) his findings...."

Christopher Wren could have known William Harvey[20], and the first edition of Harvey's De Motu Cordis in English appeared in the year 1653 when Wren became a newly elected fellow of All Souls College, Oxford. It would be surprising if a man with such a wide ranging mind did not think of intravenous infusions. Reports of conversations and letters between Robert Boyle, John Wilkins, William Petty, and Wren leave little doubt that one day in 1656 Wren injected substances into the vein of a living dog[20,21,22,23,24].

The year 1656 has now been accepted as the authoritative year for that event[23]. Like Timothy Clarke, Wren seems to have neglected making a formal report of his experiments though it is likely he continued them. In correspondence he wrote: "...I am now in further pursuit of the experiment which I take to be of great concernment, and what will give great light to the theory and practice of physick"[25]. In 1663 Robert Boyle described one of Wren's experiments in detail[23].

"Whereupon our Knowledge of his (Wren's) extraordinary Sagacity, making us very desirous to try what he proposed, I provided a large Dog, on which he made his Experiments in the Presence & with the Assistance of some eminent Physicians, & other learned Men: His Way (which is much better learn'd by Sight than Relation) was briefly this: First, to make a small and opportune Incision over that Part of the hind Leg, where the larger Vessels that carry the Blood, are most easy to be taken hold of: then to make a Ligature upon those Vessels, and to apply a certain small Plate of Brass (of above half an Inch long, and about a quarter of an Inch broad, whose Sides were bending inwards) almost of the Shape & Bigness of the Nail of a Man's Thumb, but somewhat longer. This Plate had four little Holes in the Sides, near the Corners, that by Threads pass'd through them, it might be well fasten'd to the Vessel; and in the same little Plate, there was also left an Aperture, or somewhat large Slit, parallel to the Sides of it, and almost as long as the Plate, that the Vein might be there exposed to the Lancet, and kept from starting aside. This Plate being well fastened on, he made a Slit along the Vein, from the Ligature towards the Heart, great enough to put in at it the slender Pipe of a Syringe; by which I had proposed to have injected a warm Solution of Opium in Sack, that the Effect of our Experiment might be the more quick & manifest. And accordingly our dexterous Experimenter having surmounted the Difficulties, which the tortured Dog's violent Strugglings interposed, conveyed a small Dose of the Solution or Tincture into the opened Vessel, whereby getting into the Mass of Blood, (some Quantity of which 'tis difficult to avoid shedding the Operation) it is quickly, by the circular Motion of that, carried to the Brain, and other Parts of the Body: So that we had scarce untied the Dog, (whose four Feet it had been requisite to fasten very strongly to the four Corners of the Table) before the Opium began to disclose its Narcotick Quality, and almost as soon as he was on his Feet, he began to nod with his Head, and faulter and reel in his Pace, & presently after appeared so stupified, that there were Wagers offered his Life could not be saved. But I, that was willing to reserve him for further Observation, caused him to be whipped up and down a neighbouring Garden, whereby being kept awake, and in Motion, after some Time he began to come to himself again; and being led home, and carefully tended, had not only recovered, but began to grow fat so manifestly, that 'twas admired:...Succeeding attempts informed us, that the Plate was not necessary, if the Fingers were skilfully employed to support the Vessel to be opened, & that a slender Quill fastened to a Bladder containing the Matter to be injected, was somewhat more convenient than a Syringe... The Inventor of it afterwards practised it in the Presence of that most learned Nobleman, the Marquis of Dorchester, & found that a moderate Dose of the Infusion of Crocus Metallorum did not much move the Dog to whom it was given; but once, that he injected a large Dose, (about two Ounces or more) it wrought so soon and so violently upon a fresh one, that within a few Hours after he vomited up Life and all, upon the Straw whereon they had laid him. I afterwards wished, that not only some vehemently working Drugs, but their appropriated Antidotes, (or else powerful liquid Cordials) and also some Altering Medicines might be in a plentiful Dose injected, and in Diureticks, a very ingenious Anatomist & Physician told me he try'd it with very good Success".

On a date close to his intravenous studies Wren extirpated the spleen of a dog. This was part of a physiological experiment on an organ of great interest at that time[20,23] and not a surgical whim. The operation was successful, and in two weeks the dog had regained its normal state. Wren provided a detailed description in a letter to Boyle.

"Provide a Dog, as big as a Spaniel, and having tied him in a fit Posture on the right Side, with a Cushion under him, that his Belly may turn a little up; first clip away the Hair, and mark with Ink the Place for Section, drawing a Line two Fingers breadth below the Sortribs; cross the Abdomen at right angles to the Musculus rectus, beginning short of it a Finger's breadth, & so carry it up the Length of three Finger's breadth towards the Back; then thrust in a sharp Knife, like a Sowgelder's Knife, till you feel you have just pierced thro' the Muscles and Peritonaeum, having a Care of the Guts; thence rip up freely, carrying on the Point of the Knife to the End of the Line; then put in two Fingers, and while another presses down the Abdomen, draw out the Spleen just without the Wound, having a great Care of pulling it too far out, because of disordering the adhering Vessels within, the Stomach, the Caul, the Arteries, & Veins; then either tie the Veins and Arteries with untwin'd Thread, but strong, and in three or four Places, Caul and all, and so cut them off close to the Parenchyma of the Spleen, and anointing the Ends of the Vessels and Wound of the Caul with Balsam, or Oil of Hypericon, put them in their Places, or else sear off the Vessels, and anoint them with the Juice of Sengreen and Plaintain beaten with Whites of Eggs; or else, cum Unguento Diacalcitheos dissolv'd with Vinegar and Oil of Roses, especially the Nerve; then sew up the Wound with the Suture call'd Gastrorophia, leaving at the lower End room enough for Matter to come out, first anointing the Wound with Balsam, then R. Olei Mirtini & Rosarum, ii. Cerae alb. i. Farinae hord. Boli Armeni & Terrae Sigillatae, ana vi. make a large Plaister of this to cover the Wound, and all the Muscles about; swath his Belly warm, and lay him upon his left Side in Straw; after six Hours let him Blood in the left hinder Leg, two or three Ounces, more or less, according to the Bigness of the Dog: The next Day if there seem to lye any clotted Blood in the Abdomen; out of a Glister-pipe (one holding the Dog in his Arm, or hanging over the Table, so that the Wound may be downward) inject half a Pint of Decoction of Barley with Honey of Roses and red Sugar, till you have wash'd out the clotted Blood, then tent the remaining Hole with the yellow Salve, and wrap him up in the former Plaister as before till the Wound begins to suppurate"[23]

This account of surgery and immediate post-operative care is reminiscent of recovery of an animal from sedation or general anaesthesia, though any inactivity of the animal may equally well have been due to exhaustion, or a psychological result of acute restraint.[26]

Timothy Clarke, Johanne Elsholtz, and Christopher Wren were not the only persons at that time seriously experimenting with intravenous injection as a medical method. Among them were Johannes Schmiedt (Fabritious), Michael Ettmüller, and Johannes Daniel Major. Fabritious reported his injections into human subjects to Oldenburg in 1667[27]. Ettmüller experimented with animals and humans, publishing a scholarly work in Leipzig 1668 "Dissertatio de Chirurgia Infusoria"[3] A question of priority with reference to the work of Elsholtz does not seem to have been raised.

Major came from Breslau and completed his doctorate in Padua. He practised in Hamburg and 1665 became a professor at the newly founded University of Kiel. He based his interest in intravenous injection in humans on the work of Borel who, in a publication Historiarium, et Observationium Medico-Physicarium Centuriae IV" Paris, 1656, described the anatomic injection of milk into the veins of a placenta[3]. Major, in 1664, published a book "Prodromus Inventae a Se Chirurgiae Infusoriae..." which has been described as scholarly rambling[2] and not to be compared with the presentation of the scientifically oriented Elsholtz, though Major was reputed to be an eloquent and charming speaker. Major dispatched letter with a copy of his book to Oldenburg in 1664[28]. This was acknowledged but did not elicit an editorial response beyond a statement that Dr. Timothy Clarke was "duly engaged in promoting such experiments, and is about to publish shortly his collections on this question"[29].

In conclusion, a verdict on the place in medical history of CLYSMATICA NOVA (Berlin 1665) must include comment on its scientific quality and its chronological relationship with other contributions to the subject. If priority in discovery is an issue, then that word priority can be defined, but in any disputed priority so many elements of diverse origin are merged that it is impossible to establish where the achievements of an individual discoverer begin and end. For example, this situation has been discussed with reference to William Harvey[30]. In addition, once an investigator believed circulation of blood within the body actually occurred it would not be surprising that experiments with intravenous techniques were independently begun. It is accepted that William Harvey, by repute, was the first to inject opiate and other substances into the veins of living dogs, and further writings on the subject of intravenous drug administration may yet come to light. However, Johann Sigmund Elsholtz' Clysmatica Nova 1665 is a precisely structured presentation of the author's developing series of experiments and his conclusions drawn from them. Apparently at that time it was a unique and valuable contribution to medical science.

Addendum: Recommended reading for persons seeking a broader view of Elsholtz' environment is: Lester S King. The Road to Medical Enlightenment 1650 - 1695. New York, American Elsevier Inc. 1970

Acknowledgements:

I am most grateful for the invaluable assistance of Jeannette Buckingham of the John W Scott Medical Sciences Library, University of Alberta; Michael Ward, BA, Department of Classics, University of Alberta, and Prof. Dr. med. Jürgen Plötz, Bamberg, Germany.

References:

1. Sachs M. Die Entdeckung Der Intravenösen Injektions-Und Infusiontherapie Durch Johann Sigismund Elsholtz (1623-1688). Zent. Lb. Chir. 1991; 116:1425-1432.

2. Buess H. Die Historischen Grundiagen Der Intraven6sen Injektion. Aarau. Verlag H. R. Sauerlander Und Co. 1946.

3. Elsholtz JS. Clysmatica Nova, Oder Newe Clystier. Berlin: D. Reichel 1665.

4. Elsholtz JS. Clysmatica Nova. Berlin: D. Reichel 1665.

5. Buess H. Die Injektion. Ciba Zeitschrift No 100. 9. Jahrgang Mar 2, 1946.

6. Hall AR, Hall MB. The Correspondence of Henry Oldenburg. Vol I Introduction pp XXIX-XL. University of Wisconsin Press. Madison 1962.

7. Hall AR, Hall MB. The First Human Blood Transfusion: Priority Disputes. Med Hist 1980; 24:461-5.

8. Hall AR, Hall MB. The Correspondence of Henry Oldenburg. Vol VIII 1671-1672. University of Wisconsin Press. Madison 1971.

9. Hall AR, Hall MB. The Correspondence of Henry Oldenburg. Vols I-XI. University of Wisconsin Press/Mansell.

10. Letter: Robert Boyle to Henry Oldenburg 22 October 1665. In: The Correspondence of Henry Oldenburg. Hall AR, Hall MB. Vol II Letter 439.

11. Letter: Robert Boyle to Henry Oldenburg 28 October 1665. In: The Correspondence of Henry Oldenburg. Eds Hall AR, Hall MB. Vol II. Letter 441.

12. Anon. An Account of the Rise and Attempts of a Way to Convey Liquors Immediately into the Mass of Blood. Phil Trans. Monday, December 4, 1665 pp 128-130.

13. Harvey W. Exercitatio Anatomica de Motu Cordis et Sanguinis In Animalibus. Guilielmi Fitzeri: Frankfurt 1628.

14. Chauvois L. On William Harvey At Padua And The Way In Which He Was Stimulated To Reinvestigate The Problem Of Heart And Blood Movements And On The Credit He Merits For The Discovery. J of the Hist of Med 1957; 12:175-180.

15. Weil E. The Echo of Harvey's De Motu Cordis 1628-1657. J of the Hist of Med 1957; 12:167-174.

16. Anon. An Account of Some Books. Joh Sig Eisholtii, Elector Brandenburg Medeci. Clysmatica Nova. Coloniae Brandenburgica 1667. 2nd Edn. Phil Trans. no 58 (25 April 1670) pp 1200-1201.

17. Anon. The Method Observed in Transfusing The Blood Out of One Animal Into Another. Phil Trans no 20 (17 December 1666) pp 353 358.

18. Anon. Tryals Proposed by Mr. Boyle To Dr. Lower, To Be Made By Him, For the Improvement Of Transfusing Blood Out of One Live Animal to Another. Phil Trans no 22 (11 February 1666) pp 385-388

19. Clarck (Clarke) T. Anatomical Inventions and Observations, Particularly the Origin of the Injection into Veins, the Transfusion of Blood, and the Parts of Generation. Phil Trans, no 35 (18 May 1668 672-682. (Note: The date this letter was written is unknown bu presumably not long before publication. Hall AR, Hall MB. The Correspondence of Henry Oldenburg 1667-1668 Vol IV p 367. University of Wisconsin Press 1967.)

20. Gibson WC. The Biomedical Pursuits of Christopher Wren. Med History 1970; 14:331-341.

21. Elmes J. Sir Christopher Wren and His Times. Chapman and Hall. London MDCCCL II.

22. Gunther RT. Early Medical and Biological Science. Oxford University Press. London 1926.

23. Doby T. Sir Christopher Wren and Medicine. Episteme 1973; 4:83-106.

24. Frank Jr, RG. The John Ward Diaries: Mirror of Seventeenth Century Science and Medecine. J of the Hist of Med 1974; 29:147-179.

25. Bennett JA. A Study of Parentalia, With Two Unpublished Letters of Sir Christopher Wren. Ann of Science 1973; 30:129-147.

26. Porro CA, Carli G. Immobilization and Restraint Effects on Pain Reactions in Animals, Pain 1988; 32:289-307.

27. Letter. Johannes Schmiedt (Fabritius) to Henry Oldenburg. Some New Experiments. Phil Trans no 30 (9 December 1667) pp 564-565

28. Letter. Johann Daniel Major to Oldenburg (13 December 1664) In The Correspondence of Henry Oldenburg. Eds Hall AR, Hall MB Vol 11 Letter 361.

29. Letter. Oldenburg to Johann Daniel Major (11 March 1665) In The Correspondence of Henry Oldenburg. Eds Hall AR, Hall MB. Vol II Letter 370.

30. Pazzini A. William Harvey, Disciple of the Girolamo Fabrizi D'Acquapedente and the Padual School. J of Hist of Med 1957; 12: 197-201.

* Abbreviated Title Phil Trans.
Philosophical Transactions: Giving Some Accompt of the Present Undertakings, Studies and Labours of the Ingenious in Many Considerable Parts of the World. London and Oxford 1665-1677.

The History of Anaesthesia – a Personal Perspective with a Cartesian Touch

F. Magora
Hadassah University Hospital, Jerusalem, Israel

When I started my residency in Anesthesiology forty years ago, cyclopropane was considered to be the champagne of anaesthetic agents, and its application was believed to be the most sophisticated mode of anaesthesia. The potency and the physical characteristics of cyclopropane, forced physicians to measure anaesthetic gas concentrations precisely and to careful monitor respiratory and hemodynamic parameters. These procedures can be regarded as the first steps towards modern anaesthesia.

Ever since I have stayed in anesthesiology, and thus have gone through an important period in its history. For this reason, my lecture will reflect on historical aspects of anaesthesia and characters from a personal point of view expressing my own convictions and beliefs. Thus I will omit the numerous facts and figures involved in the development of our field.

In order to give a brief overview I believe it is appropriate to summarize my thoughts as a paraphrase of the French philosopher René Descartes: Cogito ergo sum - I think, therefore I am (Fig. 1) Descartes discovered the principles of modern science: reasoning, deduction and logic, which replaced the medieval science based on contemplation and on occult and obscure argumentation.

Descartes was not the only one supporting his concept that humans were a creative able to think: famous artists such like Rodin and Van Gogh portrayed him like that. Van Gogh even painted a physician thinking.

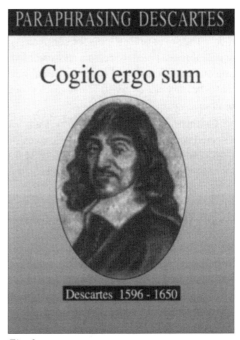

Fig. 1

Thinking was perceived as the conscious process of the mind searching for knowledge and truth. By means of thinking only, ideas can be realized and conclusions can be drawn. However, I believe that at least 10 other words can be replaced in Decartes statement justifying that humans are aware of their existence. I suggest to replace I think "think therefore I am" by: "I question, therefore I am" , "I oppose", "I change", "I modify, therefore I am", "I communicate", "I hurt", "I remember", "I love", "I imagine", "I hope", and because I care I most certainly am (Fig. 2).

Let us look at the first sentence: "I question therefore I am. "To doubt and to question are manifestations of an inborn curiosity demanding to be satisfied. By instinct we are driven to feed not only our empty stomach, but also our hungry spirit. By looking out for the right questions , we find correct solutions, we progress and ensure the continuity of our existence. To illustrate "I oppose therefore I am", I selected a painting by an Israeli artist which she named: "Face to face". The act of protest calls for controversy and dialogue, helps to refine and establish objective concepts , and more than enabling us to be, it teaches us to stand up for our opinions.

To illustrate "I change therefore I am", I selected a picture called "The three ages of man" and the cover of a book from 1884 by Dr. Carl Koller who discovered the anaesthetic effects of cocaine. This book was reprinted for the history of anaesthesia series and shows Dr. Koller in 1885 in Vienna and another photograph of him at an older age. Changing with time proves that we exist, that is why I prefer to discuss changes occurring around us, and our influence upon them in modifying ties and priorities, and in making an impact in the evolution of things.

To exemplify this, I will use the history of anaesthesia. When I began my residency, the image of an anesthetist was a person who bent over a mask putting a patient to sleep. We were also seen as physicians running around to cope with desperate situations in order to resuscitate a patient. Later, this image changed. We became the intensivist using sophisticated equipment and precise monitoring devices. We also perfected regional anaesthesia, added opioids and other drugs to local anaesthetics and applied them during surgery, as well as outside the operating theaters to treat acute and chronic pain.

"I communicate therefore I am". Since the very beginning of human race there has been an incredible striving to write down our experience. Man left messages on stones and on papyrus for future generations. When Gutenberg invented the technique of printing we increased to write and to publish. The negative connotation of cliché "publish or perish" misses an important point: writing enables us to pass frontiers and will let us in the future.

Modern techniques like computers with their software allows us to preserve and note our observations, that is why we can consider ourselfes to be very fortunate: we can take advantage of these facilities!

There probably is no need to convince an audience of physicians, that we are most aware of our body when we hurt. "I hurt therefore I am" - refers not only to a nociceptive event in for physical distress, but also to suffering.

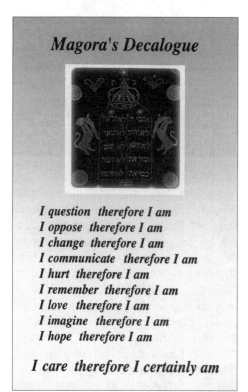

Fig. 2

Suffering unfortunately, and too often unnecessarily, remains a part of our existence.

"I remember", is the next important trait which characterizes the actions of man. I selected four celebrities of giants in anaesthesiology: Professor Bonica needs no introduction to this audience. Him, Professors P. Wall and Tony Yaksh, greatly influenced the treatment of pain with their basic and clinical research. Their findings and wisdom guided me, and are still echoed in many of the qualities that anesthesiologists present. Many of you are too young to remember Dr. Rowenstine who was director of the anaesthesiology department of the Bellevue Hospital in New-York until his death from cancer in 1960. His department was famous for its research in anaesthesiology and its special course in the anatomy, physiology and therapy of pain. Every year we honor him by dedicating a lecture to him and his contributions to anaesthesia during the ASA meeting.

This is a reproduction of John Snow's book on "The Inhalation of the Vapour of Ether" a gift to me from Dr. Rowenstine at the end of my fellowship in New-York during his last year of life (Fig. 3). By remembering, we preserve our personal and community heritage, and are able to revive important moments and significant personalities from our past. Our consciousness is enriched by the ability to remember. I take this opportunity to congratulate and thank the scientific committee for the selection of the main topic of this symposium: A history in remembrance.

It was very difficult for me to select the 8th word and a picture to represent its meaning. My decision fell on "love" because it contains and completes the previous as well as the next words. Love raises questions and, it sometimes hurts and always changes our lives, it is remembered, it makes us communicate imagine and hope. The things we accomplish through love complete our thinking process and elevate us above a bare existence. The girl in this picture by Picasso, has abandoned her toy to give tender love and care to a little bird. Our love and dedication to science, our profession and our patients has consolidated the place of anaesthesia in medicine.

... And so does our imagination which stimulates new forms of thought and plants the seeds of invention. Hence, I imagine therefore I am.

The same is also true about our hopes. The Chief Editor of the Israel Journal of Medical Sciences wrote an autobiography titled "Prisoner of hope" and in the introduction he claims that without hope life can only be incomprehensible and sterile. Many others express their hope, desires and beliefs in a prayer... Maybe we are, after all what we hope and pray for.

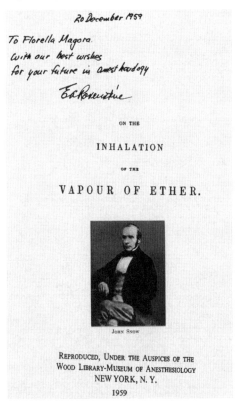

Fig. 3

But what would Descartes write today if he was me?

I wish to quote a verse written for the management of trauma:

the emergency physician	gives interview
the radiologist	takes time
the hematologist	takes blood
the surgeon	takes credit
the anesthesiologist	takes the blame

I wish to change this to:

"The anesthesiologist – takes care" concluding that we function as an important part of the team attending the patient's need, and protecting him at the same time. I think that the inspiration I received from the great mentors who preceeded us, will be transmitted to the following generations and that the wish to care will survive. With this I would like to bring my paper to an end and provide you with an anaesthesiuologist's version of Descartes' proverb: "I care, therefore I am."

An International Study of Educational Programs for Nurses Providing Anesthesia Care

W. Kelly,
Department Professional Education, Kaiser Permanente, Pasadena, California, USA

The opportunity to engage in a descriptive study about the educational processes for nurses administering anesthesia care internationally came in 1991 in Oslo, Norway, at the 3rd International Congress for Nurse Anesthetists. The study was to be an initiatory document of the educational process identifying nurses as anesthesia providers. Because of language barriers and distance, some of the data captured may be incomplete and/or may not be depicted in the complete form of the country submitting the information. The information was not presented as a conclusive report but as a beginning leading to discussion and comment at the first educational forum at the 4th World Congress for Nurse Anesthetists in Paris, France, on May 13, 1994.

History

Anesthesia was not a new state of conscious. Ether was distilled as a liquid by a Spanish chemist, Lillius, in the 13th century and named by a German, Frobenius, in 1730. A Scottish obstetrician, Sir James Simpson, probably made the continent of Europe more aware of the state of anesthesia in 1853 by using chloroform as an anesthetic for Queen Victoria's eighth delivery than any other single act during the early centuries.[1]

In was a German Catholic nursing order that established hospitals along the railroads as they spread west across the United States that brought nurse anesthesia to the North American continent.[2] Also, many lay nurses were trained by physicians to provide anesthesia care as healthcare reached out to other distant stations of the world. Each country represented at the World Congress in Paris probably had a bit of history connecting nurse anesthesia to the present. The lay nursing orders in Africa at the turn of the century, the Red Cross Ambulance Corp in France in World War I, and the MASH (mobile Army surgical hospital) units and the Catholic Nursing Orders in Korea in the police action in the 1950s were just a few examples of our early history.

Our history is rich with stories of extraordinary nurses who made a patient's care better by anesthesia. Again, in Paris, remarkable nurse anesthetists who had distinguished themselves brought together nurses to discuss the anesthesia care provided their patients.

The intent of this research was to assist the nurse providers of anesthesia care in developing a network for communicating educational needs. The 3-year research project was not a quantitative study, but rather a descriptive analysis to provide information regarding the educational process of the countries of the world providing instruction for nurses in anesthesiology.

The International Federation of Nurse Anesthetists (IFNA) was chartered in June of 1989. Eleven countries were admitted as charter members (Table I).

The host country for the first IFNA meeting in 1985, was Switzerland. The opening ceremony was held in the town hall in Lucerne.

Table I
International Federation of Nurse Anesthetists charter members

  Austria
  Germany (formerly Federal Republic of Germany)
  Finland
  France
  Iceland
  Norway
  South Korea
  Sweden
  Switzerland
  United States of America
  Yugoslavia (Slovenia)

Table II
Educators meeting in Oslo, 1991

Austria	Republic of South Korea
Denmark	Sweden
Finland	Switzerland
France	Tunisia
Netherlands	United States of America
Norway	Yugoslavia (Slovenia)
Poland	

The opportunity for interaction by educators of nurse anesthesia and for discussion of the educational process occurred at the 3rd International Congress in Oslo, Norway, in 1991. Thirteen countries were represented by 44 nurse anesthetists at the meeting (Table II).

It was at the Oslo meeting that a group of educators elected to survey the educational process of nurses providing anesthesia care in countries of the world. Ronald Caulk, Certified Registered Nurse Anesthetist (CRNA) in the United States, was the presiding president of IFNA and the presiding officer at the educational meeting. Two issues were addressed:

1. A committee was to be appointed to develop:
   a. A position on educational standards for preparing nurse anesthetists;
   b. A position on standards of practice for nurse anesthetists; and
   c. A statement on ethical standards.
2. An International Study of Educational Programs for nurses providing anesthesia care.

Having the opportunity to gather the data and present the results at the 4th World Congress in Paris was indeed one of the most rewarding activities this researcher had ever undertaken. The letters and calls were beautiful and heartwarming. Thank you for your participation. The data were presented on your behalf and with your assistance.

The survey addressed nine issues regarding the educational process. The issues were:
1. Required nurse entry level credentials and education.
2. Required experience as a nurse for entry into anesthesia.
3. Required courses for entry into an anesthesia program.
4. Required courses in an anesthesia program.
5. Academic instructor information.
6. Clinical instructor information.
7. Required examinations to practice anesthesia.
8. Anesthesia skills performed in the practice setting upon completion of the program.
9. Specify language spoken by participants in an anesthesia program.

Educational programs

The information from the educational programs for nurses in anesthesia was reviewed. The data collected were ranked into three educational groups of instructional structure provided by the individual institutions. Group I was identified as Primary, Group II as Secondary, and Group III as Advanced process of instruction (Table III).

■ *Group I - Primary*. The primary training programs did not have an affiliation with an educational institution. They commonly were part of a hospital or clinic. The nurse assisted the physician in carrying out many other nursing duties. The body of knowledge

Table III
Educational groups

Group I—Primary
 On-the-job training
 Few planned classes
 Length of program: 6 months to 9 months

Group II—Secondary
 Structured program plan
 Scheduled classroom lecture series
 Organized clinical practice (application)
 Length of program: 1 year to 2 years and 3 months

Group III—Advanced
 University program
 Academic degree (advanced)
 Scheduled classroom lecture series
 Organized clinical practice (application)
 Length of program: 2 years to 3 years and 6 months

gained regarding anesthesia was by observation. No lecture series was provided for continuity of patient care.

The training process was 6 to 9 months in length. No specific identification of license was provided for the patient anesthesia care activity.

In one of the countries the nurse was also trained to be a midwife. No structured program or process, as in anesthesia, was provided for the midwife's patient care.

■ *Group II - Secondary.* The secondary training programs were well developed and described. The group had classroom lectures in specific subjects that were listed for a defined number of hours. The clinical practice (practicum) or application outlined types of cases for which anesthesia would be provided. These programs were hospital based and educational institution affiliated.

In some of the African countries, nurses were certified as nurse anesthetists and also as nurse midwives. No data was collected on this issue, but the information of the dual role as nurse anesthetist and nurse midwife was provided for enlightenment.

A few countries gave academic degrees for the nursing educational process with the anesthesia program being a part or an extension of the nursing educational process. The majority of the countries gave technical diplomas for the anesthesia programs.

The educational training programs were 1 year to 2 years and 3 months. One program had a 3-month preentry program. Successful completion was required prior to entering the 2-year nurse anesthesia program.

A process was in place for recognition as a nurse anesthetist. A written and/or an oral examination was given in every country. Successful completion of the examination was required for nurse anesthetist recognition and participation in the patient's anesthesia care. The skills performed by the nurse anesthetist upon completion of the program were identified as preanesthesia evaluation, induction, maintenance, emergency, and postanesthesia care. Othe nursing duties were also listed. The duties most often listed were ambulance, airlift support, intravenous therapy, intensive care units, oxygen therapy, reanitiation, respiratory care, and laboratory.

■ *Group III - Advanced.* The advanced program's classroom lecture series or curriculum and application of a specific number of cases in the clinical practicum were given academic and practicum credit at a university or college. The nurses in the programs received advanced degrees from the university or college upon successful completion of the academic and clinical process. The registered nurse must have at least 1 year of nursing practice in a critical care area prior to applying for entry into an educational program of nurse anesthesia. All students must graduate from the program with a master's degree by 1998.

The programs were 24 months to 3 years and 16 months in length. The program's curriculum was presented in both semester and quarter systems. After completion of the academic degree, it was common practice for the student to complete a clinical residence (practicum) program for entry into practice that varied in length from 3 months to 1 year. Some clinical (practicums) residency programs ran concurrent to the academic programs.

The clinical skills for patient care fulfilled by the graduates were preanesthesia evaluation, induction, maintenance, emergency, and postanesthesia care. A list of other duties were also carried out. The duties most often listed were intravenous therapy and cardiopulmonary resuscitation.

A certification and license process for practice as a nurse anesthetist was required. The national written certification examination for Certified Registered Nurse Anesthetists was prepared and administered by the Council on Certification of Nurse Anesthetists. The written examination for the registered nurse was administered by the state board of nursing in each state in the United States.

Descriptive analysis by country groupings

The descriptive analysis of the data is presented by country groupings. The educational process was varied in these groupings.

- Africa. The countries responding to the questionnaire are listed in Table VI. Some countries were unable to fully complete the form because of the language barrier. The form was presented in English.

Sixteen countries in Africa responding to the questionnaire stated nurses entering the anesthesia educational programs were prepared for patient care in a 3-year diploma nursing school (Table VI). One school noted a 3-year basic science course was taught at the university. The nurses were required to have 1 to 3 years of clinical nursing experience after completion of a nursing program. Three of the participants remarked that the nurse anesthetists were promoted to supervisor status after completing the nurse anesthesia educational process. Six of the anesthesia programs surveyed confirmed the nurses were also certified midwives. The programs were 6 months to 2 years and 3 months in length. The nurse anesthetist educational processes are shown in Figure 1.

The anesthesia skills identified and performed in the practice setting upon completion of the program were preanesthesia evaluation, induction, maintenance, emergency, and postanesthesia care. Anesthesia skills included regional and epidural blocks. Other skills performed were in the intensive care unit, oxygen therapy, laboratory technician, reanitiation, respiratory care, and the postanesthesia care room.

Table VI
Countries providing data

Benin	Ivory Coast
Botswana	Kenya
Cameroon	Mali
Congo	Nigeria
Ethiopia	Togo
Gabon	Tunisia
Gambia	Uganda
Ghana	Zaire

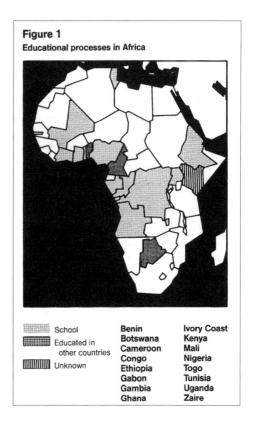

Figure 1
Educational processes in Africa

Eleven programs, included their curriculum. Similar curriculums are listed in Table VII. The respondents listed other classes that were not common among the programs such as ethics, history of anesthesia, psychology, and care of instruments.

Table VII
Responding anesthesia program's curriculum
Basic and advanced principles of anesthesia
Chemistry/physics
General and regional anesthesia pharmacology

Gabon had a 3-month prerequisite course which included anesthesia pharmacology, physiology, and social science at the university and practical work in the hospital setting. The student must successfully complete the 3-month course and examination to continue the 2-year educational process in anesthesia.

Ethiopia had a nationalized 2-year nurse anesthesia program administered by the Ministry of Health. The country had only one school which received 30 students every 2 years. The nurse anesthetists administered 97% of the anesthesia care in the 85 hospitals in the country.

Ghana nurses entering the nurse anesthesia programs were 3-year diploma nurses. The anesthesia programs were 18 months in length. Twelve months were spent in a training and educational process after which the student completed a 6 months' house job (in-house training). The formal lecture series consisted of 200 hours which included anatomy, physiology, physics, pharmacology, and equipment. The students were given both a written and oral examination prior to graduation. Successful completion was required to practice anesthesia care. The skills applied upon graduation were preanesthesia evaluation, induction, maintenance, emergency, and postanesthesia care.

Nigerian programs were 18 months in length. Students from Cameroon attended school in Nigeria. The nurse anesthesia programs were established after the Nigeria/Biafra Civil War in 1970-71. A full range of anesthesia care was provided, including preanesthesia evaluation, induction, maintenance, emergency, and postanesthesia care.

Togo and Binen shared an educational process. Mali and Gambia also shared an educational program. The programs were not identified as to length of anesthesia care provided upon completion of the educational process.

From 1954 to 1962, Tunisia provided a 2-year specialty nurse educational training program. In the years from 1962 to 1972, a 2-year anesthesia specialty nursing program was developed for nurses having completed the 2-year nursing program. In 1972, an anesthesia nursing specialty degree was granted by three universities in Tunisia. The anesthesia educational programs included a 1-year basic science course at a university with 2 years in anesthesia theory and practice at a hospital. The third year of the process was a full-time clinical practicum at a hospital.

An anesthesia educational program in Uganda was being developed by the Health Volunteers Overseas, a U.S. volunteer organization. The program was postnursing education. A full range of anesthesia care would be provided by the graduate nurse anesthetists upon successfully completing the proposed anesthesia program and examination.

■ *Southwest Asia.* Four countries were participants in the Southwest Asia group. The countries responding are listed in Table VIII.

Iran had a 9-month certificate program for registered nurses (RN) who had completed 2 years of clinical nursing experience. No scheduled classes were provided. Technical skills and observation of the anesthetized patient were supervised by physicians practicing the specialty of anesthesiology.

Table VIII
Countries providing data
Iran
Israel
Saudi Arabia
United Arab Emirates

Saudi Arabia and the United Arab Emerates utilized nurse anesthetists that were educated in other countries. Most nurse anesthetists in Saudi Arabia were educated in Europe and Korea. The clinical practice of the nurse anesthetist was supervised by a physician anesthetist. The level of the patient's anesthesia care provided by the nurse anesthetist was limited by the supervising physician anesthetist. A wide range of supervised anesthesia practice plans were reported from independent practice of delivery of the induction, maintenance, and amergence to very limited practice of delivery of the induction, maintenance, and emergence of the patient's anesthesia care. Preanesthesia evaluation or postanesthesia care was not reported as being provided by the nurse anesthetist.

Educational programs in Israel were identified by participants. No questionnaires were received regarding the educational process. Nurse anesthetist educational processes in Southwest Asia are displayed in Figure 2.

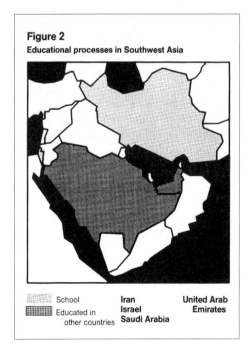

Figure 2
Educational processes in Southwest Asia

School · Iran · United Arab Emirates
Educated in other countries · Israel · Saudi Arabia

- *Europe*. Europe was addressing a standard for nursing education that would initiate a European license for registered nurses. The European Commission on Nursing was restructuring the nursing programs and processes. The nursing educational programs in the countries of Europe would then have one university level of education for Rns. Eventually there would be a European Nursing License rather than a license issued by each individual country.

The cluster groups for Europe included a range of nursing educational backgrounds. The largest group of nurses providing anesthesia care in Europe were the nurses with a 3-year diploma. Other levels of nursing education were also listed, such as the technical nurse who at the age of 16 enters a technical school for nurses with a limited scope of nursing practice. The other category of nursing listed was the university educated nurse who enters the university after 11 years of preparatory education and receives a bachelor's degree upon successfully completing a 4-year educational program.

Twelve countries presented nurse anesthesia education data. The information was collected from the countries listed in Table IX.

Table IX
Countries providing data

Austria	Poland
Czechoslovakia	Romania
France	Spain
Germany	Switzerland
Luxembourg	United Kingdom
Netherlands	Yugoslavia (Slovena)

Four years of hospital practice were required to enter the anesthesia programs in Austria. The diploma anesthesia program was 12 months in length. The anesthesia process was divided into two 6-month sequences. The first 6 months were directed to primary anesthesia education with 230 hours of theory and 460 hours of clinical anesthesia practice. The second 6 months were applied to advanced practical anesthesia experience with 250 hours of theory and 500 hours of clinical anesthesia practice. Graduates from the nurse anesthesia programs fulfilled the full scope of clinical functions in anesthesia, preanesthesia evaluation, induction, maintenance, emergency, and postanesthesia care. The Austrian National Association of Nurse Anesthetists was in the process of developing a national educational program for Austria.

The nurse anesthesia programs in France were nationalized. A nurse who had 2 years of prior nursing experience was admitted by a competitive examination to the nurse anesthesia program. The 17 programs in France were 24 months in length. The accreditation process for the anesthesia programs were nationalized and managed by the Ministry if Health. Nurse anesthetists had practiced in the country since 1947 and were unionized in 1951. The first school opened in 1949. Since 1992, the graduates have been awarded a National Diploma of Nurse Anesthesia (DEIA). The 4,500 nurse anesthetists work in 3,500 public and 1,000 private institutions in France. No liberal (independent practice) activities regarding the patient's anesthesia care were permitted. The anesthesia studies were divided into six sequences. The academic process included 4,056 hours of theory and practice. The formal studies provided general and regional anesthesia for all ages and categories of patient care and surgery. The nurse anesthetists provide preanesthesia evaluation, induction, maintenance, emergency, and postanesthesia care.

Germany had a combined program of nurse anesthesia and intensive care. The applicants were 3-year diploma registered nurses. The educational program had 480 hours of theory and practice. A written examination was given after 2 years of study. The nurses were licensed and certified as nurse anesthetists. The graduates of the programs had a full scope of practice in small hospitals, preanesthesia evaluation, induction, maintenance, emergency and postanesthesia care, while a more limited practice was provided in the larger hospital where physician anesthetists also provided anesthesia care.

The nurses providing anesthesia care in Romania were listed as nursing technical assistants. Nurses were assisting physicians as supervised assistants with the delivery of the patient's anesthesia care.

The countries of Czechoslovakia and Yugoslavia had been in a state of change during the time the survey was being conducted. Both countries listed nurse anesthesia educational programs, but the status of the programs was unknown.

Anesthesia educational programs were listed in Luxembourg, Netherlands, Poland, Spain, and Switzerland. These countries did not complete the questionnaire. Anesthesia care was reported as provided by nurse anesthetists, but no data regarding the scope of anesthesia practice were collected.

The United Kingdom had theatre nurses assisting physician anesthetists in anesthesia

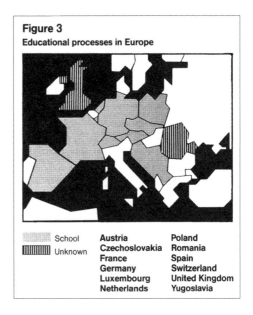

Figure 3
Educational processes in Europe

care. A certificate of anesthesia care was provided nurses leaving the United Kingdom to practice anesthesia care outside the country. No organized program was presented.

The nurse anesthetist educational processes in Europe are shown in Figure 3. Twelve countries are displayed.

- *Northern Europe.* Five countries in northern Europe provided data. These countries were generally known as the Scandinavian countries. They are listed in Table X.

Table X
Countries providing data
  Denmark
  Finland
  Iceland
  Norway
  Sweden

The educational programs for nurse anesthetists in Denmark were nationalized and directed by the Minister of Health. The registered nurse had at least 2 years of acute care nursing prior to applying for admission to the nurse anesthesia program. The anesthesia programs were two years in length. The study of anesthesia practice consisted of 150 hours of theory followed by hospital clinical instruction. Hospitals in Denmark had nurse anesthetist instructors that monitored and evaluated the clinical practice of the student nurse anesthetists. Upon completion of the 2-year program, a written examination was given. Successful completion of the examination was required to practice as a nurse anesthetist in Denmark. Full scope of anesthesia practice, preanesthesia evaluation, induction, maintenance, emergency, and postanesthesia care was provided by the graduates of the nurse anesthesia programs.

Finland was in the process of charging the anesthesia educational programs. The anesthesia programs were the fourth year of the 4-year nursing program. A specific course plan was developed for registered nurses in anesthesia. The perioperative practical program was 596 hours which included perioperative, operating, anesthesia, intensive care, and outpatient department nursing. A clinical anesthesia practice program of 6 weeks to 2 months was being added to the then program of clinical studies. The clinical program would take place at the work site postcompletion of the 1-year anesthesia program. Upon graduation from the national course plan for Rns, the nurse would work as a nurse anesthetist or an operating nurse.

The Norwegian anesthesia programs were nationalized. The Norwegian Association of Nurse Anesthetists first met in 1974 to develop a curriculum for the nurse anesthesia educational programs. National approval of the curriculum was gained in 1980. In 1989, the programs were upgraded to an 18-month academic and clinical program with a 6-month clinical practice required prior to a national examination. Students admitted to the program were licensed as registered nurses in Norway. Each student was also required to have 2 years of intensive care nursing practice prior to entering the nurse anesthesia educational program. The anesthesia lecture series included 550 hours of academic preparation in physiology, chemistry, and anesthesia principles. Anesthesia principles prepared the student to administer patient care for regional and general anesthesia and pain management. A nationalized accreditation process was in place for the anesthesia programs. Successful completion of a written and an oral examination was required to practice as a nurse anesthetist in Norway.

To enter the nurse anesthesia programs in Sweden, the applicant must have completed a university registered nursing program and hold an RN license. The applicant must have also completed 6 months of clinical practice as a registered nurse. The programs presented 40 weeks of theoretical and clinical training. The full-time study included 18 weeks of theoretical training in a university setting and a total of 24 weeks of clinical training in a hospital setting. The clinical training was mainly in the operating room as part of the Anesthesia Department, but clinical training was also conducted in the intensive care unit. Regional anesthesia was administered in cooperation with a physician anesthetist. Intravenous regional anesthesia was performed independently by CRNAs. Nurse anesthetists provided staffing for helicopter transport services and venous access for fluid administration service for the hospital. Three types of examinations were given prior to practice as a Certified Registered Nurse Anesthetist (CRNA). The examinations were written, oral, and clinical application. The CRNAs perform a full range of anesthesia skills, preanesthesia evaluation, induction, maintenance, emergency, and postanesthesia care in the anesthesia practice setting upon successful completion of the anesthesia program and the three examinations.

Anesthesia programs were indentified in Iceland, but no questionnaires were completed. It was noted that in Iceland nurse anesthetists provided a full scope of practice for patient anesthesia care (Figure 4).

Five countries presented information. The nurse anesthetist educational processes are shown in Figure 4.

■ *Northern Western Asia.* Each country in Western Asia was undergoing structural and political changes in healthcare. No questionnaires were chompleted. The countries are listed in Table XI with the information submitted outlined below.

Figure 4
Educational processes in Northern Europe

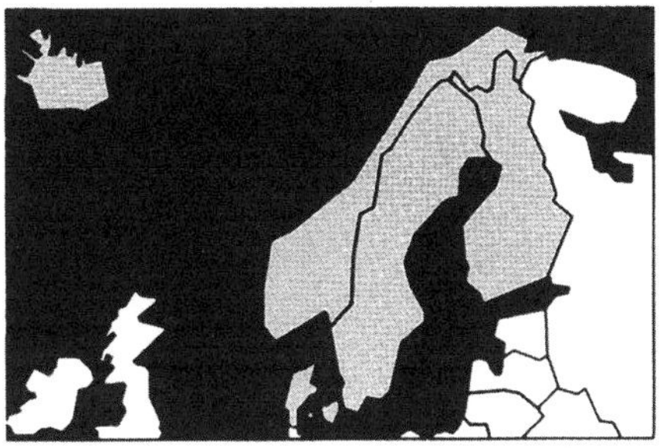

School — Denmark, Finland, Iceland — Norway, Sweden

Russia had three educational levels for nurses: the technical nurse, who entered a technical nursing school at the age of 16; a 3-year diploma nurse; and the university educated nurse. No structured anesthesia programs were identified. Each nurse would participate in the anesthesia care to the level of the individual nurse's educational background. Anesthesia equipment and agents limited the practive of anesthesia care in the hospitals. Nurses and physicians had a collaborative practice. The educational process was tutorial.

Estonia, Latvia, and Lithuania were under the same healthcare system as Russia at the time the information was received.

The nurse anesthetist educational processes are displayed in Figure 5.

■ *Southeastern Asia.* Information was received from seven countries. Questionnaires were completed by four of the countries. The countries are listed in Table XII.

Table X
Countries providing data
Denmark
Finland
Iceland
Norway
Sweden

Table XII
Countries providing data
Cambodia — Republic of South Korea
China — Thailand
Indonesia — Vietnam
Philippines

Cambodia had just completed developing an educational process for nurses in anesthesia. Academic classes and a tutorial clinical practicum was in place. The program had graduates which were prepared for a full scope of anesthesia care, preanesthesia evaluation, induction, maintenance, emergency, and postanesthesia care. No questionnaires were completed.

China had a variety of healthcare providers at different educational levels administering patient care in both eastern and western medicine. Nurses provided a full scope of anesthesia care, preanesthesia evaluation, induction, maintenance, emergency, and postanesthesia care in some areas of the country. A similar acadeic and clinical program for nurses in anesthesia was in place in larger cities. As healthcare providers progressed up the academic ladder, they were allowed to take an examination to become a physician. Physicians were prepared at the bachelor educational level in the university.

The Philippine Islands provided no educational process for nurse anesthetists, although nurse anesthetists educated in the United States were allowed to practice a full scope of patient anesthesia care including preanesthesia evaluation, induction, maintenance, emergency, and postanesthesia care.

The Republic of South Korea had a nationalized program since 1974. The licensed registered nurses were diploma nurses, 36 months, and bachelor of science in nursing nurses from the university. The accreditation process of the educational program was carried out by the Ministry of Health and Social Affairs. The academic program included 200 hours of classroom lectures. The clinical practical experience included 1,300 hours of anesthesia care. Both regional and general anesthesia were performed. The anesthesia courses were conducted in two general hospitals which were designated by the Health and Social Affairs Ministry. The Certified Registered Nurse Anesthetist (CRNA) could practice if the following four conditions were met:

1. Graduated from an approved licensed school of nursing and currently licensed as an RN.
2. Graduated from an accredited program recognized by the Korean Ministry of Health and Social Affairs in Nurse Anesthesia studies.
3. Complied with the Korean Association of Nurse Anesthetists (KANA) regulations for ongoing in-service education, prepared by KANA; also cooperated with the ongoing education requirements of the Korean Nurses Association to retain an active RN license and CRNA certification.
4. Complied with the government requirements regulating both Rns and CRNAs.

Anesthesia skills performed in practice settings upon completion of the program were preanesthesia evaluation, induction, maintenance, emergency, and postanesthesia care.

Thailand had the diploma and the university degree nurse, both of whom were admitted to the anesthesia programs after 2 years of nursing practice. The programs were 1 year in length and consisted of 6 months of classroom instruction (approximately 200 hours) and 6 months of clinical application of anesthesia practice. The nurse anesthetists received a certification after successfully completing a written, oral, and practical experience examination. The certified anesthesia nurses performed a full range of anesthesia skills, preanesthesia evaluation, induction, maintenance, emergency, and postanesthesia care upon completion of the anesthesia program.

The nurse anesthetist educational processes of Southern Asia are displayed in Figure 6. Seven countries submitted information.

■ *North America.* Two countries and one commonwealth in North America replied to the questionnaire. The countries are listed in Table XIII.

Table XIII
Countries providing data
- Canada
- Puerto Rico
- United States

The issue of nurse assistance in the field of anesthesia care was under discussion and debate on a national level in Canada. A committee had been appointed to evaluate allied healthcare providers in anesthesia. Representatives from the Canadian Anaesthetists Society, Operating Room Nurses of Canada, and Respiratory Technology were to discuss the roles in anesthesia fulfilled by nurses and to formulate a position statement on anesthetic assistants in June 1994.

Two registered nurses were presently in a program which listed a baccalaureate degree in nursing preferred for the proposed educational process for Rns in anesthesia. The areas of study in the proposed program were induction, maintenance of anesthesia, physiology, monitoring techniques, and technology of anesthesia.

In the United States, the nurses held a baccalaureate degree from a university or college and were licensed registered nurses with at least 1 year of critical care nursing experience prior to making application to the anesthesia program. The 92 anesthesia programs were to be in the master's academic framework by 1998. Eighty percent of the programs were in the master's framework at the time of the survey. A national accrediting body, the Council on Accreditation of Nurse Anesthesia Educational Programs, accredited the anesthesia educational programs. Accreditation is necessary to receive federal funding from the federal government. The accrediting body established the "Standards for Accreditation of Nurse Anesthesia Educational Programs."

The Council listed six educational standards the schools must address to be accredited:

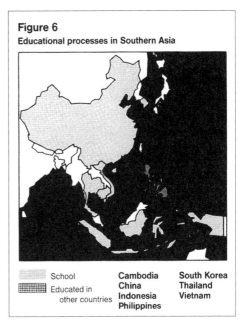

Figure 6
Educational processes in Southern Asia

Standard I. Administrative Policies and Procedures
Standard II. Institutional Support
Standard IV. Faculty
Standard V. Evaluation
Standard III. Curriculum and Instruction
Standard VI. Ethics

The university or college programs were 2-3 years in length in both the semester and quarter university academic system. The programs presented in were multidisciplinary offerings, biology, health science, nursing, and nurse anestheology. The Council on Certification of Nurse Anesthetists established criteria for the national certification examination for practice as a Certified Registered Nurse Anesthetist (CRNA) in the United States. The application for certification listed a minimum of 450 hours of specific course content for the academic curriculum and 800 hours for application of anesthesia for specific categories of clinical cases required prior to making application for the certification examination. Successful completion of the certification examination was required to practice.

Anesthesia educational programs had been providing instruction in the United States for more than 100 years. Approximately 24.000 active practicing CRNAs provided anesthesia care. Full scope of clinical practice skills were performed by the CRNAs in preanesthesia evaluation, induction, maintenance, emergency, and postanesthesia care. Application and maintenance of regional anesthesia were provided by CRNAs. Many states, however, have developed methods of recognition for CRNAs in addition to RN licensure. The methods of recognition (e.g., "licensure", "certification", "authorization") vary from state to state. Continuing education was mandatory for recertification as a CRNA.

Puerto Rico had the same regulatory practice requirements as were established by the Council on Accreditation and the Council on Certification in the United States. Nurse anesthetists were licensed Rns and certified CRNAs.

The nurse anesthetist educational processes are shown in Figure 7. Two countries and one commonwealth are displayed.

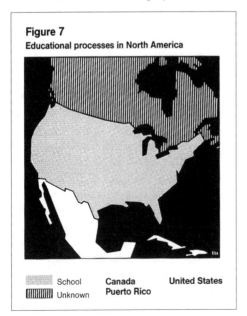

Figure 7
Educational processes in North America

School — Canada — United States
Unknown — Puerto Rico

- *Central America.* No questionnaires were completed by Central American countries. Educational processed were identified in countries listed in Table XIV.

Table XIV
Countries providing data
- Honduras
- Mexico
- Nicaragua
- Panama

Mexico had nurses assisting in patient anesthesia care in the military. The educational programs for the nurses were not standardized. The Mexican government had this year requested information regarding the educational programs for nurse anesthetists from the Council on Accreditation in the United States. Honduras, Nicaragua, and Panama had nurses providing anesthesia care. The educational processes were not identified, and no questionnaires were completed.

The nurse anesthetist educational processes are displayed in Figure 8. Four countries are shown.

- South America. Educational background of the nurse anesthesia providers was submitted by the countries listed in Table XV. No questionnaires were completed.

Health Volunteers Overseas, a U.S. volunteer agency, was in the process of organizing a school for nurse anesthetists in Guyana. The planned program was 18 months in length. Four nurse anesthetists from Guyana were the future faculty of the program. Health Volunteers Overseas would facilitate the educational process with CRNAs from the United States for the present preparing the local nurse anesthetists to continue the educational program in the future.

Table XV
Countries providing data
- Chile
- Columbia
- Guyana
- Peru

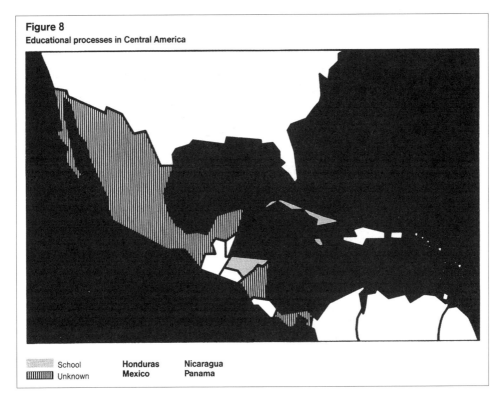

Figure 8
Educational processes in Central America

Legend: School, Unknown, Honduras, Mexico, Nicaragua, Panama

Chile, Columbia, and Peru had nurses providing anesthesia care. The level of the educational background was not provided in the questionnaire.

South American's nurse anesthetist educational processes are displayed in Figure 9. The data collected identified four countries.

- Caribbean Islands. One nurse anesthesia educational program was listed in the Caribbean Islands. The school in Jamaica provided an educational process for the nurse anesthetists supplying anesthesia care in the Caribbean Islands. The islands are listed in Table XVI.

Table XVI
Countries providing data

Belize	Grenada
Cayman	Jamaica
Costa Rica	Montserrat
Cuba	St. Lucia
Dominica	St. Vincent

The nurse anesthesia program in Jamaica was 18 months in length. The graduates from the program received a certificate upon successful completion of the academic and clinical course plan. Two of the nurse anesthetist instructors in the program were in the process of completing a baccalaureate degree in a university in Jamaica.

The nurse anesthetist educational processes are shown in Figure 10. Ten islands are displayed.

Summary

An overview of the information collected has been presented. Much gratitude is given to the many nurse anesthetists who took the time to complete the questionnaire and add anecdotal comments when the questionnaire did not meet their needs in presenting the information about the educational process in their country.

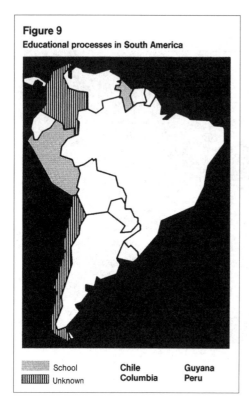

Figure 9
Educational processes in South America

School
Unknown
Chile
Columbia
Guyana
Peru

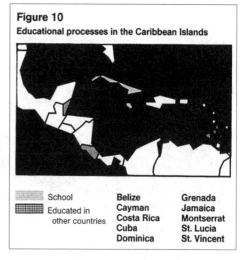

Figure 10
Educational processes in the Caribbean Islands

School
Educated in other countries

Belize
Cayman
Costa Rica
Cuba
Dominica
Grenada
Jamaica
Montserrat
St. Lucia
St. Vincent

The information compiled from this study could be a stepping stone for educators in nurse anesthesia programs to developed a network which would facilitate collecting needed information regarding the academic and clinical process for their individual students. The international study identifies countries on each continent where nurses provided anesthesia care.

References

[1] Keys TE: The History of Surgical Anesthesia. New York: Dover Publications, Inc. 1963:8; 35.

[2] Thatcher VS: History of Anesthesia with Emphasis on the Nurse Specialist. Philadelphia, Pennsylvania: J.B. Lippincott Company. 1953:63.

A Census of Copies of the Original Edition of John Snow's "On the Inhalation of the Vapour of Ether in the Surgical Operations"

A. Matsuki
Department of Anesthesiology, University of Hirosaki, School of Medicine, Hirosaki, Japan

J. W. R. McIntyre †
Department of Anesthesiology, University of Alberta Hospital, Edmonton, Alberta, Canada

Introduction

A bibliographical survey has been profoundly made on several invaluable medical classics. In 1984 Horowitz and Collins[1] tried a worldwide census of the original edition of Andreas Versalius' "De humani corporis fabrica" published in 1543 to report that 154 original copies have been preserved in the world. In 1988 Whitteridge and English revised Geoffrey Keynes[2]' "Bibliography of the writings of William Harvey[2]" to describe in detail that seventy original copies of the first edition of so-called "De motu cordis" published in 1628 are existing.

In the field of anesthesiology, John Snow's first monograph entitled with "On the inhalation of the vapour of ether in surgical operations" is the most brilliant classics as evidenced by repeated reproduction for these fifty years[3] as shown in Table 1.

Table 1: Reproduction of the original edition of John Snow's "On the inhalation of the Vapor of ether"

Editor	Year	Publisher
1. the Boston Medical Library	undated	unknown, Boston, USA?
2. the Wood Library-Museum with preface by the board of the trustees	1959	Lea and Febiger, Philadelphia, USA
3. Ole Secher (This is a reproduction of the reproduced copy by the Wood Library-Museum)	1985	Janssen pharma A/S. Birkerod, Denmark
4. Akitomo Matsuki with a preface in English and Japanese	1987	Iwanami Book Service Center, Tokyo, Japan

When the Wood Library-Museum of Anesthesiology of the United States reproduced the book by John Snow in 1958, Professor Vincent J Collins was in charge of this work and he made a census for the original edition. On our request, he wrote us on this item as follows.

When I was secretary of the board of Directions of the Wood Library-Museum of Anesthesia, I tried in 1957-58, to determine how many copies were extant. It was believed that by the rare book dealers and Drs Macintosh and Magill there were just six copies known.

They are:
1) One in the London Medical Library (now in the Welcome Institute) (Fig 1)
2) One at Oxford University
3) One in the Wood Library-Museum
4) One in the National Library of Medicine
5) One in Yale University, Cushing collection (?)
6) One in the private collection in the U.S. (not identified)

When the World Congress of Anesthesiology was held in Hamburg in 1980, I purchased by chance the original copy. The copy was autographed by John Snow to present to Mr Oppenheim, the editor of Zeitschrift für gesamte Medicine. (Fig 2) Therefore, the copy possessed by me is the seventh. (Fig 3) However, no detailed bibliographical investigation has been tried on the original copies of the first edition of Snow's book on ether anesthesia published in 1847. Thus we made an inernational census on the book.

Method

We set out to examine the likely possession of the original copy in the United States, Canada, the United Kingdom, France, Germany, Spain, Holland and Japan.

Results and Conclusion

Except for above mentioned seven copies, we found ten copies of the original edition as listed in Table 2. Therefore seventeen original copies are extant in the world so far (Fig 4).

Table 2: Ten Original Copies discovered by Our Census

1. British Museum Library (London, U.K.)
2. Library of the University of Edinburgh (Edinburgh, U.K.)
3. Medical and Biological Library, University College London (London, U.K.)
4. Library of Royal college of Physicians (London, U.K.)
5. The Bryn Thomas Memorial Library (Reading, U.K.)
6. Biblioteque Nationale (Paris, France)
7. Francis A countway Library of Medicine (Boston, U.S.A.)
8. Moody Medical Library. University of Texas at Galveston (Galveston, U.S.A.)
9. Norman Library of Science and Medicine (San Francisco, U.S.A.)
10. Catalogne 21 of Medicine and the Life Sciences (Norman Campany, U.S.A.) (presented copy to Joshua Parsons)

Acknowledgement

We would like to express our deep appreciation to the followings.

Dr. Vincent J Collins M.D., Department of Anesthesiology, University of Illinois, College of Medicine at Chicago, U.S.A

Francis A Countway Library of Medicine, Boston, U.S.A., Wellcome Institute for the History of Medicine Library, London, U.K.

Wood Library - Museum of Anesthesiology, Park Ridge, U.S.A.

Woodward Biomedical Library, Vancouver, Canada.

References:

[1] Horowitz M and Collins J: A census of copies of the first edition of Andreas Vesalius' De humani corporis (1543), with a note on the recently discovered variant issue. J Hist Med All Sci 1984; 39: 189

[2] Keynes G. Bibliography of the writings of William Harvey (3rd ed), revised by Whitteridge G and English C, Winchester, St Paul's Bibliographies, 1988

[3] Ellis RH(ed): John Snow: On Narcotism by the Inhalation of Vapours. Royal Society Medicine Services, London 1992

[4] The K Bryn Thomas Collection of Historical Books on Anaesthesia - A catalogue - Anaesthesia 1981; 36: 722

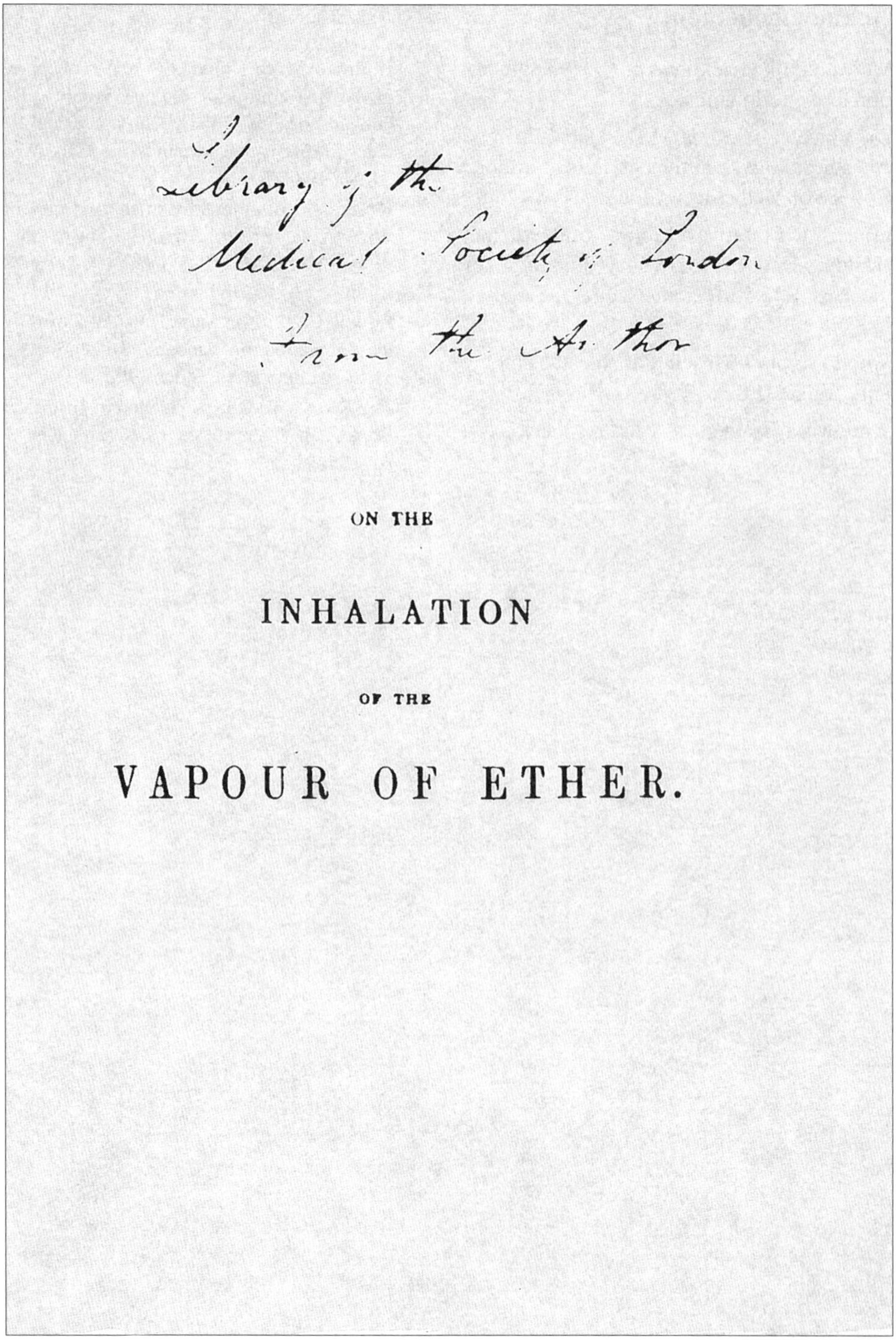

Library of the
Medical Society of London
From the Author

ON THE

INHALATION

OF THE

VAPOUR OF ETHER.

Fig. 1: Titel page of the copy in the Wellcome Institute

Zeitschrift

für die

gesammte Medicin,

mit besonderer Rücksicht

auf

Hospitalpraxis und ausländische Literatur.

Herausgegeben

von

F. W. Oppenheim.

Imperfecta, ut perfecta fiant,
id potissimum nostrum sit studium.

Siebenunddreiszigster Band.

Hamburg.
Perthes-Besser & Mauke.
1848.

Fig. 2: "Zeitschrift für die gesamte Medicin", including a review of Snow's book.

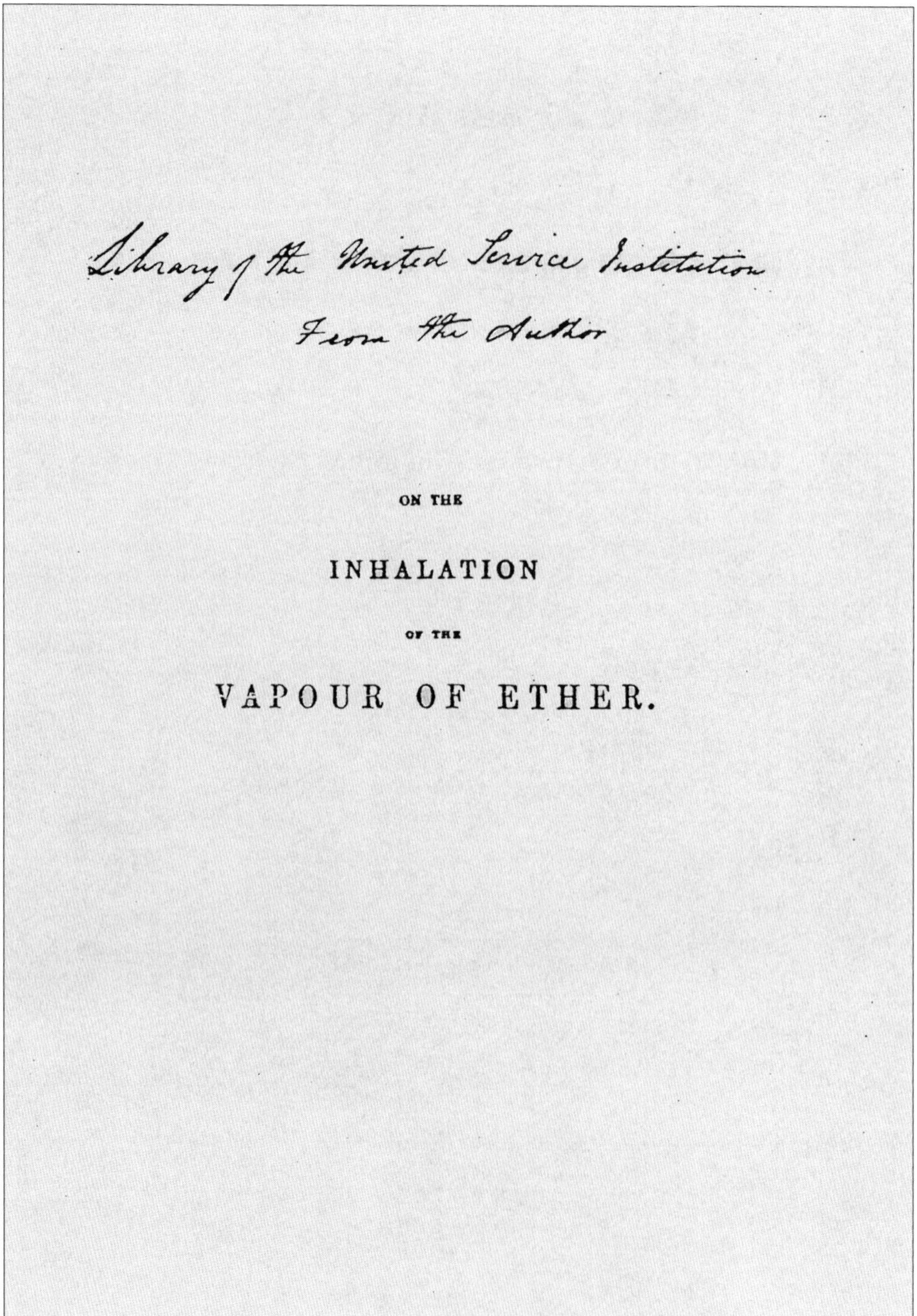

Library of the United Service Institution
From the Author

ON THE

INHALATION

OF THE

VAPOUR OF ETHER.

Fig. 3: Original copy possessed by Dr A. Matsuki presendted to Oppenheim, the editor of "Zeitschrift für die gesammte Medicin".

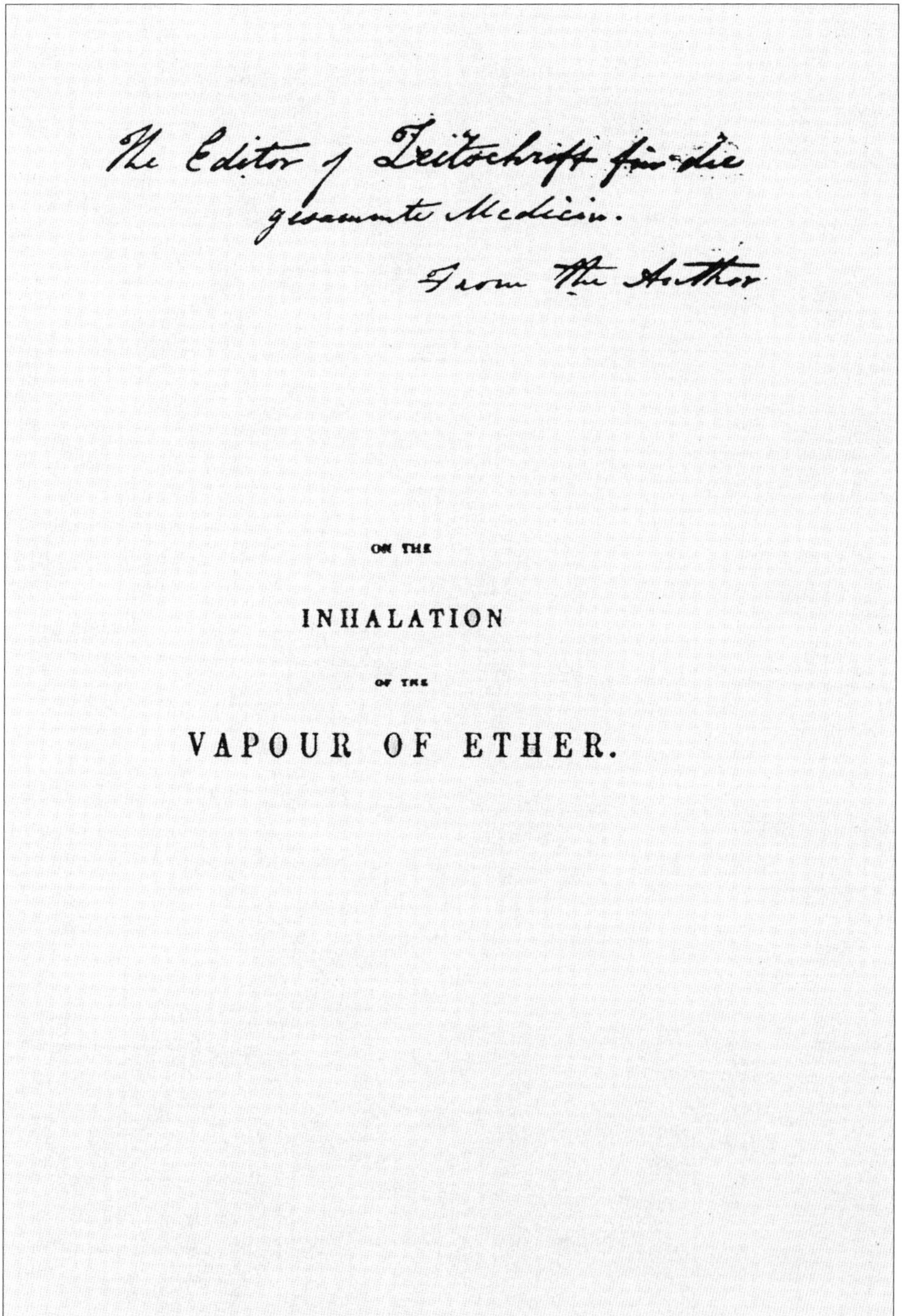

The Editor of Zeitschrift für die gesammte Medicin.

From the Author

ON THE

INHALATION

OF THE

VAPOUR OF ETHER.

Fig. 4: Title page of the copy in the Fancis A Countway Library

The Use of Curare in Poland – a Historical Outline

Szymanska-Kowalska, E. Sokól-Kobielska
Department of Anaesthesiology and Intensive Therapy
Central Clinical Hospital, Warsaw, Poland

The era of modern anaesthesiology in Poland began soon after World War II as Dr. Stanislaw (Stanley) Pokryzwnicki, the first Polish specialist in the field of anaesthesiology returned home from England in 1947.

After having graduated from CWSan (Sanitary Education Center) at the University of Warsaw, Dr. Stanislaw Pokryzwnicki became a physician in the famous Polish 302 squadron of the Royal Air Force in Great Britain during World War II with the rank of a Flying Officer).

He then turned his back to the army and specialized in anaesthesiology under the expert guidance of Professor Sir Robert Macintosh in Oxford.

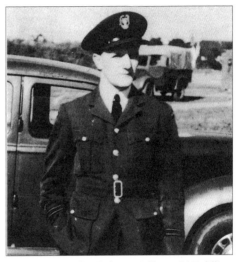

Fig.1: Dr. Stanislaw Pokryzwnicki as a RAF-Officer

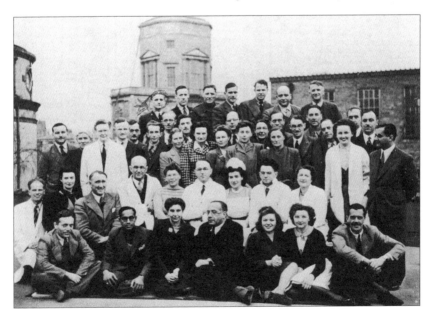

ASSOCIATION OF ANAESTHETISTS

OF

GREAT BRITAIN AND IRELAND

Founded in July, 1932

ANNUAL REPORT

1946

45 LINCOLN'S INN FIELDS,
LONDON, W.C. 2.

Telephone:
CHANCERY 6965

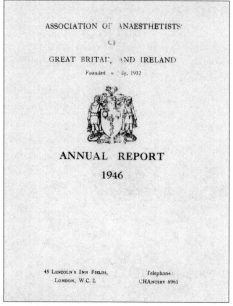

Fig. 3: Participants of the class of anaesthesia in Oxford 1946/47

22

MURRAY, Thomas Patrick, L.R.C.P. & S.I., 107 Liscard Road, Wallasey.
MUSGROVE, Alec Hugh, M.R.C.S., L.R.C.P., D.A., 1 Linden Avenue, Roath Park, Cardiff.
NAIRN, Andrew James, M.B., Ch.B., 10 Golf Road, Burnside, Rutherglen, Glasgow.
NORTHOVER, Philip Trevor, M.D., D.A., Lonach Lodge, Lansdown, Bath.
O'NEILL, Maurice Brendan, M.B., Ch.B., D.A., 11 Durham Square, Portobello, Midlothian.
ORD, John William Earling, M.D., C.M., 278 Willesden Lane, London, N.W.2.
OSBORNE, Sydney Edward, L.S.A., D.A., 2 Ansisters Road, Ferring, Worthing.
OWEN, Morus Wyn Lloyd, M.B., B.Ch., D.A., 50 Howard Road, Coulsdon, Surrey.
PARRY-PRICE, Hoel, M.R.C.S., L.R.C.P., D.A., R.N. Hospital, Plymouth.
PASK, Edgar Alexander, O.B.E., M.B., B.Ch., D.A., 6 Eddisbury Road, West Kirby, Cheshire.
PATERSON, John Carruthers, M.A., L.M.S.S.A., 11 Marsham Street, Maidstone, Kent.
PATERSON, Ursula Hamilton, M.B., B.S., D.A., 58 Beech Hill Road, London, S.E.9.
PATTERSON, William John, M.B., B.Ch., 142 Graham Road, Sheffield, 10.
PEARLMAN, Albert, M.R.C.S., L.R.C.P., D.A., Seaview, Dover Street, Folkestone, Kent.
PECK, John Portway Saville, M.B., B.Ch., 1 Lower Bridge Street, Canterbury, Kent.
PERREDES, John Felix, M.R.C.S., L.R.C.P., D.A., M.P.S., 41 Harlech Road, London, N.14.
PHILLIPS, Basil Montagu, M.R.C.S., L.R.C.P., D.A., The XVth Century Cottage, Etchilhampton, nr. Devizes, Wilts.
PHILLIPS, Edward Hamilton Dalrymple, M.R.C.S., L.R.C.P., D.A., 10 The Avenue, Worcester Park.
PILLANS, Annie Fleming, L.R.C.P. & S.E., D.A., 14 Aytoun Road, Glasgow, S.1.
POKRZYWNICKI, Stanley, M.D., 14 Chalfont Road, Oxford.
POLLEY, Stanley Frederick, M.R.C.S., L.R.C.P., D.A., 47 Tattenham Grove, Epsom Downs, Surrey.
PORTER, Norman Cunningham, M.B., Ch.B., D.A., 69 Heslington Lane, Fulford, York.
POTTER, Marie Elizabeth, M.B., Ch.B., 3 Nupton, Aylestone Hill, Hereford.
POWER, John Hale, M.B., Ch.B., 137 Binley Road, Coventry.
PRICE, Edward Newton, M.R.C.S., L.R.C.P., D.A., Old Orchard Lodge, Dane Road, St. Leonards, Sussex.
PYDDOKE, Silvia Whately, M.R.C.S., L.R.C.P., Eskbank, Tonbridge, Kent.
QUAYLE, George, M.R.C.S., L.R.C.P., D.A., 118A St. Julian's Farm Road, London, S.E.27.
RAE, William Kirk, M.R.C.S., L.R.C.P., D.A., 10 Trinity Court, Gray's Inn Road, London, W.C.1.
RAFFAN, Alfred William, M.B., Ch.B., 24 Albyn Place, Aberdeen.
RAINS, Kathleen Maude, M.R.C.S., L.R.C.P., D.A., 13 Lawton Road, Heaton Chapel, Stockport.
RANSOM, Shila Gwynne, M.R.C.S., L.R.C.P., D.A., 53 Knightwood Crescent, New Malden, Surrey.

ASSOCIATION OF ANAESTHETISTS OF GREAT BRITAIN & IRELAND.

CHAncery
6965.

45, Lincoln's Inn Fields,
London, W.C.2.

10th December, 1946.

Dear Dr. Pokrzywnicki,

I have pleasure in informing you that, at a meeting of the Council held on December 6th, you were unanimously elected a Member of the Association of Anaesthetists.

The Honorary Treasurer will be glad to receive your cheque for £2. in respect of your entrance fee and first annual subscription at your early convenience. This should be made payable to "The Association of Anaesthetists of Great Britain and Ireland", but if you prefer to use a Banker's Order, the necessary form is enclosed.

At the recent Annual Meeting it was decided that, as from July 1st, 1947, the annual subscription should be increased to £2. 10s. 0d. to cover the cost of the new journal of the Association, "Anaesthesia". Members wishing to receive the first three numbers of the journal, i.e. those that will be issued prior to July 1st, 1947, should send £1.2s.6d. to the Honorary Treasurer.

Yours sincerely,

Hon. Secretary.

Squad.Ldr.S. Pokrzywnicki,
14, Chalfont Road,
Oxford.

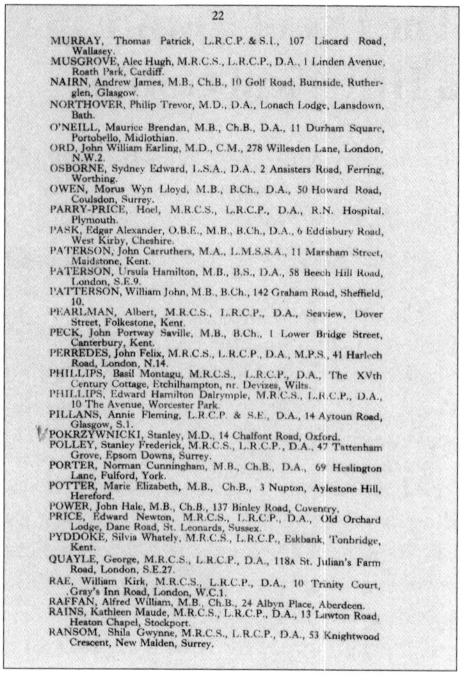

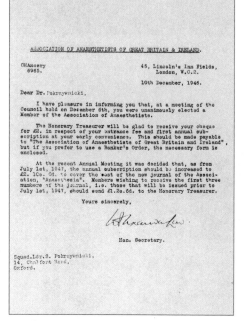

Fig. 5: Dr. Stanislaw Pokryzwnicki - a member of the Association of Anaesthesiologists of Great Britain and Ireland

From the Nuffield Department of Anaesthetics, University of Oxford

THE RADCLIFFE INFIRMARY
OXFORD

Telephone No. 48481
EXTENSION 266

5th March, 1947.

Dr. S. Pokrzywnicki has been working in this Department for the past year. Throughout this time he has proved a very pleasant, reliable and keen colleague. He has a sensible approach to the subject of anaesthetics, and I feel sure he will do extremely good work if he is afforded facilities to continue in the specialty. I regard him as a safe and sound anaesthetist, and I feel satisfied too that he can be confidently relied upon to organise an anaesthetic service to the advantage of the surgeons and hospital authorities on his return to his native country.

We are all sorry we are losing a good colleague, but I wish him happiness and every good fortune in his venture.

Nuffield Professor of Anaesthetics
University of Oxford

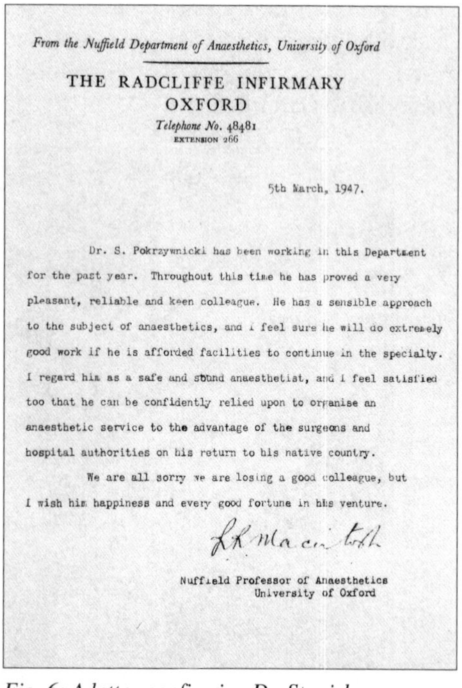

Fig. 6: A letter confirming Dr. Stanislaw Pokryzwnicki's membership

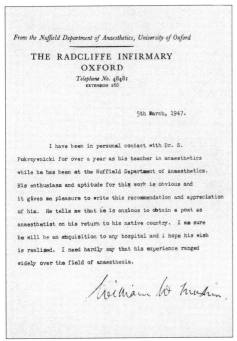

Fig. 7: Certificate of Dr. Stanislaw Pokryzwnicki's qualification as an anaesthesiologist by Professor Sir Robert Macintosh

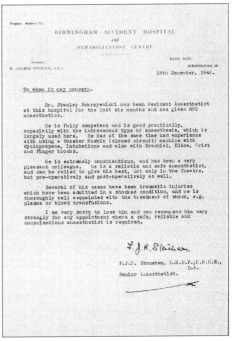

Fig. 8: Certificate by Wiliam W. Mushin

Dr. Stanislaw Pokryzwnicki later returned to his home town Kutno and performed the very first endotracheal intubation anaesthesia utilizing Curare on the 1st of December, 1947 at the St. Valentine's Hospital in Kutno on a patient undergoing cholecystectomy. This procedure took place only five years after the first application of Curare by Griffith and Johnson in Montreal, Canada, and only a year after the first European publication on its use by Gray and Halton from Great Britain.

At a celebration of the 40th anniversary of this event during a special meeting of the Polish Medical Society, the surgeon Josef Malinowski recollected his impressions of the operation as follows:

"Right from the very beginning of the procedure I was impressed by the course of the operation, especially after the peritoneum had been opened, I saw the guts as if they had been paralyzed and hence did not disturb the surgeon. As it is my habit I observed what the anaesthesiologist was doing and I stood horrified - the patient was not breathing, Dr. Stanislaw Pokryzwnicki was breathing for him! He asked me quietly if the guts had disturbed me and he advised me to proceed with the operation and not to bother with anaesthesia, since it did not fall into the surgeon's responsibility anymore. The operation seemed very easy to me. For the first time I operated in such comfort."

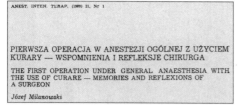

Fig. 9: Certificate of Dr. Stanislaw Pokryzwnicki's residency at the Birmingham Accident Hospital and Rehabilitation Center by F.J.R. Stoneham

From December 1947 until the 15th of January, 1949, Dr. Stanislaw Pokryzwnicki being an anaesthesiologist at the Second Clinic of Surgery at the University of Lodz, utilized Curare on 75 patients undergoing different procedures like Blalock's operation, lobectomy, pneumonectomy, esophageal resection, gastrectomy, pancreatectomy, cholecystectomy, caesarean section, hysterectomy and other minor operations and diagnostic procedures. He published his observations in the Polish Weekly Medical Magazine (Polski Tygodnik Lekarski) in 1949, Volume IV, Nr. 21, pp. 643-637.

The majority of the anaesthetized patients were in a poor general condition with a high risk for complications during anaesthesia. The duration of these operations ranged from 30 minutes to five hours (mean 3.5 hours).

As preoperative medication Dr. Stanislaw Pokryzwnicki used morphine and atropine. The induction of anaesthesia was achieved with penthotal and tubocurarine, while it was maintained with diethyl ether, penthotal, nitrous oxide or trichlorethylene. Neostigmine preceded by atropine was applied to reverse the skeletal muscle relaxation caused by tubocurarine.

Dr. Stanislaw Pokryzwnicki employed the "Oxford Vaporizer" for assisted or controlled ventilation via an endotracheal tube as well as McKesson's or Heidbrinck's apparatus.

Rodzaj przypadków operowanych z użyciem tubokuraryny lub intokostryny przedstawia się jak następuje:

Operacja	Liczba
Operatio m. Blalock	2
Lobectomia	1
Pneumonectomia	1
Thoracotomia probatoria	3
Vagotomia	1
Resectio oesophagi	7
Bronchoscopia	1
Laparatomia explorativa	4
Appendectomia	1
Cholecystectomia	
Cholecystoduodenostomia	
Cholecystectomia et omentectomia	14
Cholecystogastrostomia	
Enterocholodochostomia	
Resectio ventriculi	20
Gastrostomia	1
Operatio plastica oesophagi	2
Ca pancreatis — resectio pancreatis	1
Ca recti Op. radicalis abdomino-sacralis	3
Nephrolithiasis	1
Resectio sigmae	5
Op. varices haemorrhoidales m. Whitehead	1
Tumor ovarii, extirpatio	3
Amputatio uteri supravaginalis	1
Sectio caesarea	1
Sympaticectomia lumbalis	1
Razem	75

Fig. 10: Operations under anaesthesia performed by Dr. Stanislaw Pokryzwnicki between 1947 and 1949

Dr. Stanislaw Pokryzwnicki observed that tubocurarine helped to diminish the amount of anaesthetics used during operations, which promoted a quick recovery from anaesthesia and significantly lowered the incidence of nausea and vomiting. He also paid special attention to preventing intraoperative hypovolaemia and heat loss. In this matter he wrote the following: "I informed the surgeons that the duration of an operation from an anaesthesiologist's point of view was not as important as meticulous hemostasis and the prevention of intraoperative hypothermia."

Based on his thesis "on the Use of Curare of Anaesthesia; personal experience (75 cases)" Dr. Stanislaw Pokryzwnicki got a doctors degree (Ph.D.) at the University of Lodz in 1949.

It took five years after the invention of the drug in Canada in 1942 until the first anaesthesia utilizing Curare for muscle relaxation in Kutno, Poland, was carried out, which is quite a long period of time which has to be attributed to the terrible turmoil of World War II.)" Dr. Stanislaw Pokryzwnicki's article was published in Polish language, a language from behind the "iron curtain", which might be the reason that this publication that can be considered to be one of the first article on the clinical use of Curare in Europe, has never been mentioned in international bibliography.

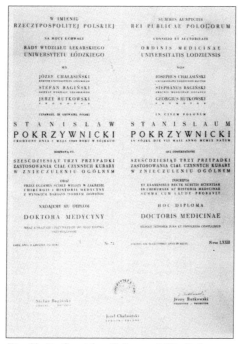

Fig. 11: Dr. Stanislaw Pokryzwnicki's diploma certifying his doctor's degree

From Tranportation to Prehospital Care – the Emergency Medical System in Hamburg 1946-1996

Paschen, H.R.*, Schallhorn, J.*, Lipp, M.,**
* *Feuerwehr Hamburg, Hamburg, Germany*
** *Klinik für Anaesthesiologie, Universität Mainz, Mainz, Germany*

Since its foundation in 1872 the professional firebrigade is in charge of the primary care for persons being involved with accidents, buried alive or trapped. On November 16th, 1945, the firebrigade of Hamburg was ordered by the British Military Government to provide transportation for street accidents which was to be "as fast as the firebrigade" itself. This project was to start immediately. Even though most of the firestations were destroyed by airraids, on April 1th, 1946, a well organized emergency system was established. The first years were dominated by a lack of adequate material and supply. The ambulances were just furnished with a stretcher, some blankets, and a very poor medical equipment. Furthermore, the training of the staff for the management of medical emergencies (EMT) was rather poor (Fig. 1).

At this time the sole purpose of the ambulances was to transfer patients to the nearest hospitals as fast as possible. Compared to todays standards, no preclinical treatment was provided on the spot or on the long way. The rapid progress in clinical emergency medicine and medical technology influenced the prehospital emergency care system. The innovations allowed to make a diagnosis and immediate adequate steps on the spot or on the way in order to help the patient. The

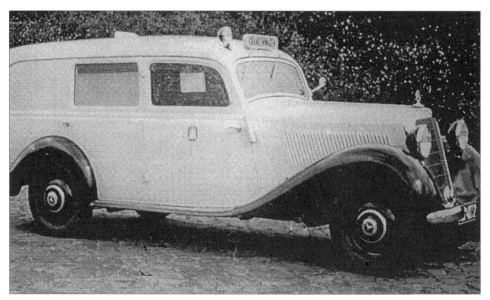

Fig. 1: Ambulance Mercedes-Benz 170 V/170 D, built in 1949

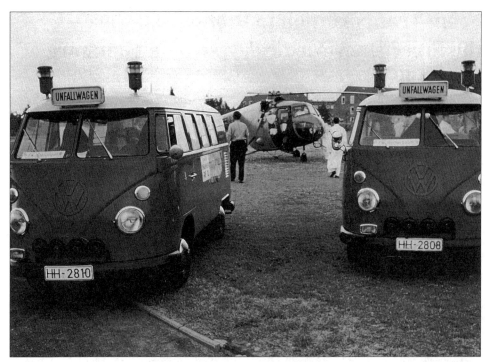

Fig. 2: Rescue helicopter type Bristol 171 Sycamore, and a standard ambulance type VV-Bus, 1960.

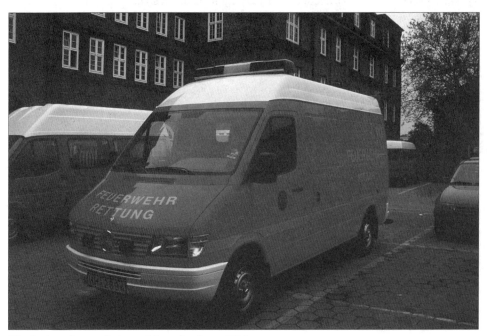

Fig. 3: A modern ambulance, Mercedes-Benz, 1996.

maxime switched from "scoop and run" to "stay and play".

In 1968 the first mobile intensive care unit (MICU) was inaugurated "bringing the physician to the emergency patient and not the patient to the emergency physician", according to the credo of the surgeon Martin Kirschner from Heidelberg (Fig. 2). As a result the training of the EMT`s was improved meeting the new situation. As the level of training of the paramedics was increasing the medical eduction of the emergcy physicians did as well. In the beginning young and unexperienced residents were appointed as emergency physicians, today´s emergency physicians have completed their training as a resident in a medical speciality and have to absolve an additional training in preclinical emergency medicine.

Today the modern ambulance is equipped with a semi-automatic defibrillator, respirator, pulsoxymetry and many other medical technical devices (Fig. 3). The staff comprises a paramedic and an EMT. It only takes 4,7 minutes from when the emergency call comes in to the ambulance arriving on the spot, which is a very short period of time. The modern equipment of the MICU allows extensive preclinical intensive care of patients in need. The emergency physician is supported by two paramedics.The MICU reaches the spot within 7,7 minutes after emergency call. In order to be able to cover all emergencies in this short time, a rescue helicopter is provided in day light in addition. The modern medical emergency system in Hamburg is equipped with a vanity of additional emergency services. For the treatment and interhospital transfer of premature newborns or severly ill neonates a special newborn MICU is available 24 hours a day. It is staffed with a neonatologist and has been especcially designed for this purpose (Fig. 4). In the presented emergency medical system the multifunctional firefighters with medical and technical education have proved to be of extreme value.

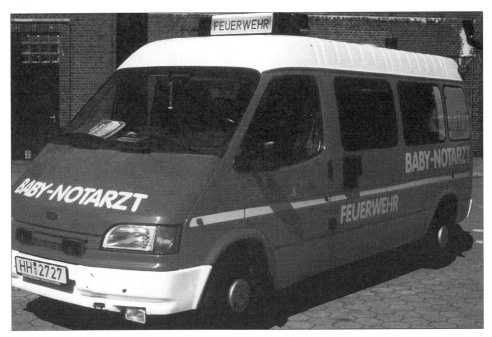

Fig. 4: Baby-MICU, especially designed for the transport of premature neonates.

Table I : Training of EMT in 1946 :

Traumatology	two hours
Internal Medicine	two hours
Venerel and Dermatological Diseases	two hours

Table II : Extent of medical education in the course of time

Year	Duration (h)	Qualification
1946	6	
1965	160	Rettungshelfer (basic EMT)
1977	520	Rettungsanitäter (EMT)
1989	2800	Rettungsassistent (Paramedic)

Table III : Special services of the EMS

- Newborn MICU
- Ambulance boat
- Ambulance for highly infectious diseases
- Chief emergency physician system

Heinz Wohlgemuth and Otto Roth: the Men behind the Technique

M. Goerig, E. Schaffner,
Department of Anaesthesiology, University Hospital Hamburg, Hamburg, Germany

When the history of anaesthetic apparatus in the German speaking area is written, the names of two surgeons should be included: Heinz Wohlgemuth and Otto Roth. Inspite of their enormous influence on the further technical development of anaesthetic apparatus at the turn of the century, little information exists on their biography.

Heinz Wohlgemuth was born to a Jewish family in 1863 in Neustettin, Pommern. In Berlin, where he was grew up, he started his medical studies in 1887. After his graduation at the University of Berlin on a topic, titled "Zur Pathologie und Therapie der scrophulös-tuberculösen Lymphadenitisgeschwulst bei Kindern bis zu 10 Jahren" in 1889 he began his surgical training under the well-respected James Israel (1850-1927) who was then chairman of the surgical department of the Hospital of the Jewish Community of Berlin. At the same time Max Michaelis (1869-1933) specialized under the reputable Ernst von Leyden (1832-1910) at

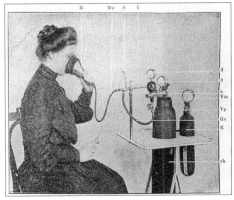

Fig 1: *Apparatus for oxygen therapy which was produced, designed and later produced by the firm "Sauerstoff-Fabrik Berlin"[2]*

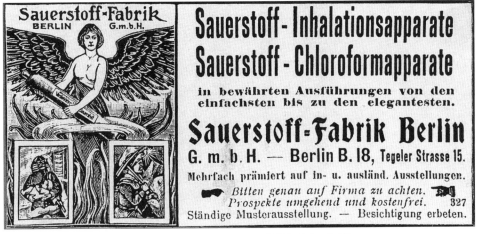

Fig. 2: *Advertisement for products of the firm "Sauerstoff-Fabrik Berlin"[13]*

the Department of Internal Medicine at the University Clinic of Berlin. As a consequence of Michaelis repeated reports on the beneficial effects of oxygen inhalation in life-threatening situations such as morphine-intoxication or extreme dyspnoea Michaelis became an early protagonist of the broad use of oxygen in the treatment of various internal diseases. The advantageous effects of the inhalation of oxygen inspired Wohlgemuth to use it in operative surgery. Under these circumstances it is understandable that Wohlgemuth (they were good friends), started to develop several sophisticated apparatus for the easy application of oxygen in surgical patients (Fig.1). He developed them in close collaboration with the firm "Sauerstoff-Fabrik Berlin" which later changed its name to "Sauerstoff Centrale Berlin" (Fig.2). Its owner was the pharmacist Ernst Silberstein (1866-1943), who, in 1906, changed his name to Ernst Silten.

As a result of his efforts Wohlgemuth developed a new anaesthetic apparatus and a mask (Fig.3). Volatile agents – usually chloroform – could be administered in a mixture with oxygen; This was a technical novelty at that time in Germany. This device of the firm "Sauerstoff-Fabrik Berlin" was equipped with some components (probably some pressure-reducing valves) originally produced by the Dräger-Company in Lübeck: the oxygen was conducted from a cylinder via a pressure reduction valve to an U-tube into which the chloroform was dripped. The volatile agent which was now enriched with

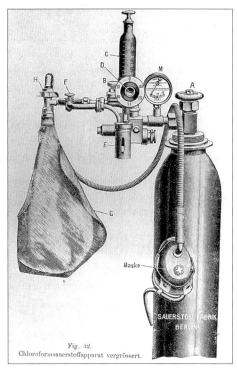

Fig 3: *Wohlgemuth´s anaesthetic device for chloroform-oxygen. Please note that the mask had a valve and that the rim of the mask was made with an inflatable rubber*[1]

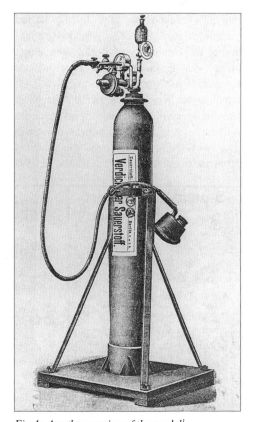

Fig 4: *Another version of the model*[1]

oxygen was led through a sponge soaked with water and then inhaled by the patient via a specially designed mask with an expiratory-valve. The mask itself had a rim made of an inflatable rubber. To guarantee the best control of the patients face Wohlgemuth initiated the production of a transparent mask made of celluloid. In 1901, during the Annual Meeting of the German Surgical Society in Berlin, Wohlgemuth reported on his first experience with the new device. He reviewed more than 180 anaesthesias which had been performed using the new apparatus (Fig.4)[1].

When in 1906 Michaelis published a well-known textbook of oxygen therapy in which the state of the art of this then new kind of therapy was discussed, Wohlgemuth was among the authors to describe the important role of oxygen therapy in operative medicine (Fig.5)[2,3]. At that time - however - Wohlgemuth's apparatus had lost its leading position among anaesthetic apparatus in Germany to the Dräger Company, Lübeck. This development was unfortunately overshadowed by legal disputes between the "Sauerstoff-Centrale Berlin" and the Dräger-Company of Lübeck (Fig. 6). Later the firm "Sauerstoff-Centrale Berlin" stopped its production of anaesthetic apparatus, but stayed in bussiness until 1938, when the Jewish owners had to sell their firms.

Unfortunately little information could be found on the further biography of Wohlgemuth. In the beginning of 1910 he worked in a private practice in Berlin as a surgeon and obstetrician but apparently he often attended surgical congresses. He wrote various articles for medical journals. It seems to us he never ceased to ask for a specialization of anaesthesiology in Germany[4,5]. Like his colleague Carl Ludwig Schleich (1859-1922) from Berlin, he praised the advantages of specialized colleagues in anaesthesia, for the patients as well as the outcome of surgery. Unfortunately a general acceptance of these ideas

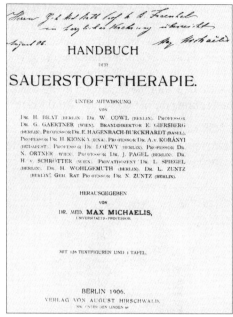

Fig 5: *Frontispiece of the well-known textbook on oxygen therapy which was edited by Michaelis in 1906*[2]

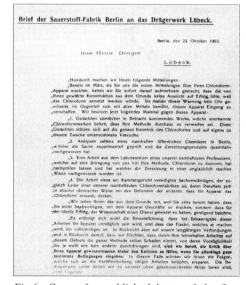

Fig 6: *Copy of a published letter of the firm "Sauerstoff-Fabrik Berlin" in which some incriminations against the "Dräger Company Lübeck", were mentioned*[13]

was not achieveable at that time and it took decades for them to be realized in Germany. When during the late twenties efforts were made to found a German anaesthesia society, Wohlgemuth died in Berlin before he was confronted with the inhumane living conditions during the period of the "Third Reich".

Otto Roth (Fig. 7) was born in 1863 in Ilsenburg, in the Harz Mountains. In 1882 he started with his medical studies in Tübingen

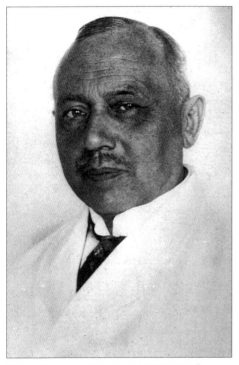

Fig 7: Portrait of Otto Roth (1863-1944)[7]

but then changed to Halle. In Leipzig, which was regarded at that time as the medical "Mecca" in Germany, he continued his studies before he returned to Tübingen where he graduated in 1891 writing about a topic titled "Ueber einen Fall von Sarkom, der mit hämorrhagischer Diathese verbunden war". He went to Berlin where he became an assistant to the well-respected surgeon Ernst von Bergmann (1836-1907) at the University Hospital. Among his surgical colleagues was Curt Schimmelbusch (1860-1895), well-known for his ingenious inventions like steam disinfection as well as his anaesthetic mask[6]. Maybe due to his contact with Schimmelbusch, Roth himself became interested in the unsolved questions of anaesthesia. In 1892 Roth went to Lübeck where – within a few years – he was renowned as an "all-round surgeon" so that in 1897 he was asked to chair the surgical clinic of the City of Lübeck. He held this position for more than 3 decades. In 1933 he retired, but still practised as a surgeon in another private hospital.

In 1911, 1921 and 1933 Roth was the president of the "Vereinigung Nordwestdeutscher Chirurgen", later he was appointed honorary member of this society for his lifelong engagement in operative medicine. Beside his interest in anaesthesia, Roth repeatedly published articles on surgical problems. The most noted were his review on fractures of the hip, the surgery of brain tumors and his experiences in the surgery of Hirschsprung's disease. Even if his contributions to the development of anaesthesia related devices were not explicitly praised by the society, Roth's name – he died highly honored in 1944 – will always be used in connection with the development of several anaesthetic devices: the "Roth-Dräger anaesthetic apparatus", the "Roth-Dräger mask" and the clinical introduction of the "Pulmotor" for the ventilation of patients[7].

We do not know if the initiative for the development of the anaesthetic apparatus came from the engineers of the Dräger firm or from Otto Roth himself, but it is evident that there was a close cooperation in the early 1900s between both[8]. The new apparatus allowed accurate measurement of drops of chloroform combined with oxygen from the storage cylinder. Roth demonstrated this device at the Annual German Congress of surgeons in

Berlin in 1902, a report of which appeared in the journal "Centralblatt für Chirurgie". In the apparatus the oxygen from the cylinder was used to operate two injectors which sucked in and vaporized drops of ether and or chloroform from separate reservoirs (Figs. 8, 9, 10).

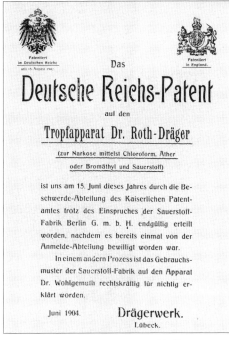

Fig 8: Patent for Roth Dräger, 1904[13]

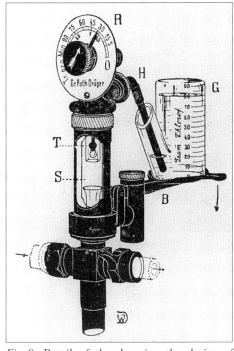

Fig. 9: Detail of the dropping the device of Dr. Roth-Dräger's apparatus[14]

The resultant mixture was inhaled from a reservoir bag through a somewhat narrow-bore tubing and a specially designed face-mask, which later became known as "Roth-Dräger's mask". The apparatus performed well and the production was started in 1903, so that the model could be sold world-wide under the name "Roth-Dräger mixed anaesthesia apparatus"[9,10]. It was shown in St. Louis during the universal exposition and the Dräger Company was awarded a diploma for it[8].

Another important development, in which Roth was involved from the early stages was the Pulmotor for the ventilation of patients via

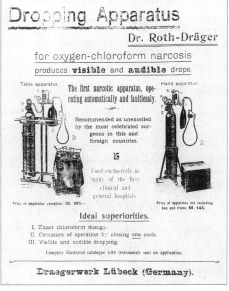

Fig. 10: Advertisement of Roth-Dräger's dropping apparatus, 1905[13]

a tight fitting mask (Fig.11). The original 1907 model had a clockwork motor that controlled the flow of oxygen from the cylinder to the positive and negative pressure venturies. The positive pressure venturi inflated the patient's lungs with the air-oxygen mixture and the other one produced a slight negative pressure to assist exhalation.

In 1910 the original model was replaced by an improved design which was both oxygen-powered and controlled11. Within a few years, fire and rescue squads rapidly adopted this model all over the world (Fig.12). Over the decades many modifications were developed[12].

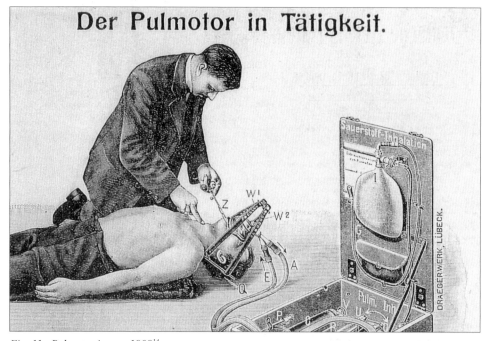

Fig. 11: Pulmotor in use, 1908[14]

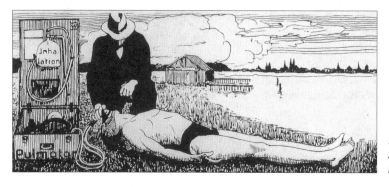

Fig. 12: Advertisement for the Pulmotor, 1920[13]

References:

[1] Wohlgemuth H: Eine neue Chloroform-Sauerstoffnarkose. Langenbeck's Arch klin Chir 1901; 64: 664-681

[2] Michaelis M: Handbuch der Sauerstofftherapie. August Hirschwald, Berlin 1906

[3] Wohlgemuth H: Der Wert des Sauerstoffs in der Chirurgie. In: M Michaelis (Hrsg): Handbuch der Sauerstofftherapie. August Hirschwald, Berlin 1906; 482-515

[4] Wohlgemuth H: Die Narkose und der Narkotiseur. Med Klin 1905; 20: 499-500

[5] Wohlgemuth H: Bessere Ausbildung in der Narkose und Anästhesie! Dtsch Med Wochenschr 1908; 37: 1595-1596

[6] Mohr W: Der Chirurg Prof. Dr. Otto Roth. 107-112. In: Der Wagen - ein lübeckisches Jahrbuch. Lübeck 1982

[7] Roedelius E: Zur Geschichte der Vereinigung Nordwestdeutscher Chirurgen. Tatsachen-Erinnerungen und Erlebnisse. Medizinhistorische Schriftenreihe Boehringer, Manheim 1967

[8] Haupt J: Die Entwicklung der Dräger Narkoseapparate. Drägerheft Nr. 280, Drägerwerk, Lübeck 1970

[9] Roth O: Zur Sauerstoff-Chloroform-Narkose. Cbl f Chir 1902; 46:1188-1190

[10] Roth O: Drägers Kombinationsapparat für Mischnarkose, Ueberdruckverfahren und künstliche Atmung. Med Klin 1911; 32: 1239-1240

[11] Roth O: Maschinelle künstliche Atmung. Bln klin Wochenschr 1911; 39:1729-1730

[12] Roth O: Wie haben wir uns die Wirkung der künstlichen Atmung vorzustellen? Zentralbl f Chir 1925; 21:1122-1123

[13] Collection Goerig, Hamburg

[14] v Brunn M: Die Allgemeinnarkose. Verlag von Ferdinand Enke, Stuttgart 1913

Did the Introduction of Anaesthesia influence the Indication for Surgical Procedures at the University of Erlangen?

W. Schwarz[1] U. v. Hintzenstern[2]
[1] Department of Anaesthesiology, University of Erlangen, FRG
[2] Department of Anaesthesiology, Municipal Hospital Forchheim, FRG

Introduction

On January 24th, 1847, Johann Ferdinand Heyfelder (1798 - 1869) (Fig. 1), who was Professor and Chairman of the Department of Surgery and Ophthalmology at the University of Erlangen from 1841 to 1854, anaesthesized a patient using sulphuric ether. By March 17th, 1847, Heyfelder had performed 121 surgical procedures under ether narcosis. He was one of the first physicians in Germany to publish his results and findings in a book in March 1847 [2].

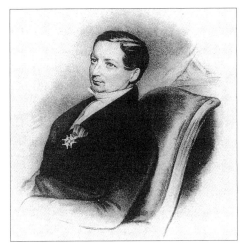

Fig. 1: Johann Ferdinand Heyfelder (1798-1869). Universitaetsbibliothek Erlangen, Portraitsammlung

Heyfelder kept a record of his clinical activities according to the so called "numeric" or "French" method established by Pierre Charles Alexandre Louis (1787-1872) [1]. From 1842 on he wrote annual reports [3] that were published as monographs or papers in medical journals.

Das chirurgische und Augenkranken-Clinicum der Universität Erlangen vom 1. October 1841 bis zum 30. September 1842

von

Herrn Dr. Heyfelder,

o. ö. Professor der Medicin u. Director der chirurgischen Klinik.

Das chirurgische Clinicum befindet sich im Universitäts-Krankenhause und besteht aus fünf geräumigen Krankenzimmern mit 27 Betten, aus einem zweckmäfsig eingerichteten Operationssaale, der zugleich als Auditorium für die Vorlesungen über Chirurgie und Augenheilkunde benutzt wird, aus einem Zimmer zur Aufbewahrung einer nicht unbedeutenden viel Interessantes enthaltenden Sammlung anatomisch-pathalogischer Präparate und aus einem Zimmer für die Assistenten.

Die Präparatensammlung wurde vom M. Jäger angelegt und enthält hauptsächlich solche Stücke, welche durch Operationen und Leichenöffnungen in der Klinik oder Poliklinik gewonnen wurden und deren Werth durch die vorhandenen Krankengeschichten erhöht ist, die über die einzelnen Fälle mit Umsicht geführt worden sind. Diese Sammlung hat in dem verflossenen Jahre manchen nicht unbedeutenden Zuwachs erhalten.

Fig. 2: Annual report 1841/42 of the Department of Surgery and Ophthalmology at the University of Erlangen

Referring to this material we would like to ask, if and how the introduction of anaesthesia influenced the indication for surgical procedures at the University Hospital at Erlangen.

Material

Data from the annual reports between 1841-1851 are listed in table 1 and presented

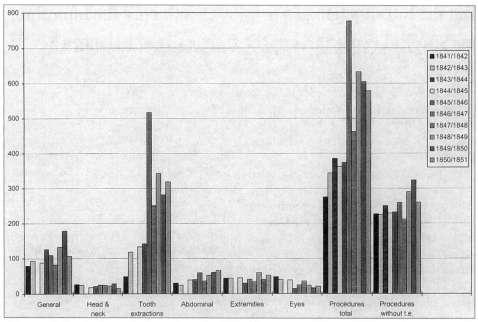

Diagram 1: Surgical procedures performed at Erlangen University Hospital 1841-1851

in diagram 1. Heyfelder classified the procedures that have been performed as "general", "head and neck", including tooth extractions, "abdominal", "extremities", and "eyes".

In diagram 2 the period prior to introduction of anaesthesia (1841-1846) is compared with the period starting with the introduction of anaesthesia (1846-1851).

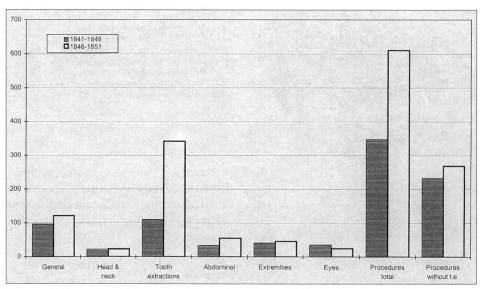

Diagram 2: Comparison of the number of operations before and after the introduction of anaesthesia at the University Hospital at Erlangen.

Diagram 2 shows the effect of anaesthesia being available, on the number of surgical interventions performed.

Results

The data from Heyfelder's annual reports suggest that:
- The number of procedures performed, increased from 348 between 1841 and 1846 to 610 between 1846 and 1851.
- The total increase of 68% is consed by an increase of in teeth-extractions by 168%.
- The number of surgical procedures increased about 15% only [3].
- A greater number of abdominal operations could be performed because of anaesthesia being invented.

Discussion

The immediate effect of anaesthesia on the development of surgery was not as outstanding as would have been expected. The introduction of anaesthesia was necessary in the development of surgery just a like few other details:
- the ability to control infection,
- knowledge about "normal" and "abnormal" organ function,
- a sense of professionalism in medicine in general and in surgery in particular, as Greene has pointed out [5,6].

This accounts for the fact that modern surgery could not experience a rapid development until the end of the 19th century.

References:

Guy MB: (1839) On the value of the numerical method as applied to science, but especially to physiology and medicine. J Statist 1839; Soc 2: 25-47

Heyfelder JF: Die Versuche mit dem Schwefeläther und die daraus gewonnenen Resultate in der chirurgischen Klinik zu Erlangen. Heyder, Erlangen 1847

Heyfelder JF: Das chirurgische und Augenkranken-Clinicum der Universität Erlangen
vom 1. Oktober 1841 bis zum 30. September 1842. Heidelberger Med Ann " 1-94, 1842
vom 1. Oktober 1842 bis zum 30. September 1843. Kunstmann, Erlangen, 1843.
vom 1. Oktober 1844 bis zum 30. September 1845. Kreuzer, Stuttgart, 1845
vom 1. Oktober 1845 bis zum 30. September 1846. Magazin für die gesammte Heilkunde 66: 233-309, 1848
vom 1. Oktober 1846 bis zum 30. September 1847. Z ges Med 37: 1-48+145-196, 1848
vom 1. Oktober 1847 bis zum 1. September 1848. Prager Vierteljahrschrift für die praktische Heilkunde 21: 1-42, 1848
vom 1. Oktober 1848 bis zum 30. September 1849. Prager Vierteljahrschrift für die praktische Heilkunde 26: 1-60, 1850

Heyfelder JF, Heyfelder O: Das chirurgische und Augenkranken-Clinicum der Universität Erlangen
vom 1. Oktober 1850 bis zum 30. September 1851. Deutsche Klinik 3: 487-490, 497-500, 506-509, 519-521, 523-527, 1851

Heyfelder O: Das chirurgische und Augenkranken-Clinicum der Universität Erlangen
vom 1. Oktober 1849 bis zum 30. September 1850. Prager Vierteljahrschrift für die praktische Heilkunde 31:1-26, 1851

Hintzenstern U v, Schwarz W: Frühe Erlanger Beiträge zur Theorie und Praxis der Äther- und Chloroformnarkose. Teil 1. Heyfelders klinische Versuche mit Äther und Chloroform. Anaesthesist 1996; 45:131-139

Greene NM: A consideration of factors in the dicovery of anesthesia and their effects on ist development. Anesthesiology 1971; 35: 515-522

Greene NM: Anesthesia and the development of surgery (1846-1896). Anesth Analg 1979; 58:5-1

Tracheotomy in Ancient Egypt - Fact or Fiction?

W. Maleck[1], U. v. Hintzenstern[2], K. P. Koetter[3]

[1] Department of Anaesthesiology, Klinikum, Ludwigshafen, Germany
[2] Department of Anaesthesiology, Municipal Hospital Forchheim, Forchheim, Germany
[3] Department of Neurological Intensive Care Unit, Leopoldina-Hospital, Schweinfurt, Germany

Introduction:

We became interested in the problem after reading Stetter[1,2]: *"Obviously the ancient [Egyptian] physicians could do much more: a picture from antiquity (First and Second Dynasties) apparently shows a tracheotomy, the surgical opening of the airway above and below the thyroid in cases of choking".*

Methods:

Stetter is vague about the original source. We tried to find the original picture and further hints about this knowledge, using Meline, new books on Ancient Egyptian Medicine and its secondary literature.

In Medline (Silverplatter 1966-1996) we looked for (ancient) AND (tracheotomy OR tracheostomy OR intubation).

Results:

Inaccurate citations

At first, our results were disappointing. We discovered several papers mentioning Ancient Egyptian Tracheotomy as a matter of fact (sometimes doubtful, though) without giving the original picture or an exact description of its contents.

Alberti[3]: *"It has been suggested that tracheotomy was practiced by the Egyptians 3,500 years before ... Christ".*

Booij and Feenstra[4]: *"Tracheotomie is een van de oudste bekende levensreddende handelingen. De techniek van en het instrumentarium voor de ingrep komen al voor op Egyptische kleitabletten en wastafels van 3600 jaar voor onze jaartelling."*

Brüssel[5]: *"Die Tracheotomie ist eine chirurgische Maßnahme, die in Indien und Ägypten schon vor 4000 Jahren durchgeführt worden ist. Die Ergebnisse dieser Eingriffe waren jedoch aus heutiger Sicht unbefriedigend."*

Frostad and Rönning-Arnesen[6]: *"Egyptian tablets (of approximately B.C. 3600) probably represent tracheostomies."*

Heurn et al.[7]: *"Het is onzeker wanneer de eerste tracheotomie werd verricht, maar waarschijnlijk werd deze ingreep reeds 3500 jaar geleden in Egypte uitgevoerd."*

Wenig and Applebaum[8]: *"References to tracheotomy describe this procedure being practiced by the ancient Egyptians and Hindus."*

Myers and Carrau[9] might also refer to Ancient Egypt with their cryptic statement: *"...there are reports of tracheotomies being performed before 2000 BC ..."* and the same applies to Zeitouni and Kost[10]: *"Although some accounts of tracheostomy date back over 4000 years, Asclepiades ... is the first person credited with the procedure."*

A very short statement is made by Russell[11]: *"Intubation has a recorded history back to Egyptian times."*

Papyrus Ebers

Some authors refer to Ancient Egyptian tracheotomy, citing an operation on the neck mentioned in Papyrus Ebers (early New Kingdom, about 1,500 B.C.)[12,13]. This, however, seems unjustified as the text in Papyrus

Ebers is about the operation of a tumour. Thus, although Papyrus Ebers proves that the Ancient Egyptians operated on the neck, it does not tell us that they performed tracheotomies.

The reason for these misinterpretations of papyrus Ebers is probably that they are based on the first translation by Joachim[14] in 1890. Here the tumour is located in the throat: *"Wenn Du ein Fett-Gewächs in seiner Kehle triffst und findest es wie ein Abcess des Fleisches, der unter Deinen Fingern erreicht ist, ... so sag Du dazu: er hat ein Fett-Gewächs in seiner Kehle. Ich werde die Krankheit mit dem Messer behandeln, indem ich mich vor den Gefässen in Acht nehme."*

Later translations locate the tumour superficially. Ebbell[15] wrote: *"If thou examinest a cystoid enlarged gland on his neck, and thou findest it like the thymus in the body, being soft to feel and its secretion being whitish ..., then thou shalt say concerning it: one suffering from cystoid enlarged gland on his neck; it is a disease which I will treat by an operation that guards the vessels."*

von Deines et al.[16]: *"Wenn du beurteilst ein Fettgeschwür an seiner Halsvorderseite, und Du findest es wie eine ... Schwellung des Fleisches, indem es weich ist unter deinen Fingern, seine Beschaffenheit ist weiß, schwach. Dann mußt du dazu sagen: einer mit einem Fettgeschwür an seiner Halsvorderseite: eine Krankheit, die ich behandle mit einer Messerbehandlung. Beachte die Gefäße."*

Bardinet[17] translated the position of the tumour as: *"dans la partie antérieure de son cou."*

Papyrus Smith

Papyrus Smith (about 1500 BC) describes another operation on the neck. Here the oesophagus and possibly the trachea are injured (resulting from trauma, not from tracheotomy).

The relevant case has been translated by Breasted[18]: *"If thou examinest a man having a gaping wound in his throat, piercing through to his gullet; if he drinks water he chokes and it comes out of the mouth of his wound; it is greatly inflamed, so that he develops fever from it; thou shouldst draw together that wound with stiching. Thou shouldst say concerning him: One having a wound in his throat, piercing through to his gullet. An ailment with which I will contend."*

In the translation of von Deines et al.[16]: *"Wenn du untersuchst einen Mann mit einer Klaff-Wunde an seiner Halsvorderseite, die aufgeweicht ist bis zu seiner Röhre. Wenn er Wasser trinkt, dann ... und es kommt aus der Öffnung seiner Wunde heraus. Sie ist sehr entzündet; infolgedessen bekommt er Hitze. Dann sollst du jene Wunde mit einem Faden zusammenfassen. Dann mußt du dazu sagen: einer mit einer Wunde an seiner Halsvorderseite, die aufgeweicht ist bis zu seiner Röhre: eine Krankheit, mit der ich kämpfe."*

Bardinet[17]: *"Si tu procèdes à l'examen d'un homme ayant une plaie béante à la partie antérieure du cou, qui transperce jusqu'au gosier, s'il boit l'eau, il défaille, alors que cela sort par l'orifice de sa plaie, alors qu'elle est chaude à l'excès et qu'il attrape la fièvre à cause de cela, tu devras maintenir ensemble cette plaie avec du fil. Tu diras à ce sujet: Un homme atteint d'une plaie à la partie antérieure du cou, qui transperce jusqu'au gosier, un mal avec lequel je combattrai."*

The labels

Finally, we could trace the source of the picture mentioned by Stetter to two labels dating back to protodynastic time (first and second dynasty, about 3,000 BC).

The first of these was discovered by Petrie in Abydos and published in 1901[19,20]. It consists of ebony wood. It consists of one part with the "tracheotomy" scene and another

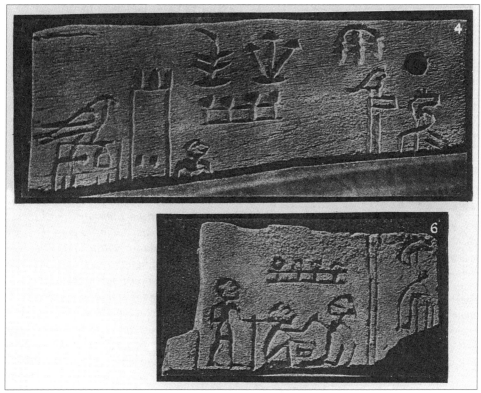

Fig. 1:
The ebony label discovered by Petrie in Abydos and dating back to the reign of Aha.
Note that the lower part is only about 5 cm long and 3 cm tall. The persons are less than 2 cm tall!

part with hieroglyphs which Petrie considers to be part of it (Figure 1).

The second was discovered by Emery and Saad in Saqqara and published in 1938[21]. It consists of unspecified wood and was found in the tomb of Hemaka (Figure 2).

The origin of the ritual sacrifice interpretation

Petrie as well as Emery and Saad interpreted their findings as pictures of a ritual sacrifice.

Petrie[19]: *"In front of the name of Aha is a building with the khaker ornament. Next is res meh shep, perhaps recieving (captives) of the south and the north. Below is a superintendent standing, and a man seated, apparently stabbing a seated captive in the breast. This suggests a scene of sacrificing captives at the royal funeral."*

Griffith[20] gave no interpretation of the picture, but a slightly different translation of the hieroglyphs above: *"Note ... [hieroglyph] in what seems to be its usual form in the Old Kingdom, and the signs for the South and North countries. One might conjecture that it means "Receiving the princes of the North and South," or "receiving the Kingdom of the North and South."*

Emery and Saad gave the following interpretation[21]: *"... the ... group ... consists of two seated human figures, both bearded. The one*

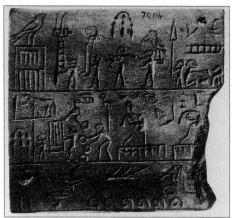

Fig. 2:
The wooden label discovered by Emery and Saad in Saqqara dating back to the reign of Zer (Djer). Note that the original label is only about 9 cm long and 8 cm tall. The persons in the "tracheotomy" scene in the upper right corner are only about 1 cm tall!
Reproduced from 23 with kind permission of the Institut Francais d'Archéologie Orientale du Caire.

on the right is apparently a captive with his arms tied behind his back ... The second ... facing him appears to be stabbing him in the breast with a knife which he holds in one hand, while with the other he holds a vase, presumably in which to catch the blood ... Above ... is a group of hieroglyphic signs ... which may perhaps be translated as receiving (or taking) from the south and north."

More than 20 years later, in a book first published in 1961, Emery repeated this interpretation[22]: *"The Sakkara label apparently records some important religious festival at which human sacrifice was performed."*

The origin of the tracheotomy interpretation

Vikentiev was the first to propose an interpretation of the labels as tracheotomies[23]. It is difficult to give a short but representative quotation from his 30-page paper dealing exclusively with the labels (the *"résumé"* is 4 pages long.) He discusses both egyptological (*"preuve lexicographique"*) and medical aspects (*"preuve epigraphique"*) of the labels.

He pleads that one of the ancient Egyptian verbs for "to breathe" was written with a lancet determinative, and thus might stand for an artificial respiration established by surgery: *"Ce qui vient d'etre dit et ce dont il sera question plus loin nous suggèrent que les cinq verbes nfi, tpi, ssn, hnp et hnm, parlent de l al respiration normale, tandis que la sixièmer, srk, déterminé, comme nous l'avons dit, par un outil piquant ou tranchant, dans lequel nous avons reconnu un instrument chirurgical, ou par la figure de l'arachnide, elle aussi munie d'un dard piquant et se lisant srk, aurait trait à la respiration, rétablie artificiellement au moyen d'une incision à la gorge."*[23 (p.188)]

He refuses to accept the idea of a violent act: *"L'impression qui se dégage de la scène n'est aucunement celle d'une action violente. L'homme que nous tenons pour le patient n'est pas frappé avec un couteau, comme le prétentent Petrie et Emery, mais l'instrument trachant est appliqué à sa gorge soigneusement et avec une attention concentrée."*[23 (p. 191)]

He translates the hieroglyphs above as *"La réception par le Sud et par le Nord du souffle de la vie".*[23 (p. 199)]

Other authors preferring the tracheotomy interpretation

The first author to support the interpretation of Vikentiev was Hussein[24] *"Je voudrais vous rappeler ici la communication extremement intéressante du Prof. Vikentief sur la trachéotomie chez les anciens Égyptiens. Je crois que le dessin est très probablement celui d'une vraie trachéotomie.1. L'instrument spécial employé permettait à l'opérateur d'en faire varier la direction afin d'ouvrir la trachée pour permettre l'introduction d'un roseau. Un simple perforateur ou un simple couteau n'aurait pas été aussi efficace que cet outil triangulaire. 2. L'attitude de l'opérateur est bien celle d'un chirurgien et rappelle très fidèlement celle de l'opérateur dans l'opération de circoncision de Sakkara. 3. L'opéré n'est pas une momie vu la difficulté extreme de mettre une momie dans la position accroupie comme dans le dessin."*

A person named something like Skody (spelling of Sercer[26]), Shody (spelling of Guerrier and Mounier-Kuhn[27]), or Shohdy (spelling of Shehata[28]) seems to have written a comment on the labels in the Medical Journal of the Egyptian Armed Forces in 1956[25]. According to both Sercer and Shehata, he argued in favour of an interpretation of the labels as tracheotomies. We were, however, unable to get a verified copy of this. We got a copy of a paper written by a "Col. Mohamed A. Shohdy" with the title "Ancient Egyptian Surgery" from Klippe[29]. But this copy, three pages long, does not mention tracheotomy. It might, however, be an incomplete copy and it neither gives the name of the journal nor the year and volume. It could also be an English summary of a longer Arabic text as the Medical Journal of Egyptian Armed Forces was a publication in Arabic language (according to SERLINE on Silverplatter 1997).

Brewer[30] seems to have supported the theory concerning a tracheotomy too: *"I had an opportunity ... to make some studies in Egypt, and I thought it might be ... interesting to take some pictures ... One was taken from hieroglyphics on the wall of the tomb at Sakkara, which is one of the oldest tombs in Egypt (3000 B.C.). Egyptian scholars believe it showed a tracheotomy being performed. Horus, the god of medicine, is watching either a surgical procedure or perhaps a sacrificial rite."*

An interesting fact here is that a mural is mentioned. If this is true, this would point to another original apart from the labels. However, as this was only a contribution to a discussion, and as Brewer is inaccurate in calling Sakkara a tomb (it is a cemetery), it should not be taken too seriously.

Drawings of the labels are included in an arabic publication of Doghaim[31]. According to Shehata[28], this also a favours the version of a tracheotomy.

Guerrier and Mounier-Kuhn[27] wrote: *"Quittons la légende pour en arriver à l'histoire. Il semblerait que la première trachéotomie eut été pratiquée par les Égyptiens, 3600 ans av. J.-C."*

As mentioned above, Shehata[28] supports the tracheotomy thesis: *"Two engravings were discovered in Abydos and Sakkara regions in Egypt, from the old predynastic time (3600 B.C.) represented the performance of a tracheostomy operation and the instruments used in its performance. ... This discovery was doubted by some authors, and confirmed by others."*

Pahor[32, 33] published two papers, in 1986 and 1992 respectively: *"Each slab depicts a seated person directing a pointed instrument to the throat of another person who is kneeling backwards with his arms tied behind his back. Petrie, Emery and Zaki Saad believed that this denotes human sacrifice whereas Vikentiev and Hussain believe it to be a tracheostomy ... The latter view is more appropriate as ... the way the scalpel is handled is more appropriately directed to the trachea than the neck vessels. The arms placed behind ... will be explained on similar grounds to our present day practice of placing a sandbag between the shoulder blades ..."*

Biefel and Pirsig[34] argued cautiously in favour of tracheotomy: *"Einzelne Autoren interpretieren bestimmte Darstellungen auf ägyptischen Tafeln aus Abydos und Saqqara aus der Zeit um 3000 v. Chr. als ... Tracheotomie. Von den drei hier gezeigten Personen wird der rechts sitzenden ein Messer an den Hals gesetzt ... Die mittlere Figur wird als Arzt gedeutet, der eine Tracheotomie durchführt.*

Daß hier keine Tötungsszene dargestellt wird, läßt sich aus der Anhäufung der vier "Anch"-Zeichen über dem Kopf des "Tracheotomierten" ablesen."

Helidonis[35] seems to support Vikentiev too: *"Emery described two tablets dating from the beginning of the dynastic period ... They show a person sitting and directing a sharp instrument towards the neck of a kneeling person. Vikentieff believes that this was a magical ceremony tracheotomy meant to insufflate life into the aged king."*

Other authors preferring the interpretation as sacrifice

Weill[36] argued from an egyptologist viewpoint in favour of human sacrifice in Ancient Egypt in general and specifically on the two labels discussed here. Interestingly, he does not mention Vikentiev, although Weill's book was published over 10 years later. He mentions the label discovered by Emery, but does not discuss the "tracheotomy" scene in the upper right corner. Concerning the label discovered by Petrie, he only briefly mentions the person with his arms tied back as *"l'homme qu'on sacrifie"*.

Sercer[26], arguing from the viewpoint of an ENT-surgeon, also clearly dismissed the tracheotomy interpretation: *"1956 überraschte Skody ... mit der Publikation zweier ägyptischer Tafeln aus der vordynastischen Zeit (etwa 3600 Jahre v.Chr.). Die eine wurde in Abydos, die andere in Sakkara gefunden; angeblich sollten sie beide eine Tracheotomie darstellen. ... Ein genaues Studium der Abbildungen läßt eher an die Darstellung eines Menschenopfers denken, denn die hockende Gestalt stößt anscheinend einen langen Dolch in das Herz des ... Opfers, und nichts deutet auf eine Operation am Halse hin."*

Taillens[37] essentially argued like Sercer: *"Pictures from the period of King Djer in Sakkarah in Egypt dating from 3600 B.C. allude to the first known tracheotomy in history. In fact it is an oft[en]-repeated error to consider this as an allusion to tracheotomy because the knife is plunged into the cardiac and not the cervical region."*

Authors preferring an open question

Some authors consider this to be an unanswered question, e.g. in two papers by Klippe et al.[29] and Sauret-Valet[38] and in the books of Ghalioungui[39, 40] and Nunn[41].

Klippe[29]: *"Im Gegensatz zu Skody verneint Sercer jedoch die Kenntnis der Tracheotomie bei den alten Ägyptern."*

Sauret-Valet[38]: *"También se ha especulado sobre si realizaron traqueostomías, basándose en unos dibujos en tablilla que muestran a un hombre (médico, sacerdote?) dirigiendo un cuchillo a la garganta de un supuesto enfermo, e incluso se ha lanzado la hipótesis de traqueostomías, para insuflar el pneuma de la vida a faraones envejecidos."*

Ghalioungui[39, 40]: *"It is impossible to be certain when the facts are so thin, but it must be added that many egyptologists firmly believe that human beings were sacrificed at least in the very earliest epochs of Egyptian history ... This drawing may, therefore, suffer many interpretations ..."*

Nunn[41]: *"Ghalioungui also drew attention to two slabs from the First Dynasty ... Each shows a kneeling figure with his arms behind his back, while another person points something looking like a dagger at the upper part of ... his chest. Petrie interpreted this as ritual sacrifice but Vikentieff ... suggested it might be a performance of a tracheostomy. This can only be surmise and seems very unlikely because the setting is that of a ritual and the point of the instrument is aimed too low for a tracheostomy."*

Finally, Nunn[42] recently reminded us of an important fact that had been overlooked so far by most authors (including himself and us), i.e. that the figures in question are very small:

"It was a shock to realize that the "patient" in the Djer label was only 9 mm tall in the original". The figures in the Abab label are only slightly larger, measuring less than 2 cm. (See figures 1 and 2.)

Authors not mentioning possible Ancient Egyptian tracheotomy

Finally, there are authors not mentioning the question of tracheotomy, e.g. the books of Bardinet[17] and Westendorf[43].

Conclusion:

We agree with Ghalioungui *"It is impossible to be certain when the facts are so thin"* and furthermore so small.

The only hard facts are two labels dating back to early dynastic time, about 3,000 BC (note the inaccuracy of several authors dating them back to predynastic time about 3,600 BC). These show a person stabbing another. The fact that the scenes on both labels (which date back to different kings) are remarkably similar points to an important ritual of some sort.

In our opinion, it is unlikely that these labels represent tracheotomies performed either as a therapy or as a public demonstration on captives. The most important argument against tracheotomies is that the tip of the instrument is pointed rather to the chest than to the neck.

This, however, does not exclude that the Ancient Egyptians performed tracheotomies, as tracheotomy does not require high-tech instruments; and as both Papyrus Ebers and Papyrus Smith report operations on the neck.

Furthermore, King Djer - whose reign one of the labels dates back to - was, according to Africanus, citing Manetho, a physician and wrote books on anatomy: *"Athotis [or Djer], his [i.e. Menes'] son, [ruled] for fifty-seven years. He built the palace at Memphis, and his anatomical works are extant, for he was a physician"*[41]. This points to a strong interest in medicine in his time. Even his anatomy books could have existed (maybe written by "ghost-writers").

Based on this, it might be that the labels represent neither a therapeutic measure nor a religious ritual but vivisection of captives for the advancement of anatomy. However, this is just another hypothesis which cannot be proven at the present state of knowledge.

References:

1. Stetter C: Denn alles steht seit Ewigkeit geschrieben. Quintessenz, München 1990, p. 43
2. Stetter C: The Secret Medicine of the Pharaohs. Edition Q, Chicago 1993, p. 36 and 41
3. Alberti PW: Tracheotomy versus Intubation. Annals of Otology, Rhinology and Laryngology 1984; 93:333-337
4. Booij LHDJ, Feenstra L: Tracheotomie en Intubatie. Nederlands Tijdschrift voor Geneeskunde 1990; 134:1205-1209
5. Brüssel T: Intubation versus Tracheotomie bei Langzeitbeatmung. Anästhesiologie, Intensivmedizin, Notfallmedizin, Schmerztherapie 1995; 30:504-506
6. Frostad AB, Rönning-Arnesen A: Tracheostomy in Acute Obstructive Laryngitis. Journal of Laryngology and Otology 1973; 87:1101-1106
7. van Heurn LWE, Brink PRG, Kootstra G: De Geschiedenis van de Tracheotomie. Nederlands Tijdschrift voor Geneeskunde 1995; 139:2674-2678
8. Wenig BL, Applebaum EL: Indications and Techniques of Tacheotomy. Clinics in Chest Medicine 1991; 12:545-553
9. Myers EN, Carrau MRL: Early Complications of Tracheotomy. Clinics in Chest Medicine 1991; 12:589-595
10. Zeitouni AG, Kost KM: Tracheostomy: a Retrospective Review of 281 Cases. Journal of Otolaryngology 1994; 23:61-66
11. Russell CA: Developments in Thermoplastic Tracheal Tubes. In: Barr AM, Boulton TB, Wilkinson DJ: Essays on the History of Anaesthesia. Royal Society of Medicine, London 1996, p. 94-97
12. Frost EAM: Tracing the Tracheostomy. Annals of Otology, Rhinology and Laryngology 1976; 85:618-624
13. McClelland RMA: Tracheostomy: its Management and Alternatives. Proceedings of the Royal Society of Medicine 1972; 65:401-404
14. Joachim H: Papyros Ebers. Verlag Georg Reimer, Berlin 1890, p. 188-189
15. Ebbell B: The Papyrus Ebers. Levin & Munksgaard, Copenhagen 1937, p. 121-122
16. von Deines H, Grapow H, Westendorf W: Grundriss der Medizin der Alten Ägypter. Vol IV,1. Übersetzung der medizinischen Texte. Akademie-Verlag, Berlin 1958, p. 188-189 and 223
17. Bardinet T: Les Papyrus Médicaux de l'Égypte Pharaonique. Fayard, 1995, p. 366 and 508
18. Breasted JH: The Edwin Smith Surgical Papyrus, Vol 1. University of Chicago Press, Chicago 1930, p. 451
19. Petrie WMF: Royal Tombs of the Earliest Dynasties. (Part II of Royal Tombs of the First Dynasty.) Egypt Exploration Fund, London 1901, p. 20 and plate III
20. Griffith FL: The Inscriptions. In: Petrie WMF: Royal Tombs of the Earliest Dynasties. (Volume II of Royal Tombs of the First Dynasty) Egypt Exploration Fund, London 1901, p. 48-54
21. Emery WB, Saad ZY: The Tomb of Hemaka. Government press, Cairo 1938, p. 35-36 and plate 17-18
22. Emery WB: Archaic Egypt. Penguin Books, London 1991, p. 59
23. Vikentiev V: Deux Rites du Jubilé Royal à l'Époque Protodynastique. I. Donation du Souffle de la Vie au Peuple, Illustrée par l'Incision dans la Trachée-Artère ("Tracheotomie") Bulletin de l'Institute d'Égypte 1949-50; 32:171-200 and Plate I
24. Hussein MK: Quelques Spécimens de Pathologie Osseuse chez les Anciens Égyptiens. Bulletin de l'Institute d'Égypte 1949-50; 32:11-17
25. Skody A, Shody or Shohdy MA: Ancient Egyptian Surgery. Medical Journal of Egyptian Armed Forces 1956. (Cited According to Sercer, Guerrier and Shehata)
26. Sercer A: 2000 Jahre Tracheotomie. Ciba-Symposium 1962;10:78-86
27. Guerrier Y, Mounier-Kuhn P: Histoire des Maladies de l'Oreille, du Nez et de la Gorge. Editions Roger Dacosta, Paris 1980, p. 397-398

[28] Shehata MA: History of Laryngeal Intubation. Middle East Journal of Anaesthesiology 1981; 6:49-55

[29] Klippe HJ, Löhr J, Kroeger C: Historische Aspekte zur Entwicklung der endotrachealen Intubation. Praxis und Klinik der Pneumologie 1981; 35:413-420

[30] Brewer LA: Discussion. In: Dugan DJ, Samson PC: Tracheostomy: Present Day Indications and Technics. American Journal of Surgery 1963; 106:290-306

[31] Doghaim NM: Surgery and Medicine of Ear, Nose and Throat in Ancient Egypt. Alexandria Medical Journal 1972;18:30-45

[32] Pahor AL: Ear, Nose and Throat in Ancient Egypt. In: David RA: Science in Egyptology. Manchester University, Manchester 1986, p. 243-250

[33] Pahor AL: Ear, Nose and Throat in Ancient Egypt, Part II. Journal of Laryngology and Otology 1992; 106:773-779

[34] Biefel K, Pirsig W: Tracheotomien vor 1800. Gesnerus 1988;45:521-539

[35] Helidonis ES: The History of Otolaryngology from Ancient to Modern Times. American Journal of Otolaryngology 1993; 14:382-393

[36] Weill R: Recherches sur la 1re Dynastie. Institut Francais d'Archéologie Orientale, Caire 1961, Vol. 2, Chapter 14

[37] Taillens JP: Modern Indications for Tracheotomy in Cases of Acute and Chronic Asphyxia. Advances in Oto-Rhino-Laryngology 1968;15:1-31

[38] Sauret-Valet J: Las Enfermedades Respiratorias en el Antiguo Egipto. Archivos de Bronconeumologia 1994; 30:506-507

[39] Ghalioungui P: Magic and Medical Science in Ancient Egypt. 1st Ed., Hodder&Stoughton, London 1963, p. 93-95

[40] Ghalioungui P: The House of Life per Ankh. Magic and Medical Science in Ancient Egypt. 2nd Ed., B.M.Israel, Amsterdam 1973, p. 90-92

[41] Nunn JF: Ancient Egyptian Medicine. University of Oklahoma, Norman 1996, p. 42 and 169

[42] Nunn JF: Personal Communication, August 1997

[43] Westendorf W: Erwachen der Heilkunst. Artemis & Winkler, Zürich 1992

Acknowledgments:

We thank Marianne Herrmann very much for helping with the translation of the French articles and Lynne Lörler for her critical revision of our English manuscript.

Management of Difficult Airways in 1898: E. Tschudy (Zurich) – Forgotten Pioneer of Orotracheal Intubation

H. Wulf, H. Gockel, J. Wawersik
Department of Anaesthesiology and Operative Intensive Care, University of Kiel, Kiel, Germany

To our current knowledge it was Sir William Macewen[1], professor of surgery in the University of Glasgow, who was the first to use orotracheal intubation instead of tracheotomy to secure the airway in 1878. These attempts were made in order to prevent the entrance of blood and secretion from the oral cavity into the larynx during surgery, to administer anaesthesia with chloroform, and to obtain a patent airway in case of oedema glottis.

Obviously, the technique was not in widespread use at the turn of the century. In Europe, professor Karl Maydl[2] from Prague reintroduced the intubation of the larynx in 1893. His intention was predominantly to prevent the aspiration of blood into the tracheopulmonary system, supplemented with a tamponade of the pharynx. The tube was connected to the anaesthesia machine. In the US, O´Dwyer[3] constructed a metal laryngeal tube for orotracheal intubation and ventilation. Last not least it was Franz Kuhn[4] who further developed the technique of endotracheal intubation and intratracheal insufflation anaesthesia at the start of this century.

On May 3rd, 1898, Eugen Tschudy[5], a surgeon in Zurich, managed a case of difficult airway during strumectomy using the technique of orotracheal intubation. To our knowledge this report from Tschudy has not been cited in literature before. We discovered this paper by chance, while looking for the preceeding article in this volume: August Bier: "Weitere Mittheilungen....".

In Tschudy's case in a 30y female patient with tracheomalacia the airway became completely obstructed during surgery and chloroform anaesthesia. Respiration ceased, the patient became cyanotic and the pulse faded. Due to the large struma attempts at immediate tracheotomy were impossible. Therefore, as an ultimate idea, a gastric tube was introduced through the mouth and guided by a finger down to the trachea. The patient was resuscitated successfully (artificial ventilation and "ether injected subcutaneously") and

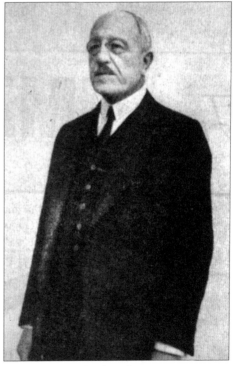

Eugen Tschudy (1866-1938)

the operation was finished after 2h under spontaneous ventilation. Afterwards the tube was removed from the trachea. Anaesthesia had been delivered via the orotracheal tube. According to Tschudy the method offered a valuable technique in case of tracheal obstruction and an alternative to short term tracheotomy. He published the case in 1901, the year of "Die perorale Intubation" by F. Kuhn. Obviously, he was not aware of former reports on the subject.

Curriculum vitae: Dr. Eugen Tschudy (13. August 1866 - 28. March 1938) Head of the department of surgery of the catholic Hospital Theodosianum in Zurich from 1. April 1897 - 28.March 1938. Tschudy received his surgical education in the Kantonsspital Münsterlingen, Swiss (Head of the surgical department was Dr. Otto Kappeler). During his time as head of the surgical department of the Theodosianum, Dr. Tschudy performed more than 20.000 operations, including more than 2000 strumectomies. (The help of Professor Rüttimann, (Head of the Institute of History of Medicine, University of Zurich, Switzerland) in providing the data of the biography of E. Tschudy is gratefully acknowledged)

Translation of the important parts:
XII: Short Communications:
Acute tracheal stenosis managed with tracheal intubation. By Dr. E. Tschudy, Head of the Surgical Department, Hospital Theodosianum, Zurich, Switzerland.

...in a case of total tracheal kinking (obstruction) during surgery for a goiter (strumectomy), when tracheatomy was impossible, we used a method that has not been used before (at least we did not find any description in the surgical literature available for us), and that could replace with some benefit – due to its simplicity – in many cases tracheotomy.

Case report: a 30 year old housewife with "struma dyspnoetica" was admitted to the hospital. She had a giant struma (goiter) "as big as a human head" with severe tracheal stenosis, significant stridor, severe dyspnoea and recurrent episodes of acute respiratory distress.

Operation on May 3rd 1898 : Chloroform anaesthesia with a Kappeler's Apparatus (see figure), the patient received morphine 0.02 subcutaneously beforehand. ...following skin incision and mobilisation of the struma .... and in this moment the patient was unable to breathe any more despite vigorous respiratory attempts. Immediate repositioning was without success, the trachea remains obstructed. ...Tracheotomy proved to be impossible ... and respiration ceased. She was cyanotic and no pulses were palpable. Fortunately, a life-saving thought came to our mind; we rapidly introduced a medium-smooth and medium-size gastric tube into the trachea and advanced it carefully down to the bifurcation; than immediate artificial ventilation and ether subcutaneously. The air was floating freely through the tube and following 10 min of artificial ventilation the patient started to breathe again spontaneously. The tube was left in place for the remainder of surgery for two hours and worked without problems, ... The further postoperative course was without significant complications.

... the kinking of the trachea was immediately and completely overcome by advancing the gastric tube down to the bifurcation ...; the introduction of the tube guided by the finger did not result in any difficulties in this asphyctic (deeply cyanotic) patient and was performed within a few seconds.

The tube allowed respiration within the normal range and anaesthesia was maintained by placing the orifice of the tube beneath the face mask of the Kappeler apparatus .... This method (resembling nothing else but an intubation of the trachea) could make tracheotomy unneccessary and replace it in all cases, in which ... a transient partial or complete obstruction of the larynx is the problem, and it is of paramount interest for all general practitioners because it allows to manage a case of imminent asphyxia without surgical help in an easy and safe manner. – That even a prolonged application for several hours is without major drawbacks is demonstrated by the present case .... If one prefers a metallic instrument, a flexible metallic tube constructed like König's tracheotomy-tube could be obtained; we will perform some trials within the next time with such an instrument and will report on it later[5].

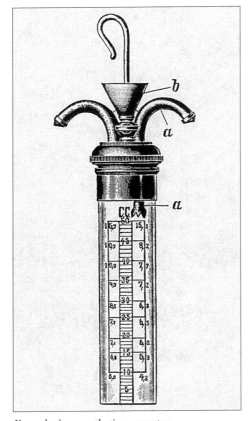

Kappeler's anaesthetic apparatus

References:

[1] Macewen W: Clinical observations on the introduction of tracheal tubes by the mouth instead of performing tracheotomy or laryngotomy. Br Med J 1880; 2:122-4

[2] Maydl: Intubation des Larynx als Mittel gegen Einfliessen von Blut in die Respirationsorgane bei Operationen. Wiener Medizinische Wochenschrift 1983; 43: 57-59, 102-106

[3] O´Dwyer J: The evolution of intubation. Trans Am Ped Soc 1896; 8: 9

[4] Kuhn F: Die perorale Intubation. Centralblatt für Chirurgie 1901; 28: 1281-1285

[5] Tschudy E: Ueber Behandlung acuter Trachealstenose durch Trachealintubation. Langenbeck´s Archiv für Klinische Chirurgie 1901; 64: 260-3

Dr. CT Jackson's Inductive Discovery

R. Patterson
University of California, Los Angeles, USA

At the Second International Symposium on the History of Anaesthesia, Dr. R.H. Ellis introduced some overlooked letters belonging to William Whewell that he had discovered lying loose in the Wren Library, Trinity College. One letter, written at the time clinicians were learning of the ether demonstration at the Massachusetts General Hospital, initiates the acclamation, (vexing and misunderstood in the materialistic society of the mid-19th C., as well as the 20th), of peers to one not personally present at the public demonstration.

A letter from Edward Everett, President of Harvard College, Cambridge Massachusetts, dated 20 Nov. 1846, addressed to the Reverend William Whewell, Master of Trinity College, Cambridge England, gave a short account of "a very curious method of producing by inhalation entire insensibility, under the most severe surgical operations." Everett went on to say that he had seen ether insensibility for himself, "It seems not easy to over-rate the importance of this discovery."[1] The letter was a means of announcing the news to the British Association for the Advancement of Science of which they both were members: additionally it directly apprised the chronicler of the history and philosophy of science of a previously unknown truth.

Everett then wrote to Dr. Charles Thomas Jackson on 26 Feb. 1847: "considering the great importance of your discovery of a mode of producing temporary insensibility to pain, during the performance of surgical operations, I have thought that it might be advisable for you, in the form of a paper addressed to the American Academy of Arts and Sciences, to place on record the most important facts connected with the discovery and its introduction into general noteriety and practice. Although these facts are known to many persons in their general outline in the neighborhood, Others at a distance do not possess that advantage, and a due regard to the interests of Science seems to require some such statement from the most authentic source."[2] The following day a letter to Jackson from John C. Warren reiterated these sentiments.[3]

Later, in Novum Organon Renovatum, the third part of his overview of human intellectual progress, Whewell specifically cited Jackson as being responsible for revealing by induction an aspect of science to be exploited in the future by the deductions (Art) of technicians. Whewell was emphatic in precisely distinguishing between the discovery of what occured and the discovery of why a phenomenon occurred.[4]

Whewell, as had previous commentators, held that there were common elements of creative thinking: ability to structure the problem; extensive background knowledge in potential relevant areas; continuing preoccupation with a problem over considerable periods of time, a process that requires strong motivation. Well documented episodes in Jackson's life epitomize such characteristics.

As early as age 14 Jackson was corresponding and exchanging mineral specimens with leading American and European naturalists. Gradually he became aware that these observers and collctors were laying the foundations for the philosophers of the future: by age 22 he was convinced that scientific investigation was of more than utilitarian value. Preceding Whewell's 1837 expressed belief that Scientific knowledge was part of Universal Truth and would lead to a Science of Morals and Religion, Jackson wrote:

"I believe that it is necessary to be acquainted with the Lower Kingdoms of nature in order to be a good physiologist. That our studies if arranged in what might be strictly called a natural manner would first make us acquainted with the mineral kingdom then the vegitable then the animal, with a consideration of the manner in which changes take place in these bodies as explained by chemistry. Then having learned the relations of these bodies to each other we should finally arrive to the consideration of intellectual and moral relations which would naturally lead us to a religion or a consideration of our connection with the world to come."[5]

During postgraduate medical study in Paris in 1829 the necessary inevitableness of pain and bodily stress accompanying the surgical procedures he was now practicing prompted Jackson to declare that any ameliorating discovery, if only a shortening of the duration of suffering, was worthy of the thanks of the world to the nation that spawned the inventor. Having familiarized himself with the technique he made plans to purchase for $500 the instruments designed by Doctor Jean Civiale to remove bladder stones without cutting. In Civiale's hands the average time was less than three minutes from introducing the instrument into the bladder through the natural orifice, grinding the stone to dust and removal by injecting water into the bladder, to removal of the instrument.

"What an improvement and substitute for that dreadful operation so horrible and so frequently fatal in its conseq. to this humane and safe and effectual operation. The name of Civiale rendered immortal by the invention of this ingenious effecient and humane operation will never be forgotten. His life will be inscribed upon the pages of philanthropy and France will be proud of the honor of giving birth to this distinguished man."[6]

His sojourn abroad initiated not only a lifelong reflection on the mitigation of pain, but also an unshakeable realization of the benefits of rational science to his homeland:

"...my national vanity must be a little humbled on comparing the state of knowledge in any of our Capitals with that of Paris. I love my country and see in her infancy a blank sheet to be filled up in time with character that will not only vie with any in Europe but at length surpass them. When man begins to think of something beyond the mere acquisition of money we may be able to make Something of a figure in the world."[7]

After Paris and before returning to America Jackson undertook a Wanderjahr which eventually took him to Naples and an ascent of Vesuvius and a night in the erupting volcano's crater. The currents of hot vapor, ejection of stones, and streams of liquid lava made a lasting impression. Upon first returning to Boston he recieved more money from lecturing on volcanoes than he did from medical practice. To close the lectures he "exhibited a magnificent display of fireworks resembling the appearance of a volcano in eruption."

During the succeeding years he gradually lessened his medical activities while making extensive geological surveys throughout the country; being employed in chemical consultations for industries; and establishing one of the first laboratories in the United States for the teaching of analytical chemistry. One among the long list of students under his tutelege was William Thomas Green Morton.

His interest in volcanoes persisted. In 1837 while perfecting the eruption demonstration with various smoke-producing chemical mixtures he accidently inhaled chlorine gas with consequent choking pain. He immediately treated himself with inhalations of ether vapor which relieved the severe strangling discomfort. Ether was not an unusual prescription for pulmonary disorders; being commonly used in cases of phthisis, asthma, whooping cough, croup, and catarrh.

"In my case it was an effective remedy for the strangling and toxic effects resulting from the inhalation of chlorine gas and it was used for that purpose in my laboratory from that time forth. Henry Sumner and William Channing, pupils working in my laboratory were similarly affected by chlorine, both relieved with ether. This discovery I made known at the time to most of the chemists with whom I was acquainted, and it was adopted extensively."[8]

Of all the innumerable other uses to which ether inhalation had been tried (for treatment of cholera when Jackson was in France during the 1832 epidemic; trials of inhalation to put hysterical women to sleep; during the fad of "ether frolics" wherein participants had roused to feel pain) and no one had the foresight to repeat the inhalation and take away the pain (no deductions were forthcoming concerning the amelioration of surgical pain.

It was Whewell's thesis that there was a "mask of theory over the whole face of nature". Therefore Francis Bacon's view of inductive generalization as a summary of a class of observations needed revision in the following manner; To understand the "truth" from observation of a phenomenon is a two part process. Apparent facts involve theoretical assumptions; therefore the mind is active in perception, giving "form", "Idea" to sensation. From an assemblage of relevant but disconnected ideas, suddenly the mind actively "superinduces" an understanding of the phenomenon.[9]

Jackson writes of a February 1842 disaster as he was again assembling a number of experiments in illustration of his theory of volcanic eruptions:

"I prepared a large quantity of chlorine gas, collecting it in gallon glass jars over boilng water. Just as one of these large jars was filled with pure chlorine it overturned and broke, and in my endeavor to save the vessel, I accidently got my lungs full of chlorine gas, which nearly suffocated me, so that my life was in imminent danger. I immediately had ether and ammonia brought and alternately inhaled them with great relief."

"The next morning my throat was severely inflamed, and very painful, and my lungs were still much oppressed. I determined therefore to make a more thorough trial of ether vapour, and for that purpose went into my laboratory. I had a large supply of perfectly pure washed sulphuric ether ... soaking a towel ... seated in a rockingchair ... began to inhale ether vapour mingled with air deeply into my lungs .... Soon entire loss of feeling ...."

Consciousness was lost, the towel fell; after some minutes he became aware of his surroundings.

"I observed that all pain had ceased in a suffering part of my body during the inhalation preceding and following the unconscious state."[10]

Jackson knew that physiological experiment and clinical observation confirmed that the nerves of sensation, motion, and of organic life were distinct, and that one system might be paralyzed without necessarily and immediately affecting the others. Judging from his own uneventful recovery from unconsciousness ether had no apparent effect on the involuntary functions of respiration and circulation. His crucial and seminal observation, the "idea-provoking" observation was "that the state of insensibility of the nerves of sensation before consciousness was lost continued for a sufficient length of time to admit of most surgical operations"; immediately, "in a flash" his mind predicted that "during the unconscious period the degree of insensibility was still greater, so that it would be impossible that any pain could be felt from a surgical operation." His mind had "sensed" the significance of the differential effect of ether vapor on the human nervous system!

"It was my intention to revisit Europe, and to bring out this discovery in the great hospitals of Paris, but I was at the time actively engaged in geological surveys so that I had not a month that could be spared for a voyage to Europe. Having confided my discovery to twelve of my friends, some of whom are gentlemen devoted to science, and some of them physicians and dentists, I considered it safe, so far as priority of discovery was considered."[11]

Since he had essentially curtailed his medical practice and had no regular patients, he resorted to telling other practitioners of his induction in order to interest them in demonstrating its efficacy. Dentist Samuel A. Bemis recalled being in conversation in Sept. 1842 with William F. Channing, Jackson, and several other gentlemen when the subject of pain and painful operations incident to dental practice came up:

"Dr. Jackson then remarked that it was his wish to alleviate or destroy all sensation of pain and suffering during operations of a surgical nature ... by the introduction of a new treatment or agent which would prevent all consciousness of pain. Dr. Jackson said that if I desired it he would give or provide me with something which he knew would effect that object and also proposed to me to introduce the same into my profession. The substance to be used viz: sulphuric ether ... that he had been induced to try its effect upon himself when suffering in consequence of some accident, and that he had been completely successful in its application."[12]

Bemis then expressed his reluctance to pioneer a novel experiment, protesting the unnecessariness (one of numerous evasions that delayed the introduction and later contributed to arguments against its use during the rest of the century:

"I replied as a reason why I should not be willing to introduce the use of the new agent into my own practice, that in such operations as came under my particular care there was seldom much suffering, and that I had more often found difficulty in impressing my patients with a belief that there was really no necessity for operations than to persuade them to submit when operations were deemed necessary."[12]

Four years later Jackson was visited in his laboratory by WTG Morton, his quondam student. Morton now had a thriving "tooth factory" providing dental plates which often required preliminary multiple tooth extractions. This day, according to assistants George Barnes and Joseph Peabody working with Jackson, Morton wanted to borrow a rubber bag which he planned to fill with room air and convince a very reluctant female patient that inhaling from this bag would prevent the pain of the extractions. Jackson remonstrated against this flimflam and told Morton what he had told others over the preceding years, that the inhalation of ether vapor was the way to eliminate pain.[13]

Morton's demonsration of the effectiveness of ether at the Massachusetts General Hospital on October 16, 1846 occured while Jackson was out of town on a geological consultation; Morton at the time acknowledging Jackson's idea and responsibility.

The ensuing personality dominated, politically and financially ridden dispute, "the ether controversy" thoroughly muddled who had priority of discovery; its reward; and what constituted the discovery. Support of Jackson was affirmation of Whewell's distinction between observer and discoverer; confirmation that the "discovery" was an induction; recognition that reward was the honor of the discovery, "a right dearer to scientific men than money or life itself".[14]

Surprised and baffled by attacks claiming that he was the usurper of the ideas of others Jackson soon became resigned; a condition expressed by Ralph Waldo Emerson in a letter to Louis Agassiz:

"He has run the gauntlet so often, and has come at last to see that there is a power in facts against all opposition, that he has become perfectly peaceable and amiable on the subject, and quite willing to say nothing, and let his claim rest on the very testimony offered by his opponents."[15]

References:

[1] Everett E: Letter of 20 Nov. 1846 to William Whewell. The Whewell Papers. The Wren Library, Trinity College, Cambridge England

[2] Everett E: Letter of 26 Feb. 1847 to Dr. Charles Thomas Jackson. CT Jackson Archives, Massachusetts Historical Society, Boston

[3] Warren JC: Letter of 27 Feb 1847 to Dr. Charles Thomas Jackson. CT Jackson Archives, Massachusetts Historical Society, Boston

[4] Whewell W: Novum Organum Renovatum. 3rd ed. JW Parker, London 1858

[5] Jackson CT: Letter of 1827 to Charles Brown. CT Jackson Archive. Houghton Library, Harvard University, Cambridge, Massachusetts

[6] Jackson CT: Letter of 18 Feb. 1830 to Charles Brown. CT Jackson Manuscript Collection, Library of Congress, Washington, DC

[7] Jackson CT: Letter of 23 July 1832 to Lydia Jackson. CT Jackson Manuscript Collection, Library of Congress, Washington, DC

[8] Jackson CT: A Manual of Etherization. JB Mansfield, Boston. 1861 p.16

[9] Yeo R: Defning Science, Cambridge University Press 1993

[10] Jackson CT: (op, cit, ref 8)

[11] Jackson CT: (op. cit. ref 8) p.48

[12] Bemis SA: Deposition 20 May 1847. CT Jackson Archives. Countway Library of Medicine, Boston

[13] Barnes G: Deposition 11 Nov. 1846. CT Jackson Archives, Massachusetts Historical Society, Boston

[14] Lord J l: A defence of Dr. Charles T. Jackson's claims to the discovery of etherization. Office of Littell's Living Age. 1848

[15] Emerson RW: Letter 1 May 1859 to Louis Agassiz. CT Jackson Archive. Massachusetts Historical Society, Boston

The "Coughing Pistol", Hustenpistole or Tussomat

J. Stoffregen, Husterstraße Hagen, Hagen, Germany

With the help of Heinz Oehmig, I developed the Hustenpistole (the coughing-pistol) in Heidelberg in 1955. This piece of apparatus simulates coughing and helps to remove retained or aspirated material - secretions, blood, gastric contents or foreign bodies - from the lungs (Fig. 1). The device consists of a vacuum-container connected via a pistol-like rotating valve (or artificial glottis) to the endotracheal tube. By pressing the trigger, the valve closes firstly the opening to atmosphere (or ventilator) and, within 0.03seconds, connects the trachea and bronchi with the evacuated vacuum-container (5.0ml at -600mbar). In this way, a small amount of air is suddenly aspirated at high velocity (ca. 8L/sec) from the lungs with any aspirated material. The technique provides a close imitation of a spontaneous cough, the purpose, of course, being to assist the removal of aspirates from patients suffering from respiratory insufficiency or paralysis due to unconsciousness or anaesthesia. After obtaining a licence, the Dräger Company of Lübeck produced and sold the device for some ten years under the name "Tussomat" but it was expen-

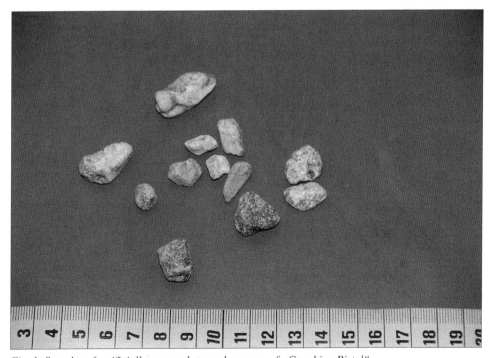

Fig. 1: Samples of artificially removed stones by means of „Coughing Pistol"

sive and poorly promoted and was finally taken off the market (Fig. 2). This seems a pity because it could have saved lives. Later, in 1981, I asked a small firm - Wagonbrett of Bremen - to make a new version at a reasonable price, and they did this, but I have yet to find a distributor.

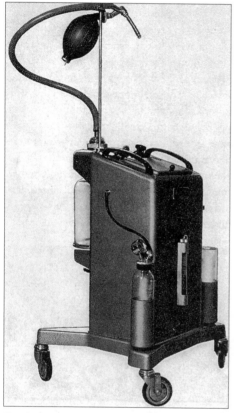

Fig. 2: Dräger's "Tussomat"

In 1956, with Professor Janker of Bad Godesberg, who had cine-X-ray facilities, I made a short film demonstrating the effectiveness of the coughing-pistol in an anaesthetised German-shepherd dog. With the help of my friend Ernst Kolb, the anaesthetised dog was paralysed with suxamethonium, intubated and ventilated with oxygen for some minutes. Liquid contrast medium was then instilled into the left lower lobe. The efficiency of the device was clearly demonstrated when two or three artificial coughs completely cleared the contrast medium from the bronchial tree down to the smallest bronchioli. The dog was unharmed by this hour-long procedure and 20 minutes later woke up, waved its tail in a friendly manner and drank water. Examples of the use of the device in clinical practice follow:

Case I:

In 1958 in Göttingen, a 7 month-old infant weighing 4kg, needed bronchography for the diagnosis of an oesophageal fistula. This would not have been practical previously due to total filling of the bronchi of the infant by the contrast medium. With the cough-pistol this did not happen, the contrast was completely removed. A baby was anaesthetised with halothane, intubated after suxamethonium and manually ventilated. The tube connector was removed and replaced by a 20ml syringe filled with Bronchografin, a viscous liquid which had to be warmed to become injectable. This was instilled via the endotracheal tube to obtain a complete tracheobronchogram of both lung fields

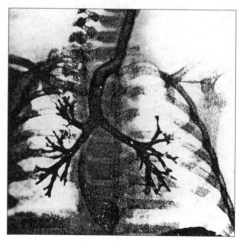

Fig. 3a: Complete filling bronchogram in a 4000 g succling infant before

(Fig. 3a). The baby's gaseous exchange was completely blocked, but after the X-rays had been taken, the cough-pistol was connected to the tube and the Bronchografin removed (Fig. 3b). After four coughs, virtually nothing remained. The whole procedure lasted about 45 seconds.

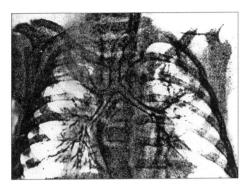

Fig. 3b: and after the first first artificial cough

Case II:

In 1970, near Göttingen, a 70 year-old farmer fell with his tractor into a gravel pit and was nearly drowned. Face down, he aspirated water and gravel. He was rescued and resuscitated with difficulty due to the stones impacted in his trachea. In the clinic he was reintubated with the largest tube possible and then, with the coughing-pistol, two hand-fulls of stones were retrieved from the trachea and bronchi. Figure 1 shows some of the stones, the largest measuring 22 mm. Three weeks later, after standard intensive care, the patient left the hospital in excellent condition.

Case III :

In 1978, late on a Saturday evening, a woman who had undoubtedly had her last meal some 10 hours previously, had to be anaesthetised for caesarean section. After the usual precautions, including the anti-Trendelenburg position to about 35°, anaesthesia was induced with methohexitone and suxamethonium. Immediately, a large quantity of brown-coloured gastric contents was regurgitated and seen to quickly disappear through the wide-open glottis. She was intubated blindly and the infant delivered within 60 seconds. Anaesthesia was maintained and attention given to clearing the mother's lungs. Normal saline was squeezed from plastic bags down the endotracheal tube and cleared by several artificial coughs. The process was repeated until the lavage fluid was absolutely clear and auscultation of the chest, using an electronic amplifier, was normal. The post-operative period was uneventful, the patient leaving hospital 11 days later without being aware of any abnormal occurrence.

A non-rebreathing System used with the Takaoka-Ventilator
("Modell Göttingen", "ANE 2000")

J. Stoffregen, Husterstraße Hagen, Hagen Germany

With few, but well-defined exceptions, we have used this little ventilator developed by K.S. Takaoka of Sao Paulo in 1957, for anaesthesia since 1965. The machines are widely available in South America, but rarely in Germany and were originally invented for resuscitation of the new-born but later found to be suitable for ventilation of a wide range of patients. The Takaoka-Respirator is technically a pressure-cycled flow generator delivering a constant laminar flow. It may be considered an improvement on other ventilators in that it was designed to ventilate the lungs without gas turbulence and therefore without additional resistance, even under extreme conditions such as in status asthmaticus or during cardio-pulmonary resuscitation. In addition it is small and easy to handle. Its I:E = 1 ratio is fixed and, due to the constant laminar flow, the arterial respiratory pressure waves are similar to those found during spontaneous breathing. The ventilator has to be used with a non-rebreathing system, e.g. the "Model Göttingen" which has many advantages in comparison with conventional semi-closed circle systems. It makes anaesthesia less dangerous, simpler to carry out and easily controllable. These factors are compatible with St. Exupery's definition of progress: "Progress means to make what is imperfectly complicated as far as possible perfectly uncomplicated".

A number of authors have put forward their own and other people's futuristic views of cockpit-like anaesthetist's working places and of ways to improve the rather awful current situation. Too complicated machinery, with its ever increasing number of buttons, valves, tubes, dials, gauges and monitoring devices overtaxes the anaesthetist - and also the patient, instead of reducing the risk to the latter.

This situation must change, not by the development of a "pilots cockpit" approach,

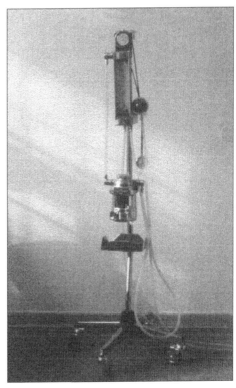

Non-rebreathing anaesthetic apparatus – "Model Göttingen" with Takaoka-Respirator

but by simplification rather than sophistication. The basic evil is the apparent necessity - since Water's introduction in 1923 of CO_2 absorption to reduce the cost of cyclopropane - to have the anaesthetised patient rebreathe his own expired air. This is both senseless and dangerous.

Since that time, manufacturers of anaesthetic apparatus have steadily made their equipment more complex, more unreliable and therefore more dangerous for the patient. In the author's opinion the time is now overdue for this generally hazardous trend to be reversed by using:
- non-rebreathing compact anaesthetic machines
- which are stripped of unnecessary parts,
- easy to handle ("user-friendly"),
- out of surgeon's field by 1 m or more, eg. for intracranial surgery, with minimal necessity for maintenance and minimal cost.

This would include
- simply constructed pressure-cycled ventilators - preferably of the Takaoka type
- audibly alarmed monitors - in this sequence of importance:
- disconnection, inspired O_2 concentration, SAP, ECG, and nothing else.

As was shown in a film, the author believes that the ANE 2000 combined with the Takaoka Ventilator (respectively, the Magill/Kuhn spontaneous breathing system) fulfils all the above criteria. It is uncomplicated and inexpensive and has been used in the author's clinics without problems for 25 years - from 1964 to 1989 - for approximately 1 million cases. To quote Georg Christoph Lichtenberg, (1772-1799 Göttingen doctor and philosopher), "Es ist unmöglich die Fackel der Wahrheit durch ein Gedränge zu tragen, ohne jemand dabei den Bart zu verbrennen". [It is impossible to carry the torch of truth amidst a crowd without burning somebody's beard.]

Stanislaw Przybyszewski's Drawing that was an Inspiration for Carl Schleich's Discovery

J. L. Kroll, W. Jurczyk, P. Kroll
Department of Anaesthesiology and Intensive Therapy of the
Karol Marcinkowski University of Medical Sciences in Poznan, Poland

This paper is based on Carl Ludwig Schleich's memoirs "Besonnte Vergangenheit". Schleich was born in Szczecin in 1859 being the son of a reputed physician. He studied in Zurich and Berlin. He was a very eager and talented artist, but was not as much enthusiastic concerning his medical studies. As he puts it in his autobiography, he preferred to play violoncello, compose, paint, write poems, short stories, dramas and philosophical dissertations, he was an actor and singer and just like loads of geniuses he was far from abstaining from alcohol. While studying he had the opportunity to become an assistant of Rudolf Virchow (1821-1902) for several years, which accounts for his medical experience and education. In spite of this he finally managed to pass his exams and improved his surgical skills while working with Prof. Heinrich Helferich (1851-1946) in Greifswald and the famous Prof. Ernst von Bergmann (1836-1907). Later he opened his own surgical clinic in Berlin with the strong support of his father. At that time Schleich met Stanislaw Przybyszewski (1868-1927) in one of the pubs that Bohemian artists used to go to. Stanislaw Przybyszewski was a famous author not only in Poland and Germany, his publications were translated into several different languages. He was writing stories and his philosophical thesis in German that year. Schleich described him as follows: About 1890 among other Bohemian personalities I met a Pole Stanislaw Przybyszewski, whom we used to call a bloody physiologist. He was a very talented poet, genius with a subtle mind ... he played Chopin extremely beautifully ... he had no extraordinary painting skills etc.

It is evident, that both of them had a similar taste concerning arts, but they differed profoundly concerning their personality. The German Schleich had a vivid imagination as is typical for the Polish, whereas Stanislaw Przybyszewski was a Pole with a thoroughness which is very distinctive for Germans. His remarkable essays and stories showed immense philosophical depth. He adopted problems of the battle of sexes from the German literature, but most of all he concentrated on describing the naked soul and the sufferings on torments caused by lust in both sexes. These torments were often related to problems and aspects of the soul as well as to the brains influence on the soul. In order to find out more about the relationship between the soul and the mind, the mind and the brains, as well as between the brain and nerves and in order to get some scientific background into his philosophical studies, he started to attend lectures in anatomy and psychiatry at the University of Berlin. Wilhelm von Waldeyer (1836-1921) was among his lecturers. Stanislaw Przybyszewski was particularly interested in specific topics of medicine like anatomy and especially in subjects associated with the brain, ganglions, nerves and neurons familiarizing himself with details much further than Schleich. One day both of them met each other after Prof. Waldeyers lecture, Stanislaw Przybyszewski carrying his lecture notes and drawings with

853

him that attracted Schleichs attention. Schleich found detailed anatomical drawings of ganglions and neural cells that were delineated them as meticulously as he had never seen them before. As he puts it, he was engrossed in studying those minute wonders of nature and started thinking about the function of neuroglia in those complicated structures. Suddenly he jumped on his feet shouting: Stanislaw, my friend! The neuroglia is a mute of the piano strings! The apparatus that switches registers (of organs), the control of inhibition! Schleich came to the conclusion, that some amount of fluid, i.e. blood, when injected into the tissues should - exerting the pressure through the neuroglia - inhibit or suppress the conducting abilities of sensory nerves.

The same night Schleich went to his clinic and injected various solutions of saline into his body in the presence of his assistant Wittkowski. He noticed that they acted as a very good local anaesthetic even though the injection was painful. Trying to avoid the initial pain he added a tiny amount of cocaine to 0.5 promille saline. He write This was it became conclusive. The efficacy of anaesthesia increased manifold. In situations when others could administer only one Pravaz syringe of cocaine due to its toxicity, I could give thousands of them. In hundreds of experiments he carried out on himself, it appeared that tissues anaesthetized this way were completely insensitive to cutting, pressure, burning and scratching.

That was how regional anaesthesia with the use of low concentrations of local anaesthetic agents made a fundamental contribution to the progress of surgery, ENT and maxillo-facial surgery at the end of the 19th century.

Schleich considered the elaboration of regional anaesthesia to be his lifes major success, stressing that the lighting spark was Stanislaw Przybyszewski, his expositions and magnificent anatomical drawings.

References:

Schleich CL: Besonnte Vergangenheit. Lebenserinnerungen 1859-1919. Vier Falken Verlag Berlin, 1920, pp 245, 253-254, 309

Przybyszewski S: Der grosse Brockhaus Band 15, 15. Auflage, 1935, p 196

List of Contributors

Adams, A., Dr.
12 Redwood Lodge, Grange Road
CB39 AR Cambridge, U. K.

Ahrens, P., Dr.
Zentrum Anaesthesiologie, Rettungs-
und Intensivmedizin, Universitätsklinik
Göttingen
Robert-Koch-Straße 40, 37075 Göttingen,
Germany

Alvarez, J., Professor Dr.
Servicio de Anesthesiología, Hospital
General de Galicia, c/ Geleras s/n,
15705 Santiago (La Coruña), Spain

Andreen Sachs, M., Professor Dr.
Department of Anaesthesia and Intensive
Care, Danderyd Hospital, 18288 Danderyd,
Sweden

Astrup, P., Professor Dr.
Department of Clinical Chemistry,
University of Copenhagen, Copenhagen,
Denmark

Atkinson, R., Dr.
Southend General, 75 High Cliff Drive,
01702 74932 Leigh on Sea, Essex, U. K.

Baar, H. Dr.
Woldsenweg 3, 20249 Hamburg, Germany

Bacon, D., Professor Dr.
Department of Anaesthesia, Western New
York Health Care System, Medical Center,
3495 Bailey Avenue, Buffalo N.Y. 1425,
USA

Baker, A.B., Professor Dr.
Department of Anaesthetics,
The University of Sydney University,
Sydney, N.S.W. 2006 Australia

Baum, J., Professor Dr.
Abteilung für Anästhesie und Intensiv-
medizin, Krankenhaus St.-Elisabeth-Stift,
Lindenstraße 3-7, 49401 Damme, Germany

Bause, G., Dr.,
Wood Library-Museum of Anesthesiology,
520 Northwest Highway, Park Ridge,
Illinois, USA

Benzer, H., Professor Dr.
Universitätsklinik für Anästhesie und
Allgemeine Intensivmedizin,
Leopold-Franzens-Universität Innsbruck,
Arnichstraße 35, 6020 Innsbruck,
Austria

Böhrer, H., Priv.-Doz. Dr.
Klinik für Anästhesiologie,
Ruprecht-Karls-Universität Heidelberg,
Im Neuenheimer Feld 110,
69120 Heidelberg, Germany

Boulton, T. B., Dr.
Townsend Farm, Streatley-on-Thames,
Berkshire RG8 9JX, U.K.

Braun, U., Professor Dr.
Zentrum Anästhesiologie, Rettungs- und
Intensivmedizin,
Georg August-Universität Göttingen,
Robert-Koch-Straße 40, 37075 Göttingen,
Germany

Buroš, M., Dr.
Department of Anaesthesiology,
University Hospital, Jihlavska 20,
63900 Brno, Czech Republic

Carter, A., Dr.
Department of Anaesthetics,
North Staffordshire, Newcastle Road,
ST46Q G Stoke-on-Trent, U.K.

Connor, H., Dr.
Department of Medicine, County Hospital,
Union Walk, HH 12 ER Hereford, U.K.

Cope, D., Professor Dr.
Pain Evaluation and Treatment Institute,
University of Pittsbburgh,
Medical Center, 4601 Bacon Boulevard,
Pittsburgh, Pennsylvania 15213-1217,
USA

Cortéz, J. , Dr.
Servicio de Anesthesiología, Hospital
General de Galicia, c/ Geleras s/n,
15705 Santiago (La Coruña), Spain

Cousin, M., Dr.
Department d'Anesthésie et Réanimation,
Inst. Broussais, 9, rue du Haros, 78530 Buc,
France

Cundrle, I., Dr.
Department of Anaesthesiology,
University Hospital, Jihlavska 20,
63900 Brno, Czech Republic

Davies, Ch. K., Dr.
Rockyview Hospital Calgery, Canada

Defalque, R. J., Professor Dr.
Department of Anesthesiology,
University of Alabama-Birmingham,
619 South 19th Street, 6810 Birmingham,
Alabama, USA

Desbarax, P., Dr.
Alfred Coolsstraat 13, 2020 Antwerpen,
Belgium

Diz, J.C., Dr.
Servicio de Anesthesiología,
Hospital General de Galicia, c/ Geleras s/n,
15705 Santiago (La Coruña), Spain

Duda, K., Professor Dr.
Department of Anesthesiology,
Center of Oncology, M. Sklodowska-Curie
Institute Carcow, Ul. Garncarska 11,
31-115 Krakow, Poland

Dressler, P. Dr.
Klinik für Anästhesiologie,
Ruprecht-Karls-Universität Heidelberg,
Im Neuenheimer Feld 110,
69120 Heidelberg, Germany

Dworacek, B., Dr.
Department of Anaesthesiology, University
Hospital, Jihlavska 20, 63900 Brno,
Czech Republic

Eiblmayr, H., Dr.
Institut für Anästhesie und Intensivmedizin,
Landesfrauenklinik OÖ, Lederergasse 47,
4020 Linz, Austria

Erdmann, Professor Dr.
Department of Anaesthesiology,
Erasmus University Rotterdam,
Ziekenhaus Dijkzigt, Dr. Molewaterplein
40, 3015 GD Rotterdam,
The Netherlands

Espinheira, A. Dr.
Museu Anesthesiolgia, Rua José Duro,
17-3. Dto., 1700 Lisboa, Portugal

Fleischer, Priv. Doz. Dr.
Klinik für Anästhesiologie,
Ruprecht-Karls-Universität Heidelberg,
Im Neuenheimer Feld 110,
69120 Heidelberg, Germany

Franco, A., Professor Dr.
Servicio de Anesthesiología, Hospital
General de Galicia, c/ Geleras s/n,
15705 Santiago (La Coruña), Spain

Frost, E., Professor Dr.
Department of Anesthesiology New York
Medical College New York, Marcy Pavilion
Valhalla, NY 10595, USA

Ghişoiu, S., Dr.
Department of Anaesthesia, Spitalul Clinic
Judetean, Nr. 1, A. Odobescu Nr. 19,
1900 Timisoara, Romania

Giese, C, Dr.
Abteilung für Anästhesiologie und Operative
Intensivmedizin der Universität Gießen,
Rudolf Buchheim Straße 7, 35385 Gießen,
Germany

Gockel, H., Dr.
Klinik für Anästhesiologie und Operative
Intensivmedizin,
Christian-Albrechts-Universität zu Kiel,
Schwanenweg 21, 24105 Kiel, Germany

Goerig, M., Dr.
Klinik für Anästhesiologie, Universitäts-
Krankenhaus Eppendorf, Martinistr. 52,
20246 Hamburg, Germany

Gunga, H.-C., Priv.-Doz. Dr.
Institut für Physiologie, Fachbereich Human-
medizin, Klinikum Benjamin Franklin,
Arnimallee 22, 14195 Berlin, Germany

Haridas, R. P., Dr.
Department of Anaesthetics, Faculty of
Medicine, University of Natal Durban,
Private Beg 7, Congella,
4013 South Africa

Harrison-Calmes, S., Professor Dr.
Department of Anesthesiology, Olive View,
UCLS Medical Centre, 14445 Olive View
Drive, 91342 Sylmar, California, USA

Hempelmann, G., Professor Dr.
Abteilung für Anästhesiologie und Operative Intensivmedizin der Universität
Gießen, Rudolf Buchheim Straße 7,
35385 Gießen, Germany

Holmes, C.Mc., Dr.
Department of Anaesthetics,
The University of Sydney University,
Sydney, N.S.W. 2006 Australia

Horton, J., Dr.
18 Amhurst Court, Grange Road, CB3 9 BH
Cambridge, U.K.

Hughes, R., Dr.
Bella Vista, 19 A Warren Drive, Deganwy,
Gwyned LL31 9ST, U.K.

Hutter, C., Dr.
City Hospital Nottingham, UK

Jurczyk, W., Professor Dr.
Instytutu Anesthezjologii j, Intensywnej
Terapii AM, ul. Sw. Marii Magdaleny 14,
61861 Poznan, Poland

Kelly, J., Professor Dr.
Department of Professional Education,
Kaiser Permanente, 311 East Glenarm 7,
Pasadena 91106, California, USA

Kernbauer, A., Dr.
Klinik für Anästhesiologie und Intensivtherapie LKH Graz, Auenbruggerplatz 29,
8036 Graz, Austria

Kiss, I., Priv.-Doz. Dr.
Klinik für Anaesthesie und Schmerz-
therapie, Alfred-Krupp-Krankenhaus,
Alfred-Krupp-Straße 21, 45117 Essen,
Germany

Klippe, H.-J., Dr.
Abteilung für Anästhesiologie,
Zentrum für Pneumologie und Thorax-
chirurgie, LVA Freie und Hansestadt
Hamburg, Wöhrendamm 80,
22927 Großhansdorf, Germany

Kloes, H.G., Dr.
Zoologischer Garten Berlin,
Hardenbergpaltz 1, 10787 Berlin,
Germany

Kötter, K., Dr.
Abteilung für Neurologie,
Lepoldina Krankenhaus Schweinfurt,
Gustav Adolf Straße, 97422 Schweinfurt,
Germany

Kohlweyer, B., Dr.
Klinik für Anästhesiologie,
Städtisches Klinikum St. Georg,
Delitzscher Straße. 141, 04129 Leipzig,
Germany

Krause, T., Dr.
Klinik für Anästhesiologie,
Städtisches Klinikum St. Georg,
Delitzscher Straße 141, 04129 Leipzig,
Germany

Kroll, J., Dr.
Department of Anaesthesiology,
Academy of Medicine, Przybyszewski 49,
60355 Poznan, Poland

Kroll, P. Dr.
Department of Anaesthesiology,
Academy of Medicine, Przybyszewski 49,
60355 Poznan, Poland

Kubisz,A., Dr.
Department of Anaesthesiology,
Center of Oncology, M. Sklodowska-Curie
Institute Carcow, Ul. Garncarska 11,
31-115 Krakow, Poland

Kus, M., Professor Dr.
Collegium Medicum UJ, Anesthezjologii i
Intensywnej Terapii AM, Kierownik,
Katedry i Zakladu, ul. Kopernik,
31501 Krakow, Poland

Lipp, M., Dr.
Einsatzabteilung Hamburger Feuerwehr,
Wendenstr. 251, 20537 Hamburg, Germany

List, W. F., Professor Dr.
Klinik für Anästhesiologie und Intensivtherapie LKH Graz, Auenbruggerplatz 29,
8036 Graz, Austria

Magora, F., Professor Dr.
Hadassah University Hospital,
Jerusalem, Israel

Maier, C., Priv. Doz. Dr.
Klinik für Anästhesiologie und Operative
Intensivmedizin,
Christian-Albrechts-Universität zu Kiel,
Schwanenweg 21, 24105 Kiel,
Germany

Maleck, W. , Dr.
Abteilung für Anästhesiologie,
Klinikum Ludwigshafen,
67063 Ludwigshafen, Germany

Maltby, J. R., Professor Dr.
Department of Anaesthesia,
University of Calgary, Foothills Hospital,
1403-29 Street N.W., Calgary,
Alberta, T2N 2T9, Canada

Matsuki, A., Professor Dr.
Department of Anaesthesia,
University of Hirosaki School of Medicine,
Hirosaki, Japan

Mayer, J. A., Dr.
Loma Linda University Medical Center,
Loma Linda University Children's
Hospital, P.O. BOX 2000, Loma Linda,
California, 92354 USA

Mc Kenzie, A., Dr.
Department of Anaesthesia,
Eastern General Hospital,
Seafield Street, Edinburgh EH67LN,
U.K.

McIntyre, J., Professor Dr.
Deptartment of Anaesthesia,
University of Alberta,
8440-112 Street, Edmonton,
Alberta T6G2B7, Canada

McLaren, C. A., Dr.
12 Brohdacres, Road Town, Wootton,
Bassett, Wiltshire SN4 7RP, U.K.

Menzel, H., Dr.
Senner Hellweg 5, 33659 Bielefeld,
Germany

Morris, L.E., Professor Dr.
Department of Anesthesiology,
University of Washington,
15670 Point Monroe Drive NE,
Bainbridge Island, WA 98110, USA

Muschaweck, R., Dr.
Heinichenweg 39, 65929 Frankfurt/M.,
Germany

Nemes, C., Dr.
Abeilung für Anästhesie,
Kreiskrankenhaus Pfaffenhofen a.d. Ilm,
Krankenhausstraße 70,
85276 Pfaffenhofen/Ilm, Germany

Nolte, N., Professor Dr.
Alte Poststraße 110,
32457 Porta Westfalica, Germany

Notcutt, W. G., Dr.
James Paget Hospital, Lowestoft Road,
Gorleston, Norfolk GT Yarmouth NR316
LA, USA

Ocklitz, A., Dr.
Geißbergstraße 31, 10777 Berlin,
Germany

Padfield, A., Dr.
Department of Anaesthesia,
C-Floor, Royal Hallamshire,
Glossop Road, S102JF Sheffield, U.K.

Panning, B., Professor Dr.
Abteilung für Anästhesiologie I,
Medizinische Hochschule Hannover,
Carl-Neuberg-Straße 1, 30625 Hannover,
Germany

Parascandola, J., Professor Dr.
Public Health Service Historian, 18-23,
Parklawn Building, 56 Fishers Lane,
Rockeville, Maryland 20857, USA

Parsloe, C., Professor Dr.
Department of Anesthesia, Hospital Samaritano, Rua Conselheiro Brotero 1486,
01232-010 Sao Paulo, SP Brasil, Brasilia

Paschen, H.-R., Dr.
Einsatzabteilung Hamburger Feuerwehr,
Wendenstraße 251, 20537 Hamburg,
Germany

Patterson, R., Professor Dr.
143 Greenfield Avenue,
90049 Los Angeles, CA, USA

Petermann, H.
Schronfeld 63a, 91054 Erlangen, Germany

Petrioanu, G.A. Dr.
Institut für Pharmakologie und Toxikologie,
Fakultät für klinische Medizin Mannheim
der Universität Heidelberg,
Theodor Kutzer Ufer, 68135 Mannheim,
Germany

Piepenbrock, S., Professor Dr.
Abteilung für Anästhesiologie,
Medizinische Hochschule Hannover,
Carl-Neuberg-Straße 1, 30625 Hannover

Plötz, J., Professor Dr.
Institut für Anaesthesiologie,
Klinikum Bamberg, Buger Straße 80,
96049 Bamberg, Germany

Pokorný, J., Professor Dr.
Department of Anesthesiology,
University Hospital, Jihlavska 20,
63900 Brno, Czech Republic

Rendell-Baker, L., Professor Dr.
Loma Linda University Medical Center,
Loma Linda University Children's Hospital,
P.O. BOX 2000, Loma Linda, California,
92354 USA

Richardson, J., Professor Dr.
Department of Anaesthetics,
Royal Infirmary, BD96RJ Bradford, U.K.

Riedl, Th., Dr.
Zentrum Anästhesiologie,
Rettungs- und Intensivmedizin,
Georg August-Universität Göttingen,
Robert-Koch-Straße 40, 37075 Göttingen,
Germany

Röse, W., Professor Dr.
Klinik für Anästhesie und Intensivtherapie,
Otto-von-Guericke Universität Magdeburg,
Leipziger Straße 44, 39210 Magdeburg,
Germany

Rupreht, J., Professor Dr.
Department of Anaesthesiology,
Erasmus University Rotterdam,
Ziekenhaus Dijkzigt,
Dr. Molewaterplein 40, 3015 GD Rotterdam,
The Netherlands

Safar, P., Professor Dr.
Safar Center for Resuscitation Research,
University of Pittsburgh, Medical Center,
3434 Fifth Avenue, 15260 Pittsburgh,
Pennsylvania, USA

Schaffner, E., Dr.
Klinik für Anästhesiologie,
Universitäts-Krankenhaus Eppendorf,
Martinistraße 52, 20246 Hamburg,
Germany

Schallhorn, J., Dr.,
Einsatzabteilung Hamburger Feuerwehr,
Wendenstr. 251, 20537 Hamburg,
Germany

Schulte am Esch, J., Professor Dr.
Klinik für Anästhesiologie, Universitäts-
Krankenhaus Eppendorf, Martinistraße 52,
20246 Hamburg, Germany

Schwarz, W.
Klinik für Anästhesiologie,
Friedrich Alexander-Universität
Erlangen-Nürnberg,
Krankenhausstraße 12, 91054 Erlangen,
Germany

Sear, J., Professor Dr.
The John Radcliff Hospital, Level I,
Nuffield Departments of Anesthetics,
University of Oxford, Headington Oxford
9DU OC3, U.K.

Severinghaus, J., Professor Dr.
Department of Anesthesia, UCSP,
0542 San Francisco, CA 94132 USA

Standl, Th., Priv. Doz. Dr.
Klinik für Anästhesiologie,
Universitäts-Krankenhaus Eppendorf,
Martinistraße 52, 20246 Hamburg,
Germany

Stinshoff, K., Dr.
Brunnenstraße 181, 10119 Berlin, Germany

Stoffregen, J., Professor Dr.
Husterstraße 3a, 58093 Hagen, Germany

Straimer, A., Dr.
Abeilung für Anästhesie,
Kreiskrankenhaus Pfaffenhofen a. d. Ilm,
Krankenhausstraße 70,
85276 Pfaffenhofen/Ilm, Germany

Szymanska-Kowalska, M., Professor Dr.
Department of Anaesthesiology and Intensive Therapy, Central Clinical Hospital,
Szaserow 128, 00-909 Warsaw, Poland

Takrouri, M.S.M., Professor Dr.
Department of Anaesthesia and SICU
(451), King Khalid University,
P.O. Box 17805, Riyadh 11472,
Saudi Arabia

Terekes, M., Professor Dr.
Department of Anaesthesia and Intensive
Therapy, Medical University of Pecs,
P.O. Box 99, 7643 Pecs, Hungary

Van Wijhe, M., Dr.
Department of Anaesthesia,
Acad. Groningen, Greekerrinekskamp 6,
7491 BW, Delden, The Netherlands

Von Hintzenstern, U., Dr.
Abteilung für Anästhesiologie, Städtisches Krankenhaus Forchheim, Spitalstraße 4, 91299 Forchheim, Germany

Wawersik, J., Professor Dr.,
Klinik für Anästhesiologie und Operative Intensivmedizin,
Christian-Albrechts-Universität zu Kiel, Schwanenweg 21, 24105 Kiel, Germany

Weaver, B. M. Q., Dr.
Quarmain, 79, Sanford Road, Wiscombe, Avon BS2 51JJ, U.K.

Weißer, Ch., Dr.
Chirurgische Universitätsklinik Würzburg, Josef-Schneider Straße 2, 97080 Würzburg Germany

Wendl, J.K., Dr.
Spitzerdorf 18, 22280 Wedel, Germany

Wessinghage, D., Professor Dr.
I. Orthopädische Klinik,
Rheuma-Zentrum Bad Abbach,
Am Markt 2, 93077 Bad Abbach, Germany

Westhorpe, R., Dr.
Department of Anaesthesia,
Royal Children's Hospital,
Parkville 3052, Victoria, Australia

Wiedemann, B., Priv. Doz. Dr.
Klinik für Anästhesiologie,
Städtisches Klinikum St. Georg,
Delitzscher Straße 141, 04129 Leipzig, Germany

Wiedemann, K. Professor Dr.
Abteilung für Anaesthesie, Thoraxklinik Heidelberg-Rohrbach, Amalienstraße 5, 69126 Heidelberg, Germany

Wilhelm, St., Dr.
Klinik für Anästhesiologie, Universitäts-Krankenhaus Eppendorf, Martinistraße 52, 20246 Hamburg, Germany

Williams, S., Dr.
Institute of Education, History and Philosophy, University of London,
20 Bedford Way, London OAL WC1H, U.K.

Wilkinson, D., Dr.
Department of Anaesthesia,
St. Bartholmew's Hospital,
West Smithfield, London ECIA 7B, U.K.

Wollbrück, M., Dr.,
Abteilung für Anästhesiologie und Operative Intensivmedizin der Universität Gießen, Rudolf Buchheim Straße 7, 35385 Gießen, Germany

Wulf, H., Priv. Doz. Dr.
Klinik für Anästhesiologie und Operative Intensivmedizin,
Christian-Albrechts-Universität zu Kiel, Schwanenweg 21, 24105 Kiel, Germany

Wright, A.J., MLS
Department of Anesthesiology,
University of Alabama-Birmingham,
619 South 19th Street, 6810 Birmingham, Alabama, USA

Zeitlin, G., Dr.
Department of Anesthesiology,
Brigham Women's Hospitaal,
104 Plainfied Street, 02168 Newton, Massachussetts, USA

Ziegler, U., Dr.
Klinik für Anästhesiologie, Städtisches Klinikum St. Georg, Delitzscher Straße 141, 04129 Leipzig, Germany

Ziętkiewicz, M., Dr.
Department of Anaesthesiology,
Center of Oncology,
M. Sklodowska-Curie Institute Carcow,
Ul. Garncarska 11, 31-115 Krakow, Poland

Zimmer, M., Dr.
55, rue de Sélestat, 67100 Strasbourg, France

Index of Persons

Abbot, Gilbert 47
Abel, John Jacob 600, 627
Adriani 452, 720
Aegina, Paul von 311
Ahnefeld, Friedrich 296
Alant 608
Albert, Eduard 477
Amersbach, Karl 554
Andrews, Edmund 67, 179
Anrep, Vassily von 323
Aoyagi, Takuo 595
Apgar, Virginia 58, 293, 710
Arányi, Lajos 231
Arnot, James 40
Arrhenius, Svante 139, 591
Artusio, Joseph 64, 266
Astrup, Poul 592, 712
Atherstone, William Guybon 73
Auer, John 727

Babcock, Wayne W. 631
Bainbrigge 475
Balassa, János 231
Baldwin, Lucy 483
Bancroft, Joseph 422
Bannister, Roger 145
Barany, Robert 727
Barcroft, Joseph 458, 594
Bark, Richard Heinz Joachim 117ff
Basta 611
Baumberger, Percy 593
Bause, George, S. L. 723
Bayliss, William 207
Beaumont, Elie de 97
Beaumont, William 579
Beck, Claude S. 291
Beddoes, Thomas 39, 44, 313, 658
Beecher, Henry K. 593

Bell, Alexander Graham 414
Bell, Jointly 353
Benda, Carl 745
Bennett, Horace 659
Berend, Hermann 251
Bergmann, Ernst von 819, 853
Bergson, J. 661
Berla, Ernst 556
Bernard, Claude 66, 127, 154, 518, 599
Bert, Paul 317ff
Berthoud, Henri 91
Bettini 273
Bey, Abdullah 224
Bibra, Ernst Freiherr von 603
Bichat, Marie François Xavier 127
Bier, August 62, 274, 329, 505, 631
Bierkowski, Ludwig 273
Bigelow, Henry 47, 235, 270
Bigelow, Jacob 50, 82, 87
Billroth, Theodor 273
Binswanger Ludwig 237
Bird, Forrest M. 703
Björk, Viking 526
Blackwell, Elizabeth 693
Blackwell, Emily 693
Blake, James 601
Blandin, P. F. 649
Blinks, Lawrence R. 593
Bloch, Oscar Thorwald 265
Boccacio, Giovanni 751
Böhm, Rudolf 290, 390, 725
Bois-Reymond, Emil du 683
Boit 540
Bolase, John Bingham 314
Bonica, John 111, 437, 583
Boot, Francis 51, 59, 649, 683
Borchardt, Moritz 556
Bouisson, Etienne F. 344

863

Boulier, Jaque 279
Bourne, Wesley 58
Boyer, Alexis 79
Boyle, Robert 591, 598
Braddock, John 87
Brain, Archie I. J. 707
Brauer, Ludolph 745
Braun, Heinrich 62, 330, 725
Breitner, Burghardt 109
Brettauer, Josef 274
Brickley, William 211
Brink, Frank 593
Brinkmann, Robert 595
Broca, Paul 356
Broca, Pierre Paul 242
Brodie, Benjamin 66
Bronk, Detlef W. 593
Brook, Geoffrey 427
Brown, Alexander Crum 601
Brown, Allan 132, 452
Brown, Gilbert 58
Brücke, Ludwig 683
Brunn, Max von 392
Bruns, Viktor von 242, 251
Brunton, Thomas Lauder 600
Bryce-Smith, Roger 526
Brynschwieg, Hieronymus 279
Buchheim, Rudolf 599
Buckett, W. R. 607
Bunte, Hans 560
Burfitt, Albinus 157
Burkhardt, Ludwig 600
Buros, M. 588
Buxton, Dudley W. 579

Caglieri, Guido 62
Cairns, Hugh 131
Calmes, Selma, H. 723
Calverley, Rod K. 22, 723
Carlens, Eric 526, 733, 737ff
Carrearas 432
Castellano, José Sancho 690
Cathélin, Fernand 564, 726
Caux, F. P. de 66
Caventou 323
Cemer, Max 592
Chalmers, Thomas 474
Charcoat, Jean Martin 242

Charriede 650
Chatelier, Henri Louis Le 591
Chauliac, Guy de 279, 751
Churchill, Frederick 157, 227
Clark, Leland 593
Clarke, Timothy 774
Clarke, William E. 35, 41
Clover, Joseph Thomas 93, 431
Clutton-Brock, John 428
Cnevale, Isdore 652
Codman, E. A. 225
Cogswell, A. G. 88
Cohen 556
Cohen, Maurice 562
Coleman, Alfred 93, 443ff
Colton, Quincey 43, 61 ,87
Connell, Karl 210
Cordus, Valerius 61, 636ff, 658
Corning, James Leonhard 61, 493, 631
Crafoord, Clarence 521, 733
Crane, John W. 88
Credé, Karl S. 737
Crile, George 291, 329
Crowfoot, E. E. 87
Cullen, Stuart 109, 359
Cunningham, John Henry 690
Cushing, Harvey 131, 135

Dale, Henry 594
Dalziel 414
Dam, Willy 102
Danneel, Heinrich Ludwig 591
Davies, Philip W. 593
Davy, Humphry 35, 39, 44, 313, 339ff, 599, 658
Dax, Marc 356
De Sola, Abraham 475
Decartes, René 779
Del Gericio 294
Delpech, Jaques 79 118
Demme, Hermann 171, 251, 650
Dick, Wolfgang 296
Dickins, Charles 313
Dieffenbach, Johann Friedrich 79ff, 172, 238, 251
Dihet, Pierre 649
Dioscorides, Pedanius 79, 279
Domenech, Francisco 664

Dönhardt, Axel 671
Dott, Norman 131
Dräger, Bernhard 447
Drapka, Miloslav 146
Dripps, Robert Dunning 292
Dumas, Jean-Baptiste 343
Duncan, James Mathew 649, 663
Dupuy, Marc 689
Dupuytren, Guillaume 238
Durig, Arnold 457
Dwaoracek, B. 588

Eastment 159
Eaton, William 161
Eberhardt, Patrick 594
Eck, C.R. Ritsema van 120
Ehrlich, Paul 395, 555
Eichholtz, Fritz 624
Einhorn, Alfred 62, 140, 275, 623
Einthoven, Willem 207
Eiselsberg, Anton von 109, 273
Eisenberg, M. S. 292, 296
Eisenmenger, Rudolf 405ff
Eisleb, Otto 618
Elam, James O. 292, 487, 452
Elliotson, John 41, 313
Ellis, R. H. 841
Elsberg, Charles 727
Elschnig, Anton 554
Elsholtz, Johann Sigismund 771ff
Emerson, John H. 701, 714
Engstrom, Carl-Gunnar 712
Epstein, Hans G. 717
Erdmann, Adolph 63
Erdtman, Holger 63, 139
Escherich, Theodor 242
Esmarch, Friedrich von 242
Estana, Mur 434
Euler, Hand von 139
Evans, John Henry 375
Evans, Thomas 61, 89, 93
Everett, Edward 50, 841
Eversole, Urban 209

Fallopius, Gabriel 752
Faraday, Michael 659
Filehne, Wilhelm 620ff
Finsterer, Hans 276

Fischer, Emil 549
Fischer, Otto 620
Fisher, Willis 649
Flagg, Josuah Foster B. 88
Flór, Franz 231
Foldes, Francis F. 709
Forbes, John 50, 571
Foregger, Richard von 65, 275, 449
Fothergill, John 671
Fraenkel, Eugen 561
Franklin, Benjamin 312
Fraser, Thomas 601
Fraser, William Baillies Thomas 50
Frenckner, Paul 519, 733ff
Freud, Sigmund 274, 323
Frey, Rudolf 24, 101, 296, 437
Frneckner, Paul 737
Frost, Eben 46
Frumin, M. Jack 701
Fürth, Otto von 627

Gaedicke, Friedrich 61
Gaeln 279
Galí, Rubio y 689
Gauss, Carl Joseph 447ff, 563, 621
Gavieso, Carreras 434
Gay-Lussac, Louis Joseph 617
Gegner, Michael 247
Geppert, Julius 455, 563
Gerbershagen, Hans-Ulrich 437, 583
Gersch, L.Y. 547
Gerster, Hans 686
Gerstorff, Hans von 279
Gibbs, Josiah Willard 591
Giers, Knut Harald 737
Gillies, Harold 141
Gillingham, John 133
Glover, Robert Mortimer 163
Godoy, José 690
Goldberg, Leonard 141
Gómez, Vicente Guarnerio 665
Gordh, Torsten 62, 70, 139
Gordon, Archer 290
Gordon, Emeric 133
Gottlieb, Rudolf 561
Gradenwitz 410
Graefe, Albrecht von 82, 195
Graham, Malcolm 214

Gravenstein,, Joachim 572
Gray, T. Cecil 721
Greene 631
Greener, Hannah 157, 344
Griffith, Harold 66
Gross, Dieter 438
Gross, Erwin 359
Gruby, David 242
Guarnerio, Vincente 664
Guedel, Arthur 58, 224, 427
Guérin, Jules 345
Gurlt, Ernst Julius 199
Gusserow, Adolf Ludwig 737
Guthrie, Samuel 343, 663
Gwathmey, Taylor 265, 317, 690

Haber, Fritz Jacob 592
Habs, Rudolf 745
Haid, Bruno 72, 109, 120
Haidinger, W. 323
Halász, 231
Hales, Stephen 426, 443
Hall, Marshall 290
Hall, Richard 61
Halla, Joseph 272
Halsted, William 62, 274
Hammer, Adam 242, 251
Hammerschmidt, Karl Eduard 223
Hanaoka, Seishu 38
Harcourt, Vernon 135
Harden, Arthur 139
Harless, Emil 603
Harris 294
Harvey, William 289, 599, 772
Hasselbalch, Karl Albert 592
Hata, Sachahiro 556
Hauke 414
Hedersson, Yandell 544
Heiberg, Jacob 290
Heim, Ernst Ludwig 80
Heinz, Robert 623
Heister, Lorenz 279
Hejduk, B. 147, 647
Helferich, Heinrich 853
Helmholtz, Hermann 683
Henderson, Lawrence J. 592
Henderson, Velyien 568
Henkel, Max 540

Herbert, Thomas 157
Hering, C. E. 229
Hermann 519
Herold 289
Herparth, William 649
Herxheimer, Gotthold 554
Hewitt, Frederick 60, 63
Heyfelder, Johann Ferdinand 83, 173, 650, 685, 825
Heyrovsky, Jaroslav 593
Heyse, Paul 196
Hickl, Theodor 549
Hickman, Henry Hill 40, 270, 315ff, 426, 658
Hildebrand, Otto 745
Hildebrandt, August 631
Hildebrandt, Jan 584
Hilden, Fabricius 279
Hinckley, Robert 47
Hingson, Robert A. 118, 718
Hinterthür, Anton 225, 272ff
Hirsch, Cesar 554, 559
Hirsch, Julius 558
Hirsch, Maximilian 564
Hochenegg, Julius von 275
Hoder, Joseph 146
Hoffa 291
Hofmeister, Franz 228, 272
Holmes 505
Holmgren, Gunnar 733
Holzknecht, Guido 555
Honigsbaum, Frank 489
Hooke, Robert 671
Hopgood, Richard Cooper 88
Hoppe-Seyler, Felix 594
Hörlein, Heinrich 617
Horseley, Victor 135
Horton, J. Warren 210
Hosemann, Hans 549ff
Hossli, Georg 120
Hottel, Hoyt 211
Howardt, William Lee 290
Hoyt 631
Hrdlica, M. 147, 647
Huch, Albert 594
Huch, Renate 594
Hügin, Werner 120, 531
Humboldt, Alexander von 242

Hunter, John 289, 671
Huygens, Christian 667

Ibsen, Bjorn 588, 592, 711
Israel, James 815
Iterson, Jan Egens van 205

Jackson, Charles Thomas 44, 45, 49, 235, 244, 353ff, 841ff
Jackson, Chevalier 733
Jackson, Dennis 58, 443ff, 719
Jacobaeus, Hans Christian 523, 733, 737
Janssen, Paul A. 709
Jarman, Ronald 65
Jeger, Ernst 727ff
Jones, Henry Bence 591
Jones, Oliver 58, 414
Jude, C. 294
Juliá, José Soler 690
Jüngken Christian 195

Kadlic, T. 147
Kaiser Karl VI 267
Kaiser Maximilian 267
Kaiserin Maria Theresia 267
Kane 572
Kapesser 452
Kappeler, Otto 838
Kappus, Adolf 558
Kausch, Walther 153ff
Kaye, Geoffrey 58
Keith 663
Kerridge, Phyllis 592
Keszler, Hugo 148, 587
Kety 135
Kewney, George 160
Keys, Thomas E.
Killian, Gustav 733
Killian, Hans 24, 65, 118, 368, 445
King Chalres II of England 771
King Friedrich Wilhelm von Brandenburg 771
King George II of England 321
King Louis XVI 312
King Ludwig I 262
King Ludwig I of Bavaria 686
King, A. Charles 486
Kingsley, Norman W. 89

Kirby, Major 713
Kirk, John 350, 572
Kirschner, Martin 333ff, 368, 583, 763
Kirschner, Martin 333ff
Klain, Mirislav 714
Klaschik, Eberhard 584
Klemensiewicz, Zygamunt 592
Knickerbocker, Guy 294
Knight 572
Knorr, Ludwig 617
Kocher, Theodor 135
Koenig, Franz 389
Kolb, Ernst 848
Koller, Carl 36, 61, 140, 274, 559
Kömm, Johan Nepumuk 225, 273
König, Franz 220
Koss, Ferdinand 368
Kouwenhoven, William 292, 391
Krackowiczer, Ernst 224
Kramer, Kurt 594
Kraske 390
Krause, Fedor 153
Kreiselman, J. 671
Kreitmaier, H. 763
Krezler 291
Krieger 195
Kroeff-Pires, Flavio 505ff
Kronacker, Hugo 265, 558
Kronschwitz, Helmut 118
Kuhn, Franz 136, 443ff, 745, 838
Kulenkampff, Diedrich 265
Kulmus, Adam, J. 656
Kümmell, Hermann 63, 291, 367
Küppers, Karl 563

Laennec, René Théophile Hyacinth 571
Laer, B. 296
Lahey, Frank Howard 209, 690
Lamballe, Joseph Jobert de 51, 97, 236, 649
Landerer, Albert 154
Landsteiner, Carl 275
Langenbeck, Bernhardt von 242, 273
Langenbuch, Carl 389
Laorden, Andrés 664
Larrey, Baron Philippe 40, 79, 93
Laskownicki 331
Lauzer, Martin 91
Lavosier, Antoine-Laurent 312

Läwen, Arthur 66, 330, 725ff
Le Brun, Alexander 273
Leigh, Digby 58
Leroy, d`Etoile 671
Levy, Goodman A. 207, 45
Lewelin, J. H. 649
Leyden, Ernst von 815
Liano, Diaz de 432
Liebig, Justus von 42, 322, 343, 663
Liebreich, Oskar 557, 600
Liljestrand, Gunnar 523
Lingstone, Marie 347ff
Liston, Robert 27, 50, 227, 273
Little, William John 80
Livingstone, David 347 ff
Loefgren, Nils 139ff
Loewe, Siegfried 555
Loewy, Adolf 456, 518
Long 683
Long, William Crawford 659
Lorenz 323
Lotsch, Fritz 745ff
Louis, Charles Alexandre 825
Lübbers, Dietrich 594
Lucas, G. H. W. 568
Ludwig, Carl 291, 683
Luer, Wülfing 241
Lumninter, Sándor 231
Lundquist, Bengt 141
Lunkenheimer, Peter-Paul 714
Lyman, Henry 579
L`Obel, Mathieu de 397

Maass, Friedrich 290, 389
MacEwen, William 135
Macintosh, Robert Reynolds 22, 58, 68, 110, 123, 145, 716
MacIver, George 211
Magill, Ivan 63, 79, 113, 127, 236, 323, 522, 599, 650, 698
Mainzer, Jacob 723
Maissoneuve, Jaques G. T. 650
Malgaigne, Joseph François 236, 344, 649
Mapleson, William M. 702
Marcinkowski, K. 743
Marcy, E. E. 87
Martin, Alexis 572
Martin, Aloys 235, 249ff, 661

Mathieu 519
Matthes, Karl 594
Maydl, Karl 837
Mayrhofer, Otto 110, 291
Mck. Holmes 62
McMechan, Francis Hoeffer 63, 402ff, 652
Mehring, Joseph von 153
Meissner, Traugott 653
Meissner, Traugott 653
Meltzer, Samuel James 558, 727
Mendel, Felix 556
Mendelsson, C. L. 579
Mendoza, Antonia 191
Mennel, Zebuton 135
Mesmer, Franz Friedrich 41, 311
Meyer, Felix 561
Meyer, Hans Horst 603
Meynert, Theodor 365
Michaelis, Max 815
Mikisch, Eduard 272
Mikulicz, Johannes von 154, 392
Milikan, Glen 594
Minár, J. 147
Minkowski, Oskar 153
Minnitt, R. J. 486ff
Moffat, Robert 348
Mollière, Daniel 689
Monod, Robert 544
Moore, Charles 313
Moore, James 40
Morales, Antonio 431ff
Morch, Trier 102
Morris, Lucien 452, 703
Morris, William Lord 68, 535, 720
Morton, Thomas Green 35, 58, 82, 97, 157, 235, 270, 441, 473, 649, 683, 844
Mosso, Angelo 457
Most 275
Mueller, Baron Ferdinand von 422
Muir 608
Müller, Otto 593
Muschaweck, Roman 626
Mushin, William 58, 722
Musil, Mathias 272, 652
Musil, Robert von 650

Naegeli, Theodor 118
Nathan, Leopold 273

Navratil, J. 647
Neff, William B. 714
Negowski 291
Nernst, Hermann Walther 591
Nesi 545
Neu, Maximilian 63, 560
Nicolai, Ludwig 594
Niehans, Paul 389
Niehaus 389
Nielsen, Holger 290
Niemann, Albert 61, 274, 321ff
Northfield, Douglas 131
Nunn, J. F. 676
Nunn, Robert 157
Nussbaum, Nepomuk 242, 617

Obenaus, Carl F. E. 171, 249, 251, 650
Oberst, Maximilian 274
Oehmig, Heinz 847
Oliffe, Joseph 93
Olivares, José González 665
Ombrédanne, Louis 543, 547ff
Opitz, Coelestin 227, 272
Ostwald, Wilhelm 591
Oré, Cyprien 557
Organe, Geoffrey 58
Overton, Charles 603
O`Dwyer, Joseph 837
O`Shaughnessy, William 591

Paár 231
Packard B. John H. 265
Paracelsus 636ff
Paracelsus, Aurelius Philipp Theophrast
  Bombast von Hohenheim 41, 268, 279,
  289, 636
Paré, Ambroise 37, 276
Parkinson, Ann 157
Parmly, George Washington 92
Parmly, Henry Clay 92
Parmly, Samuel Pleasan 92
Pascha, Ali 224
Pass, Ten 452
Patorová, J. 114, 146
Paul Bert 182
Pauli, Emil Theodor 236
Pelletier 323
Pérez, Antonio Morales 434

Pettenkofer, Max von 242
Pflüger, Eduard 242, 455, 5517, 55
Pfolsprunt, Heinrich von 279
Philippe, Adrien 343
Pirogoff, Nicilai I. 757
Piskacek, Ludwig 477
Pitha, Franz 227, 273
Pitkin, George 373ff
Plomley, Francis 649
Pokorny 291
Pokrzywnicki, Stanislaw 805
Pollard, B. J. 675
Pooler 215
Pope Pius XII 110
Pope, Elijah 42
Porten, Ernst von der 554, 562
Posselt, 323
Préterre, Apolloni 90
Préterre, Eugène 90
Préterre, Peter 89
Préterre, Pierre 89
Priestley, Joseph 35, 38, 313, 658
Przybyszeski, Stanislaw 853ff

Quincke, Heinrich 62, 493

Rafn 289
Raventos, James 708
Réclus, Paul 274
Rees, Gordo Jackson 705
Rehn, Eduard 117, 370
Reid, John 422
Reimann 323
Rendell-Baker, Leslie 705
Reston, James 318
Rhign, Arnoldus van 356
Rich, John B. 94
Richardson, Bejawmin Ward 181,184, 601,
  753
Richardson, Elliott 36
Ricord, Philippe 90, 649
Rigg, John 43
Ringer, Sidney 291, 395
Rippel, PR. 626
Ritsert, K. 622
Rivett, Louis 487
Robert 350
Roberts, Robert Bryan 707

Robertshaw, Frank 526
Robinson 572, 649, 683
Rodrigo, Antonio Casares 664
Rodzinski, Ryszard 329ff
Roe, Cecil 213, 219
Romberg, Moritz 196
Rominger, Ernst 554
Röntgen, Conrad 83
Rosendfeld, Josef 231
Rosenfeld, Max 555
Rost, Eugen 618
Roth, Otto 819
Rothmund 171, 242, 249, 262, 686
Rottenstein, Jean Baptiste 92, 241
Rouelle, Hilaire Marin 591
Roughton, Francis John Worsley 594
Roux Philibert Joseph 127, 236, 238, 650
Rovenstine, Emery Andrew 68, 568
Rowbotham, Edgar St. 114, 145
Ruben, Henning 293, 671, 699
Rudea, Antonio Mendoza 664
Runge 323
Rust, Johann Nepumuk 79
Rymer, Lee 88

Sabarth 265
Sadevenko, G.Y. 547
Saez, Antonio 191, 689
Safar, Peter 290
Sághy 231
Sahli, Hermann 205
Sartorius, Johann Friedrich 80
Sauer, Carl 443
Sauerbruch, Ferdinand 206, 745
Savage 607
Savarese 611
Schäfer, E. A. 290
Schaumann, Otto 618
Scheele, Carl Wilhelm 658
Scherzer, Karl 323
Schiff, Moritz 290
Schimmelbusch, Curt 757, 821
Schleich, Carl Ludwig 62, 195, 274, 557, 819
Schlesinger, J. 656
Schmidt, Albrecht 367
Schmidt, Helmut Carl Detlef 65, 367 ff, 448, 633

Schmiedeberg, Oswald 591, 597
Schönlein, Johann Lucas 195
Schreiber, Peter J. 704
Schröder, Karl 737
Schroetter, Hermann von 274, 455ff, 518
Schueck, Franz 557
Schuh, Franz 224, 271, 650
Schultze, Bernhard 737
Schwann, Theodor 683
Schwarz, Emil 555
Scudamore, Charles 571
Sebrecht, Joseph 493ff
Secher, Ole 22, 52
Sédillot, Charles E. 344
Semmelweis, Ignaz Philippe 271
Sertürner, Friedrich Wilhelm 274, 322, 617
Severinghaus, John W. 452, 700
Shaw, Robert 595
Sheridan, David S. 698
Sherrington, Charles 594
Shields, Harry 58
Shipman, Robert 161
Siehs, Joseph 650
Sievers, Roderich 726
Silberstein, Ernst 815
Silk, Fredrick 63
Silten, Ernst 815
Silva, J. Theotnio da 230
Sim, Patrick 723
Simenauer, Erich 557
Simpson James Young 51-52, 225, 265, 347ff, 473, 663, 693ff
Sims, James Marion 88
Sjostrand, Ulf H. 714
Skramlik, Emil Ritter von 555
Smith, Papyrus 311, 383ff
Smith, R. B. 714
Smith-Clarke, George Thomas 535
Snow, John 38, 188, 441, 572
Soban, D. 22
Soehring, Klaus 627
Solis-Cohen 572
Soubeiran, Eugène 343, 663
Soucek, Donald H. 706
Spaeth, Joseph 477
Spinadel, Lev 145, 587

Sprague, A. W. 88
Squire, James 157, 227
Starling, Ernest 291
Stenlake 608
Stoeckel, Walter 726
Stokes, Georg Gabriel 594
Stolz, Friedrich 620
Stow, Richard Walcott 593
Straub, Walther 600, 618
Strauss, Hermann 556
Strode, Cicely Mary
Stromeyer, Georg Friedrich 242
Stromeyer, Louis 80
Stürtzbecher, Fritz 522
Suckling, Charles 708
Sudeck, Paul 65, 265, 367ff, 448, 562
Sugita, Seikei 655
Swiecicki, Heliodor 741ff
Sword, Brian C. 449

Tait, Dudley 62, 431
Takaoka, K. S. 452, 851
Tarrow 572
Tatum, Arthur L. 568
Taylor, Thomas 158
Terry, John B. 87
Textor, Kajetan 242, 251, 260
Ther, Leopold 627
Thiersch, Carl 242, 265
Topping, Audrey 318
Tossach 289
Trendelenburg, Friedrich 330, 725
Trendelenburg, Paul 540
Tschirner, M. 584
Tschudy, Eugen 837

Uhlfelder 275, 623
Underwood, Arthur 93
Unger, Ernst 558

van Slyke, Donald 591
van`t Hoff, Jacobus Hendricus 591
Velpeau, Alfred Louis 97, 236, 345, 650
Vesalius, Andreas 268, 289, 636ff
Vierordt, Karl von 594, 683
Virchow, Rudolf 237, 853
Visser, M. J. 207
Voertel, Wilhelm 652

Volwiler, E. H. 65
Vose-Bell, Luther 353

Wade, Reubens 115
Waine 537
Waldeyer, Wilhelm von 853
Waldie, David 663
Waller, Augustus Desiré 426
Walter, Friedrich 591
Walther, Philipp Franz von 79
Wanscher, Oscar 689
Warren, John Collins 44, 47, 97, 184, 235, 270
Waters, Ralph 66, 211, 427, 445ff, 567ff
Waterton, Charles 66
Watmann-Malcamp-Beaulieu, Joseph Freiherr von 225, 271, 650
Wee, M.Y. K. 676
Weese, Hellmut 65, 368, 557
Weickert, Heinrich Eduard 171, 249ff, 650
Weiger, Jospeph 223
Wells, Horace 35, 42, 49, 61, 97, 244, 659
Welz, Robert Ritter von 251, 259ff,
Wendl, H. K. 531ff
Weninger, A. Edward 713
Werigo 519
Wernicke, Carl 356
Whewell, William 841
White, Samuel S. 87
Wieland, Hermann 447ff, 563
Wieland, Theodor 140
Wierda 609
Wiggers, C. J. 291
Wiiliams, Rhys 483
Winckel, Franz Wilhelm von 322, 737
Wohlgemuth, Heinz 556, 815
Woillez, Eugen Joseph 414
Wolff, Albert 195
Wolff, Julius 82
Wolffberg, Siegfried 517
Wood, Earl 595
Wood, Paul 63, 402, 723
Woodbridge, Phil 210
Woolley, Albert 213, 219
Wren, Christoph 425, 772
Wright, John George 426
Wunderlich, Reinhold 242

Yamamura, Hideo 24
Yversen, Axel 689

Zaaijer, Hendrik 207, 371
Zech, D. 584
Zilstra, Willem 595

Zimmermann, Ferdinand 653
Zindler, Martin 368
Zoellner, Fritz 117
Zoll, P. M. 295
Zutz, Nathan 455ff
Zweifel, Paul 737

Index of Topics

Aboringines 421ff
Academic anaesthesia 68
Academic anaesthesiology 567ff
Académie de Médicine 97
Académie des Sciences 97, 127
Active-Compression-Decompression 405
Acupuncture anaesthesia 318
Adrenaline 397
Airway and anaesthesia 114
Airway- separation during anaesthesia 517ff
Alternative analgesic and anaesthetic techniques - use in Australia 421
Ambubag manual resuscitator 671, 699
Amerian Society of Regional Anesthesia 402
American Medical Association 401
American Society of Anesthesiologists 63
Anaesthesia charts 375
Anaesthesia during Austro-Hungarian Monarchy 267ff
Anaesthesia for animals 425ff
Anaesthesia for cardiac surgery 647
Anaesthesia for plastic surgery 114
Anaesthesia in Innsbruck 109
Anaesthesia in Japan - early steps of 655
Anaesthesia in Lisbon - early use in 229
Anaesthesia in military surgery - early use in 231
Anaesthesia in operative gynecology 477
Anaesthesia in Romania - early steps 649ff
Anaesthesia in the Czech countries - early use in 227
Anaesthesia in the Middle Ages 279ff
Anaesthesia machine - early models 63
Anaesthesia per rectum 689ff
Anaesthesiology - development in Czechoslovakia 145ff

Anaesthetic equipment - construction faults in 461ff
Analeptic agents 395
Analgesia for delivery 741
Anemic syncope 207
Anesthesia Patient Safety Foundation 705
Anoci- association 329
Antiinflammatory drugs 620
Antipyretic drugs 620
Apgar Score 711
Apnoic oxygenation 558
Apparatus - early devices for chloroform 683ff
Apparatus - early devices for ether 683ff
Arterenol 628
Artificial respiration 636
Aspiration pneumonitis 707
Aspiration syndrome 580
Associated Anaesthetists of Great Britain and Ireland 64
Association for the Study of Pain 583
Astrup apparatus 712
Atlanta meeting 29
Atracurium, development of 608

Benzocaine, development of 622
Biomotor 409
Bird ventilator 704
Blood bank 558
Blood gas analysis 591ff
Boot's apparatus 685
Brain protection 132
British College of Obstetricians and Gynecologists 485
Bronchial catherization 733
Bronchology 733
Bronchspirometry 523

CO₂ electrode 592
Caffein 397
Camphor 395
Capnometry 679ff
Carbon dioxide absortion 443ff
Carbonic acid puffer system 592
Cardiac massage - closed chest 390
Cardiac massage - open chest 389
Cardiac syncope 207
Cardiazol 396
Cardic surgery - early steps 647
Cardiopulmonary resuscitation - development of modern 290ff
Cardiovent 672
Carlens' double lumen tube 526
Cerebral resusciatation research 297ff
Charrière's apparatus 685
Childbirth - pain relief concepts in UK 483ff
Chloral hydrate 600ff
Chloralhydrate - intravenously used 557
Chloroform - early publications 665
Chloroform anaesthesia - early use in France 343ff
Chloroform anaesthesia - early use in Spain 663
Chloroformists 59
Chloroprocaine 710
Cicuta minor 749
Circulatory risk under anaesthesia 205ff
Cisatracurium, development of 611
Clark's electrode 594, 700
Closed rebreathing system 443ff, 451
CO₂ absorber 721
CO₂ circle absorption apparatus 697
Cocaine research 321ff
Cocaine- numbing effects 61
CODIC 767
Combibag 672
Commission of Neuroanaesthesia 137
Complication under spinal anaesthesia 213ff, 219
Concentration camps 556
Continuous caudal anesthesia 718
Contralateral therapeutic local anaesthesia 438
Contribution of dentists for anaesthesia 42, 60

Controlled hypotension 132
Controlled ventilation in neurosurgery 131
Copenhagen Anaesthesiology Centre 587
Coramin 396
Corbasil 628
Cornecain, development of 625
Cough remedies 619
Coughing Pistol 847
County Nursing Associations 487
Cuirasse-ventilator 536
Cunard Line 97
Curare - early use in Poland 805
Cyclopropane - its explosive properties 451

Datura stramonium
Death under anaesthesia 157ff
Death under anaesthesia in Spain 191ff
Death under anaesthesia in the German speaking countries 171
Death under anaesthesia in the Middle East 167ff
Death under Chloroform 195
Dendrocnide excelsa 421
Der Schmerz 554
Deutsche Arbeitsgemeinschaft für Anaesthesiologie 118
Deutsche Gesellschaft für Anaesthesie 118
Deutsche Rotawerke 561
Development of analgesics 617ff
Difficult airway 837ff
Discussion on the priority of the invention of ether anaesthesia 660
District Nursing Associations 487
Dolantin 618
Double-lumen bronchoscope 519
Doxacurium, development of 611
Dräger Company Lübeck 816
Dräger Resutator 671
Dräger's Modell A 449
Dräger's Pulmotor 820
Dräger's Tussomat 848
Dubbelbronchoskop av Frenckner 733
Duboisia Leichhardtii 422
Duboisia myoporoides 422

Economising apparatus 443
Edo period 655
Education in anaesthesiology 401ff

EEG 118
EEG under Xenon anaesthesia 369ff
Effects of ether, early descriptions 636
Eisenmenger's biomotor 405ff
Electric thermic ether inhaler 432
Electrocardiography under Xenon anaesthesia 364
Endobronchial catheterisation 518
Engstrom ventilator 713
Ephedrine 397
Erythrophleum chlorostadis 421
Erythrophleum laboucherii 422
Ether - early use in the UK 51
Ether - its introduction into Japan 655ff
Ether anaesthesia in Würzburg - early use of 259ff
Ether Day 45ff
Ether frolics 659
Ether- its intravenous use 556
Etherists 59
Etherization in Germany - early use 247ff
Ethic considerations in anaesthesia 71
Eucalyptus prunosa 421
Euodia vitiflora 421
Euphorbia drummondii 422
Experimental pharmacologie 127
Experiments with chloroform in animals 664
Explosion under anaesthesia 209ff
External cardiopulmonary resuscitation - development of modern 292ff

Fasting preoperatively 579ff
First insensitivity 265
Frenckner's bronchoscope 524
Frenckner's Spiropulsator 735
Frumin inflating valve 702
Frumin positive pressure ventilator 702

Geppert's apparatus 564
German publications on anaesthesia - early 251ff
German Society for Anaesthesia 118
Göttinger Modell 549

Hamburg - congress in 370
Hamburg meeting 30
Head injuries 132

Hexeton 396
Heyfelder's apparatus 685
High altitude physiology 456
High frequency ventilation 701, 713
Hostacaine, development of 625
Hustenpistole 847
Hyoscymus niger 749
Hyperosmolar diuretics 132
Hyperventilation 136
Hypnosis of surgical pain 41
Hypodermic syringes 395

Infusion cannula 395
Infusion therapy 555
Intensive Therapy - development in Czechoslovakia 145ff
Interdisciplinary Association of Pain Therapy 584
International Anesthesia Research Society 63
International Federation of Nurse Anesthetists (IFNA) 783
International Symposia on the History of Anaesthesia (ISHA) 21
Intraoperative monitoring 374
Intratracheal insufflation technique 727
Intravenous barbiturates 65
Intravenous injection technique 395
Intravenous regional anaesthesia 505
Iron lung 536
Iron lung 701
Iron lung 720
Isolation of alkaloids 322

Jackson Rees breathing system 706
Jackson's aphasia 353ff
Jackson's apparatus 444
Jackson's claim 49
Jewish pioneers in anaesthesia 553ff
Journal de Physiologie Éxperimentale 121
Journal of Neurosurgical Anesthesia 138

Kalipatrone 443
Kappeler's anaesthetic apparatus 839
Kendall Cardiovent 672
Kirschner's spinal needle 335
Koenig's technique 391
Koupierte Narkose 266

Krankenbehandler 555
Krypton gas 359
Kuhn's apparatus for local anaesthesia 759

Laryngeal mask airway 707
Laryngosope - use of in anaesthesiology 115
Letheon 659
Levallorphane 710
Lidocain, development of 139
Lipid solubility 603
LL30 141
Lobeline 396
Local anaesthetics 617ff
Local anaesthetics, development of 622ff
Local anesthesia - its use in neurosurgery 135
London meeting 29
Long Island College of Medicine 401
Long Island Society of Anesthetists 63
Long term artificial respiration 726
Lotsch's anaesthesia apparatus 747
Lotsch's canula 747

Magill's tracheoscope 521
Mandragora 36, 597
Mandrake 36, 281ff
Mapleson breathing system 706
Medianoscopy 738
Medical School of Hamburg 64
Meltzer-Auer's device for artificial respiration 728
Mesmerism 311ff
Meyer-Overton hypothesis 603
Minneapolis - congress in 369
Minnitts's apparatus 486
Misleading developments in anaesthesia 311ff
Mivacurium, development of 611
Mobile intensive care unit 813
Modification of Ombrédanne's inhaler 543ff
Moody's endobronchial blocker 521
Morphine 600
Morphine structure 618
Mortality form general anaesthesia 179ff
Morton's fate 48
Morton's inhaler 48

Morton's patent 48
Mouth opening instrument - Egypt device 507ff
Muscle relaxants - development of 607ff

Naloxone 710
Narcylene 447
Narkose und Anaesthesie 563
Nasal tubes 115
National Birthday Trust Fund 483
Naturhistorisch-Medizinischer Verein in Heidelberg 561
Neonatal respiratory deficiency syndrome 706
Neuroanaesthesia 131
New York Dental Institute 44
New York Society of Anesthetists 401
New York State Society of Anesthetists 63
News of etherizaion - its spread to the UK 50
Newspapers reports on the introduction of anaesthesia 641ff
Nitrous oxide - early use of 43ff
Nitrous oxide - early use of in France 87
Nitrous oxide anaesthesia 89ff, 181ff
Nitrous oxide frolics 659
Nitrous-oxide anaesthesia 371ff
Non-aryan 555
Novalgin 621
Novocain, development of 623ff
Nurse anesthesia care 783ff

O_2 electrode 592
Obstetric anaesthesia 473ff
Oesophageal Detector Device 675ff
Oil of vitriol 636
Ombrédanne's inhaler 539ff
Oral herbal preparations 36
Osmotic pressure 602
Out- patient surgery 71
Outcome studies in anaesthesiology 182
Oxford inflating bellow 671
Oximetry 594
Oygen - early use of during anaesthesia 66ff

Pain management 69
Pain therapy 583

Palliative care 583ff
Pancuronium, development of 607
Pantocaine 559
Paper somniferum 281
Papyrus Ebers 827
Papyrus Smith 828
Paravertebral injection 726
Parenteral nutritition 153
Patient safety 71
pCO$_2$ equipment
PEEP 702
Perioperative care 69
ph indicator 721
pH- analysis 591
Pharmacology and anaesthesia 597ff
Pharyngeal airway 372
Pharyngeal tube 556
Physicochemical characteristic of cells 602
Physioflex 453
Pioneer of anaesthesia in Austria 233ff
Pipercuronium, development of 608
Pituitary extracts 397
Plastic disposable anesthesia breathing system 707
Pneumatic Institute 39ff, 658
Pneumatic medicine 314ff
Pneumatische Kammer 457
Polamidon 619
Polio respiratory care unit 712
Postdural puncture headache 631
Postspinal headache 631ff
Precordial auscultation 135
Prehospital care 811
Preparation of oil of vitriol 636ff
Préterre's gas regulator 90
Préterre's mask 90
Primäre Narkose 265
Primary anaesthesia 265
Priority discussion between Morton and Jackson 46
Protagonist of specialization in anaesthesiology in Germany 369
Pulmonary surgery and anaesthesia 521ff
PVC- tubings 698
Pyrazolone derivates 620

Quality assurance in anaesthesia - an early contribution 199

Rapacuronium, development of 609
Rausch-Narkose 265
RBS pediatric facemask 706
Rebreathing system 441ff
Record keeping - early use in anaesthesiology 179
Rectal herbal preparation 36
Relaxometry 118
Replica of a Papyrus Hunefer "Laryngoscope" 511ff
Rescue apparatus 697
Respiratory devices 671ff
Respiratory resuscitation - development of modern 288ff
Resusci Annie 699
Resuscitation - an early description of 84
Resuscitation - development of modern 287ff
Resuscitation in Egypt 379ff, 383ff
Revell circulator 452
Revell circulator 703
Rocuronium, development of 608
Rotameters 560
Roth-Dräger's anaesthesia apparatus 818ff
Roth-Dräger's mask 819
Rotterdam meeting 22ff
Rubenbag 671
Russian modifications of Ombrédanne's inhaler 547ff

S.E.E. 757, 763ff
Safety bellow 671
Salvarsan 395
Sauerstoff-Centrale Berlin 816
Sauerstoff-Fabrik Berlin 815
Schimmelbusch's mask 757
Schockcalorose 557
Self experiments in anaesthesia 244
Self experiments with chloroform 664
Small-volume resuscitation 557
Smeeth's apparatus 686
Societas Medicorum Germanicorum Parisiensis 235
Society of German Medical Practitioners in Paris 238
Society of German physicians in Paris 238
Soda lime 721
Solanaceae family 36

Solanum nigrum 749
South Africa - early anaesthetic pioneer in 73
Southern Moravia 647
Spasmolytics 618
Speciality organizations - early attempts 63
Spinal anaesthesia 61, 327, 373ff
Spinal anaesthesia - its use in Belgium 493ff
Spinal anaesthesia - Kirschner's technique 333ff
Spinal needle 631ff
Spinal-epidural anaesthesia - combination of 329ff
Spiropulsator 733, 737
Spongia sominefera 750
Spongia somnifera 38ff
Sterbeklinik 583
Stethoscopy during anaesthesia 571ff
Stow's electrode 700
Strauss'cannula 556
Strophantin 398, 561
Structure-activity relationship 601
Strychnine 396
Stürtzbecher's tube 522
Succinylcholin 710
Suprarenin 395, 628
Swiecicki's apparatus 742

Takaoka's ventilator 851
Takaoka's venturi circulating device 452
Temesvarer Wochenblatt 272, 650
Theory of narcosis 603
Therapeutic hypothermia 298
Therapeutic nerve block 437
Thermoetherization 431ff
Thoracic surgery under spinal anaesthesia 327ff
Thoracoscopy 737

To and fro ventilation technique 443ff, 720
Tokugawa shogunate 655
Tracheal catherization 733
Tracheotomy 827ff
Trancutaneous PO_2 equipment
Trichloroethylene -vaporizer 549
Triggerpoint 437
Tussomat 847
Tutocaine 559
Twilight sleep 753

U.S. Anesthesia Standard System 707
Ultracaine, development of 626
Universal filter 452
University of Wisconsin 402

Vaporizer 452, 716
Vasoconstrictor, development of 627ff
Vecuronium, development of 607
Verein deutscher Aerzte in Paris 238
Veronal 745
Volatile anaesthetics, development of 621

Weal therapy 437
Wells' fate 49
Wendl-tube 531ff
Wohlgemuth's anaesthesia apparatus 815
Women in medicine 693ff
Woolley and Roe trial 219ff
World Congress of Anaesthesiologists in Hamburg 101
World Federation of Societies for Anesthesiologists 70

Xenon 359ff
Xylocain, development of 139

Zuntz-Geppert's respiration apparatus 455
Zuntz-Lehmann's Laufband 457